Emergency Management of Infectious Diseases

The diagnosis and management of infectious disease is a key component of contemporary emergency medicine, ranging from the definitive treatment and discharge of a patient with a simple abscess, to the recognition of a rare infection in a traveler, and to the resuscitation and stabilization of a patient with septic shock. The changing epidemiology of infectious diseases presents a considerable challenge. Acute care practitioners are sentinels for emerging outbreaks and must rapidly synthesize history and exam findings with laboratory studies, imaging results, and epidemiology. Time-dependent morbidity requires practitioners to balance a high degree of suspicion for deadly diagnoses with the precision needed for high-yield diagnostic testing and appropriate care. This book provides a practical, clinically oriented, systems-based overview of infectious disease with an emphasis on emergent diagnosis and treatment. It offers broad coverage of viral, bacterial, fungal, and parasitic diseases in a narrative supplemented by explanatory photos, diagnostic tables, and treatment charts. It should prove an invaluable reference for practitioners confronting the spectrum of infectious disease in the acute care setting.

Emergency Management of Infectious Diseases

Edited by

Rachel L. Chin, MD
University of California, San Francisco School of Medicine
San Francisco General Hospital

Associate Editors

Michael S. Diamond, MD, PhD
Washington University School of Medicine

Teri A. Reynolds, MD, PhD
Alameda County Medical Center–Highland Campus

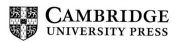
CAMBRIDGE
UNIVERSITY PRESS

CAMBRIDGE UNIVERSITY PRESS
Cambridge, New York, Melbourne, Madrid, Cape Town, Singapore, São Paulo, Delhi

Cambridge University Press
32 Avenue of the Americas, New York, NY 10013-2473, USA

www.cambridge.org
Information on this title: www.cambridge.org/9780521871761

First published 2008

Printed in Hong Kong by Golden Cup

A catalog record for this publication is available from the British Library.

Library of Congress Cataloging in Publication Data

Emergency management of infectious diseases / [edited by] Rachel L. Chin, Michael S. Diamond, and Teri A. Reynolds
　　p. ; cm.
Includes bibliographical references and index.
ISBN 978-0-521-87176-1 (hardback)
1. Communicable diseases – Treatment. 　2. Infection – Treatment. 　3. Emergency physicians. 　4. Emergency medicine.
I. Chin, Rachel L., 1965– 　II. Diamond, Michael S. 　III. Reynolds, Teri A.
[DNLM: 1. Communicable Diseases – diagnosis. 　2. Communicable Diseases – therapy. 　3. Emergency Medicine – methods.
WC 100 E53 　2008]
RC111.E34 　2008
616.02′5 – dc22
　　2007041078

ISBN 978-0-521-87176-1 hardback

To my mother, who taught me that I can do anything; my husband,
Tom; and my wonderful daughters – the queens, Elizabeth and
Katherine – who give me more than I could ever wish for
– RLC

For my wife, Susan, and daughter, Thisbe
– MSD

For Franco, who understands about work and the sound of the sea
– TAR

Contents

Part III. Special Populations   *307*

Part IV. Current Topics   *419*

Section A. Bioterrorism

Section B. Emerging Infection

Preface

The diagnosis and treatment of infectious disease is a key component of contemporary emergency medicine, ranging from the definitive treatment and discharge of a patient with a simple abscess, to the recognition of a rare infection in a traveler, and to the resuscitation and stabilization of a patient with septic shock.

We aimed to produce a practical, clinically oriented, systems-based overview of infectious disease with an emphasis on emergent diagnosis and treatment. Our text covers a broad range of viral, bacterial, fungal, and parasitic diseases, in a narrative supplemented by explanatory photos, diagnostic tables, and treatment charts.

Practitioners in the acute care setting are sentinels for emerging outbreaks and must rapidly synthesize history and exam findings with laboratory studies, imaging results, and epidemiology. We hope that our book will serve emergency physicians, primary care physicians and specialists, nurse practitioners, physician assistants, residents, and medical students who care for patients with infectious diseases.

We thank the many nationally and internationally respected clinicians, educators, and researchers who have contributed, and we hope that *Emergency Management of Infectious Diseases* will prove an invaluable reference for practitioners confronting the spectrum of infectious disease.

Rachel L. Chin, MD
Michael S. Diamond, MD, PhD
Teri A. Reynolds, MD, PhD

Contributors

Fredrick M. Abrahamian, DO
Associate Professor of Medicine
David Geffen School of Medicine at UCLA
Director of Education
Department of Emergency Medicine
Olive View–UCLA Medical Center
Los Angeles, CA

Rebeka Barth, MD
Stanford University School of Medicine
Stanford, CA
Kaiser Permanente Medical Center
Santa Clara, CA

George Beatty, MD, MPH
Associate Clinical Professor of Medicine
University of California, San Francisco School of Medicine
Positive Health Program at San Francisco General Hospital
San Francisco, CA

Diane Birnbaumer, MD
Professor of Clinical Medicine
David Geffen School of Medicine at UCLA
Associate Program Director
Department of Emergency Medicine
Harbor–UCLA Medical Center
Torrance, CA

Alex Blau
University of California, San Francisco School of Medicine
San Francisco, CA

Olivia Bruch, MSc
Health Program Coordinator
Communicable Disease Control and Prevention Section
San Francisco Department of Public Health
San Francisco, CA

Jessica A. Casey, MD
David Geffen School of Medicine at UCLA
Los Angeles, CA

Adithya Cattamanchi, MD
Fellow in Pulmonary and Critical Care Medicine
University of California, San Francisco School of Medicine
San Francisco General Hospital
San Francisco, CA

Rachel L. Chin, MD
Editor in Chief
Professor of Emergency Medicine
University of California, San Francisco School of Medicine
San Francisco General Hospital
San Francisco, CA

Paul D. Choi, MD
Assistant Clinical Professor of Orthopaedic Surgery
Keck School of Medicine
University of Southern California
Childrens Hospital Los Angeles
Los Angeles, CA

Esther K. Choo, MD
Fellow and Clinical Instructor
Department of Emergency Medicine
Oregon Health and Science University
Portland, OR

Deborah Cohan, MD, MPH
Associate Clinical Professor of Obstetrics,
    Gynecology, and Reproductive Sciences
University of California, San Francisco School of Medicine
Medical Director
Bay Area Perinatal AIDS Center
Assistant Director
National Perinatal HIV Consultation and Referral Service
San Francisco General Hospital
San Francisco, CA

Deborah Colina, MD
Michigan State University/Sparrow Hospital
Lansing, MI

Jeffery Critchfield, MD
Associate Professor of Clinical Medicine
University of California, San Francisco School
    of Medicine
San Francisco General Hospital
San Francisco, CA

Shani Delaney, MD
University of California, San Francisco School of Medicine
San Francisco General Hospital
San Francisco, CA

Heather K. DeVore, MD
Clinical Instructor of Emergency Medicine
Georgetown University School of Medicine
Washington Hospital Center
Washington, DC

Michael S. Diamond, MD, PhD
Associate Editor
Associate Professor of Medicine
Molecular Microbiology, Pathology, and Immunology
    Division of Infectious Diseases
Washington University School of Medicine
St. Louis, MO

Erik R. Dubberke, MD
Assistant Professor of Medicine
Division of Infectious Diseases
Washington University School of Medicine
St. Louis, MO

Matthew Fei, MD
Pulmonary/Critical Care Fellow
University of California, San Francisco School of Medicine
San Francisco General Hospital
San Francisco, CA

Jorge A. Fernandez, MD
Assistant Professor of Clinical Emergency Medicine
Keck School of Medicine
University of Southern California
Director of Medical Student Education
Department of Emergency Medicine
Los Angeles County–USC Medical Center
Los Angeles, CA

Alexander C. Flint, MD, PhD
Neurocritical Care and Stroke
Department of Neuroscience
Kaiser Permanente Medical Center
Redwood City, CA

Bradley W. Frazee, MD
Associate Clinical Professor of Medicine
University of California, San Francisco School of Medicine
San Francisco, CA
Alameda County Medical Center–Highland Campus
Oakland, CA

Gus M. Garmel, MD
Clinical Associate Professor of Surgery, Emergency Medicine
Stanford University School of Medicine
Stanford, CA
Co-Program Director, Stanford/Kaiser Emergency
    Medicine Residency Program
Senior Staff Emergency Physician, The Permanente
    Medical Group
Santa Clara, CA

B. Joseph Guglielmo, PharmD
Professor, and Chair of Clinical Pharmacy
Department of Clinical Pharmacy
University of California, San Francisco School of Pharmacy
San Francisco, CA

Theresa A. Gurney, MD
Department of Otolaryngology–Head and Neck Surgery
University of California, San Francisco School of Medicine
San Francisco General Hospital
San Francisco, CA

Barbara L. Haller, MD, PhD
Associate Clinical Professor of Laboratory Medicine
University of California, San Francisco School of Medicine
Chief of Microbiology
San Francisco General Hospital
San Francisco, CA

Hobart Harris, MD, MPH
Professor of Surgery
Chief, Division of General Surgery
Vice Chair, Department of Surgery
University of California, San Francisco School of Medicine
San Francisco, CA

Karen A. Holbrook, MD, MPH
Medical Epidemiologist
Communicable Disease Control and Prevention Section
San Francisco Department of Public Health
San Francisco, CA

Renee Y. Hsia, MD, MSc
Clinical Instructor of Emergency Medicine
University of California, San Francisco School of Medicine
San Francisco General Hospital
San Francisco, CA

Serena S. Hu, MD
Professor of Orthopaedic Surgery
Co-Director, UCSF Spine Care Center
University of California, San Francisco School of Medicine
San Francisco, CA

Laurence Huang, MD
Professor of Medicine
University of California, San Francisco School of Medicine
Chief, AIDS Chest Clinic
Division of Pulmonary and Critical Care Medicine and
    HIV/AIDS Division
San Francisco General Hospital
San Francisco, CA

Jennifer C. Hunter, MPH
Research Assistant
Communicable Disease Control and Prevention Section
San Francisco Department of Public Health
San Francisco, CA

Paul Ishimine, MD
Associate Clinical Professor of Medicine and Pediatrics
University of California, San Diego School of Medicine
Director, Pediatric Emergency Medicine
Department of Emergency Medicine
Associate Director, Pediatric Emergency Medicine
    Fellowship
San Diego Rady Children's Hosptial and Health Center
San Diego, CA

Ramin Jamshidi, MD
Adjunct Professor of Physics
University of San Francisco
University of California, San Francisco School of Medicine
San Francisco, CA

Asim A. Jani, MD, MPH
Assistant Director
Infectious Diseases Fellowship Program
Orlando Regional Healthcare
Orlando, FL

Cheryl A. Jay, MD
Clinical Professor of Neurology
University of California, San Francisco School of Medicine
San Francisco General Hospital
San Francisco, CA

Yeva Johnson, MD
Associate Clinical Professor of Family and Community
    Medicine
University of California, San Francisco School of Medicine
Medical Epidemiologist
Bioterrorism and Infectious Disease Emergencies Unit
Communicable Disease Control and Prevention Section
San Francisco Department of Public Health
San Francisco, CA

Laura W. Kates, MD
Clinical Instructor of Emergency Medicine
University of California, San Francisco School of Medicine
San Francisco General Hospital
San Francisco, CA

Janel Kittredge-Sterling, DO
St. Vincent Mercy Medical Center
Perrysburg, OH

Michael Kohn, MD, MPP
Associate Clinical Professor of Epidemiology and
    Biostatistics
University of California, San Francisco School of Medicine
San Francisco, CA
Attending Emergency Physician
Mills-Peninsula Medical Center
Burlingame, CA

Anita Koshy, MD
Department of Medicine (Infectious Diseases) and
    Microbiology and Immunology
Stanford University School of Medicine
Stanford, CA

Thomas S. T. Lai, MD
Consultant and Chief of Infectious Disease
Department of Medicine and Geriatrics
Princess Margaret Hospital
Lai Chi Kok
Kowloon, Hong Kong

Chi Wai Leung, MD
Consultant Pediatrician and Chief of Pediatric Infectious
    Diseases
Princess Margaret Hospital
Lai Chi Kok
Kowloon, Hong Kong

Pancy Leung, RN, MPA
Infection Control Nurse Manager
Bioterrorism and Infectious Disease Emergencies
    Unit
Communicable Disease Control and Prevention
    Section
San Francisco Department of Public Health
San Francisco, CA

Matthew Lewin, MD, PhD
Assistant Clinical Professor of Emergency Medicine
University of California, San Francisco School of Medicine
San Francisco, CA
Expedition Doctor
American Museum of Natural History
New York, NY

Suzanne Lippert, MD, MS
Alameda County Medical Center–Highland Campus
Oakland, CA

Conan MacDougall, PharmD
Assistant Professor of Clinical Pharmacy
University of California, San Francisco School of Pharmacy
San Francisco, CA

William Mallon, MD
Associate Professor of Emergency Medicine
Keck School of Medicine
University of Southern California
Los Angeles County–USC Medical Center
Los Angeles, CA

Catherine A. Marco, MD
Professor of Surgery
Division of Emergency Medicine
University of Toledo College of Medicine
Toledo, OH

Preston C. Maxim, MD
Associate Clinical Professor of Emergency Medicine
University of California, San Francisco School of Medicine
San Francisco General Hospital
San Francisco, CA

Maureen McCollough, MD, MPH
Associate Professor of Emergency Medicine and
    Pediatrics
Keck School of Medicine
University of Southern California
Director, Pediatric Emergency Department
Department of Pediatrics
Medical Director, Department of Emergency Medicine
Los Angeles County–USC Medical Center
Los Angeles, CA

Roland C. Merchant, MD, MPH, ScD
Assistant Professor of Emergency Medicine and Community
    Health
Warren Alpert Medical School
Brown University
Rhode Island Hospital
Providence, RI

James M. Mok, MD
Department of Orthopaedic Surgery
University of California, San Francisco School of Medicine
San Francisco General Hospital
San Francisco, CA

Gregory J. Moran, MD
Professor of Medicine
David Geffen School of Medicine at UCLA
Department of Emergency Medicine and Division
of Infectious Diseases
Olive View–UCLA Medical Center
Los Angeles, CA

Andrew H. Murr, MD
Professor of Clinical Otolaryngology–Head and Neck Surgery
University of California, San Francisco School of Medicine
Chief of Service
San Francisco General Hospital
San Francisco, CA

Payam Nahid, MD, MPH
Assistant Professor of Medicine
Division of Pulmonary and Critical Care
University of California, San Francisco School of Medicine
San Francisco General Hospital
San Francisco, CA

Parveen K. Parmar, MD
International Emergency Medicine Fellow
Division of International Health and Humanitarian Programs
Department of Emergency Medicine
Brigham and Women's Hospital
Boston, MA

Nikkita Patel, MPH
Research Assistant
Communicable Disease Control and Prevention Section
San Francisco Department of Public Health
San Francisco, CA

Lisa Rahangdale, MD, MPH
Instructor of Obstetrics and Gynecology
Department of Obstetrics and Gynecology
Stanford University School of Medicine
Stanford, CA

Teri A. Reynolds, MD, PhD
Associate Editor
Alameda County Medical Center–Highland Campus
Oakland, CA

Patricia A. Robertson, MD
Professor of Clinical Obstetrics, Gynecology, and
Reproductive Sciences
Division of Perinatal Medicine and Genetics
University of California, San Francisco School of Medicine
San Francisco, CA

Robert Rodriguez, MD
Professor of Medicine
University of California, San Francisco School of Medicine
San Francisco General Hospital
San Francisco, CA

Michelle E. Roland, MD
Associate Professor of Medicine
University of California, San Francisco School of Medicine
San Francisco, CA

Positive Health Program at San Francisco General Hospital
Chief, Office of AIDS, California Department of Public Health
Sacramento, CA

William Schecter, MD
Professor and Chief of Clinical Surgery
University of California, San Francisco School of Medicine
San Francisco General Hospital
San Francisco, CA

Kimberly Schertzer, MD
Simulation Fellow
Stanford University School of Medicine
Stanford, CA
Kaiser Permanente Medical Center
Santa Clara, CA

Seema Shah, MD
Attending Emergency Physician
University of California, San Diego School of Medicine
San Diego Rady Children's Hospital and Health Center
San Diego, CA

Ghazala Q. Sharieff, MD
Associate Clinical Professor of Pediatrics
University of California, San Diego School of Medicine
Medical Director
San Diego Rady Children's Hospital and Health Center
Director of Pediatric Emergency Medicine
Palomar-Pomerado Health System/California Emergency
Physicians
San Diego, CA

Melinda Sharkey, MD
Department of Orthopaedic Surgery
University of California, San Francisco School of Medicine
San Francisco General Hospital
San Francisco, CA

Jan M. Shoenberger, MD
Assistant Professor of Clinical Emergency Medicine
Keck School of Medicine
University of Southern California
Associate Residency Director
Los Angeles County–USC Medical Center
Los Angeles, CA

Aparajita Sohoni, MD
Alameda County Medical Center–Highland Campus
Oakland, CA

Serena S. Spudich, MD
Assistant Adjunct Professor of Neurology
University of California, San Francisco School of Medicine
San Francisco General Hospital
San Francisco, CA

David M. Stier, MD
Medical Epidemiologist
Medical Director
Adult Immunization and Travel Clinic
Communicable Disease Control and Prevention Section
San Francisco Department of Public Health
San Francisco, CA

Stuart P. Swadron, MD
Associate Professor of Emergency Medicine
Keck School of Medicine
University of Southern California
Residency Program Director
Los Angeles County–USC Medical Center
Los Angeles, CA

Sukhjit S. Takhar, MD
Assistant Clinical Professor of Emergency Medicine
Faculty Division of Infectious Diseases
University of California, San Francisco
UCSF Fresno Medical Education Program
Fresno, CA

Timothy M. Uyeki, MD, MPH, MPP
Assistant Clinical Professor of Pediatrics
University of California, San Francisco School of Medicine
San Francisco, CA
Deputy Chief
Epidemiology and Prevention Branch
Influenza Division
National Center for Immunization and Respiratory Diseases
Centers for Disease Control and Prevention
Atlanta, GA

Amy E. Vinther, MD
Clinical Instructor
Stanford University School of Medicine
Stanford, CA

Lan Vu, MD
University of California, San Francisco School of
    Medicine
San Francisco General Hospital
San Francisco, CA

Ralph Wang, MD
Assistant Clinical Professor of Emergency Medicine
University of California, San Francisco School of
    Medicine
San Francisco, CA

Derek Ward
University of California, San Francisco School of
    Medicine
San Francisco, CA

Francis Yao, MD
Professor of Clinical Medicine and Surgery
Associate Medical Director, Liver Transplantation
University of California, San Francisco School of
    Medicine
San Francisco, CA

Clement Yeh, MD
Clinical Instructor of Emergency Medicine
University of California, San Francisco School of
    Medicine
San Francisco General Hospital
San Francisco, CA

PART I

Systems

1. Infective Endocarditis

Jorge A. Fernandez and Stuart P. Swadron

Outline   Introduction
             Epidemiology and Pathophysiology
             Clinical Features
             Differential Diagnosis
             Laboratory and Radiographic Findings
             Treatment and Prophylaxis
             Complications and Admission Criteria
             Pearls and Pitfalls
             References
             Additional Readings

INTRODUCTION

Cardiac infections are classified by the affected site: endocardium, myocardium, or pericardium. Although the terms *pericarditis*, *myocarditis*, and *endocarditis* refer to inflammation in general, most cases are secondary to infectious disease.

EPIDEMIOLOGY AND PATHOPHYSIOLOGY

Infective endocarditis (IE) affects the endocardium, though inflammation may damage the cardiac valves themselves, as well as the underlying myocardium. IE more commonly affects the left side of the heart, more commonly affects males (2:1), and increases in incidence with age. The pathogenic agent is usually bacterial but may also be fungal, rickettsial, or protozoan, particularly in immunocompromised patients.

Infective endocarditis occurs when circulating pathogens adhere to the endocardium in areas of turbulent flow, particularly around cardiac valves. Host susceptibility is an integral part of the pathophysiology. Several decades ago, rheumatic fever was the most common cause of valvular lesions, and bacterial adherence to these damaged valves could occur in any age group. Now, congenital heart disease and degenerative valvular disease are the most common predisposing factors to IE, in children and the elderly, respectively. An increasing percentage of cases arise from prosthetic heart valves, which have enhanced susceptibility to infection.

When bacteremia is frequent, adherence to the endocardium may occur even in the absence of a valvular lesion, and intravenous drug users, immunocompromised patients, and those with indwelling vascular catheters or poor dental hygiene are at greater risk for IE.

The most common pathogens found in IE are gram-positive cocci, such as *Staphylococcus* species, both coagulase positive (e.g., *S. aureus*) and negative (e.g., *Staphylococcus epidermidis*), and the viridans group streptococci (*Streptococcus sanguis*, *bovis*, and *mutans*). Enterococci are also becoming increasingly common causes of IE. The clinical scenario may suggest the pathogen involved: *S. aureus* is common in intravenous drug users, viridans streptococci in patients with recent dental procedures, and gram-negative bacilli in patients following invasive genitourinary procedures.

Pathogens that are much less commonly implicated in IE include the HACEK (*Haemophilus aphrophilus, Haemophilus paraphrophilus, Haemophilus parainfluenzae, Actinobacillus actinomycetemcomitans, Cardiobacterium hominis, Eikenella corrodens*, and *Kingella kingae*) group of slow-growing gram-negative bacteria, *Bartonella*, and atypical organisms such as *Chlamydia, Legionella*, and fungi. Infections with these organisms may be especially difficult to detect in the acute care setting because they do not always cause fever or grow in routine blood cultures.

Once bacteria adhere to the endocardium, infection spreads toward the valves, resulting in stenotic and/or regurgitant function, and toward the myocardium, resulting in mural endocarditis, which may result in septic emboli.

CLINICAL FEATURES

The presentation of IE (Table 1.1, Figure 1.1) ranges from the well-appearing patient with nonspecific symptoms to the toxic patient in severe septic shock with multiorgan failure.

Patients with mild symptoms are often misdiagnosed with viral syndromes. Symptoms may include low-grade fever, headache, malaise, and anorexia. The presence of a new murmur may be helpful, especially in a young person, but its importance in making the diagnosis is often overemphasized. The high prevalence of a baseline murmur in older adults makes this finding rather nonspecific. Patients with a more indolent or subacute presentation may display physical findings that result from the deposition of immune complexes in end-vessels throughout the body: hematuria (due to glomerulonephritis), subungual splinter hemorrhages, or petechiae of the palate and conjunctiva. They also include the so-called classic stigmata of IE: *Roth spots* (exudative lesions on the retina), *Janeway lesions* (painless erythematous lesions on the palms and soles), and *Osler nodes* (painful violet lesions on the fingers or toes). These signs are present in the minority of patients with IE; they should be sought on examination, but their absence does not rule out the diagnosis.

As the clinical presentation becomes more severe, it is characterized by the septic and mechanical complications of endocarditis. In left-sided endocarditis, this may include signs of systemic embolization, which may occur in any organ system. Infections that initially appear to be focal or localized may, in fact, be a result of septic emboli. Examples include stroke and spinal cord syndromes, mycotic aneurysms, osteomyelitis,

Table 1.1 Clinical Features: Infective Endocarditis

Organisms	• *Staphylococcus aureus* • *Streptococcus viridans* • *Enterococcus* • *Staphylococcus epidermidis* • *Streptococcus bovis* • HACEK
Signs and Symptoms	Fever, malaise, chest/back pain, cough, dyspnea, arthralgias, myalgia, neurologic symptoms, weight loss, night sweats
Laboratory and Radiologic Findings	**Duke Clinical Criteria** 2 Major *or* 1 Major + 3 Minor *or* 5 Minor **Major (Microbiology):** • Typical organisms × 2 blood cultures (*S. viridans, S. bovis*, HACEK, *S. aureus*, or enterococcus) with no primary • Persistent bacteremia (≥12 hours) 3/3 or 3/4 positive blood cultures **Major (Valve):** • Positive echocardiogram • New valve regurgitation **Minor:** • Predisposing heart condition or IDU • Fever ≥ 38°C (100.4°F) • Vascular phenomenon (arterial embolism, mycotic aneurysm, intracerebral bleed, conjunctival hemorrhage, Janeway lesions) • Immune phenomenon (glomerulonephritis, Osler node, Roth spot, rheumatoid factor) • Positive blood culture not meeting above criteria • Echocardiogram – abnormal but not diagnostic
IDU, injection drug use.	

epidural abscesses, septic arthropathies, necrotic skin lesions, and cold, pulseless extremities. Mycotic aneurysms most often occur in the middle cerebral artery and may cause meningitis, headaches, or focal neurological deficits. When significant mechanical failure of the mitral or aortic valve occurs, signs and symptoms of severe acute left-sided heart failure, such as pulmonary edema and hypotension, may occur.

Right-sided endocarditis is frequently associated with septic pulmonary emboli. These may cause respiratory symptoms that mimic the presentation of pneumonia or pulmonary embolism. Mechanical failure of the valves usually results in regurgitant disease with signs and symptoms of acute right-sided heart failure.

Other serious sequelae of endocarditis include intravascular hemolysis, which results in hemoglobinemia, hemoglobinuria, and jaundice. In patients with mural endocarditis, abscesses around the annulae of the cardiac valves may result in conduction blocks and bradydysrhythmias. Finally, ventricular wall rupture may lead to cardiac tamponade or hemorrhagic shock.

DIFFERENTIAL DIAGNOSIS

The differential diagnosis of IE is vast, especially in its more indolent presentations. It includes both acute and chronic infections, malignancies, and a wide spectrum of inflammatory and autoimmune disorders. IE should be suspected in any febrile patient with a history of:

• injection drug use
• rheumatic heart disease
• valvular insufficiency
• indwelling catheters
• pacemakers
• prosthetic heart valves
• congenital heart disease
• prior endocarditis

In patients with more severe signs and symptoms, the differential diagnosis includes other life-threatening causes of:

• severe sepsis with end-organ dysfunction (pneumonia, urinary tract infection, peritonitis, or soft-tissue infections)
• left- and right-sided heart failure (myocardial infarction, valvular incompetence or stenosis, pulmonary embolism, or aortic dissection)
• systemic embolization (carotid stenosis, vascular dissection, or cardiac dysrhythmias)

When these complications occur in febrile patients, the diagnosis of IE should be suspected, particularly in those patients at risk. Alternatively, when these complications occur in the absence of fever or risk factors, the underlying diagnosis of IE is highly unlikely.

LABORATORY AND RADIOGRAPHIC FINDINGS

The majority of tests available in an acute care setting are insufficient to confirm or eliminate a suspected diagnosis of IE. Results of routine blood tests, including inflammatory markers (complete blood count [CBC], erythrocyte sedimentation rate [ESR], C-reactive protein [CRP]) lack specificity. The definitive diagnosis is made, in large part, by blood culture. It is important that blood cultures be drawn with good technique and sufficient volume (10 mL) and at multiple sites to enhance diagnostic sensitivity.

The administration of empiric antibiotics in ill-appearing patients with suspected IE should not be unduly delayed, though it is essential to obtain blood cultures prior to giving antibiotics. Special cultures are necessary for the following organisms: HACEK, *Legionella, Mycoplasma*, nutritionally variant strep (*Abiotrophia*), *Bartonella, Coxiella, Brucella*, gonococci, *Listeria, Nocardia*, corynebacteria, and mycobacteria.

Many of the positive findings in diagnostic evaluation may mislead clinicians toward a focal process, rather than direct them toward a unifying diagnosis. For example, an abnormal urinalysis may lead to a diagnosis of cystitis or glomerulonephritis, infiltrates on a chest x-ray may be interpreted as consistent with pneumonia, or findings on a lumbar puncture may lead to a diagnosis of meningitis.

Electrocardiography is seldom helpful in establishing the diagnosis of IE. The most common electrocardiogram abnormality in IE is sinus tachycardia. Signs of acute right heart strain, such as right bundle branch block and rightward axis, may accompany right-sided endocarditis and pulmonary emboli. Severe heart blocks may represent an infection that has moved into the myocardium and around the valvular annulae.

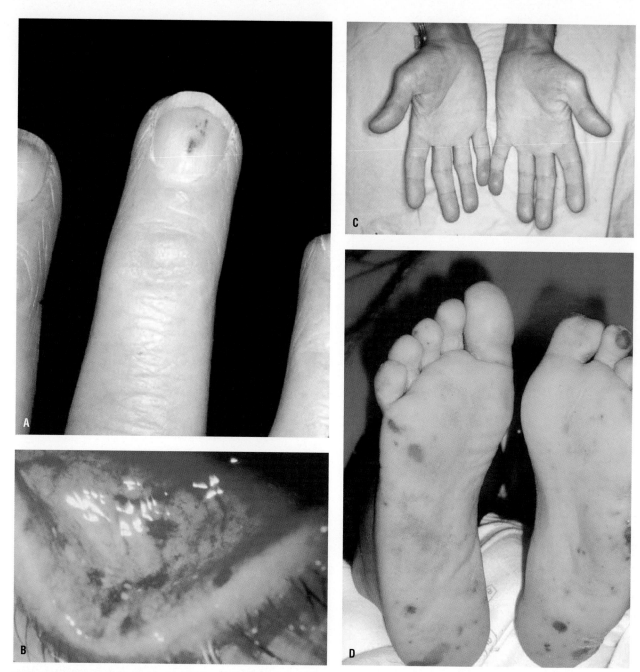

Figure 1.1 Classic physical examination findings in IE. (A) Splinter hemorrhages. (B) Conjunctival petechiae. (C) Osler's nodes. (D) Janeway lesions. Images from Mylonakis E and Calderwood SB. Infective endocarditis in adults. N Engl J Med, 2001;345(18):1318–30. Copyright © 2008 Massachusetts Medical Society. All rights reserved.

Echocardiography is essential in establishing the definitive diagnosis of IE; however, its utility in the emergency department (ED) is more related to its ability to detect life-threatening complications such as pericardial effusion, cardiac tamponade, and valvular rupture.

TREATMENT AND PROPHYLAXIS

Empiric therapy toward likely bacterial pathogens is indicated when the diagnosis of endocarditis is strongly suspected, and antibiotic selection should occur with current and local patterns of sensitivity in mind (Table 1.2). The duration of ther-apy is typically long, up to and, in some cases, exceeding 6 weeks. It may be appropriate to withhold antibiotics pending culture results in patients with chronic, intermittent fevers who otherwise appear well, provided that close follow-up is available.

Antibiotic prophylaxis should be administered to patients at risk for IE prior to certain invasive procedures (Table 1.3). Fortunately, most procedures routinely performed in the ED do not require prophylaxis, except for emergent upper endoscopy (only if sclerotherapy of esophageal varices is performed), incision and drainage of gingival abscesses, and urethral catheterization in the setting of urinary tract infections. In these situations, patients with known valvular

Table 1.2 Empiric Treatment for Infective Endocarditis

Patient Category	Therapy Recommendation
Adults	nafcillin 2 g IV q4h *or* vancomycin 1 g IV q12h (if high prevalence of resistant staph or PCN allergy) *and* gentamicin 1–1.7 mg/kg IV q8h
Children	nafcillin 50 mg/kg IV q6h *or* vancomycin 10–15 mg/kg IV q12h (if high prevalence of resistant staph or PCN allergy) *and* gentamicin 1.5–2.5 mg/kg IV q8h
Pregnant Women	nafcillin 2 g IV q4h *or* vancomycin 1 g IV q12h (if high prevalence of resistant staph or PCN allergy) *and* ceftriaxone 2 g IV q12h
Immunocompromised	As above, depending on age and pregnancy status

PCN, penicillin.

Table 1.3 Antibiotic Prophylaxis for Invasive Procedures in High Risk Patients

Patient Category	Recommended Antibiotics Prophylaxis
Adults	ampicillin 2 g IV/IM × 1 *or* vancomycin (if PCN allergic) 1 g IV × 1 *and* gentamicin 1.5 mg/kg IM/IV × 1
Children	ampicillin 50 mg/kg IV/IM × 1 *or* vancomycin (if PCN allergic) 20 mg/kg IV × 1 *and* gentamicin 1.5 mg/kg IM/IV × 1
Pregnant Women	ampicillin 2 g IV/IM ×1 *or* vancomycin (if PCN allergic) 1 g IV × 1 *and* ceftriaxone 2 g IV × 1
Immunocompromised	As above, depending on age and pregnancy status

PCN, penicillin.

disease or a prior history of IE should be given prophylaxis tailored to the typical pathogens associated with the organ system involved.

COMPLICATIONS AND ADMISSION CRITERIA

The treatment of septic and mechanical complications of endocarditis can be challenging. Cardiac dysrhythmias can be treated according to advanced cardiovascular life support (ACLS) guidelines. In cases of suspected acute valvular dysfunction, emergent echocardiography and consultation with a cardiothoracic surgeon and cardiologist are indicated. In cases of septic emboli, anticoagulation with heparin is not recommended because it has no effect on decreasing the rate of subsequent embolization and because the risk of hemorrhagic transformation is particularly high in these patients. Limb-threatening emboli (e.g., a cold, pulseless extremity) may require revascularization with interventional or surgical techniques, such as the administration of local fibrinolytics.

Patients for whom the diagnosis of IE is being considered should generally be admitted for further evaluation and parenteral antibiotics. In cases in which suspicion for IE is lower, it may be appropriate to discharge certain febrile but otherwise well-appearing patients home with blood cultures pending, provided that follow-up is available within 48 hours. Patients with septic or mechanical complications of IE should be managed in a monitored setting, preferably one in which cardiothoracic surgical intervention is readily available.

PEARLS AND PITFALLS

1. Echocardiography is recommended prior to discharge in all cases of suspected myocarditis, pericarditis, endocarditis, and acute rheumatic fever.
2. Endocarditis is important to consider in any febrile patient with a preexisting valvular abnormality.
3. Mechanical complications of IE may require emergent surgical intervention. Diagnosis of such complications should be made by echocardiography.

REFERENCES

Alexiou C, Langley SM, Stafford H, et al. Surgery for active culture-positive endocarditis: determinants of early and late outcome. Ann Thorac Surg 2000;69(5):1448–54.

Barbaro G, Fisher SD, Gaincaspro G, Lipshultz SE. HIV-associated cardiovascular complications: a new challenge for emergency physicians. Am J Emerg Med 2001 Nov;19(7):566–74.

Cabell CH, Jollis JG, Peterson GE, et al. Changing patient characteristics and the effect on mortality in endocarditis. Arch Intern Med 2002;162(1):90–4.

Calder KK, Severyn FA. Surgical emergencies in the intravenous drug user. Emerg Med Clin North Am 2003;21(4):1089–116.

Olaison L, Pettersson G. Current best practices and guidelines indications for surgical intervention in infective endocarditis. Infect Dis Clin North Am 2002;16(2):453–75.

Pawsat DE, Lee JY. Inflammatory disorders for the heart. Pericarditis, myocarditis, and endocarditis. Emerg Med Clin North Am 1998 Aug;16(3):665–81.

Samet JH, Shevitz A, Fowle J. Hospitalization decision in febrile intravenous drug users. Am J Med 1990;89(1):53–7.

Sandre RM, Shafran SD. Infective endocarditis: review of 135 cases over 9 years. Clin Infect Dis 1996;22(2):276–86.

Sexton DJ, Spelman D. Current best practices and guidelines. Assessment and management of complications in infective endocarditis. Infect Dis Clin North Am 2002;16(2):507–21.

Towns ML, Reller LB. Diagnostic methods current best practices and guidelines for isolation of bacteria and fungi in infective endocarditis. Infect Dis Clin North Am 2002;16(2):363–76.

Wilson LE, Thomas DL, Astemborski J, et al. Prospective study of infective endocarditis among injection drug users. J Infect Dis 2002;185(12):1761–6.

Young GP, Hedges JR, Dixon L, et al. Inability to validate a predictive score for infective endocarditis in intravenous drug users. J Emerg Med 1993:11(1):1–7.

ADDITIONAL READINGS

Fernandez J, Swadron S. Infective endocarditis. In: Stone S, Slavin S, eds, Infectious diseases. Burr Ridge, IL: McGraw-Hill, 2006:255–87.

Mylonakis E, Calderwood SB. Infective endocarditis in adults. N Engl J Med 2001;345(18):1318–30.

2. Myocarditis and Pericarditis

Jorge A. Fernandez and Stuart P. Swadron

INTRODUCTION

Cardiac infections are classified by the affected site: endocardium, myocardium, or pericardium. As the pathophysiology, clinical presentation, differential diagnosis, and treatment of myocarditis and pericarditis overlap significantly, these will be discussed together.

EPIDEMIOLOGY AND PATHOPHYSIOLOGY

Myocarditis is an inflammation of the myocardium; the term myopericarditis describes the frequent additional involvement of the pericardium. Pericarditis involves only the pericardium. Isolated myocarditis is often relatively asymptomatic and therefore frequently misdiagnosed. Thus, the true incidence is unknown, although autopsy studies have demonstrated occult myocarditis in up to 1% of the general population. For unclear reasons, young men more frequently develop myocarditis as well as pericarditis.

The pericardium provides a protective barrier and is composed of two layers: visceral and parietal. The visceral layer is firmly attached to the epicardium, whereas the parietal layer moves freely within the mediastinum. Approximately 20 mL of fluid is normally present within the pericardial sac. Fluid accumulation within the pericardial sac may result in cardiac tamponade if the pericardium does not have sufficient time to stretch, as compliance increases slowly over time. Thus, the rate rather than the absolute amount of fluid accumulation in the pericardial sac is the most important determinant of tamponade physiology.

Cardiac infections may spread directly from one intracardiac region to another (from endocardium toward pericardium or vice versa). Alternatively, pleural or mediastinal infections can extend into the pericardium and cause cardiac infections.

Infectious Causes of Myocarditis

Infectious causes of myocarditis include viruses, bacteria, fungi, rickettsia, spirochetes, and parasites. In all types of infection, myocardial damage may result from destructive effects of the invasive pathogen or from immune-mediated lysis of infected cells. In developed nations, viruses represent the most common infectious cause. Several viruses cause myocarditis, with coxsackieviruses representing more than 50% of confirmed cases of viral myocarditis. Other common agents include influenza virus, echovirus, herpes simplex virus (HSV), varicella-zoster virus (VZV), Epstein-Barr virus (EBV), cytomegalovirus (CMV), and the hepatitis viruses. Human immunodeficiency virus (HIV) infection may also cause myocarditis, either directly from HIV-induced cytotoxicity during any phase of the infection, or indirectly as a result of other opportunistic infections. Most cases of viral myocarditis are preceded by an upper respiratory infection by 1–2 weeks.

Bacterial myocarditis is often caused by direct extension from infected endocardial or pericardial tissue. The most common causative organisms in these cases mirror those most commonly causing bacterial endocarditis or pericarditis. Certain exotoxin-mediated bacterial illnesses, such as diphtheria, may also cause myocarditis.

Other pathogenic organisms associated with myocarditis include rickettsia, spirochetes, and parasites. Tick-borne illnesses caused by rickettsia (Rocky Mountain spotted fever, Q fever, and scrub typhus) and spirochetes (Lyme disease) have all been associated with myocarditis. Immunocompromised patients may develop myocarditis secondary to toxoplasmosis. Parasitic causes of myocarditis in immigrant populations include Chagas disease and trichinosis.

Noninfectious Causes of Myocarditis

There are a variety of noninfectious causes of myocarditis, including autoimmune disorders, medications, and environmental toxins. Autoimmune causes include systemic lupus erythematosus (SLE), rheumatoid arthritis (RA), sarcoidosis, and various vasculitides (Kawasaki disease and giant cell arteritis). A variety of drugs and chemotherapeutics can directly induce myocardial inflammation, including cocaine, amphetamines, lithium, phenothiazines, zidovudine (AZT), chloroquine, and doxorubicin. Hypersensitivity reactions to penicillin and sulfonamides may trigger inflammatory changes in the myocardium, resulting in myocarditis. Environmental toxins such as carbon monoxide, lead, and arsenic, as well as stings from spiders, scorpions, and wasps, can also result in myocardial inflammation.

Table 2.1 Important Causes of Myocarditis and Pericarditis

Idiopathic Viral Infections	Mycobacterial Infections	Malignancy Medications
Coxsackievirus A and B	*Mycobacterium tuberculosis*	Penicillin
Echoviruses	**Parasitic Infections**	Sulfa drugs
Adenoviruses	Chagas disease	Procainamide
HIV	Trichinosis	Hydralazine
Bacterial Infections	Toxoplasmosis	Isoniazid
Gram-positive species	**Fungal Infections**	Phenytoin
Gram-negative species	*Histoplasma capsulatum*	Chemotherapeutic agents
Anaerobes	*Aspergillus* species	**Environmental/Toxins**
Mycoplasma	**Autoimmune Mediated**	Cocaine
Rickettsial Infections	Acute rheumatic fever	Amphetamines
RMSF	Dressler's syndrome	Carbon monoxide
Q fever	Systemic lupus erythematosus	Lead
Scrub typhus	Rheumatoid arthritis	Stings/bites
Spirochetes	Vasculitis (e.g., Kawasaki)	**Radiation Exposure**
Lyme disease	Sarcoidosis	**Metabolic Disorders**
Syphilis	Postvaccination	Hypothyroidism
	Trauma or Surgery	Uremia (dialysis-related)
	Postpericardiotomy syndrome	

Adapted from Ross AM, Grauer SE. Acute pericarditis. Evaluation and treatment of infectious and other causes. Postgrad Med. 2004 Mar;115(3):67–75. RMSF, Rocky Mountain spotted fever.

Table 2.2 Clinical Features: Myocarditis and Pericarditis

Signs and Symptoms: Adults	• Nonspecific – fever, malaise, night sweats
	• Chest pain (substernal, sharp, stabbing, squeezing, or pleuritic)
	• Friction rub (only if pericarditis)
	• Congestive heart failure
	  L-sided: DOE, near syncope, rales
	  R-sided: JVD, HSM, peripheral edema
	• Tamponade: Syncope, Beck's triad, pulsus paradoxus
	• Dysrhythmia or conduction disturbance – palpitations, light-headedness, or syncope
	• Bacterial:
	  Pneumonia – cough, dyspnea, hemoptysis
	  Mediastinitis – odyno/dysphagia, sepsis
	  Endocarditis – murmur, septic emboli, rash
	• Tuberculous – TB exposure, cachexia, pleurisy
	• Lyme/Rickettsial – tick exposure, rash, arthritis

Signs and Symptoms: Infants	• As above • Nonspecific – lethargy, poor feeding, cyanosis

Laboratory and ECG Findings	• Leukocytosis, elevated C-reactive protein level, ESR, and cardiac enzymes
	• ECG findings include:
	  Sinus tachycardia and nonspecific ST-T changes
	  Diffuse ST-segment elevation
	  Decreased QRS amplitude and Q waves
	  Ventricular ectopy
	• Occasional conduction disturbances, BBB, or tachydysrhythmias

DOE, dyspnea on exertion; HSM, hepatosplenomegaly; TB, tuberculosis.

Infectious Causes of Pericarditis

Acute pericarditis, like myocarditis, is most frequently caused by viruses, including coxsackieviruses, echoviruses, influenza, EBV, VZV, HIV, mumps, and hepatitis (Table 2.1). Again, upper respiratory infection generally precedes pericardial involvement, and males older than 50 years are at highest risk.

Tuberculous pericarditis is prevalent in developing nations and in immigrant populations. It is caused by hematogenous or lymphatic spread of mycobacteria.

Bacterial pericarditis is fortunately rare. It most often results from direct extension of adjacent pulmonary, mediastinal, or endocardial infection, or iatrogenic inoculation following cardiac surgery. These patients usually appear toxic, unlike most patients with viral pericarditis.

Noninfectious Causes of Pericarditis

Noninfectious causes of acute pericarditis include uremia, trauma, malignancy (lymphoma or cancers of the breast, lung, or kidney), radiation, chemotherapy, drug reactions (penicillin or minoxidil), and autoimmune disorders (SLE, RA, or Dressler's syndrome after myocardial infarction or cardiac surgery). See Table 2.1.

CLINICAL FEATURES

The clinical presentation of infectious myocarditis and pericarditis varies depending on the virulence of the infective agent and the severity of the host immune response (Table 2.2). Most patients with acute myocarditis or pericarditis have mild symptoms, which include low-grade fever, malaise, and substernal chest pain. The pain is often described as sharp, stabbing, squeezing, or pleuritic. The pain is commonly postural: lying supine exacerbates the pain, whereas sitting relieves it. Patients may complain of dyspnea on exertion, particularly when presenting in heart failure or with cardiac tamponade. Patients with pericarditis may also complain of cough, odynophagia, or dysphagia, presumably secondary to the spread of the inflammatory process to adjacent structures. In the event of associated dysrhythmia, patients may complain of palpitations, light-headedness, or syncope. Neonates and infants frequently present with nonspecific symptoms, such as fever, respiratory distress, cyanosis, or poor feeding.

Physical exam findings in myocarditis and pericarditis depend on the severity of illness and presence of complications. The classic finding in acute pericarditis is a pericardial friction rub, which is best heard at the apex while the patient leans forward or lies prone. Insensitive findings for cardiac tamponade include pulsus paradoxus (>10 mm Hg decline in systolic blood pressure with inspiration) and Beck's triad (jugular-venous distension [JVD], distant heart sounds, and hypotension). In cases of myocarditis, signs of left-sided heart failure may include tachypnea, hypoxia, and pulmonary rales. Right-sided heart failure may present with JVD, hepatosplenomegaly, and peripheral edema. Occasionally, patients with acute myocarditis present in acute heart failure without associated fever or chest pain.

Bacterial Myopericarditis

Patients with bacterial myopericarditis generally appear toxic and frequently have evidence of lower respiratory, endocardial, or mediastinal infection. The diagnosis should be suspected whenever septic-appearing patients have a history of cardiac surgery, or present with chest pain, congestive heart failure (CHF), or tamponade.

In contrast, tuberculous pericarditis generally presents as an indolent illness with nonspecific symptoms such as fever, night sweats, weight loss, and fatigue. However, these patients occasionally appear toxic. This diagnosis should be suspected in all cases of pericarditis associated with possible exposure to tuberculosis.

Spirochete and Rickettsial Myopericarditis

Lyme or rickettsial myopericarditis should be considered in all symptomatic patients living in endemic regions, as most patients do not recall a history of tick exposure. Any cardiac inflammation associated with rash and arthritis should heighten the suspicion of tick-borne illness.

Clinical Course of Myocarditis and Pericarditis

Most cases of acute myocarditis resolve spontaneously without sequelae. Recurrent or chronic myocarditis, however, can progressively damage the myocardium, leading to dilated cardiomyopathy and chronic congestive heart failure in up to 30% of patients. If symptomatic heart failure results from myocardial infection, the 5-year mortality exceeds 50%.

The prognosis of acute pericarditis depends on the etiology: viral pericarditis is frequently benign and transient, whereas malignant pericardial effusions carry an exceedingly poor prognosis. In cases of recurrent pericarditis, prognosis is worsened by chronic fibrosis and thickening, which cause constrictive pericarditis and diminished cardiac output.

DIFFERENTIAL DIAGNOSIS

The differential diagnosis of a patient complaining of chest pain or dyspnea in an emergent or urgent setting should include:

- aortic dissection
- pulmonary embolism
- pneumothorax and tension pneumothorax
- acute coronary syndrome
- cardiac dysrhythmias
- esophageal perforation
- myopericarditis
- mediastinitis
- pneumonia
- bronchitis
- gastroesophageal reflux disease
- costochondritis
- panic attack
- herpes zoster
- pleurisy

The diagnosis of myopericarditis should be strongly considered whenever chest pain, dyspnea, dysrhythmias, heart failure, or cardiac tamponade accompanies recent upper respiratory symptoms or in association with risk factors for myopericarditis (autoimmune disorders, malignancy, renal failure, recent cardiac surgery, or exposure to toxins, tuberculosis, or ticks).

Misdiagnosis of acute myopericarditis as ST-segment elevation myocardial infarction may result in inappropriate administration of fibrinolytic agents, beta-blockers, and heparin. The differentiation of myopericarditis and acute coronary syndrome should not be made on historical features alone, as fever, cough, and pleuritic chest pain may be seen in both conditions. Electrocardiographic findings are more reliable because myopericarditis generally occurs diffusely, unlike acute coronary syndrome, which involves the territory of a specific coronary artery.

Differentiating myopericarditis from adjacent infectious or inflammatory processes is frequently difficult. In fact, bacterial myopericarditis frequently occurs in conjunction with endocarditis, pneumonia, empyema, or mediastinitis. Furthermore, inflammatory conditions (such as SLE, RA, or vasculitis) and toxins (including medications and environmental exposures) may cause cardiac, pulmonary, or aortic disease. Electrocardiography, echocardiography, and advanced imaging are frequently necessary to differentiate these conditions.

LABORATORY AND RADIOGRAPHIC FINDINGS

In the acute care setting, routine studies in patients presenting with chest pain or dyspnea include pulse oximetry, chest x-ray, and electrocardiography. Unfortunately, these tests are insensitive and nonspecific in acute myocarditis. Electrocardiography (ECG) is useful in detecting early cases of pericarditis.

Laboratory findings in acute myocarditis and pericarditis may include leukocytosis, elevated C-reactive protein levels, and increased erythrocyte sedimentation rate (ESR). Elevated cardiac markers may be seen in severe cases of myocarditis; this may cause difficulty in distinguishing cases of acute myocarditis from acute coronary syndrome. Fortunately, ECG findings are usually distinct in each entity. Although viral serology may reveal a causative agent, these results will rarely be available acutely (with the possible exception of rapid influenza or mononucleosis tests). Skin testing and acid-fast bacilli testing of the sputum should be performed in suspected tuberculous pericarditis, and blood cultures should be obtained in all toxic-appearing patients.

Common ECG findings in myocarditis include sinus tachycardia and nonspecific ST-T changes (Figure 2.1). When present, ST-segment elevation is frequently diffuse. Other characteristic findings include decreased QRS amplitude and the development of Q waves. Ventricular ectopy is common. Occasionally, conduction system disturbances, bundle branch blocks, or tachydysrhythmias may develop as well.

Electrocardiography findings can be diagnostic of pericarditis (Figure 2.2). Acute pericarditis causes a characteristic progression of ECG findings through four distinct phases. The first stage may last for days and is characterized by diffuse ST elevation in all leads except avR and V1. PR segment depression is another common finding during the first stage and may precede the ST elevation. The second stage, which occurs days to weeks after the first, involves normalization of the ST segment with T wave flattening. The third stage involves diffuse T wave inversion without Q wave formation, and the fourth stage is characterized by ECG normalization. Electrical alternans, characterized by alternating voltage of the P wave, QRS segment, and T wave, is a rare but pathognomonic finding of cardiac tamponade. Other ECG findings in tamponade

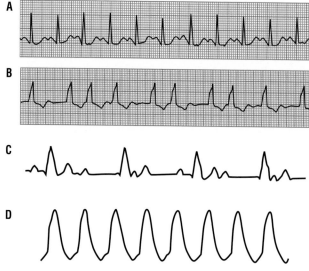

Figure 2.1 Rhythm disturbances in acute myocarditis. (A) Sinus tachycardia. (B) Atrial fibrillation with bundle-branch block morphology. (C) Third-degree (complete) atrioventricular block with wide QRS complex escape. (D) Wide QRS complex tachycardia. Reprinted with permission from Brady WJ, Ferguson JD, Ullman EA, Perron AD. Myocarditis: emergency department recognition and management. Emerg Med Clin North Am 2004 Nov;22(4):865–85.

uncertain. Echocardiographic evidence of cardiac tamponade includes inadequate ventricular filling with diastolic collapse of the right atrium or ventricle. Furthermore, a dilated inferior vena cava without inspiratory collapse strongly suggests tamponade (Figure 2.4).

Computed tomography (CT) scanning is able to reliably detect small pericardial effusions, though echocardiography and magnetic resonance (MR) imaging are better tests. The sensitivity and specificity of MR in myocarditis and pericarditis approach 100%. MR is increasingly being used to detect occult myocarditis in younger patients who present with idiopathic dysrhythmias and have normal electrophysiology testing. Diagnostic pericardiocentesis or myocardial biopsy may be performed in cases of pericarditis and myocarditis in cases of unclear etiology.

TREATMENT

After ruling out potentially life-threatening complications, such as pericardial effusion, congestive heart failure, conduction disturbances, or dysrhythmias, treatment of myocarditis and pericarditis consists of symptomatic relief (Table 2.3). Some studies recommend that patients with suspected or diagnosed myocarditis should limit activity for 6 months. For pericarditis, nonsteroidal agents such as aspirin, ibuprofen, or indomethacin are effective in reducing associated inflammation; however, some studies suggest that these drugs are potentially harmful in cases of isolated myocarditis. In refractory cases of pericarditis, colchicine has been successfully used. No definitive treatment benefit of corticosteroids or intravenous gamma globulin has been documented with myocarditis or pericarditis, except when caused by specific collagen vascular diseases such as SLE or RA. Additionally, the use of steroids in acute pericarditis has been shown in some studies to increase the risk of recurrent or chronic pericarditis and thus is not recommended for routine treatment. Inciting medications should be discontinued when hypersensitivity is suspected.

include low-voltage QRS and nonspecific T wave changes. Constrictive pericarditis is frequently associated with atrial fibrillation.

Chest x-ray findings in myocarditis and pericarditis may include cardiomegaly or pulmonary vascular congestion secondary to heart failure; however, a normal x-ray does not rule out these diagnoses. Associated pleural effusions are frequently seen (Figure 2.3).

Echocardiography is recommended in all cases of suspected myocarditis. In well-appearing patients with a clear diagnosis of pericarditis, echocardiography is not always necessary; however, echocardiography is recommended in all complicated cases of pericarditis or when the diagnosis is

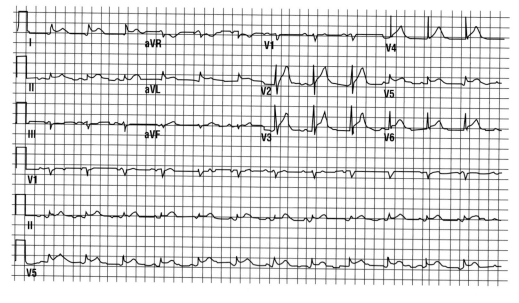

Figure 2.2 Electrocardiography demonstrating characteristic findings of acute pericarditis (stage 1). Reprinted with permission from Ross AM, Grauer SE. Acute pericarditis. Evaluation and treatment of infections and other causes. Postgrad Med 2004 Mar;115(3):67–75.

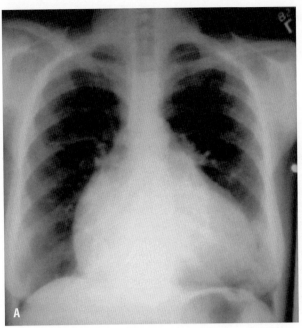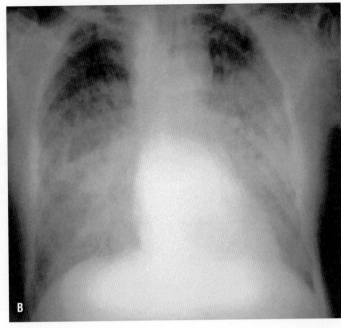

Figure 2.3 Chest x-ray findings in myocarditis. (A) Cardiomegaly without pulmonary edema. (B) Another patient with early myocarditis demonstrating pulmonary edema without cardiomegaly. Reprinted with permission from Brady WJ, Ferguson JD, Ullman EA, Perron AD. Myocarditis: emergency department recognition and management. Emerg Med Clin North Am 2004 Nov;22(4):865–85.

COMPLICATIONS AND ADMISSION CRITERIA

Standard advanced cardiovascular life support (ACLS) protocols should be followed in cases complicated by bradycardia or tachydysrhythmias. Because conduction disturbances are generally transient, insertion of a transvenous pacemaker is usually not necessary in cases of myocarditis-induced bradycardia.

Congestive heart failure with acute pulmonary edema may require aggressive treatment with vasodilators such as nitrates and angiotensin-converting enzyme inhibitors. Beta-blockers should be avoided, as they not only are contraindicated in acute congestive heart failure, but also have been shown to worsen cardiac inflammation in animal models.

Cardiac tamponade requires aggressive fluid resuscitation accompanied by emergent pericardiocentesis if a patient is unstable and does not immediately improve with a fluid bolus. Emergent thoracotomy with pericardiotomy may be necessary in refractory cases. Cardiac transplantation may be

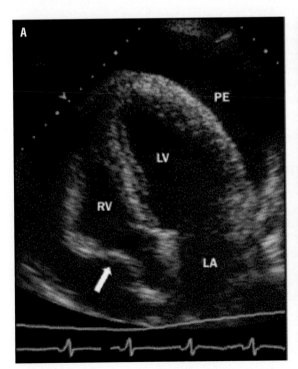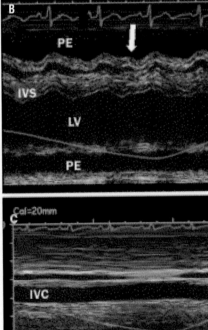

Figure 2.4 Echocardiographic evidence of cardiac tamponade. Echocardiographic images of a large pericardial effusion with features of tamponade. PE, pericardial effusion; LV, left ventricle; RV, right ventricle; LA, left atrium; IVS, interventricular septum; IVC, inferior vena cava. (A) Apical four-chamber view of LV, LA, and RV that shows large PE with diastolic right-atrial collapse (arrow). (B) M-mode image with cursor placed through RV, IVS, and LV in parasternal long axis. The view shows circumferential PE with diastolic collapse of RV free wall (arrow) during expiration. (C) M-mode image from subcostal window in same patient that shows IVC plethora without inspiratory collapse. Reprinted with permission from Elsevier (*The Lancet*, 2004, Vol. 363, pp. 717–27).

Table 2.3 Initial Treatment for Pericarditis and Myopericarditis

Patient Category	Therapy Recommendation
Adults	Nonsteroidal anti-inflammatories: (avoid if isolated myocarditis) ibuprofen 600 mg PO tid *or* naproxen 500 mg PO qd *and/or* colchicine 0.6 mg PO bid or qd (for refractory pericarditis only)
Children	Nonsteroidal anti-inflammatories: (avoid if isolated myocarditis) ibuprofen 5–10 mg/kg PO qid *or* naproxen 5–10 mg/kg PO bid *and/or* colchicine 0.6 mg PO qd (for refractory pericarditis only)
Pregnant Women	acetaminophen 500 mg PO qid
Immunocompromised	As above, depending on age and pregnancy status

Table 2.4 Complications of Myopericarditis and Recommended Treatment

Complication	Recommended Therapy
Congestive Heart Failure	Nitroglycerin 0.25–3 mcg/kg/min IV Enalaprilat 0.005–0.01 mg/kg IV q8 Captopril 0.01–0.2 mg/kg PO q12 Furosemide 0.5–1 mg/kg IV q6 BiPAP Note: Beta-blockers are contraindicated.
Cardiac Tamponade	Aggressive fluid resuscitation Pericardiocentesis
Heart Block and Tachydysrhythmias	As per ACLS or APLS protocols
Cardiogenic Shock	Dobutamine 2–20 mcg/kg/min IV Dopamine 1–20 mcg/kg/min IV Intra-aortic balloon pump Ventricular assist device Cardiac transplantation

APLS, advanced pulmonary life support; BiPAP, bilevel positive airway pressure.

life saving in cases of fulminant myocarditis associated with cardiogenic shock; however, these patients are at high-risk of recurrent myocarditis or rejection. Emergent placement of an intra-aortic balloon pump or left-ventricular assist device may serve as a bridge to transplantation.

All cases of suspected myocarditis should be admitted, preferably to a telemetry or intensive care unit setting. In cases of pericarditis, echocardiography assists with appropriate disposition. In the setting of a normal echocardiogram, patients with acute pericarditis who are well appearing may be safely discharged. In cases of pericarditis with associated pericardial effusion, hospitalization is recommended. Small or moderate effusions can be followed with serial echocardiograms; large effusions require urgent pericardiocentesis or placement of a pericardial window. See Table 2.4.

PEARLS AND PITFALLS

1. Most cases of myocarditis and pericarditis are viral and generally have a benign course.
2. Misdiagnosis of acute pericarditis as ST segment elevation myocardial infarction (STEMI) may result in inappropriate administration of fibrinolytic agents.
3. Serious complications of any form of carditis include congestive heart failure, conduction disturbances, tachydysrhythmias, and pericardial tamponade.

REFERENCES

Acker MA. Mechanical circulatory support for patients with acute-fulminant myocarditis. Ann Thorac Surg 2001 Mar;71(3 Suppl):S73–6.

Barbaro G, Fisher SD, Gaincaspro G, Lipshultz SE. HIV-associated cardiovascular complications: a new challenge for emergency physicians. Am J Emerg Med 2001 Nov;19(7):566–74.

Carapetis JR, McDonald M, Wilson NJ. Acute rheumatic fever. Lancet 2005; Jul 9–15;366(9480):155–68.

Cilliers AM, Manyemba J, Saloojee H. Anti-inflammatory treatment for carditis in acute rheumatic fever. Cochrane Database Syst Rev 2003;(2):CD003176.

Meune C, Spaulding C, Lebon P, Bergman JF. Risks versus benefits of NSAIDs including aspirin in myocarditis: a review of the evidence from animal studies. Drug Saf 2003;26(13):975–81.

Pawsat DE, Lee JY. Inflammatory disorders for the heart. Pericarditis, myocarditis, and endocarditis. Emerg Med Clin North Am 1998 Aug;16(3):665–81.

Ross AM, Grauer SE. Acute pericarditis. Evaluation and treatment of infectious and other causes. Postgrad Med 2004 Mar;115(3):67–75.

Stollerman GH. Rheumatic fever in the 21st century. Clin Infect Dis 2001 Sep 15;33(6):806–14.

Trautner BW, Darouiche RO. Tuberculous pericarditis: optimal diagnosis and management. Clin Infect Dis 2001 Oct 1;33(7):954–61.

ADDITIONAL READINGS

Brady WJ, Ferguson JD, Ullman EA, Perron AD. Myocarditis: emergency department recognition and management. Emerg Med Clin North Am 2004 Nov;22(4):865–85.

Chan TC, Brady WJ, Pollack M. Electrocardiographic manifestations: acute myopericarditis. J Emerg Med. 1999 Sep–Oct;17(5):865–72.

Troughton RW, Asher CR, Klein AL, Pericarditis. Lancet 2004 Feb 28;363(9410):717–27.

3. Dental and Odontogenic Infections

Preston C. Maxim

INTRODUCTION

Infections of the oral cavity are a common presenting complaint in the acute care setting and represent a diverse spectrum of disease ranging from dental caries to Ludwig's angina and retropharyngeal abscess. Odontogenic infections are generally due to normal mouth flora, specifically aerobic and anaerobic *Streptococcus* species, *Bacteroides fragilis*, and *Prevotella intermedia*.

EPIDEMIOLOGY

Dental infections are common in the general population, afflicting 40% of children by age 6 and 85% by age 17. The incidence approaches 100% by age 45, with approximately 50% having modest to severe periodontal disease. Comorbidities including diabetes, smoking, injection drug use, and poor oral hygiene increase the risk and severity of patients' periodontal disease. Fortunately, the incidence of secondary odontogenic infections has declined with the use of antibiotics, as has their morbidity and mortality. For example, although deep mandibular space abscesses, or Ludwig's angina, still represent 13% of the deep space infections of the neck, its mortality has declined from greater than 50% in the 1940s to approximately 5% currently.

CLINICAL FEATURES

Dentoalveolar Infections

Patients with dentoalveolar infections present to the acute care setting with a spectrum of disease ranging from caries to periapical abscesses. The persistent presence of dental plaque leads to the breakdown of the enamel and dentin layers that protect the dental pulp. Once the pulp is exposed, bacteria cause inflammation and subsequent necrosis. Most patients with dentoalveolar infections present with an acute episode of pain due to pulpitis (Table 3.1). This is inflammation of the structures confined within the dental pulp and is usually caused by infection, although thermal, chem-

ical, and traumatic injuries are other causes. The primary pathogens in an acute exacerbation of pulpitis are *Streptococcus mutans* species. On physical exam, patients with pulpitis have carious teeth without significant focal tenderness to percussion.

As the pulpal abscess extends it will erode out of the pulpal space and decompress into the oral cavity, the alveolar ridge, the apex of the tooth, or the fascial planes of the face, forming a periapical abscess (Table 3.2). Although the most common initial bacterial pathogen is *Streptococcus mutans* species, up to 60% of subsequent abscesses are polymicrobial and include *Staphylococcus* species, *Prevotella intermedia*, and *Actinomyces* species. Patients with a periapical abscess present with an acute episode of persistent localized tooth pain and thermal sensitivity. On clinical exam, the tooth is exquisitely tender to percussion. The buccal and/or lingual gingiva supporting the tooth will be swollen and erythematous and usually has an area of fluctuance. Bite-wing radiographs of the teeth can help differentiate pulpitis and periapical abscess; pulpitis shows carious erosion of the dentin, whereas periapical abscess exhibits erosion through the dentin below the gum line. As these radiographs may not be available in most acute care settings, diagnosis is generally made on clinical examination.

Table 3.1 Clinical Features: Pulpitis

Organisms	• *Streptococcus mutans* • *Actinomyces* • *Corynebacterium*
Signs and Symptoms	• Acute onset of dental pain • Evidence of a decayed tooth • Minimal focal tenderness to palpation • No evidence of swelling or fluctuance on the buccal or lingual gingiva
Laboratory and Radiographic Findings	• No role for blood work • Bite-wing radiographs may show carious erosion of the dentin

Table 3.2 Clinical Features: Periapical Abscess

Organism	• *Streptococcus mutans* • *Actinomyces* species • *Corynebacterium* • 60% are polymicrobial with *Staphylococcus* and *Streptococcus mutans* species and *Prevotella intermedia*
Signs and Symptoms	• Acute onset of dental pain • Evidence of a decayed tooth • Significant focal tenderness to palpation • Swelling or fluctuance on the buccal or lingual gingiva
Laboratory and Radiographic Findings	• No role for blood work • Bite wing radiographs may show carious erosion through the dentin below the gum line

Periodontal Infections

The persistent presence of dental plaque causes the gingiva to retract slightly from the base of the tooth, exposing the cementum and alveolar bone. This leads to further gingival retraction, plaque formation, and calcification. Healthy gingiva has scant bacterial flora, though what is present is primarily *Streptococcus* and *Actinomyces* species; however, as the gingiva becomes diseased the absolute bacteria count increases and shifts toward anaerobic gram-negative bacilli, primarily *Prevotella intermedia*. Patients with periodontal infections present with acute onset of localized tooth and gum pain and have a history suggestive of gum disease and periodontitis (i.e., bleeding gums with brushing) (Table 3.3). On physical exam, the gingiva is swollen and erythematous but the associated teeth are not tender to palpation (unlike a periapical abscess) and may not have caries (Figure 3.1).

Pericoronitis

Pericoronitis is a variant of periodontal infections in which the gingiva overlying a tooth becomes inflamed and painful (Table 3.4). Whereas this can happen in the primary and permanent teeth in children, in adults it usually happens in the gingiva overlying the crown of an impacted third molar. Often a fragment of food acts as a nidus for infection with anaerobic gram-negative bacilli (e.g., *Prevotella intermedia*) as in periodontal infections. On physical exam, there is pain and erythema of the gingival flap overlying a partially erupted tooth. Occasionally, purulent material and a small amount of inspissated food can be expressed from under the flap. There may also be generalized swelling and erythema of the adjacent gingiva, reactive cervical adenopathy, and trismus.

Table 3.3 Clinical Features: Periodontal Infections

Organism	• *Streptococcus mutans* • *Actinomyces* species • *Prevotella intermedia* and other anaerobic gram-negative bacilli
Signs and Symptoms	• Acute onset of tooth and gum pain • Diffusely receding gums • Focal gingival erythema and swelling • Absence of tenderness to palpation of the tooth
Laboratory and Radiographic Findings	• No role for blood work or radiographs

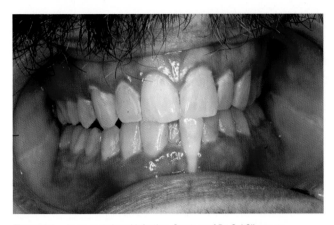

Figure 3.1 Acute periodontal infection. Courtesy of Dr. Sol Silverman.

Table 3.4 Clinical Features: Pericoronitis

Organisms	• *Streptococcus mutans* • *Actinomyces* species • *Prevotella intermedia* and other anaerobic gram-negative bacilli
Signs and Symptoms	• History of recurrent pain in the area • Trismus and pain with mastication or swallowing • Focal pain and swelling over an erupting tooth • Erythematous and swollen flap of gingiva on crown of tooth • May be able to express pus or food from under the gingival flap
Laboratory and Radiographic Findings	• Generally no role for blood work or radiographs • Consider WBC and facial CT for patients with systemic toxicity or severe trismus

CT, computed tomography; WBC, white blood (cell) count.

Acute Necrotizing Ulcerative Gingivostomatitis

This disease was relatively unknown until World War I, when approximately 25% of all troops in the European theater were afflicted, thereby leading to the name *trench mouth*. This progressive, necrotizing gum inflammation occurs in young adults and is correlated with stress, smoking, lack of adequate hygiene, and immune suppression (Table 3.5). Although trench mouth begins in infected gingiva, it rapidly extends to healthy gingival and dental tissue (Figure 3.2). *Streptococcus* and *Actinomyces* species are the primary initial pathogens, but as the infection evolves and becomes necrotizing, the microbiologic spectrum expands to include *Bacteroides*, *Fusobacterium*, and spirochetes (*Treponema vincenti* and *Borrelia* species). Interestingly, most of these pathogens exist as

Table 3.5 Clinical Features: Acute Necrotizing Ulcerative Gingivostomatitis

Organisms	• *Streptococcus mutans* • *Actinomyces* species • *Bacteroides fragilis* • *Fusobacterium* • Spirochetes (*Treponema vincenti* and *Borrelia* species)
Signs and Symptoms	• Fever and cervical lymphadenopathy • Fetid breath • Diffusely erythematous and edematous gingiva • Necrosis and ulceration of the interdental gingival papilla • Gray pseudomembrane may overlie the interdental papilla
Laboratory and Radiographic Tests	• May have an elevated WBC and ESR • Bite-wing radiographs or facial CT may help delineate the degree of alveolar bone destruction

CT, computed tomography; ESR, erythrocyte sedimentation rate; WBC, white blood (cell) count.

Table 3.6 Clinical Features: Deep Mandibular Space Infections

Organisms	• *Streptococcus mutans* • *Actinomyces* species • *Bacteroides fragilis* and *Prevotella intermedia* • Other gram-negative anaerobes
Signs and Symptoms	• Fever and cervical lymphadenopathy • Swelling over the chin extending posteriorly to the level of the hyoid • Carious anterior mandibular teeth • No difficulty breathing • No elevation of tongue within the floor of the mouth
Laboratory and Radiographic Findings	• Elevated WBC and ESR • Soft-tissue neck CT required to delineate position and extent of abscess

CT, computed tomography; ESR, erythrocyte sedimentation rate; WBC, white blood (cell) count.

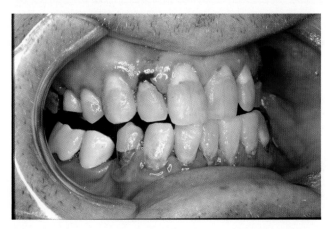

Figure 3.2 Acute necrotizing ulcerative gingivitis in an HIV patient. Courtesy of Dr. Sol Silverman.

normal oral flora and develop a fulminant form in the stressed patient. These patients present with acute onset of malaise, fever, fetid breath, dysphagia, and generalized mouth pain. Physical exam is characterized by cervical lymphadenopathy, hyperemic painful gingiva with erosion of the interdental papilla, and the development of a light gray pseudomembrane over the gingival ulcerations.

Deep Mandibular Space Infections

These infections are odontogenic in origin with decompression of the necrotic dental pulp into the sublingual, submandibular, and submental potential spaces within the mandible. All deep mandibular space infections are due to mixed bacteria including *Streptococcus*, *Actinomyces*, and β-lactamase producing gram-negative anaerobes such as *Bacteroides fragilis*.

Of the three potential deep mandibular spaces, the submental space is the least likely to communicate with the other spaces. Infections of the submental space are due to carious anterior mandibular teeth in which abscesses decompress

below the insertion of the mentalis muscle (Table 3.6). These patients present with pain and swelling extending from the chin posteriorly to the hyoid bone. Patients should not complain of difficulty breathing, the presence of which suggests the infection has extended posteriorly into the submandibular space.

Submandibular infections arise from mandibular molars in which a pulpal abscess perforates below the mylohyoid muscle (Table 3.7). Patients present with pain and swelling beneath the mandible and are at risk for airway compromise. Physical exam reveals submandibular edema extending posteriorly onto the neck; however, the tongue should have a normal lie in the floor of the mouth, unless the infection has extended into the sublingual space.

Sublingual infections arise from the mandibular molars when a pulpal abscess perforates above the mylohyoid muscle (Table 3.8). Patients present with pain, drooling, and swelling under the tongue. The tongue is usually elevated in the mouth

Table 3.7 Clinical Features: Submandibular Infections

Organisms	• *Streptococcus mutans* • *Actinomyces* species • *Bacteroides fragilis* and *Prevotella intermedia* • Other gram-negative anaerobes
Signs and Symptoms	• Fever and cervical lymphadenopathy • Trismus • Swelling under the chin, which may extend down the neck • Carious mandibular molars • May have difficulty breathing • No elevation of tongue within the floor of the mouth
Laboratory and Radiographic Tests	• Elevated WBC and ESR • Soft-tissue neck CT required to delineate position and extent of abscess

CT, computed tomography; ESR, erythrocyte sedimentation rate; WBC, white blood (cell) count.

Table 3.8 Clinical Features: Sublingual Infections

Organisms	• *Streptococcus mutans* • *Actinomyces* species • *Bacteroides fragilis* and *Prevotella intermedia* • Other gram-negative anaerobes
Signs and Symptoms	• Fever and cervical lymphadenopathy • Trismus and difficulty swallowing secretions • Swelling under the tongue, which is held elevated above the floor of the mouth • Carious mandibular molars • Majority have impending airway compromise
Laboratory and Radiographic Findings	• Elevated WBC and ESR • Soft-tissue neck CT required to delineate position and extent of abscess

CT, computed tomography; ESR, erythrocyte sedimentation rate; WBC, white blood (cell) count.

Table 3.9 Clinical Features: Ludwig's Angina

Organisms	• *Streptococcus mutans* • *Actinomyces* species • *Bacteroides fragilis* and *Prevotella intermedia* • Other gram-negative anaerobes
Signs and Symptoms	• Fever and cervical lymphadenopathy • Trismus and difficulty controlling secretions • Elevation of tongue within the floor of the mouth • Tense edema both sublingual and submandibular • Generally due to carious mandibular molars • All have impending airway compromise
Laboratory and Radiographic Tests	• Elevated WBC and ESR • Soft-tissue neck CT required to delineate position and extent of abscess

CT, computed tomography; ESR, erythrocyte sedimentation rate; WBC, white blood (cell) count.

and slightly protuberant between the teeth. By themselves, sublingual infections should not produce any extraoral swelling. Most of these patients have an element of airway compromise and need emergent airway control, preferably in the operating room.

Classically, Ludwig's angina refers to patients with bilateral infections of the submental, sublingual, and submandibular spaces, who can then develop chest pain as the infection descends into the mediastinum (Table 3.9). More commonly, these patients present with pain, difficulty breathing, and inability to control their own secretions. On physical examination, the patients are drooling and the tongue is elevated in the mouth. Palpation of the sublingual gingiva will reveal tense induration of that space. Bilateral swelling, brawny induration, and tenderness to palpation over the submandibular space will also be present. This condition is uniformly fatal if untreated, mostly because of airway compromise.

DIFFERENTIAL DIAGNOSIS

Distinguishing features of dental infections are:

- **Dentoalveolar Infections**
  - Pulpitis – Minimal focal tenderness to palpation and no gingival swelling.
  - Periapical Abscess – Significant tenderness to palpation and gingival swelling and erythema.
- **Periodontal Infections** – A history of bleeding gums and acute onset of gingival pain and erythema at the base of the teeth. No focal tooth pain.
- **Pericoronitis** – A swollen erythematous flap of gingiva overlying a partially erupted tooth.
- **Acute Necrotizing Ulcerative Gingivostomatitis** – Evidence of systemic infection with generalized erythema and ulceration of the interdental papilla with a gray overlying pseudomembrane. The only dentoalveolar infection that invades previously healthy tissue.

- **Deep Mandibular Space Infection**
  - Submental Infection – Swelling primarily over the chin without elevation of the tongue in the floor of the mouth or respiratory difficulty.
  - Submandibular Infection – Trismus and swelling under the chin without elevation of the tongue in the floor of the mouth or respiratory difficulty.
  - Sublingual Infection – Trismus and drooling with elevation of the tongue above the floor of the mouth.
  - Ludwig's Angina – Trismus, drooling, and tense edema under the chin with elevation of the tongue and difficulty breathing.

LABORATORY AND RADIOLOGIC FINDINGS

For the vast majority of patients with dental infections, a focused history and physical exam are sufficient to ascertain the diagnosis, and laboratory and radiologic testing do not change management. Laboratory testing usually does not offer additional information, although consultants may request a white blood cell (WBC) count and erythrocyte sedimentation rate (ESR). An ESR greater than 100 mm/hr is highly sensitive, but not specific for osteomyelitis, which is a concern in patients with severe pericoronitis and acute necrotizing ulcerative gingivostomatitis.

Although the majority of patients with dental infections do not require radiographs, all patients with either severe pericoronitis or deep mandibular space infections will need a computed tomographic (CT) scan. These patients require careful airway assessment prior to CT. For patients with severe pericoronitis, systemic toxicity, inability to control secretions, or severe trismus, a facial CT with intravenous (IV) contrast is required to evaluate for a complicating parapharyngeal abscess. Patients with evidence of a deep mandibular space infection should undergo soft-tissue neck CT with IV contrast in order to delineate purulent fluid collections and proximity of significant vascular structures.

TREATMENT AND ADMISSION CRITERIA
Dentoalveolar Infections

Patients presenting with an acute pulpitis without evidence of periapical abscess should be given penicillin VK or clindamycin as a first-line agent to cover *Streptococcus mutans* and *Actinomyces* species. These patients need semiurgent referral to a dentist within 48–72 hours to prevent further destruction or loss of the tooth.

Patients with periapical abscesses require incision and drainage of any clinically evident abscesses while in the acute care setting. The area can be anesthetized by performing a supraperiosteal block on both of the teeth adjacent to the abscess and placing gauze impregnated with 5% lidocaine jelly over the abscess site. The incision can be made with the edge of an 18-gauge needle if the abscess is small, or a no. 11 blade scalpel for larger abscesses. Patients should be discharged on penicillin VK or clindamycin, which seem to remain clinically active against *Streptococcus* and *Bacteroides* in spite of increasing antibiotic resistance patterns. The abscesses rarely require drain placement, and follow-up with a dentist or oral surgeon should occur within 24 hours.

Periodontal Infections

Isolated periodontal disease is usually an incidental finding because abscesses in the periodontal pocket generally spontaneously drain through the gingival sulcus. If spontaneous drainage does not occur, the abscesses should be drained and the patient should be discharged with penicillin VK or clindamycin, as well as Peridex (chlorhexidine gluconate 0.12%) oral wash. Patients require referral to a dentist within 5–7 days for periodontal disease or 2–3 days for periodontal abscess. Although these patients rarely have acute complications, periodontal infections and chronic periodontal disease increase the likelihood of other infections with significant complications.

Pericoronitis

Most cases are mild and only require curettage and irrigation of the overlying gingival flap to remove any purulent material or trapped food, a procedure that can generally be performed with a topical anesthetic alone. Patients are discharged with penicillin VK or clindamycin and Peridex (chlorhexidine gluconate 0.12%) oral wash. They need to follow up with an oral and maxillofacial surgeon in 48 to 72 hours. Rare patients with severe trismus, facial swelling, or systemic signs of toxicity need urgent evaluation by the oral and maxillofacial surgeons for possible admission and treatment with intravenous antibiotics. Similarly, patients may rarely have medial extension of the infection and develop parapharyngeal abscesses and airway obstruction.

Acute Necrotizing Ulcerative Gingivostomatitis

Historically, patients could be treated with analgesics, oral rehydration, antibiotics, and close follow-up; however, as most patients with this disease now present with underlying immunosuppression and deconditioning, they will likely need admission. Moreover, in more severe cases, the rate of alveolar ridge osteomyelitis is up to 20%. Patients should be treated with penicillin VK or erythromycin and Peridex (cholohexidine gluconate 0.12%) solution in addition to good oral hygiene. Treatment with "Magic Mouthwash," a mild anesthetic solution composed of equal parts Kaopectate, viscous lidocaine, and diphenhydramine, may offer symptomatic relief.

Deep Mandibular Space Infections

Regardless of the location of the infection (submental, sublingual, submandibular, or Ludwig's), the vast majority of these patients will require operative incision and drainage; however, there is a small subset who can be successfully treated with parenteral antibiotics and close observation in the intensive care unit.

All of the deep mandibular space infections are due to mixed bacterial infections of *Streptococcus mutans* and often anaerobes such as *Bacteroides fragilis*, with up to 50% of cultures showing resistance to penicillin. As a result, the antibiotics of choice are extended spectrum penicillins, such as ampicillin/sulbactam or penicillin G plus metronidazole. For penicillin-allergic patients, clindamycin and metronidazole provide good coverage.

COMPLICATIONS
Loss of Teeth

All patients with dentoalveolar infections are at increased risk of tooth loss; they differ in the rate at which the teeth are lost and the options for salvage. Patients with chronically untreated pulpitis or periapical abscess can often have these teeth saved after a root canal or the placement of a crown. Pericoronitis in adults usually involves the third molar, which is commonly carious and needs removal after the acute inflammation/infection has resolved. Similarly, deep mandibular space infections generally originate from nonsalvageable teeth. Acute necrotizing ulcerative gingivostomatitis causes recession of the alveolar ridge, which then leads to the loss of an otherwise healthy tooth.

Osteomyelitis

Osteomyelitis is a complication of all these dentoalveolar infections with an incidence ranging from less than 5% in patients with dental caries to 15–20% in patients with acute necrotizing ulcerative gingivostomatitis or deep mandibular space infections. The majority of these cases of osteomyelitis are due to local extension of the infection, rather than hematogenous spread, and involve the alveolar ridge or mandible.

Parapharyngeal Abscess

The parapharyngeal space is a potential space shaped like a cone with the base of the cone at the base of the skull and the apex at the hyoid. Dentoalveolar infections of the mandible, whether periapical abscess, pericoronitis, or submandibular abscess, can extend into the parapharyngeal space. It is imperative to recognize this complication because it can lead to airway obstruction, septic jugular venous thrombophlebitis, and rarely erosion of the carotid artery. These patients complain of fever, trismus, and pain with movement of the mandible, but also pain at the angle of the mandible. On clinical exam, they have swelling externally at the angle of the mandible and intraorally of the lateral oropharyngeal wall. Soft-tissue CT of the neck with IV contrast is useful to determine the location of purulent material as well as demonstrate intact carotid and jugular blood flow.

Airway Compromise

Airway compromise is the primary cause of death in patients with deep mandibular space infections, in which overall mortality remains 5–10% (down from 50% prior to the advent of antibiotics). Similarly, it is the leading cause of death in patients with parapharyngeal abscess, for which the overall mortality is also about 5–10%. Patients with these infections require thorough initial and frequently repeated airway evaluation. In fact, regardless of whether their infections are treated surgically, a majority of these patients require a tracheotomy to secure the airway during treatment.

PEARLS AND PITFALLS

1. The majority of patients with dentoalveolar infections do not require blood work or radiographs, just a good clinical exam.
2. Patients with pericoronitis should not have severe trismus or signs of systemic toxicity. If these are present, a complicating parapharyngeal abscess should be suspected and aggressively evaluated by soft-tissue neck CT with IV contrast.
3. Airway impingement remains the primary cause of mortality in patients with deep mandibular space infections. They will often require a surgical airway.
4. Of the dentoalveolar infections, only acute necrotizing ulcerative gingivostomatitis presents with diffuse (rather than localized) mouth pain. Although this condition is rare, it is associated with a high rate of alveolar ridge osteomyelitis and requires admission or very close outpatient follow-up.

REFERENCES

Cummings CW, et al. Otolaryngology head and neck surgery, 4th ed. 2005. Elsevier Mosby.

Kurian M, Mathew J, Job A, et al. Ludwig's angina. Clin Otolaryngol Allied Sci 1997;22(3):263–5.

Moyer GP, Millon JM, Martinez-Vidal A. Is conservative treatment of deep neck space infections appropriate? Head Neck 2001;23(2):126–33.

Mandell GL, Bennett JE, Dolin R. Principles and practice of infectious disease, 6th ed. 2005.

Rudolph, AM, Hoffman JIE, Rudolph CD. Rudolph's pediatrics, 20th ed. 1996. Appleton and Lange.

4. Systemic Diseases Causing Fever and Rash

Catherine A. Marco, Janel Kittredge-Sterling, and Rachel L. Chin

INTRODUCTION – AGENTS

The clinical picture of fever and rash may be caused by a variety of agents, including bacterial, viral, rickettsial, or fungal infections, immunocompromised states, autoimmune conditions, and other systemic diseases. Knowledge of the epidemiology, pathophysiology, clinical presentations, and management of these conditions is essential for the acute care physician, as some of these conditions have significant time-dependent morbidity and mortality.

HISTORY AND PHYSICAL EXAMINATION

Crucial elements of the history and physical in the patient presenting with fever and rash are listed in Table 4.1.

SYSTEMIC BACTERIAL INFECTIONS

Secondary Syphilis

Syphilis is caused by the spirochete *Treponema pallidum*, which typically enters the body through mucous membranes or nonintact skin (Table 4.2). Syphilis is the third most common reportable sexually transmitted disease in the United States (after chlamydia and gonorrhea) and is spread almost exclusively through sexual contact, with some rare cases of transplacental transmission. Syphilis affects all ethnicities

equally but has a male predilection. The incubation period is 2–90 days from exposure.

Primary syphilis presents as a painless genital chancre. (See Chapter 17, Ulcerative Sexually Transmitted Diseases.) Medical care is often delayed or not sought because the lesion is painless and usually resolves spontaneously though latent disease persists. Up to 50% of patients do not recall any lesions. Secondary syphilis occurs 5–12 weeks after the chancre, and symptoms may include fever, headache, and adenopathy. Additional symptoms may include sore throat, weight loss, and splenomegaly. Skin findings may include macules, papules, follicular lesions, nodules, pustules, and annular or serpiginous lesions. Inflammatory lesions of oral and genital mucosa may occur. The trunk, extremities, and genitalia may be affected and lesions usually occur symmetrically (Figure 4.1). Alopecia and nail changes may also be seen. Secondary syphilis should be considered in the differential diagnosis of any maculopapular lesion involving the trunk, palms, or soles. Condyloma lata is the term for soft, flat-topped, red to pale papules, nodules, or plaques seen in intertriginous or mucous membranes, such as the anogenital region, the mouth, interdigital spaces, or the axillae. If untreated, secondary syphilis may progress to tertiary syphilis, with meningitis, dementia, neuropathy, or thoracic aneurysm.

Treatment of secondary syphilis may be undertaken prior to establishment of the definitive diagnosis (Table 4.3). The treatment of choice is benzathine penicillin G (Bicillin-LA, BPG), 2.4 million units intramuscular. It is important to note

Table 4.1 History and Examination for Fever and Rash

History
- Duration of symptoms
- Associated symptoms (such as fever, headache, gastrointestinal symptoms, pruritus)
- Evolution of lesions
- Distribution
- History of animal or arthropod bites
- Exacerbating and relieving factors (such as environmental exposures, foods, medications)
- Medical, occupational, and sexual history, medications, illicit drug history, travel, and allergies may be relevant

Physical Examination
Type of lesions, size, color, secondary findings (such as scale, excoriations), and distribution. Primary lesions may include the following:
- *Macules* are flat lesions defined by an area of changed color (i.e., a blanchable erythema).
- *Papules* are raised, solid lesions <5 mm in diameter.
- *Plaques* are lesions >5 mm in diameter with a flat, plateau-like surface.
- *Nodules* are lesions >5 mm in diameter with a more rounded configuration.
- *Wheals* (urticaria, hives) are papules or plaques that are pale pink and may appear annular (ringlike) as they enlarge; classic (nonvasculitic) wheals are transient, lasting only 24 to 48 hours in any defined area.
- *Vesicles* (<5 mm) and *bullae* (>5 mm) are circumscribed, elevated lesions containing fluid.
- *Pustules* are raised lesions containing purulent exudates. Vesicular processes such as varicella or herpes simplex may evolve to pustules.
- *Nonpalpable purpura* is a flat lesion that is due to bleeding into the skin. If <3 mm in diameter, the purpuric lesions are termed *petechiae*. If >3 mm, they are termed *ecchymoses*. *Palpable purpura* is a raised lesion that is due to inflammation of the vessel wall (vasculitis) with subsequent hemorrhage.
- An *ulcer* is a defect in the skin extending at least into the upper layer of the dermis.
- *Eschar* is a necrotic lesion covered with a black crust.

Secondary lesions may include:
- Scale
- Crust
- Fissure
- Erosions
- Ulcer
- Scar
- Excoriation
- Infection
- Pigment changes
- Lichenification

Color may be:
- Normal
- Erythematous
- Violaceous
- Hyperpigmented
- Hypopigmented

Patterns of lesions should be established as:
- Single
- Grouped
- Scattered
- Linear
- Annular
- Symmetric
- Dermatomal
- Central or peripheral
- Along Blaschko's lines (linear skin patterns thought to be of embryonic origin, usually forming a "V" shape over the spine and "S" shapes over the chest, stomach, and sides)

Table 4.2 Clinical Features: Syphilis

Organism	*Treponema pallidum*
Incubation Period	- Primary (chancre) lesion appears 10–90 days after contact. - Secondary (rash) occurs within 6 months of primary lesion.
Signs and Symptoms	- Mucocutaneous: usually one lesion, may be more. Untreated lasts several weeks. - Secondary: within 6 months of primary lesion; palmar-plantar copper coin rash classic; many other rash forms, condyloma latum. Other secondary symptoms include alopecia areata, fever. - CNS: meningitis (1–2 years after infection), meningovascular (5–7 years), general paresis and tabes dorsalis (10–20 years), gummatous neurosyphilis. - Ocular: uveitis, iridocyclitis, Argyll-Robertson pupils. - Cardiovascular system: ascending aortitis. - Bone: arthritis, osteitis, periostitis. - Liver: hepatitis.
Laboratory Findings	Diagnosis is made by dark-field microscopy, nontreponemal serology, or treponemal antibody tests. Nontreponemal serologic tests, including RPR and VDRL, typically correlate with disease progress and become positive 14 days after a chancre appears. Titers are expected to decline or disappear after treatment, although they may remain positive in some patients indefinitely. Treponemal antibody tests, such as FTA-ABS, do not correlate with disease activity, and many patients will remain positive indefinitely. **Primary syphilis**: - May be dark-field positive but serologically negative; TP-specific test (FTA) may be positive before RPR. **Secondary syphilis**: - RPR positive in 99%.

CNS, central nervous system; FTA-ABS, fluorescent treponemal antibody absorbed; RPR, rapid plasma reagin; TP, *Treponema pallidum*; VDRL, venereal disease research laboratory.

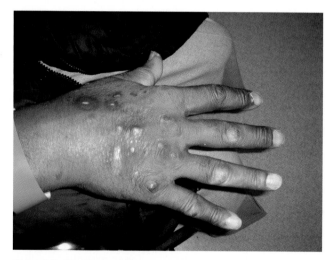

Figure 4.1 Secondary syphilis.

Table 4.3 Treatment for Syphilis

Primary and Secondary Syphilis	benzathine PCN G 2.4 million units IM × 1 PCN allergy (nonpregnant, preferred): doxycycline 100 mg PO bid × 14 days *or* tetracycline 500 mg PO qid × 14 days *or* ceftriaxone 1 g IM or IV × 8–10 days
Latent Syphilis	All treatments require well-documented close follow-up. Early latent [<1 year duration] (normal CSF exam, if done): BPG 2.4 million units IM × 1. Late latent or latent of unknown duration (normal CSF exam, if done): BPG 2.4 million units per week × 3 weeks. If any dose >2 days late, must recommence prescription from first dose. PCN allergy recommended: (1) doxycycline 100 mg PO bid × 4 weeks *or* (2) tetracycline 500 mg PO qid × 4 weeks.
Neurosyphilis	Only penicillin is currently recommended; allergic persons should be desensitized and treated with penicillin. Recommended: aqueous crystalline penicillin G 18–24 million units/day IV, administer as 3–4 million units IV q4h × 10–14 days. Alternative: procaine penicillin 2.4 million units IM qd, plus probenecid 500 mg PO qid × 10–14 days.
Syphilis in HIV-Infected	Penicillin is the highly preferred regimen for all stages of syphilis in HIV-infected persons. Primary, secondary, and early latent syphilis: use BPG as for immunocompetent persons; some experts recommend three weekly doses (i.e., as for late latent syphilis). PCN-allergic HIV-positive, primary, secondary, or early latent syphilis: can be treated as allergic HIV-negative person. Late latent syphilis or syphilis of unknown duration requires LP to rule out neurosyphilis. All require PCN-based treatment. Desensitization required.
Syphilis in Pregnancy	Only penicillin is currently recommended. Treatment during pregnancy should be the penicillin regimen appropriate to the stage of syphilis diagnosis; desensitization required for PCN-allergic pregnant patients. Some experts recommend a second dose of BPG 2.4 million units IM 1 week after the initial dose for primary, secondary, early latent syphilis in pregnancy.

CSF, cerebrospinal fluid; HIV, human immunodeficiency virus; LP, lumbar puncture; PCN, penicillin; BPG, benzathine PCN G.

Table 4.4 Clinical Features: Meningococcemia

Organism	*Neisseria meningitidis*
Signs and Symptoms	• Kernig's/Brudzinski's sign (present <5%), nuchal rigidity (30%), headache, cranial nerve palsies or other focal neurologic findings, headache, seizures, myalgia. • Rash: petechiae (50% of patients), papules, purpura, mottling, or morbilliform lesions.
Laboratory Findings	• CSF: typical results OP >30 cm, WBC >500/mm^3 with >80% neutrophils, glucose <40 mg/dL (or <2/3 plasma), and protein >200 mg/dL. • Gram-negative, diplococcus, from CSF, blood cultures, or skin lesions.
Treatment	penicillin 18–24 million units IV divided doses q4h *or* ceftriaxone 2 g IV q12h *or* cefotaxime 2 g IV q4–6h × 7–10 days Alternatives: chloramphenicol 100 mg/kg divided doses q6h (max 4 g/day) × 7–10 days Prophylaxis: household or intimate contact, medical personnel in contact with oral secretions: rifampin 600 mg PO bid × 2 days *or* ciprofloxacin 500 mg PO × 1 *or* ceftriaxone 250 mg IM × 1

CSF, cerebrospinal fluid; IM, intramuscular; OP, opening pressure; WBC, white blood (cell) count.

that the similar combination benzathine-procaine penicillin G (Bicillin-CR) is not appropriate therapy for secondary syphilis. Effective alternatives include doxycycline or ceftriaxone.

Meningococcemia

Meningococcal disease, caused by a gram-negative diplococcus *Neisseria meningitidis*, presents with a spectrum of disease (see Chapter 39, Fever and Headache). Approximately 2500 cases occur annually in the United States, and 10–14% are fatal. Over 98% of cases are sporadic, although some localized outbreaks occur. The highest incidence occurs in children 3 months to 3 years, although there has been an increasing incidence in 12- to 29-year-olds. The risk of meningococcal disease is increased among infants, asplenic patients, alcoholics, and patients with a terminal (C6-C9) complement deficiency. Meningococcal disease has a peak incidence in midwinter and early spring, and the disease is transmitted by direct respiratory secretion contact.

Clinical presentations may include respiratory tract infection, focal infection, meningitis, meningococcal bacteremia, and meningococcemia (Table 4.4). Meningococcal bacteremia and meningococcemia are associated with high morbidity and mortality and are often accompanied by characteristic hemorrhagic cutaneous findings. Typically, patients present with a systemic illness including fever, malaise, coryza, pharyngitis, headache, vomiting, myalgias, and/or arthralgias.

Acute fulminant meningococcemia (Waterhouse-Friderichsen syndrome) occurs in 10% of cases, presenting with shock, hypotension, intracutaneous hemorrhage, and multiorgan failure.

Cutaneous lesions may be varied in appearance. Lesions may include petechiae (50% of patients), papules, purpura, mottling, or morbilliform lesions. The eruption often begins on extremities and becomes generalized. Early lesions may appear as nonspecific pink macules and papules. Later lesions may display the classic intracutaneous hemorrhage of petechiae and purpura (Figure 4.2).

Disseminated Gonococcal Infection

Gonococcal infections are caused by the gram-negative diplococcus species *Neisseria gonorrhoeae*. Approximately 600,000

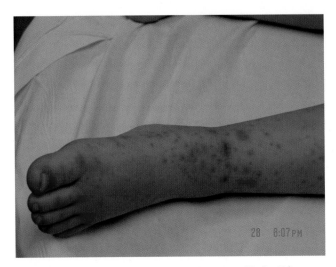

Figure 4.2 Meningococcal disease. Photograph courtesy of Dr. David C. Brancati.

Table 4.5 Clinical Features: Disseminated Gonococcal Infection

Signs and Symptoms	• Fever, mono- or polyarthralgias, tenosynovitis, endocarditis, and meningitis • Skin lesions may appear as tender erythematous or hemorrhagic papules that evolve into pustules and vesicles, with predilection for periarticular regions of distal extremities
Laboratory Findings	Gram stains: urethral and accessory gland secretions (95% sensitive); female cervical secretions (50%) immunofluorescent staining of pustule contents, blood cultures
Treatment	Recommended regimen: ceftriaxone 1 g IM or IV q24h Alternative regimens: cefotaxime 1 g IV q8h *or* ceftizoxime 1 g IV q8h spectinomycin 2 g IM q12h

*Fluoroquinolones (FQs) are no longer recommended due to high rates of developing resistance.

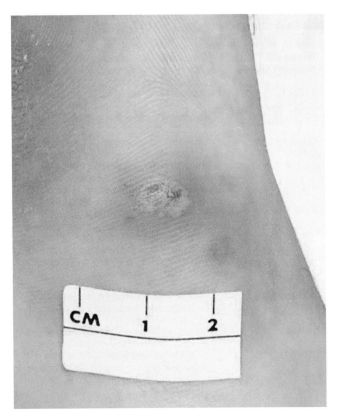

Figure 4.3 Disseminated gonococcal infection. Photograph courtesy of Centers for Disease Control Public Health Image Library, Dr. S. E. Thompson, http://phil.cdc.gov/phil/home.asp.

cases occur annually in the United States. Disseminated gonococcal infection occurs in 1–3% of patients with gonococcal infection and occurs disproportionately in women. (See Chapter 21, Adult Septic Arthritis.)

Systemic symptoms may include fever, mono- or polyarthralgias, tenosynovitis, endocarditis, and meningitis. Skin lesions may appear as tender erythematous or hemorrhagic papules that evolve into pustules and vesicles, with predilection for periarticular regions of distal extremities (Table 4.5; Figure 4.3).

Diagnostic tests may include cervical or urethral cultures (80–90% sensitive), cultures of joint or skin lesions (20–50% sensitive), immunofluorescent staining of pustule contents, and blood cultures.

Treatment should include hospital admission, for supportive care, such as intravenous hydration and antipyretics, as well as antibiotic therapy, such as ceftriaxone 1 g IV qd for 7–10 days. Alternative regimens include cefotaxime, ceftizoxime, or spectinomycin. Quinolone-resistant *Neisseria gonorrhea* (QRNG) continues to be an emerging treatment problem in the United States, and quinolones are no longer recommended. The rate of co-infection with chlamydia is high, and all patients should also be treated with azithromycin or doxycycline.

Toxic Shock Syndrome

Toxic shock syndrome is a clinical syndrome associated with *Staphylococcus aureus* infection. Historically, the disease was associated with high-absorbency tampon use, but it has also been documented in association with intravaginal contraceptive devices, nasal packing, postoperative wound infections, and other foreign bodies. Over 5000 cases have been reported since 1979, although the annual incidence has declined following tampon redesign and public education.

Patients with toxic shock syndrome present with a constellation of symptoms (Table 4.6). Typically, patients have high fever and an erythematous macular rash, often with extensive desquamation (Figure 4.4). Hypotension and tachycardia may be present. Other potential diagnoses must be ruled out, including sepsis, Rocky Mountain spotted fever (RMSF), leptospirosis, measles, hepatitis, mononucleosis, and syphilis.

Diagnostic criteria include involvement of at least three organ systems among the following: gastrointestinal (nausea, vomiting, diarrhea), muscular, renal, hepatic, hematologic, CNS, or mucosal. Abnormal laboratory values that indicate multi-system involvement include elevated creatinine kinase, blood urea nitrogen (BUN)/creatinine, bilirubin, aspartate transaminase (AST), alanine aminotransferase (ALT), platelets, and sterile pyuria. Chest radiographic findings may be consistent with acute respiratory distress syndrome secondary to sepsis.

Table 4.6 Clinical Features: Toxic Shock Syndrome

Organism	*Staphylococcus aureus* enterotoxins, TSST-1, SEB, and SEC

Signs and Symptoms and Laboratory Findings	• Fever: >38.9°C
	• Hypotension and tachycardia
	• Rash: diffuse erythematous macular rash and desquamation of palms and soles
	• Multisystem involvement (three or more of following):
	  a. GI: vomiting, diarrhea at onset
	  b. musculoskeletal: CPK > 2× normal or severe myalgia
	  c. renal: BUN/creatinine > 2× normal or sterile pyuria
	  d. hepatic: bilirubin, AST, or ALT >2× normal
	  e. Hematologic: platelets <100,000/mm³
	  f. CNS: altered mental status without focal neurologic signs

Treatment	Supportive with ICU monitoring Clindamycin 900 mg IV q8h + oxacillin 2 g IV q4h for methicillin-sensitive *S. aureus* Clindamycin 900 mg IV q8h plus vancomycin 1 g IV q12h for methicillin-resistant *S. aureus* Some favor linezolid instead of vancomycin if MRSA concerns, mainly because of protein synthesis inhibition Consider IVIG: 2 g/kg IV × 1, repeat in 48 hours if patient remains unstable

CPK, creatine phosphokinase; GI, gastrointestinal; MRSA, methicillin-resistant *Staphylococcus aureus*.

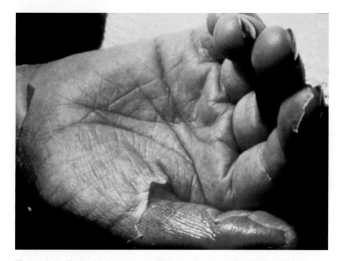

Figure 4.4 Toxic shock syndrome. Photograph source: Centers for Disease Control Public Health Image Library, http://phil.cdc.gov/phil/home.asp.

Management is primarily supportive, though removing any possible toxin source, including tampons, wound or nasal packing, contraceptive devices, indwelling lines, or any other foreign body, is crucial to initial management. *S. aureus* produces the enterotoxins toxic shock syndrome toxin-1 (TSST-1), staphylococcal enterotoxins B (SEB), and staphylococcal enterotoxins C (SEC). Therapy is guided at stopping toxin production and killing bacteria. Clindamycin inhibits toxin elaboration and is the drug of choice. Antibiotics include clindamycin and oxacillin for methicillin-sensitive *S. aureus* and clindamycin and vancomycin for methicillin-resistant *S. aureus*. Airway management and treatment of shock with pressors may be indicated. High-volume crystalloid infusion is often required; some patients require up to 20 L in the first 24 hours. If coagulation is abnormal, fresh frozen plasma may be administered. There has been no demonstrated benefit of antibiotics. Most patients with *S. aureus* toxic shock syndrome have been shown to lack antibodies to the toxin; intravenous immune globulin (IVIG) contains antibodies to this common antigen and is often used.

RICKETTSIAL INFECTIONS

Rocky Mountain Spotted Fever

Rocky Mountain spotted fever is caused by the organism *Rickettsia rickettsii* (see Chapter 54, Fever in the Returning Traveler). It is the most common rickettsial infection in the United States. The organism is transmitted by ticks, especially wood and dog ticks. Annually, there are 500–1000 cases in the United States, and RMSF is a misnomer, as less than 5% of cases occur in Rocky Mountain states, with more than 50% of cases occurring in the south Atlantic states. RMSF is more common in the summer months and in children between the ages of 5 and 9. Most patients (70%) have a history of tick bite or exposure. The incubation period is 3–12 days. If untreated, the disease may be fatal in 25% of cases.

The clinical presentation is typically one of systemic illness and may include fever, headache, muscle tenderness (especially of the gastrocnemius), photophobia, conjunctival infection, pulmonary symptoms, and gastrointestinal symptoms, including nausea, vomiting, abdominal pain, and splenomegaly (Table 4.7). Skin lesions occur in 85–95% of patients and typically appear at days 2–6. Lesions are typically macular rose-colored blanching lesions, petechiae, or ecchymoses on the extremities with centripetal spread (Figure 4.5). The lesions are not pathognomonic and the diagnosis should be made clinically based on the constellation of symptoms.

Diagnostic tests may include fluorescent antibody testing on biopsy and serologic tests, though high clinical suspicion warrants immediate treatment, pending test results.

Management should include antibiotics, such as doxycycline or tetracycline, for 5–7 days. Chloramphenicol may be used as alternative therapy.

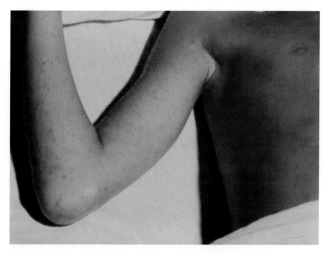

Figure 4.5 Rocky Mountain spotted fever. Photograph source: Centers for Disease Control Public Health Image Library, http://phil.cdc.gov/phil/home.asp.

Table 4.7 Clinical Features: Rocky Mountain Spotted Fever

Organism	*Rickettsia rickettsii*
Signs and Symptoms	• General: fever, myalgia, sepsis syndrome • Skin: petechial rash, begins on extremities, moves toward trunk (centripetal); endothelial cell dysfunction leads to edema of hands and feet; 50% of rashes begin after 3 days of fever • Neurological: vasculitis; headache, focal neurological deficits, deafness, meningismus (sometimes with CSF mononuclear/polynuclear pleocytosis), delirium • Renal: acute renal failure–ATN and/or intravascular volume depletion; may require hemodialysis • Pulmonary: pneumonia (alveolar infiltrates); noncardiogenic pulmonary edema; ARDS
Laboratory Findings	• Normal to low WBC; thrombocytopenia characteristic; occasionally mild anemia; coagulopathy (DIC); hyponatremia in 50%; high CK, LDH with tissue injury in severe cases • Diagnosis is made by: skin biopsy, direct fluorescent antibody; or serum IFA to detect antibodies to spotted fever group *Rickettsia*
Treatment	doxycycline (drug of choice in children as well as adults given potential fatal outcome): Adult: 100 mg PO or IV q12h, × 7 days or 3 days after defervescence Children*: tetracycline 25 to 50 mg/kg/day PO in four divided doses Alternative: chloramphenicol: Adult: 500 mg PO qid, 7 days or 3 days after defervescence Child: 50–75 mg/kg/day PO in four divided doses Adjunctive steroids not recommended

*Doxycycline or tetracycline recommended for children for two reasons: RMSF can be life threatening, and a brief course of one of these drugs is unlikely to lead to tooth problems or staining.
ARDS, acute respiratory distress syndrome; ATN, acute tubular necrosis; CK, creatine kinase; CSF, cerebrospinal fluid; DIC, disseminated intravascular coagulation; IFA, indirect fluorescence assay; LDH, lactate dehydrogenase.

Table 4.8 Clinical Features: Lyme Disease

Organism	*Borrelia burgdorferi*
Signs and Symptoms	• Stage I occurs early (3–30 days after tick bite): erythema migrans, malaise, headache, fever, and arthralgias • Stage II has secondary annular lesions, fever, neurologic manifestations (weakness, lethargy), and cardiac manifestations (AV block) • Stage III has chronic arthritis, neurologic manifestations (cranial nerve palsy including Bell's palsy, lymphocytic meningitis, or radiculopathy with pain, paresis, or paresthesias), encephalopathy, and dermatitis
Laboratory Findings	Laboratory conformation not typically necessary. Elevated ESR. EIA or IFA and Western blot – takes 4–6 weeks for seroconversion

AV, atrioventricular; EIA, enzyme immunoassay. Diagnostic tests may include a nonspecific elevated erythrocyte sedimentation rate and serologic tests, which are helpful in establishing the definitive diagnosis but are not available acutely.

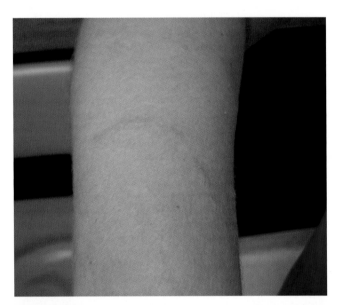

Figure 4.6 Erythema migrans associated with Lyme disease. Photograph courtesy of Dr. David C. Brancati.

Lyme Disease

Lyme disease is caused by the organism *Borrelia burgdorferi* and is transmitted by the deer tick bite (see Chapter 52, Ectoparasites). Most cases occur in the spring and early summer. Endemic areas in the United States include the Northeast, Midwest, West, and scattered other areas. Although 36–48 hours of tick attachment is necessary to transmit disease, less than 33% of patients recall a tick bite.

Clinical presentations include three disease stages (Table 4.8). Stage I occurs early and is manifested by malaise, headache, fever, and arthralgias. Stage I typically resolves in 4 weeks. Erythema migrans occurs in 60–80% of cases and manifests as erythematous annular, nonscaling lesion with central clearing (Figure 4.6). Stage II presents with secondary annular lesions, fever, neurologic manifestations, and/or AV block and may last weeks to months. Stage III manifests as chronic arthritis, CNS disease, and dermatitis.

Management should include appropriate antibiotic administration (Table 4.9). The antibiotic regimen may include doxycycline for 10–21 days, or as alternates, cefuroxime, ceftriax-one, or penicillin G. Amoxicillin may be used in pediatric and pregnant patients.

SYSTEMIC VIRAL INFECTIONS

Systemic viral infections may cause fever and rash. Common organisms include enterovirus, adenovirus, rotavirus, coxsackievirus, roseola, and numerous others. In many cases, the viral infection is brief and self-limited. Specific viruses of clinical importance, including measles and rubella, are discussed here.

Measles

Measles, or rubeola, caused by a single-stranded RNA paramyxovirus, occurs commonly in the winter months, though the number of reported cases of measles has dropped

Table 4.9 Treatment of Lyme Disease

Tick Exposure	Prompt tick removal. Single dose doxycycline 200 mg if <72 hours in epidemic area
Erythema Migrans	doxycycline 100 mg PO bid × 10–14 days Alternatives: amoxicillin 500 mg PO tid × 14–21 days *or* cefuroxime axetil 500 mg PO bid × 14–21 days
Bell's Palsy	doxycycline 100 mg PO bid × 21–28 days *or* amoxicillin 500 mg PO tid × 21–28 days
CNS (Other)	ceftriaxone 2 g IV q12h × 14–28 days *or* cefotaxime 2 g IV q6h × 14–28 days *or* PCN G 4 million units IV q4h × 14–28 days
Cardiac First-Degree Block	doxycycline 100 mg PO bid × 21–28 days *or* amoxicillin 500 mg PO tid × 21–28 days
Cardiac Second- or Third-Degree Block	ceftriaxone 2 g IV qd × 14–28 days *or* PCN G 3–4 million units IV q4h × 14–21 days
Arthritis	doxycycline 100 mg PO bid × 28 days *or* amoxicillin 500 mg PO tid × 28 days *or* cefotaxime 2 g IV q8h × 14–28 days *or* PCN G 18–24 million units IV divided q4h × 14–28 days

Table 4.10 Clinical Features: Measles

Organism	Morbillivirus, RNA virus of paramyxoviridae group
Signs and Symptoms	• Fever, cough, coryza, conjunctivitis preceding the dermatologic findings • Skin lesions: erythematous macules and papules, often beginning on the scalp and head and spreading caudally to neck, trunk, and extremities • Koplik's spots are pathognomonic
Laboratory Findings	• Laboratory conformation not typically necessary • If necessary, measles EIA IgM helpful for acute infection • IgG to screen immune status • Tissue/secretions may be cultured for virus and/or identified by IFA • Nasopharyngeal aspirate IFA offers rapid diagnosis
Treatment	Supportive care. Disease tends to be more severe in pediatric populations.

EIA, enzyme immunoassay; IFA, immunofluorescent antibodies.

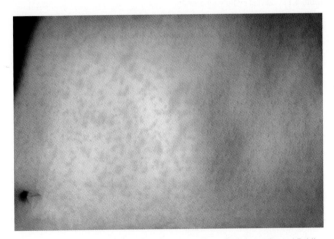

Figure 4.7 Measles. Photograph courtesy of Centers for Disease Control Public Health Image Library, Dr. Heinz F. Eichenwald, http://phil.cdc.gov/phil/home.asp.

dramatically in the United States since the advent of the measles vaccine. In recent years, typically <100 cases are seen annually in the United States, compared to the 4–5 million annual cases prior to immunization. Measles is most likely to infect unvaccinated individuals, often including preschoolers in low-income homes or in heavily populated areas. Worldwide, measles is the primary cause of death that is preventable by vaccination. Patients are considered to be contagious from 5 days prior to onset of symptoms until 5–6 days after the onset of dermatologic involvement.

Common symptoms preceding the dermatologic finding include fever, cough, coryza, and conjunctivitis (Table 4.10). Other symptoms include nausea, vomiting, diarrhea, headache, and malaise. Lymphadenopathy and splenomegaly may be found on exam. Skin lesions are erythematous macules and papules, often beginning on the scalp and head and spreading caudally to neck, trunk, and extremities (Figure 4.7). Purpura may occur in association with thrombocytopenia. Koplik's spots are small white or blue lesions on an erythematous base found opposite the second molars on the buccal mucosa (Figure 4.8).

The diagnosis is usually made clinically. Complete blood count will often reveal leukopenia with lymphocytopenia. Complement fixing detection of antibodies can be performed to confirm the diagnosis.

Complications may include pneumonia, otitis media, diarrhea, hepatitis, thrombocytopenia, and encephalitis. Children younger than age 5 are at highest risk for complications. Pneu-

monia is the most common cause of death in children with measles.

Supportive therapy, including rest, hydration, and antipyretics, is usually sufficient. Immune globulin may shorten the course if given within 6 days of exposure. Prevention of measles by immunization is the primary measure of disease control.

Rubella

Rubella, or German measles, caused by a single-stranded RNA togavirus, occurs commonly in the spring months and is more common among unvaccinated individuals.

Rubella typically presents with fever, conjunctivitis, and lymphadenopathy, followed by a rash 1–7 days after onset of symptoms (Table 4.11). Tender suboccipital, posterior cervical, and postauricular lymphadenopathy are common.

The rash typically persists for 2–3 days (hence the term "3-day measles"). Lesions appear as erythematous macules with confluence, often beginning in the head and neck and spreading to the trunk and extremities (Figure 4.9).

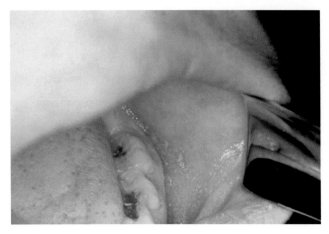

Figure 4.8 Koplik's spots. Photograph source: Centers for Disease Control Public Health Image Library, http://phil.cdc.gov/phil/home.asp.

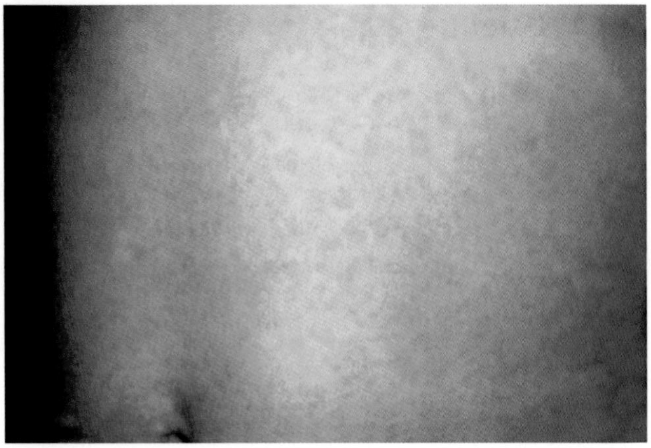

Figure 4.9 Rubella. Photograph source: Centers for Disease Control Public Health Image Library, http://phil.cdc.gov/phil/home.asp.

Table 4.11 Clinical Features: Rubella

Organism	RNA togavirus, genus Rubivirus
Incubation period	12–23 days, and 20–50% of cases may be subclinical
Signs and Symptoms	• Erythematous macules, confluence, caudal spread • Soft palate petechiae
Laboratory Findings	• Laboratory conformation not typically necessary • Virus can be cultured from respiratory tract or CSF • False positive IgM has occurred with parvovirus, EBV infections, or patients positive for rheumatoid factor • Positive hemagglutination inhibiting antibody test
Treatment	Supportive care Often mild illness, necessitates no therapy Fever, arthritic complaints may be treated with acetaminophen or other NSAIDs

CSF, cerebrospinal fluid; EBV, Epstein-Barr virus; NSAID, nonsteroidal anti-inflammatory drug. Although the clinical diagnosis is sufficient in most cases, the rubella hemagglutination inhibiting antibody test may be performed at the time of appearance of the rash and repeated 2 weeks later for comparison.

Forchheimer's sign, seen in 20% of rubella cases, is the eruption of petechiae over the soft palate. Pruritus is common with the rash, and mild desquamation often occurs.

Rare complications include encephalitis, arthritis, thrombocytopenic purpura, and peripheral neuritis. Complications are more prevalent in adolescents and adults. Congenital rubella is a serious condition occurring in utero and is manifest by multiple congenital defects, including deafness, heart disease, and cataracts.

Management includes supportive care, hydration, and antipyretics. Prevention by immunization is the mainstay of disease control.

HIV INFECTION AND ACQUIRED IMMUNODEFICIENCY SYNDROME

Common cutaneous manifestations of HIV infection and acquired immunodeficiency syndrome (AIDS) include exacerbations of preexisting dermatologic conditions and atypical presentations of common dermatological infections in the setting of immunocompromise. The coexistence of fever and rash may signify a systemic bacterial or viral infection, rising HIV antigen load, an autoimmune disorder, or a drug reaction. Selected examples of conditions causing fever and rash in the HIV-infected patient are discussed in this section.

Bacterial infections causing fever and rash in HIV-infected patients include a wide variety of soft-tissue infections, bacteremia, and other serious systemic infections, such as sexually transmitted diseases and meningitis.

Other sexually transmitted diseases occur with increased frequency in HIV-infected patients. In addition to testing for common STDs such as gonorrhea, *Chlamydia*, and herpes infections, serologic testing for syphilis should be performed in all patients. The prevalence of syphilis in the United States has recently increased, and syphilis has been associated with increased susceptibility to HIV seroconversion, as well as aggressive and atypical disease courses. Because a normal antibody response may be absent in HIV-infected individuals, heightened vigilance is important to identify potential cases of syphilis, even with negative serologies. The recommended treatment of primary or secondary syphilis is benzathine penicillin, 2.4 million units IM. For latent syphilis or secondary syphilis of unknown duration (possibly over 12 months), three weekly injections are recommended. Patients with neurosyphilis should be admitted for treatment with 12 to 24 million units penicillin G, IV, daily for 10 to 14 days. Follow-up care to ensure adequate treatment is essential, as some cases are resistant to traditional therapies and high-dose intravenous penicillin may be required to adequately manage resistant cases.

Acute seroconversion syndrome (acute retroviral syndrome) commonly occurs 2–6 weeks after primary exposure. This syndrome is often undiagnosed because of the nonspecific nature of its symptoms, which may include fever, adenopathy, fatigue, pharyngitis, diarrhea, weight loss, and rash. Myopathy, peripheral neuropathy, or other neurologic or immunologic manifestations may also be seen. Symptoms may be present for 1 to 3 weeks.

Varicella-zoster infection often presents atypically in the HIV-infected patients. Eruptions involving several dermatomes are commonly seen in patients with AIDS. Although varicella seropositivity is common among adults (90%), reactivation causing clinical disease is more common in the HIV-infected population, who are 17 times more likely than the general population to develop dermatomal zoster reactivation. Multidermatomal involvement and recurrent episodes occur with increased frequency. In the HIV-infected patient with routine dermatomal zoster infection, outpatient management should include oral famciclovir (5 mg, PO, bid or tid, for 7 days), acyclovir (800 mg, 5 times daily), or valacyclovir (1000 mg, bid, for 7 days). Admission is indicated if there is evidence of systemic involvement, ophthalmic zoster, or severe multidermatomal zoster. IV acyclovir may be administered at a dosage of 10 mg/kg every 8 hours. Varicella immune globulin may be administered to patients with primary infection and visceral involvement. The use of capsaicin, which causes depletion of substance P, steroids, topical lidocaine patch, or transcutaneous electrical nerve stimulation (TENS) unit may be useful for the treatment of postherpetic neuralgia. The varicella-zoster virus (VZV) vaccine has demonstrated efficacy among geriatric patients in leading to reduced incidence of herpes zoster infections and reduction of incidence of postherpetic neuralgia. The safety and efficacy of its use among HIV-infected patients has not been established.

Drug Reactions

Adverse drug reactions are common among HIV-infected patients, both because these patients are commonly treated with drugs known to produce adverse effects, such as antiretroviral agents, and because, for unclear reasons, HIV-infected individuals seem to have more frequent or more severe reactions to commonly used medications. Dermatologic reactions are particularly prevalent, and fever may also be seen. Antimicrobial drugs are the most commonly implicated. Potential drug interactions should always be considered when prescribing new medications. Common reactions include drug hypersensitivity, Stevens-Johnson syndrome, and toxic epidermal necrolysis. Among antiretroviral agents, the nucleoside reverse transcriptase inhibitors (NRTIs; zidovudine, lamivudine, etc.) cause hypersensitivity reactions in 5–10% of patients. The nonnucleoside reverse transcriptase inhibitors (NNRTIs; efavirenz, etc.) may cause rash and hypersensitivity reactions in up to 17% of patients. Protease inhibitors (indinavir, saquinavir, etc.) cause skin reactions less commonly than the NRTIs and NNRTIs.

SYSTEMIC DISEASES CAUSING FEVER AND RASH (AUTOIMMUNE SYNDROMES)

Disseminated Intravascular Coagulation

Disseminated intravascular coagulation (DIC) is associated with severe systemic stress, such as systemic infection, obstetric complications, hemolysis, metabolic disorders, malignancies, trauma, or burns.

Systemic symptoms may include hypotension, tachycardia, and altered mental status (Table 4.12). Skin lesions

Table 4.12 Clinical Features: Disseminated Intravascular Coagulation

Signs and Symptoms	Hypotension, tachycardia, and altered mental status. Skin lesions may include petechiae, purpura, ecchymoses, bullae, and cutaneous necrosis. Lesions are typically disseminated.
Laboratory Findings	Fragmented RBCs on peripheral smear, prolonged prothrombin time, activated partial thromboplastin time, reduced fibrinogen, and elevated fibrin degradation products.
Treatment	Treat underlying disease. Supportive care. Transfusion, anticoagulation, vitamin K replacement, fresh frozen plasma, and platelet transfusion are often necessary.

RBC, red blood cell.

may include petechiae, purpura, ecchymoses, bullae, and cutaneous necrosis. Lesions are typically disseminated (Figure 4.10).

The diagnosis is supported by laboratory evaluation demonstrating thrombocytopenia, fragmented RBCs on peripheral smear, prolonged prothrombin time, activated partial thromboplastin time, reduced fibrinogen, and elevated fibrin degradation products.

The primary treatment modality is to treat the underlying disease. Other treatment strategies have varied reports of success, including transfusion, anticoagulation, vitamin K replacement, fresh frozen plasma, and platelet transfusion.

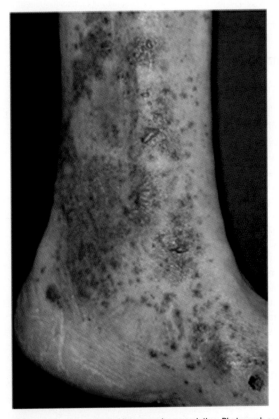

Figure 4.10 Disseminated intravascular coagulation. Photograph source: www.derm101.com, with permission.

Table 4.13 Clinical Features: Erythema Multiforme

Signs and Symptoms	Fever, arthralgias, headache, diffuse burning, and diffuse pruritus. Skin lesions are classically described as "target lesions" and may be macular, papular, or bullous with a central area that may be clear, hemorrhagic, or necrotic. Extremities and mucous membranes are commonly involved.
Laboratory Findings	Laboratory conformation not typically necessary. Clinical diagnosis but may be confirmed by skin biopsy.
Treatment	Supportive treatment. Management includes discontinuing the causal drug and treating underlying disease.

Table 4.14 Clinical Features: Toxic Epidermal Necrolysis

Signs and Symptoms	Fever, malaise, and myalgias. Dermatologic findings may include erythema, warmth, bullae, and extensive desquamation. Mucous membranes may be involved. Nikolsky's sign is positive. Epidermal detachment occurs in >30% BSA. If <10% BSA is involved, the diagnosis of Stevens-Johnson syndrome is made.
Laboratory Findings	Clinical diagnosis but may be confirmed by skin biopsy.
Treatment	Supportive treatment. Management includes discontinuing the causal drug and treating underlying disease. Treatment in burn unit is recommended.

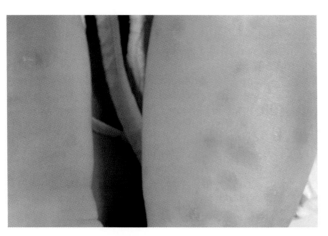

Figure 4.11 Erythema multiforme. Photograph courtesy of Centers for Disease Control Public Health Image Library, Allen W. Mathies, MD, http://phil.cdc.gov/phil/home.asp.

Erythema Multiforme

Erythema multiforme (EM) is a systemic hypersensitivity reaction, commonly associated with bacterial infection, herpes simplex infection, medications (especially sulfa, anticonvulsants), collagen vascular disease, malignancy, and toxic plants such as poison ivy, poison oak, and poison sumac. In up to 50% of cases, no etiology is found. EM commonly occurs in young adults and adolescents, and mortality may be as high as 5–10%. EM forms part of a continuum with the more severe Stevens-Johnson syndrome and toxic epidermal necrolysis, discussed in the next section.

Associated systemic symptoms may include fever, arthralgias, headache, diffuse burning, and diffuse pruritus (Table 4.13). Skin lesions are classically described as "target lesions" (hence the name "erythema multiforme") and may be macular, papular, or bullous with a central area that may be clear, hemorrhagic, or necrotic (Figure 4.11). Extremities and mucous membranes are commonly involved. The course of EM is most often benign and self-limited, resolving within 3–6 weeks.

Diagnosis is usually made by history and physical examination, but may be confirmed by skin biopsy.

Management of EM includes discontinuing the causal agent, if known, and treating any known underlying condition. Empiric treatment with antiviral agents, such as acyclovir and valacyclovir, has demonstrated benefits in small

studies, but their efficacy has not yet been definitively established. Systemic steroids may have some benefit. If more than 10% of the body surface area (BSA) is involved, admission for aggressive skin care and hydration management is considered.

Toxic Epidermal Necrolysis

Toxic epidermal necrolysis (TEN) is an acute life-threatening eruption caused primarily by transfusions and drugs, such as phenytoin, sulfa, penicillins, NSAIDs. Other etiologies may include infection and malignancy. Stevens-Johnson syndrome is a variant where both skin and mucous membranes are extensively involved. Females are affected more than males, and an increased incidence is seen among HIV-infected patients. Mortality can be up to 30%.

Clinical symptoms may include fever, malaise, and myalgias (Table 4.14). Dermatologic findings may include erythema, warmth, bullae, and extensive desquamation, and Nikolsky's sign (superficial layers of skin slipping free from the lower layers with slight pressure) is present. Epidermal detachment occurs in more than 30% BSA in TEN. If less than 10% BSA is involved, the diagnosis of Stevens-Johnson syndrome is made.

The diagnosis is based on history and physical examination and may be confirmed by skin biopsy.

Treatment includes supportive care, preferably in a burn unit, removal of the offending agent, and the use of steroids (controversial). Serum plasmapheresis may also be considered.

Erythema Nodosum

Erythema nodosum is associated with inflammatory bowel disease, streptococcal infections, drugs (sulfa, penicillins, oral contraceptives), sarcoidosis, and tuberculosis and is idiopathic in 20%. It is more common in women, in the third and fourth decades of life.

Lesions are painful, erythematous or violaceous, firm nodules that result from subcutaneous panniculitis (Table 4.15). Lesions typically are found on the pretibial areas and forearms (Figure 4.12).

Management includes treatment of the underlying disease, NSAIDs, systemic steroids, bed rest, limb elevation, and treatment with potassium iodide, 400–900 mg/day.

Table 4.15 Clinical Features: Erythema Nodosum

Signs and Symptoms	Painful, erythematous or violaceous firm nodules. Lesions typically are found on the pretibial areas and forearms.
Treatment	Management includes treatment of the underlying disease, NSAIDs, systemic steroids, bed rest, leg elevation, and treatment with potassium iodide, 400–900 mg/day.

Table 4.16 Clinical Features: Systemic Lupus Erythematosus

Signs and Symptoms	• Fever, fatigue, weight loss, malaise, arthritis, renal involvement, hemolytic anemia, pericarditis, thrombocytopenia, arthritis, pneumonitis, pleuritis, neurologic disorders, hepatomegaly, splenomegaly, and lymphadenopathy • Dermatologic findings are seen in 75% of patients and are typically erythematous macular lesions in light-exposed facial areas, or scattered papules on forearms and hands • Patients may also present with alopecia, photosensitivity, discoid lesions, or vasculitis
Laboratory Findings	Skin biopsy, ANA titers, or lupus anticoagulant (which may lead to false positive serology for syphilis)
Treatment	Supportive therapy, topical steroids, sunblock, systemic steroids, or antimalarial agents

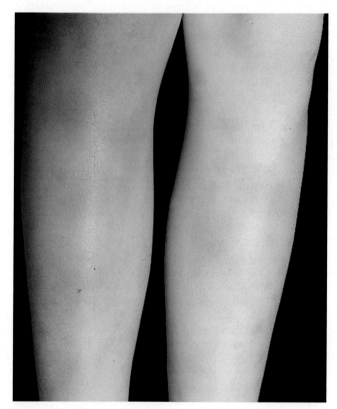

Figure 4.12 Erythema nodosum. Photograph source: www.derm101.com, with permission.

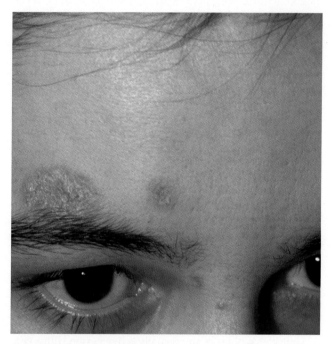

Figure 4.13 Systemic lupus erythematosus. Photograph source: www.derm101.com, with permission.

Systemic Lupus Erythematosus

Systemic lupus erythematosus (SLE) is an immune complex–mediated disorder involving connective tissue and blood vessels. It is more common in females (10:1) and in African Americans.

A multitude of clinical signs and symptoms may be seen, including fever, fatigue, weight loss, malaise, arthritis, renal involvement, hemolytic anemia, pericarditis, thrombocytopenia, arthritis, pneumonitis, pleuritis, neurologic disorders, hepatomegaly, splenomegaly, and lymphadenopathy (Table 4.16). Dermatologic findings are seen in 75% of patients and are typically erythematous macular lesions in light-exposed facial areas, or scattered papules on forearms and hands (Figure 4.13). The characteristic "butterfly rash" presents with erythema and macular or papular edema over the malar eminences and nose. Patients may also present with alopecia, photosensitivity, discoid lesions, or vasculitis.

The diagnosis is made by skin biopsy, antinuclear antibody (ANA) titers, or lupus anticoagulant (which may lead to false positive serology for syphilis).

Management includes supportive therapy, topical steroids, sunblock, systemic steroids, or antimalarial agents and should be undertaken in consultation with a dermatologist or rheumatologist.

Drug Reactions

Adverse drug reactions commonly cause dermatologic symptoms and signs. Commonly seen patterns include morbilliform rash, urticaria, EM, and vasculitis. (See the earlier sections on erythema multiforme and toxic epidermal necrolysis.) Commonly implicated medications include antibiotics, antifungal agents, and antiepileptic agents. Immunosuppressed patients, including HIV-infected patients, patients with SLE, and those with malignancy, are at increased risk for adverse drug reactions.

LABORATORY DIAGNOSIS

Many laboratory tests are discussed above with specific diagnoses. Selected patients with fever and rash should be evaluated with a complete blood count, serologic tests, skin biopsy, and cultures of blood or skin lesions.

COMPLICATIONS AND ADMISSION CRITERIA

Many patients with fever and rash can be safely discharged home with close follow-up, following the appropriate physical and laboratory evaluation. Patients with immunosuppression, unstable vital signs, or other evidence of systemic bacterial infection or sepsis should be admitted.

INFECTION CONTROL

Patients with fever and rash often do not have a definitive diagnosis made while in the acute care setting, and should be considered contagious. Standard precautions should be used at all times.

Appropriate management of sexually transmitted diseases includes treatment of the primary patient, as well as notification of and treatment of sexual contacts. Barrier contraceptive methods are important in reducing the spread of sexually transmitted diseases. Disease reporting is an important component of public health. Gonorrhea and syphilis are reportable diseases in all states. Chlamydia is a reportable disease in most states.

Close contacts of possible cases of meningococcal disease (including household contacts, child care contacts, and health care providers) should undergo prophylactic treatment with rifampin (600 mg PO bid for four doses), ceftriaxone (250 mg IM), or ciprofloxacin (500 mg PO).

PEARLS AND PITFALLS

1. Consider life-threatening infections for patients presenting with fever and rash.
2. Administer antibiotics early, even if the definitive diagnosis is not established.
3. Consider syphilis in any sexually active person with a generalized rash or painless genital ulcer.
4. Search and remove any possible toxin source in cases of toxic shock syndrome (i.e., tampons, nasal packing).

REFERENCES

American College of Physicians. Guidelines for laboratory evaluation in the diagnosis of Lyme disease. Ann Intern Med 1997;127:1106.

Banatvala JE, Brown DW. Rubella. Lancet 2004 Apr 3;363(9415):1127–37.

Brady WJ, DeBehnke D, Crosby DL. Dermatological emergencies. Am J Emerg Med 1994;12:217–37.

Brady WJ, Perron AD, DeBehnke DJ. Serious generalized skin disorders. In: Tintinalli JE, Kelen GD, Stapdzynski JS, eds, Emergency medicine: A comprehensive study guide, 6th ed. New York: McGraw-Hill Medical Publishing Division, 2004.

Centers for Disease Control and Prevention (CDC). Lyme disease – US 2001–02. MMWR 2004;53:365.

Centers for Disease Control and Prevention (CDC). Prevention and control of meningococcal disease. MMWR 2005;54(RR07):1–21.

Centers for Disease Control and Prevention (CDC). Sexually transmitted diseases treatment guidelines 2006. MMWR 2006;55.

Cunha BA. Rocky Mountain spotted fever revisited. Arch Intern Med 2004;164:221–3.

Dourmishev LA, Dourmishev AL. Syphilis: uncommon presentations in adults. Clin Dermatol 2005;23:555–64.

Duke T, Mgone CS. Measles: not just another viral exanthem. Lancet 2003 March 1;36(9359):763–73.

Fleischer AB, Feldman SR, McConnell CF, et al. Emergency dermatology: A rapid treatment guide. New York: McGraw-Hill, 2002.

Gardner P. Clinical practice: prevention of meningococcal disease. N Engl J Med 2006;355:1466–73.

Hajjeh RA, Reingold A, Weil A, et al. Toxic shock syndrome in the United States: surveillance update, 1979–1996. Emerg Infect Dis J 1999;5(6):807–10.

Hazelzet JA. Diagnosing meningococcemia as a cause of sepsis. Pediatr Crit Care Med 2005;6:S50–4.

Hernandez-Salazar A, Rosales SP, Rangel-Frausto S, et al. Epidemiology of adverse cutaneous drug reactions. A prospective study in hospitalized patients. Arch Med Res 2006;37:899–902.

Lamoreux MR, Sternbach MR, Hsu WT. Erythema multiforme. Am Fam Physician 2006;74:1883–8.

Masters EJ Olson GS, Weiner SJ, et al. Rocky Mountain spotted fever: a clinician's dilemma. Arch Intern Med 2003;163:769–74.

McCann DJ, Nadel ES, Brown DF. Rash and fever. J Emerg Med 2006;31:293–7.

Pitambe HV, Schulz EJ. Life-threatening dermatoses due to metabolic and endocrine disorders. Clin Dermatol 2005;23:258–66.

Quagliarello V, Scheld M. Treatment of bacterial meningitis. N Engl J Med 1997;336:708.

Reidner G, Rusizoka M, Todd J, et al. Single-dose azithromycin versus penicillin G benzathine for the treatment of early syphilis. N Engl J Med 2005;353:1236–44.

Robson KJ, Piette WW. Cutaneous manifestations of systemic disease. Med Clin North Am 1998;82:1359–79.

Rosenstein NE, Perkins BA, Stephens DS, et al. Meningococcal disease. N Engl J Med 2001;344:1378–88.

Singh-Behl D, La Rosa SP, Tomecki KJ. Tick-borne infections. Dermatol Clin 2003; 21:237–44.

Steere A. Lyme disease. N Engl J Med 2001;345:115.

Young N, Brown K. Mechanisms of disease: parvovirus B19. N Engl J Med 2004;350:586–97.

5. Otitis Media

Theresa A. Gurney and Andrew H. Murr

INTRODUCTION – AGENTS

The majority of otitis media (OM) infections are caused by organisms commonly found in the upper aerodigestive tract, including the ears, nose, sinuses, oral cavity, oropharynx, hypopharynx, and larynx. These agents include *Streptococcus pneumoniae*, *Haemophilus influenzae*, and less commonly, *Moraxella catarrhalis*, *Streptococcus pyogenes*, and *Staphylococcus aureus*. Anaerobic bacteria may play a role in OM in the neonatal period. Viruses that infect the upper respiratory tract also frequently cause OM.

EPIDEMIOLOGY

Young children compromise the majority of cases of OM. Children with craniofacial syndromes or trisomy 21 (Down syndrome) may be particularly prone to OM. Children with a cleft palate or submucous cleft palate are at high risk for persistent or recurrent acute OM.

Some adults also may be predisposed to OM, including those with HIV and concomitant adenoid hypertrophy that obstructs the eustachian tube orifice, as well as recipients of head and neck radiation. Additionally, certain ethnic groups, including Native Americans, have a higher incidence of OM. An otherwise healthy adult with persistent unilateral OM warrants additional work-up for a possible underlying malignancy.

CLINICAL FEATURES

Acute OM is one of the most frequently encountered otologic infections in children (Table 5.1). Young children may be inconsolable and will sometimes tug or pull on the affected ear, though this sign is very nonspecific in children under 2. They will often complain of pain or otalgia as a prominent symptom. Fever and elevated white blood counts with a left shift may be present. An otoscopic exam is essential, albeit difficult in the irritable child. If the external auditory canal is not occluded with cerumen, one usually sees a dull tympanic membrane that is not mobile with air insufflation, or pneumotoscopy. It may be possible to see bubbles or a fluid level behind the eardrum on magnified examination. Occasionally, the infection may result in a perforation in the tympanic membrane and drainage of purulent and/or bloody material may be seen.

DIFFERENTIAL DIAGNOSIS

Acute OM should be distinguished from a persistent ear effusion, which is termed serous otitis media or persistent otitis media. Acute otitis media is an acute illness that may be manifested by fever, elevated white blood cell count, otalgia, and/or an eardrum that may be erythematous and bulging, perhaps with a fluid level.

Serous OM can be present in a patient without particular discomfort or symptoms other than hearing loss. Fluid is present behind the eardrum, but there is no acute infectious illness. Multiple prior infections may cause myringosclerosis of the tympanic membrane making it appear dull on visualization; however, pneumotoscopy should reveal a mobile, albeit stiff, tympanic membrane. Cholesteatoma, abnormal squamous deposition, in the middle ear may also

Table 5.1 Clinical Features: Otitis Media

Organisms	• *Streptococcus pneumoniae* • *Haemophilus influenzae* • *Moraxella catarrhalis* • *Streptococcus pyogenes* • *Staphylococcus aureus* • Anaerobic bacteria* • Viruses

Signs and Symptoms	In children:
	• Fever
	• Tugging at one ear
	• Inconsolability
	• Otorrhea if perforation of TM has occurred
	  ○ red or bulging eardrum
	  ○ possible fluid behind TM
	In adults:
	• Fever
	• Otalgia
	• Decreased conductive hearing
	• Otorrhea if perforation of TM has occurred

Laboratory and Radiographic Findings	• Elevated white blood count • Refractory OM may require culture directed therapy • Imaging (CT or MRI) may be indicated in evaluating complications

*May play a role in OM in the neonatal period.
CT, computed tomography; MRI, magnetic resonance imaging; TM, tympanic membrane.

present as a dull immobile tympanic membrane with foul discharge and possibly a superior retraction pocket.

LABORATORY AND RADIOGRAPHIC FINDINGS

Diagnosis is usually made on clinical exam. In cases in which the tympanic membrane is perforated, with draining fluid, cultures can be sent. Treatment-directed cultures are most useful in refractory recurrent OM that has failed traditional antibiotic therapy.

Middle ear fluid can be collected with a suction trap and subsequent culture may identify the organism and yield antibiotic sensitivities. A white blood cell count with differential, though nonspecific, may suggest acute bacterial infection. In the neonate less than 6 weeks of age with fever of unknown origin or meningitis, tympanocentesis may be considered.

TREATMENT AND PROPHYLAXIS

Treatment usually consists of a 7- to 10-day course of antibiotics (Table 5.2). High-dose amoxicillin is an appropriate first-line antibiotic because of its coverage of some *Streptococcus* sp., *H. influenzae*, and *M. catarrhalis*. Recurrent cases may benefit from broadening the coverage to treat resistant organisms. Amoxicillin-clavulanate has excellent cover-

Table 5.2 Treatment of Otitis Media

Patient Category	Therapy Recommendations
Preferred Choices	amoxicillin 500 mg PO tid × 7–10 days *or* cefuroxime (Ceftin) 500 mg PO bid × 7–14 days *or* ceftriaxone 1 g IM (Rocephin) qd × 3 doses
Alternative Choices	Alternative (beta-lactam allergy or fails initial prescription): clindamycin 300 mg PO tid/qid, *or* gatifloxacin (Tequin) 400 mg PO qd, *or* levofloxacin (Levaquin) 500 mg PO qd, *or* moxifloxacin (Avelox) 400 mg PO qd – all × 7–10 days
Preferred Choices: Immunocompromised or Diabetic Patients	amoxicillin/clavulanate (Augmentin) 875 mg PO bid (or 500 mg PO tid) × 10–14 days, or use as primary therapy for immunocompromised or diabetic patient
Alternative Choices: Immunocompromised or Diabetic Patients	Alternative: clindamycin 300 mg tid × 7–10 days (PCN allergy) Referral to specialist to rule out cholesteatoma in setting of chronicity
Adjunctive Therapies	• Nasal decongestants: pseudoephedrine 120 mg qd plus topical vasoconstrictors – oxymetazoline nasal sprays 2 puffs tid × 3 days only • Antihistamines: loratadine (Claritin) 10 mg PO qd or fexofenadine (Allegra) 60 mg PO bid • NSAIDs or Tylenol
Persistent Infections	For persistent infection, intractable pain, or complications listed above, specialist referral essential

NSAID, nonsteroidal anti-inflammatory drug; OTC, over-the-counter; PCN, penicillin.

age against beta lactamase–producing bacteria, which may be present in refractory cases. Rarely, culture-directed therapy from tympanocentesis may be needed to guide effective antimicrobial treatment. Analgesics and antipyretics are also recommended.

Children with recurrent OM may benefit from pressure equalization tubes. An audiogram with tympanograms is needed prior to placement to document the amount of conductive hearing loss and formally evaluate tympanic membrane mobility.

Syndromic children, such as those with trisomy 21 (Down syndrome) or cleft palate, tend to have frequent infections, likely due to eustachian tube dysfunction. These children need close clinical care and may require pressure equalization tubes (PETs) for long-term care.

Close care of immunosuppressed (e.g., HIV and diabetic) patients is warranted as these patients are at higher risk for the development of complications.

COMPLICATIONS AND ADMISSION CRITERIA

The most common complication of OM is a simple perforated tympanic membrane that usually heals on its own. It is important for the patient to keep the ear dry until it is healed. Large perforations that do not close on their own may require subsequent tympanoplasty, a microsurgical closure of the eardrum perforation using graft material.

Acute mastoiditis is a more serious complication with clinical findings including postauricular erythema, edema, fever, proptosis of the auricle and mastoid tenderness. Antimicrobial and surgical treatments are indicated to prevent progression to meningitis.

Meningitis can be a rare complication of acute OM, either from septicemia or possibly via direct extension from the middle ear or mastoid space to the dura. Also rare, epidural abscess, subdural abscess, brain abscess, and sigmoid sinus thrombosis may all complicate acute OM. Persistent high fever with meningeal signs such as neck stiffness suggest the need for lumbar puncture or imaging.

PEARLS AND PITFALLS

1. An adult with unilateral persistent OM should be worked up for a possible underlying head and neck malignancy such as nasopharyngeal carcinoma.
2. Examination should differentiate between acute OM and serous OM.
3. Refractory treatment may warrant culture-guided antibiotics.
4. Tympanic membrane perforation usually heals on its own.
5. Mastoiditis and meningitis are more serious complications of acute OM.
6. Topical steroid or antibiotic ear drops are not helpful in acute OM unless tympanic perforation is present.

REFERENCES

Bluestone CD. Studies in otitis media: Children's Hospital of Pittsburgh – University of Pittsburgh progress report – 2004. Laryngoscope 2004;114(11):1–26.

Celin SE, Bluestone CD, Stephenson J, et al. Bacteriology of acute otitis media in adults. JAMA 1991 Oct;266(16):2249–52.

Culpepper L, Froom J, Bartelds AI, et al. Acute otitis media in adults: a report from the International Primary Care Network. J Am Board Fam Pract 1993 Jul–Aug;6(4):333–9.

Fairbanks DNF. Pocket guide to antimicrobial therapy in otolaryngology – head and neck surgery, 12th ed. Washington, DC: American Academy of Otolaryngology, 2005.

Pichichero ME, Casey JR. Otitis media. Expert Opin Pharmacother 2002 Aug;3(8):1073–90.

6. Otitis Externa

Theresa A. Gurney and Andrew H. Murr

INTRODUCTION – AGENTS

Otitis externa (OE) or "swimmer's ear" is a relatively common infection of the pinna and/or external auditory canal. Most episodes of OE are caused by *Pseudomonas aeruginosa*. Other bacterial etiologies include *Staphylococcus aureus*, other *Staphylococcus* spp., *Streptococcus*, *Proteus*, and *Klebsiella*.

OE can occasionally be caused by fungi, most often *Aspergillus* species such as *Aspergillus niger*, *flavus*, and *fumigatus*. *Candida albicans* can also cause OE.

Less commonly, a herpetic viral etiology can cause OE, or an eruption of herpetic vesicles can become secondarily infected by bacteria.

EPIDEMIOLOGY

Otitis externa occurs in both children and adults, and is often seen in months when swimming is a popular activity. This association may result from injury to the ear canal skin in the process of drying ears after swimming, which facilitates bacterial infection. Patients with chronic moisture in their ears are more susceptible to OE, and increased incidence is seen in warm, humid environments and seasons. Hearing aid wearers or frequent ear-plug users may also be at increased risk.

A history of trauma, laceration, or a recent intra-aural foreign body may be an inciting event. Overaggressive Q-tip users are frequent OE patients because of abrasion and subsequent infection of the ear canal. A careful history must be elicited in refractory cases, because although patients may have claimed that they have ceased using Q-tips, other objects such as pins, paper clips, and the ends of eyeglasses are often substituted. This behavior is exacerbated by the fact that OE often begins as an itching of the ear canal, which may result in increased scratching and skin injury.

CLINICAL FEATURES

Patients with OE commonly complain of severe local pain or uncontrollable itching, which may be accompanied by purulent ear drainage and a foul smell (Table 6.1). If debris builds up, the patient may also complain of aural fullness and decreased hearing due to a conductive component.

On examination, the external auditory canal may appear erythematous and inflamed, with occasional skin desquamation. In severe cases, the infection may extend to the tragus or pinna. The ear canal may contain whitish foul-smelling debris, especially in bacterial infections. Edema may be so severe that the tympanic membrane cannot be visualized.

Vesicles suggest a herpetic viral etiology (herpes zoster). Ramsey-Hunt syndrome is facial nerve (CN VII) paresis with vesicular viral eruption in the dermatome of the sensory portion of the facial nerve, including the ear canal. Any eye involvement should prompt ophthalmologic consultation. Auditory nerve (CN VIII) involvement may result in sensorineural hearing loss and/or vertigo.

Malignant OE is a type of skull-base osteomyelitis that presents as a very severe and progressive infection in immunocompromised patients. This process is classically noted in diabetics with poor glucose control. The diagnosis should be considered in any patient presenting with cranial

Table 6.1 Clinical Features: Otitis Externa

Organisms	• *Pseudomonas aeruginosa* • *Staphylococcus aureus* • *Staphylococcus* spp. • *Streptococcus* • *Corynebacterium* • *Proteus* • *Klebsiella* • *Aspergillus* sp. • *Candida albicans* • Herpes virus
Signs and Symptoms	• Otalgia (ear pain) • Pruritis (ear itching) • Otorrhea (ear drainage), usually foul smelling • Aural fullness • Conductive hearing loss • Vesicles may suggest a herpetic etiology • Hyphae may suggest a fungal etiology
Laboratory and Radiographic Findings	• Usually not indicated • Refractory OE may require culture-directed therapy • Imaging may be indicated if progression to malignant OE is suspected
Treatment	• Aural hygiene • Dry ear precautions • Topical antibiotic drops such as Cortisporin otic or Floxin otic

nerve palsies and OE, and a bone scan is often indicated. The treatment consists of intravenous antibiotics, often directed at *Pseudomonas* and *Streptococcus* species.

DIFFERENTIAL DIAGNOSIS

The differential diagnosis of acute OE includes bacterial, fungal, and viral causes, often distinguishable on physical examination. Bacterial infection is usually associated with whitish purulent debris, fungal infection with spore formation, and viral infection with a vesicular eruption in a dermatomal pattern.

An alternative diagnosis is an allergic dermatitis reaction in patients using topical eardrops. Many patients demonstrate a reaction to neomycin, which is a component of a commonly used eardrop (Cortisporin). The treatment is cessation of the offending agent.

LABORATORY AND RADIOGRAPHIC FINDINGS

Diagnosis is usually made on clinical examination. Rarely, a diagnostic culture is needed to direct therapy in refractory cases. In Ramsey-Hunt syndrome caused by herpes viral infection, a Tzank preparation may be helpful. Although usually not indicated, a complete blood count (CBC) may be helpful if there is a concern for bacterial dissemination or in an immunocompromised patient. Imaging studies such as a computed tomographic (CT) temporal bone or bone scan should be ordered in a patient suspected of having malignant OE.

TREATMENT AND PROPHYLAXIS

The mainstays of treatment are aural hygiene and topical antimicrobials. Aural hygiene is usually performed by an otolaryngologist using a microscope to remove purulent debris with microsuction. If the edema of the external auditory canal is so severe that the space is obliterated, a small wick or sponge can be placed in the canal to deliver the antimicrobial drops effectively and to keep the ear canal patent.

A variety of topical ear drops are utilized. Most include antibacterial coverage against *Pseudomonas*. Some also include a corticosteroid to decrease inflammation and pruritis and, occasionally, an antifungal. Care should be taken in using topical neomycin-based products because as much as 5% of the population may have allergic reactions to this antibiotic. Ironically, some agents used to treat OE (neomycin and polymyxin B) are ototoxic if administered systemically. Nevertheless, exceedingly few cases of hearing loss can be traced to these drugs when used topically in the ear canal.

Patients must also be counseled to discontinue procedures that cause auricular trauma. Instrumentation of the ear must be absolutely avoided. Dry ear precautions are also essential to the resolution of the disease. This consists of placing cotton with Vaseline in the external ear canal for showering and wearing earplugs for swimming. If swimming is continued, rinsing the ear canal afterwards with a 50:50 ratio of clean water and rubbing alcohol can promote drying.

If the infection has progressed to an auricular chondritis of the pinna, admission and intravenous antibiotics are indicated.

COMPLICATIONS AND ADMISSION CRITERIA

Tympanic membrane perforation may occur. These perforations usually heal after clearance of the infection but may require tympanoplasty.

Progression of the infection may lead to cellulitis or chondritis. Chondritis is especially concerning as the infection may result in an auricular deformity from cartilage necrosis and requires long-term antibiotics.

Patients with repeated chronic OE infections may develop granulation tissue in the external auditory canal, fibrosis, or stenosis. Stenosis of the ear canal may lead to a conductive hearing loss and require surgical intervention.

Care must be taken in the poorly controlled diabetic or immunocompromised patient because there is a risk of progression to malignant OE, involving the skull base and ultimately spreading intracranially. Clinical findings include granulation tissue at the floor of the ear canal, paresis or paralysis of cranial nerves, and central neurologic findings. Treatment includes hospital admission, intravenous antibiotics, and imaging such as gallium/technetium bone scans or CT scans to evaluate possible skull base involvement.

PEARLS AND PITFALLS

1. Aural hygiene and topical antimicrobials are the mainstay of treatment.
2. Antimicrobials are often directed at *Pseudomonas* or gram-negative organisms.
3. A careful history of any instrumentation of the ear canal is always warranted. The patient who denies Q-tips may be using other objects to alleviate itching.
4. A high degree of vigilance is warranted in patients with diabetes, uncontrolled HIV, and other immunosuppression. These patients are at higher risk for complications. Diabetic patients must maintain tight glucose control.
5. Nonbacterial etiologies of OE include fungal and viral.
6. Stenotic canals impairing administration of drops require temporary wick placement. Strict dry ear precautions while showering should be followed.

REFERENCES

Fairbanks DNF. Pocket guide to antimicrobial therapy in otolaryngology – head and neck surgery, 12th ed. Washington, DC: American Academy of Otolaryngology, 2005.

Roland PS, Pien FD, Schultz CC, et al. Efficacy and safety of topical ciprofloxacin/dexamethasone versus neomycin/polymyxin B/hydrocortisone for otitis externa. Curr Med Res Opin 2004 Aug;20(8):1175–83.

Roland PS, Stroman DW. Microbiology of acute otitis externa. Laryngoscope 2002;112(7 Pt 1):1166–77.

Rosenfeld RM, Singer M, Wasserman JM, et al. Systematic review of topical antimicrobial therapy for acute otitis externa. Otolaryngol Head Neck Surg 2006;134(4):S24–48.

van Balen FA, Smit WM, Zuithoff NP, et al. Clinical efficacy of three common treatments in acute otitis externa in primary care: randomised controlled trial. Evid Based Nurs 2004 Apr;7(2):43.

7. Sinusitis

Theresa A. Gurney and Andrew H. Murr

INTRODUCTION – AGENTS

Causative agents of acute bacterial sinusitis are similar to those seen in other infections of the head and neck and include *Streptococcus pneumoniae*, *Haemophilus influenzae*, and *Moraxella catarrhalis*. Anaerobes are less frequently encountered in acute sinusitis but play a role in chronic sinusitis. Viruses can also cause acute rhinosinusitis.

EPIDEMIOLOGY

Sinusitis is a common chronic condition for which patients seek physician attention in the United States. There are more than 25 million patient visits per year pertaining to sinus problems, including allergic rhinitis, viral upper respiratory infections, vasomotor rhinitis, bacterial rhinosinusitis, and nasal polyposis. Sinusitis occurs in patients of all ages but is more common in adults. Children with cystic fibrosis, however, are a unique population at much higher risk for sinus disease caused by atypical organisms, especially *Pseudomonas*.

CLINICAL FEATURES

The spectrum of acute to chronic sinusitis is mostly dependent on the duration of signs and symptoms. Acute sinusitis is defined as an infection that generally clears within 4 weeks. Chronic sinusitis is an infection that has been present for about 12 weeks despite treatment. Subacute sinusitis lasts longer than 4 weeks but less than 12 weeks. Recurrent acute sinusitis may be referred to as chronic (recurrent) sinusitis if a patient is afflicted with more than four infections in a year, each clearing completely (Tables 7.1 and 7.2).

Sinusitis presents with symptoms of facial pressure, headache, rhinorrhea, and smell disturbances (Table 7.3). The technical definition of sinusitis splits symptomatology into major and minor symptoms. Sinusitis is suggested by the presence of two major factors or one major and one minor factor, or by the presence of pus on nasal examination. Patients may have a history of a precedent viral upper respiratory infection (Table 7.2).

History of aspirin sensitivity may suggest underlying polypoid disease consistent with Samter's triad. The repetitive abuse of inhaled substances such as methamphetamines or cocaine may predispose to altered nasal and sinus architecture. The patient's dentition should be checked carefully. A maxillary tooth infection can be responsible for unilateral maxillary sinusitis.

Table 7.1 Major and Minor Sinusitis Factors

Major Factors	Minor Factors
Facial pain/pressure (in conjunction with other nasal symptoms)	Headache
	Halitosis
	Fatigue
Facial fullness	Dental pain
Nasal obstruction	Fever (in nonacute rhinosinusitis)
Nasal discharge/purulence	Cough
Fever (in acute rhinosinusitis)	Ear pressure/fullness

From Rosenfeld RM, Andes D, Bhattacharyya N, et al. Clinical practice guideline: adult sinusitis. Otolaryngol Head Neck Surg 2007;137(3 Suppl): S1–31.

Table 7.2 Rhinosinusitis Definitions

Type Rhinosinusitis	Duration	History (See also Table 7.1)
Acute	≤4 weeks	≥2 major factors *or* 1 major factor and 1 minor factor *or* nasal purulence on exam
Subacute	4–12 weeks	Same
Recurrent Acute	≥4 episodes/year, each episode 7–10 days; clears between episodes	Same
Chronic	≥12 weeks	Same Note: Facial pain in the absence of other nasal symptoms is *not* suggestive of chronic sinusitis!

From Rosenfeld RM, Andes D, Bhattacharyya N, et al. Clinical practice guideline: adult sinusitis. Otolaryngol Head Neck Surg 2007;137(3 Suppl): S1–31.

Table 7.3 Clinical Features: Sinusitis

Organisms	• *Streptococcus* sp. • *Haemophilus influenzae* • *Moraxella catarrhalis* • Anaerobic bacteria • Viruses
Signs and Symptoms	• Facial pressure • Headache • Purulent drainage, often unilateral • Otorrhea if perforation of TM has occurred • Smell disturbances
Laboratory and Radiographic Findings	• Usually not indicated • Refractory sinusitis may require culture-directed therapy • A sinus CT (without contrast) is usually warranted *after* a trial of medical therapy, unless clinical examination suggests an anatomic etiology or a complication of sinusitis, or if there is a diagnostic dilemma

Treatment	• Saline nasal irrigation, best with bulb syringe
	• Decongestants, oral or topical
	• Antibiotics
	  amoxicillin 0.5–1.5 g PO tid × 10–14 days
	  or
	  amoxicillin/clavulanate 825/125 mg PO bid × 10–14 days
	  or
	  azithromycin 2 g × 1 dose or 500 mg PO qd × 3 days
	  or
	  clarithromycin 500 mg PO bid × 14 days
	  Severe, nonresponsive or history of recent antibiotic use:
	    levofloxacin 500 mg PO qd × 5–10 days
	    or
	    moxifloxacin 400 mg PO qd × 5–10 days
	• Corticosteroids, in certain circumstances
	• Surgical treatment if medical treatment fails

CT, computed tomography; TM, tympanic membrane.

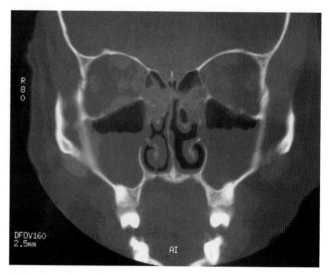

Figure 7.1 Acute sinusitis.

DIFFERENTIAL DIAGNOSIS

It is difficult to distinguish among chronic bacterial rhinosinusitis, viral rhinitis (the common cold), allergic rhinitis, vasomotor rhinitis, and migraine headache. An allergy history is often helpful. Migraines are frequently misdiagnosed as sinusitis. An endoscopic nasal examination and a computed tomography (CT) scan can be instrumental in separating bacterial rhinosinusitis from other diagnoses (Figure 7.1).

Functional obstruction by polyps or other lesions may cause sinusitis. This should be evident on nasal examination. Dental infections may cause a unilateral maxillary sinusitis and therefore all dentition should be carefully examined.

Allergic fungal sinusitis is usually caused by *Aspergillus*. Patients will characteristically have an elevated IgE level, and Charcot-Leyden crystals are noted on pathological examination. Cultures are positive for fungi, and CT imaging demonstrates a unilateral opacification of the involved sinuses, often with a stippled appearance and bone erosion. Treatment is corticosteroids and surgical debridement, and possibly immunotherapy.

Much less common is invasive fungal sinusitis. These patients are usually immunocompromised, from infection with human immunodeficiency virus (HIV), from poorly con-

trolled diabetes, or from immunosuppressive therapy such as treatment of blood malignancies or post–bone marrow transplant. Emergent evaluation of the sinus with endoscopy and biopsy of any necrotic or ulcerative tissue is required. Magnetic resonance imaging (MRI) is the study of choice to demonstrate the extent of the disease, which is usually unilateral and invades bone, but can destroy other tissues. Most patients with invasive fungal sinusitis require emergent debridement in the operating room.

LABORATORY AND RADIOGRAPHIC FINDINGS

Diagnosis is usually made on history and clinical exam. An appropriate clinical history, combined with findings such as purulent localized drainage, is usually sufficient. Endoscopic examination of the nose has become a mainstay of rhinology practices because the examination can be accomplished under topical anesthesia in the office setting. In situations in which treatment is refractory, culture-directed medical therapy may be useful.

In the majority of patients, CT sinus imaging consisting of direct coronal and axial views is more informative after the patient has completed 3–4 weeks of optimal medical therapy. This is because a certain amount of mucosal thickening and fluid can be found in healthy asymptomatic patients. Abnormal imaging findings are more reliable after medical treatment and may indicate a need for surgery. Exceptions to this would include patients with polypoid disease, unilateral disease that is suspected of neoplasm, indications of a complication of sinus disease, and in a suspected case of invasive fungal sinusitis.

TREATMENT AND PROPHYLAXIS

Medical treatment consists of nasal saline irrigation, decongestants (topical or oral), antibiotics, and sometimes mucolytics. Nasal saline rinsing is best achieved with a volume of 10–20 mL irrigated through the nasal cavity with a bulb syringe three to four times a day. The patient must be educated not to use topical decongestants, such as oxymetazoline (Afrin), for more than a few days, as chronic use causes an addictive type pattern in which cessation of the oxymetazoline results in rebound inflammation and edema (rhinitis medicamentosa). Antibiotic therapy directed at a bacterial infection is warranted. Direct visualization with a rigid endoscope may reveal a specific draining sinus, which may be cultured. Corticosteroid medication, either via topical sprays or in oral form, is indicated for some types of infection or for nasal polyposis. Antihistamines are recommended when the history is suggestive of an allergic component.

After conservative medical treatment, imaging and surgical treatment may be warranted. Coronal sinus CT scans without contrast are the most common imaging modality. Surgical intervention may include localized drainage, creation of a middle meatal maxillary antrostomy, or other sinus surgery, often performed endoscopically.

COMPLICATIONS AND ADMISSION CRITERIA

Complications can range from preseptal cellulitis of the orbit to cavernous sinus thrombosis with intracranial extension and death. Edema of the eyelid, restriction of extraocular movements, or vision change should warrant urgent imaging and ophthalmologic consultation. Rare complications of sinusitis include meningitis, epidural abscess, subdural abscess, brain abscess, or isolated cavernous sinus thrombosis.

The patient with suspected invasive fungal sinusitis warrants immediate treatment, because complications can include orbital invasion, resulting in loss of vision and/or the globe, intracranial extension, and death.

PEARLS AND PITFALLS

1. Medical therapy is usually the first-line of treatment and includes irrigation, decongestants, and antibiotics.
2. Eyelid edema, vision changes, or cranial nerve involvement may indicate serious complications and should be evaluated immediately.

3. Mucosal changes in the sinuses can be associated with viral upper respiratory infections.
4. Diagnosis is usually made clinically. CT imaging or culture is useful in refractory cases.
5. If sinusitis is unresponsive to first-line antibiotics, practitioners can consider broadening coverage, obtaining direct cultures, or CT imaging.

REFERENCES

Bhattacharyya N. Clinical and symptom criteria for the accurate diagnosis of chronic rhinosinusitis. Laryngoscope 2006;116(July 2006 suppl):1–22.

Brook I. The role of bacterial interference in otitis, sinusitis and tonsillitis. Otolaryngol Head Neck Surg 2005;133(1):139–46.

Chandler JR, Langenbrunner DJ, Stevens ER. The pathogenesis of orbital complications in acute sinusitis. Laryngoscope 1970:80(9):1414–28.

Fairbanks DNF. Pocket guide to antimicrobial therapy in otolaryngology – head and neck surgery, 12th ed. Washington, DC: American Academy of Otolaryngology, 2005.

Hickner JM, Bartlett JG, Besser R, et al. Principles of acute antibiotic use for acute rhinosinusitis in adults: background. Ann Intern Med 2001;134:498.

Piccirillo JR. Acute bacterial sinusitis. N Engl J Med 2004;351:902–10.

Remmler D, Boles R. Intracranial complications of frontal sinusitis. Laryngoscope 1980;90(11):1814–24.

Snow V, Mottur-Pilson C, Hickner JM. Principles of appropriate antibiotic use for acute sinusitis. Ann Intern Med 2001;134:495.

8. Supraglottitis

Theresa A. Gurney and Andrew H. Murr

INTRODUCTION – AGENTS

Patients with supraglottitis may present to the acute care setting with complaints of a sore throat and difficulty breathing. These symptoms may reflect a self-limited upper respiratory infection (URI) or, infrequently, an impending airway emergency.

Supraglottitis describes inflammation of the supraglottic structures, which include the epiglottis, the false vocal cords and arytenoids, and the aryepiglottic folds. In the past these infections were all called epiglottitis, but supraglottitis is a more anatomically accurate description as the surrounding supraglottic structures are usually involved. The vallecula and tongue base, technically part of the oropharynx, may also be affected.

Haemophilus influenzae was previously the primary organism responsible for epiglottitis/supraglottitis. With the advent of the *H. influenzae* type B (HIB) vaccine and its widespread use, the overall incidence of supraglottitis and *H. influenza* as a causative organism has decreased significantly. Other causative etiologies include *Streptococcus pneumoniae, Streptococcus pyogenes Staphylococcus species*, and other *Haemophilus* species, such as *Haemophilus parainfluenzae*. Less commonly involved are bacteria such as *Klebsiella* or *Pseudomonas*, viruses, or *Candida*.

EPIDEMIOLOGY

In the past, young children made up the majority of cases of epiglottitis (see Chapter 49, Pediatric Respiratory Infections). With widespread HIB vaccination of the pediatric population, however, the disease is now more common in adults than children in the United States. Although the overall incidence is decreased, the annual incidence among adults has remained constant, and cases still occur in children who have not developed immunity after vaccination or in those who have not been vaccinated. Immigrants, both young and old, from regions that do not have access to the vaccine are more vulnerable to infection. Additionally, cigarette smoking and the use of inhaled illicit substances (e.g., crack cocaine) appear to be risk factors in adult supraglottitis.

CLINICAL FEATURES

Patients with supraglottitis are usually very ill-appearing, with difficulty handling secretions, a sore throat, and complaints of shortness of breath. Most patients will have a fever. Voice changes may be noted and have been described as "muffled" or a "hot-potato voice." Stridor is a critical diagnostic sign, classically greater with inspiration, but can be at any phase of respiration. The absence of stridor, however, in the presence of other indications of supraglottitis is not necessarily reassuring and may portend imminent airway collapse.

Patients may have had a recent URI or may not have a history of any inciting event. Symptoms may be gradual in onset or may rapidly progress in a few hours. The classic *H. influenzae* epiglottitis in the pediatric population has a tendency to progress rapidly whereas adult epiglottitis is often more gradual (Table 8.1).

Visualization of the larynx is ultimately indicated, by either fiberoptic or direct visualization. Although lateral and anteroposterior (AP) soft-tissue radiographs of the neck may be helpful in differentiating the cause of stridor in children (foreign body is a common cause in this population), they are not a substitute for direct laryngeal examination and airway control. In pediatric epiglottitis, direct laryngeal examination is almost always performed in the operating room setting with anesthesia and personnel prepared to perform bronchoscopy and/or tracheotomy if necessary.

It is ill advised, and potentially fatal, to send a patient with suspected supraglottitis to the computed tomographic (CT) scanner without a protected airway. A CT scan will not make the diagnosis – only direct visualization will. In children, the goal is to keep them calm and breathing on their own until they can be anesthetized. Any gagging induced by bedside evaluation or increase in anxiety could potentially escalate the situation to respiratory obstruction and arrest.

In the adult population, the decision must be made whether it is safe to accomplish fiberoptic endoscopy in the emergency-room setting. An adult patient has a larger airway and is often more able to permit tolerate examination than young pediatric patients. An advanced case of adult epiglottitis will likely also require airway control in the operating-room setting.

DIFFERENTIAL DIAGNOSIS

The complaint of a sore throat can be a symptom of many disease processes. The differential includes viral URI, viral laryngotracheobronchitis (also known as croup), and *Streptococcus* pharyngitis. Abscess of the upper aerodigestive tract,

Table 8.1 Clinical Features: Supraglottitis

Organisms	• *Haemophilus* spp. • *Streptococcus pneumoniae* • *Streptococcus* spp. • *Staphylococcus* spp. • *Klebsiella* • *Pseudomonas* • *Candida* • Viruses
Signs and Symptoms	• Ill-appearing patient • Drooling • Voice change, "hot potato voice" • Sore throat • Difficulty breathing and/or stridor
Laboratory and Radiographic Findings	• May have elevated CBC • May be rapid *Streptococcus* positive • Lateral neck x-ray with thickening of the epiglottis, the "thumb sign," and adjacent aryepiglottic folds
Treatment	• Ampicillin–sulbactam 1.5–3 g IV q6h • Cefuroxime 750–1500 mg IV q8h • Ceftriaxone 1–2 g IV q24h • Cefotaxime 2 g IV q4–8h If PCN allergic Chloramphenicol: 50–100 mg/kg/d IV divided qid

CBC, complete blood count.

such as a peritonsillar, retropharyngeal, or deep neck abscess, may also present in a similar manner. Ludwig's angina, an abscess of the sublingual and submental space, will present with elevation of the oral tongue and edema or erythema of the skin directly underneath the mandible.

Other disease processes of the epiglottis that may cause thickening include hematoma, cyst, and abscess. Angioedema may present with stridor and hot-potato voice, though usually without the fever and pain of supraglottitis.

Other etiologies of edema and inflammation of the supraglottis include thermal injury, chemical inhalation (in particular, of illicit substances), and allergic reactions to food. A good history will help differentiate these causes.

LABORATORY AND RADIOGRAPHIC FINDINGS

Diagnosis is usually made on physical exam; however, laboratory studies such as a complete blood count may be helpful. A rapid *Streptococcus* swab of the posterior oropharynx may be indicated.

Imaging studies may be suggestive, but, to reiterate, *a patient should never be sent away from close monitoring for an imaging study unless the airway has been secured.* Although soft tissue lateral and AP views of the neck can provide substantial information, they are not as sensitive as direct visualization of the supraglottis. The "thumbprint sign" is a classic finding of the thickened epiglottis due to edema and inflammation on the lateral plain film. The aryepiglottic folds may also appear thickened.

CT or magnetic resonance (MR) imaging may also be useful. These modalities would be helpful when ruling out other disease processes in the differential, such as deep neck abscess.

TREATMENT AND PROPHYLAXIS

First and foremost, the airway must be assessed. Patients with supraglottitis may require intubation or even emergent tracheotomy or cricothyrotomy.

Broad-spectrum intravenous antibiotics should be initiated. Appropriate choices include ceftriaxone, cefotaxime, cefuroxime, or ampicillin/sulbactam. Often corticosteroids are concomitantly administered to decrease airway edema. The patient will usually warrant observation in an intensive care unit setting and intubation typically is maintained for 48 to 72 hours.

COMPLICATIONS AND ADMISSION CRITERIA

The most devastating complication is airway compromise and death. Severe pulmonary edema may also occur, including flash pulmonary edema from the sudden relief of airway obstruction. Positive end-expiratory pressure (PEEP) ventilation is usually recommended. If the infection spreads, the patient may develop pneumonia, meningitis, or sepsis.

PEARLS AND PITFALLS

1. Always consider evaluation of the airway the first priority.
2. Imaging studies, if needed, are only pursued after the airway is secure.
3. Widespread *H. influenzae* type B vaccination has significantly decreased the incidence of epiglottitis in children.
4. If indicated, a history of inhalation of illicit substances should be considered.

REFERENCES

Cantrell RW, Bell RA, Morioka WT. Acute epiglottitis: intubation versus tracheostomy. Laryngoscope 1978;88(6):994–1005.

Fairbanks DNF. Pocket guide to antimicrobial therapy in otolaryngology – head and neck surgery, 12th ed. Washington, DC: American Academy of Otolaryngology, 2005.

Osborne R, Avitia S, Zandifar H, Brown J. Adult supraglottitis subsequent to smoking crack cocaine. Ear Nose Throat J 2003;82(1):53–5.

Rodgers GK, Galos RS, Johnson JT. Hereditary angioedema: case report and review of management. Otolaryngol Head Neck Surg 1991;104(3):394–8.

9. Pharyngitis and Tonsillitis

Theresa A. Gurney and Andrew H. Murr

Outline   Introduction – Agents
Epidemiology
Clinical Features
Differential Diagnosis
Laboratory and Radiographic Findings
Treatment and Prophylaxis
Complications and Admission Criteria
Pearls and Pitfalls
References

INTRODUCTION – AGENTS

Pharyngitis and tonsillitis both are most frequently caused by *Streptococcus pyogenes* (group A beta-hemolytic streptococcus). However, many other organisms have been cultured in pharyngitis and tonsillitis, including viridans group *Streptococci*, *Staphylococcus aureus*, and *Haemophilus influenzae*. Oral flora such as *Actinomyces* can also be a bacterial etiology. It is not uncommon for the infection to be caused by a mix of aerobic and anaerobic flora.

Viruses with a predilection for the upper respiratory tract can also be causative and are, in fact, more prevalent. These include rhinoviruses, influenza viruses, adenovirus, enteroviruses, reovirus, respiratory syncytial virus, parainfluenza viruses, and coronaviruses. Infection with the Epstein-Barr virus (EBV) is common and may be accompanied by extensive tonsillar exudates. Other etiologies include toxoplasmosis, candida, tularemia, and cytomegalovirus.

EPIDEMIOLOGY

Pharyngitis and tonsillitis are most commonly seen in children and teenagers (though rarely in children under 2), and are not unusual in adults. In general, it is more likely for children than for adults to have a bacterial etiology of a sore throat. There is a peak incidence in *Streptococcus* pharyngitis from November to May.

CLINICAL FEATURES

Pharyngitis and tonsillitis both present with dysphagia, odynophagia, and a low-grade fever (Table 9.1). There may be erythema of the pharynx. In a tonsillar infection in which the many crevices (or crypts) harbor bacterial infection, patients may complain of bad breath and foul-tasting whitish lumps on the tonsils. Patients may also have tender cervical lymphadenopathy. If the infectious etiology is group A beta-hemolytic *Streptococcus*, the palate may demonstrate patches, and a diffuse scarlatiniform rash may develop. If the infectious etiology is *Corynebacterium diphtheriae*, grayish exudates forming a pseudomembrane may be present.

DIFFERENTIAL DIAGNOSIS

The differential diagnosis of pharyngitis or tonsillitis is broad. Other infectious etiologies such as supraglottitis or epiglotti-

tis can present with a severe sore throat. Sexually transmitted organisms, such as *Chlamydia pneumoniae*, *Neisseria gonorrhoeae*, and *Treponema pallidum*, may also cause a sore throat. Coxsackievirus herpangina characteristically presents with small vesicles on an erythematous base that can ulcerate.

Noninfectious etiologies of a sore throat include postnasal drip and laryngopharyngeal reflux. Exposure to environmental allergens or toxins may also cause throat discomfort. Even malignancies (such as squamous cell carcinoma or

Table 9.1 Clinical Features: Pharyngitis and Tonsillitis

Organisms	<ul><li>*Streptococcus* spp.</li><li>*Staphylococcus* spp.</li><li>*Haemophilus influenzae*</li><li>Anaerobes</li><li>Viruses such as rhinovirus, influenza virus, adenovirus, enterovirus, reovirus, respiratory syncytial virus, parainfluenza virus, and coronavirus</li></ul>
Signs and Symptoms	<ul><li>Low-grade fever</li><li>Sore throat</li><li>Exudates or enlarged tonsils if tonsillitis</li><li>Dysphagia</li><li>Odynophagia</li></ul>
Laboratory and Radiographic Findings	<ul><li>May consider CBC</li><li>Rapid strep test is an appropriate screening tool but is not always sensitive</li><li>Throat culture is the goal standard</li></ul>
Treatment	<ul><li>Penicillin V 500 mg qid × 10 days (pediatric dose: <27.3 kg: 125 mg PO tid/qid × 10 days >27.3 kg: 250 mg PO tid/qid × 10 days) *or*</li><li>Amoxicillin 500–875 mg PO bid × 7–10 days *or* Erthromycin 500 mg qid × 10 days (pediatric dose: 40 mg/kg/d PO divided tid/qid × 10 days) *or*</li><li>Amoxicillin/clavulanate 500–875 mg PO bid × 7–10 days *or*</li><li>Azithromycin 12 mg/kg up to 500 mg PO qd × 5 days (pediatric dose 12 mg/kg/d PO qd × 5 days; not to exceed 500 mg) *or*</li><li>Cephalexin 500 mg PO tid × 7–10 days (pediatric dose: 50 mg/kg/d PO qid × 10 days) *or*</li><li>Clindamycin 150–450 mg PO qid × 5 days (pediatric dose 20 mg/kg/d PO divided tid × 10 days) *or*</li><li>Benzathine penicillin G 1.2 million units IM × 1</li></ul>

CBC, complete blood count.

lymphoma) of the oropharynx and hypopharynx can present with throat discomfort. Foreign bodies and trauma may be considered given the appropriate history.

LABORATORY AND RADIOGRAPHIC FINDINGS

Diagnosis is usually made on clinical exam. When there is a concern for a bacterial etiology, rapid strep testing is commonly utilized. These tests are very specific, but not always sensitive (false negative results range from 10% to 20%). Traditional throat cultures are more sensitive. The pre-test probability for bacterial infections may be so high in some patients, that it is appropriate to treat without testing (see below).

TREATMENT AND PROPHYLAXIS

Treatment usually consists of analgesia and antibiotic therapy, either a single dose of Benzathine penicillin G 1.2 million units IM, or a 7- to 10-day course of oral antibiotics. Cephalexin (Keflex) or another first-generation cephalosporin is an appropriate first choice. Some practitioners choose amoxicillin or amoxicillin/clavulanate. Choices for those with a penicillin allergy include clindamycin, azithromycin, or clarithromycin. Antibiotic therapy is primarily aimed at the prevention of complications (see Complications and Admission Criteria below), as the pharyngitis itself is usually self-limited, resolving in 3–4 days even without antibiotic therapy. For patients whose tonsils are prone to crevasses and crypts, irrigation with a water-pick device may be helpful in controlling this chronic predisposing condition. Patients with recurrent tonsillar infections, especially those documented as *Streptococcus* positive, may warrant tonsillectomy.

If the patient is having difficulty maintaining sufficient oral intake because of discomfort, intravenous fluids may be indicated. Imaging is not indicated unless ruling out a complication, such as a peritonsillar or other deep neck infection abscess.

COMPLICATIONS AND ADMISSION CRITERIA

Untreated tonsillitis can progress to a peritonsillar or parapharyngeal abscess. Symptoms of a peritonsillar abscess include unilateral throat discomfort, ipsilateral otalgia, dysphagia, and odynophagia. On exam, the patient may have trismus and a bulge in the soft palate and uvular deviation to the contralat-

eral side. The treatment is either needle aspiration or incision and drainage.

A serious, but much less common, complication of *Streptococcus pyogenes* (group A beta-hemolytic streptococcus) is rheumatic fever and its heart valve effects. Other complications include scarlet fever, glomerulonephritis, and pediatric autoimmune neuropsychiatric disorders associated with *Streptococcal* infections (PANDAS). Notably, while prevention of rheumatic fever is one of the principal motivations for antibiotic therapy, and there is some evidence that antibiotics may improve the symptoms of PANDAS, the incidence of post-streptococcal glomerulonephritis is not affected by antibiotic therapy. Admission may be indicated for young children, toxic-appearing adults, and immunocompromised individuals.

PEARLS AND PITFALLS

1. *Streptococcus pyogenes* (group A beta-hemolytic streptococcus) is the most common bacterial infectious agent in pharyngitis and tonsillitis, and is still highly susceptible to penicillin or amoxicillin.
2. Rapid strep cultures are a quick diagnostic test; however, they may provide a false negative result. A throat culture is more sensitive.
3. Complications include rheumatic fever, glomerulonephritis, and PANDAS.

REFERENCES

Bisno AL, Gerber MA, Gwaltney JM Jr, et al. Practice guidelines for the diagnosis and management of group A streptococcal pharyngitis: Infectious Diseases Society of America. Clin Infect Dis 2002;35:113–25.

Cooper RJ, Hoffman JR, Bartlett JG. Principles of appropriate antibiotic use for acute pharyngitis in adults: background. Ann Intern Med 2001;134:509.

Fairbanks DNF. Pocket guide to antimicrobial therapy in otolaryngology – head and neck surgery, 12th ed. Washington, DC: American Academy of Otolaryngology, 2005.

Orvidas LJ, Slattery MJ. Pediatric autoimmune neuropsychiatric disorders and streptococcal infections: role of otolaryngologist. Laryngoscope 2001;111(9):1515–9.

10. Deep Neck Space Infections

Theresa A. Gurney and Andrew H. Murr

INTRODUCTION – AGENTS

The head and neck contain a variety of fascial planes forming potential spaces for the spread of infection. If these spaces are seeded, infection may travel to vital structures such as the carotid artery, jugular vein, or mediastinum. Deep neck spaces include the submandibular, peritonsillar, parapharyngeal, retropharyngeal, and prevertebral spaces.

The majority of deep neck space infections are caused by the organisms that frequently infect or colonize the upper aerodigestive tract. These include *Streptococcus* and *Staphylococcus* species, as well as bacteria commonly found in the oral cavity such as *Bacteroides* species, *Klebsiella*, *Escherichia coli*, *Enterobacter*, *Actinomyces*, and *Eikenella corrodens*. Often these infections involve mixed flora.

EPIDEMIOLOGY

Both adults and young children can develop deep neck space infections. Teenagers and young adults present with peritonsillar space abscesses more commonly than other age groups. A recent dental infection or procedure may be a predisposing factor for a submental or submandibular space infection (see Chapter 3, Dental and Odontogenic Infections). Intravenous or subcutaneous injection of illicit substances into neck veins or tissue also predisposes to neck infections.

CLINICAL FEATURES

The clinical features of a particular deep neck space infection will reflect the anatomic characteristics of the deep neck space involved (Table 10.1). A submandibular space infection may reveal a concomitant infection of the submandibular duct. Odontogenic infections can progress to submental or sublingual infections, and therefore a through dental examination is always indicated.

If the infection is superficial to the mylohyoid muscle, one should suspect Ludwig's angina. The resultant erythema, edema, and induration of the floor of the mouth may progress to such an extent that the tongue is displaced posteriorly and may result in airway obstruction and death. Frequently the patient is dysarthric and has difficulty handling secretions. Intubation is challenging because the tongue edema makes it difficult to visualize the vocal folds.

Infection of the parapharyngeal space may be associated with a recent tonsil or dental infection. In addition to pain and dysphagia, the patient may also have ipsilateral otalgia, odynophagia, a muffled voice, and neck stiffness. The parapharyngeal space extends from the hyoid bone to the skull base. The space abuts the peritonsillar space and is separated from it by the superior constrictor muscle. A parapharyngeal space infection may cause airway compromise or may rapidly progress to the mediastinum.

A peritonsillar abscess is confined on the oral cavity side of the superior pharyngeal constrictor muscle in a potential space between the tonsil and the constrictor. Symptoms

Table 10.1 Clinical Features: Deep Neck Space Infections

Organisms	• *Streptococcus* spp. • *Staphylococcus* spp. • *Bacteroides* spp. • *Klebsiella* • *E. coli* • *Enterobacter* • *Actinomyces* • *Eikenella*
Signs and Symptoms	• Fever • Otalgia • Trismus • Neck stiffness • Muffled voice quality • Dysarthria • Dysphagia • Odynophagia • Drooling
Laboratory and Radiographic Findings	• Leukocytosis • CT with contrast demonstrates rim-enhancing fluid collection consistent with that of an abscess • Culture of the abscess is usually a mixture of aerobes and anaerobes
Treatment	Antibiotics: • amoxicillin 500–875 mg PO bid • amoxicillin/clavulanate 500–875 mg PO bid • piperacillin-tazobactam 3.375–4.5 g IV q6h • clindamycin 150–450 mg PO qid Incision and drainage if there is an abscess Supplemental oxygen may be indicated The airway must be secured if any concern for compromise

of this infection include otalgia, trismus (difficulty opening the mouth), uvular deviation, and a bulge in the soft palate. A muffled "hot potato" voice is often noted. Lymph nodes in the neck at the level of the jugular foramen may be palpable.

Retropharyngeal space infections may develop from nasal, sinus, adenoid, or scalp infections (see Chapter 49, Pediatric Respiratory Infections). As noted before, pain, dysphagia, a muffled voice, and neck stiffness are common presenting signs and symptoms. The neck stiffness due to the irritation of the prevertebral fascia may mimic that of meningitis. Adenoiditis leading to a retropharyngeal space infection in young children may present with high fever, neck discomfort, and an elevated white blood count.

Although lateral soft-tissue x-rays will be suggestive, a computed tomographic (CT) scan with contrast will be more definitive if the diagnosis is questionable.

DIFFERENTIAL DIAGNOSIS

The differential diagnosis of a deep neck space infection includes other infections of the head and neck such as tonsillitis, sinusitis, and dental infections. The neck stiffness seen in deep neck space infections that irritate the prevertebral fascia may mimic meningitis. Fever and otalgia can also occur in otitis media and otitis externa. Supraglottitis and epiglottitis may also present with drooling, odynophagia, and muffled voice quality. Trauma from foreign-body ingestion or from injection of illicit drugs may also present with similar symptoms.

"Cold" infections of the neck may in some cases present similarly. This includes etiologies such as mycobacterial infection, which, although rare, may present as a deep neck or retropharyngeal abscess. The patient, however, is usually less acutely ill, without severe pain and high fever. These abscesses should not necessarily be drained, as the risk of fistula formation on the nonhealing wound track may occur. Medical therapy target to the offending organism is indicated.

LABORATORY AND RADIOGRAPHIC FINDINGS

Diagnosis is usually made by physical exam and imaging. The signs and symptoms of deep neck space infections are discussed above and can help differentiate the deep neck space that is likely involved.

Computed tomography with contrast is the imaging modality of choice and usually will demonstrate a rim-enhancing fluid filled collection in the affected space (Figure 10.1).

In early infection, fat stranding and asymmetry in the fascial planes of the neck may be subtle findings. Concomitant tonsillitis, sinusitis, dental infection, recent trauma, or evidence of a recent procedure may also be noted.

A complete blood count (CBC) usually demonstrates a leukocytosis, though this is a nonspecific finding. Cultures of the affected fluid may reveal the offending organisms, and subsequent sensitivities may guide antimicrobial selection.

TREATMENT AND PROPHYLAXIS

An abscess requires immediate incision and drainage. The procedure is both diagnostic and therapeutic. Sometimes a

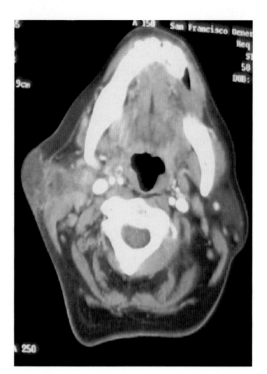

Figure 10.1 Neck infection.

simple, uncomplicated abscess, such as a peritonsillar abscess in an otherwise healthy patient, may be incised and drained transorally at the bedside or in the clinic. However, in patients with a concern of airway compromise, treatment should be performed in the controlled setting of the operating room. Protection of the airway may require intubation, or even a tracheotomy. Parapharyngeal neck infections and Ludwig's angina, are usually drained through the neck in the operating room, sometimes with a concomitant tracheotomy for airway control.

As deep neck infections are commonly of mixed flora, a broad-spectrum antibiotic with both aerobic and anaerobic coverage is indicated. Appropriate choices include ampicillin-sulbactam, piperacillin-tazobactam, or clindamycin (especially in patients with a penicillin allergy).

COMPLICATIONS AND ADMISSION CRITERIA

Complications can include airway compromise, necrotizing fasciitis, septic thrombophlebitis of the internal jugular vein, erosion of the carotid artery, mediastinitis, meningitis, disseminated sepsis, septic shock, and death.

PEARLS AND PITFALLS

1. Management of the airway is the first priority.
2. Infection of the floor of the mouth may result in Ludwig's angina, in which the tongue is retrodisplaced posteriorly and may occlude the airway.
3. Neck stiffness due to infectious irritation or involvement of the prevertebral fascia may mimic meningitis.
4. Broad-spectrum antibiotics should cover both aerobes and anaerobes.
5. CT with contrast is the imaging study of choice.

REFERENCES

Fairbanks DNF. Pocket guide to antimicrobial therapy in otolaryngology – head and neck surgery, 12th ed. Washington, DC: American Academy of Otolaryngology, 2005.

Herzon FS. Peritonsillar abscess: incidence, current management practices and a proposal for treatment guidelines. Laryngoscope 1995;105(8):1–17.

Herzon FS, Martin AD. Medical and surgical treatment of peritonsillar, retropharyngeal and parapharyngeal abscesses. Curr Infect Dis Rep 2006;8(3):196–202.

Lin D, Reeck JB, Murr AH. Internal jugular vein thrombosis and deep neck infection from intravenous drug use: management strategy. Laryngoscope 2004;114(1):56–60.

Myers EN. Deep neck abscesses. In: Operative otolaryngology head and neck surgery. 1997:667–75., Saunders; 1st edition. http://www.amazon.com/Operative-Otolaryngology-Head-Surgery-Two/dp/0721638414.

11. Mumps

Theresa A. Gurney and Andrew H. Murr

INTRODUCTION

Once considered a common childhood illness, mumps has dramatically declined in incidence with the widespread usage of the mumps vaccine, though there have been significant sporadic outbreaks in the United States recently. Mumps is still a common disease in countries without widespread vaccination programs.

EPIDEMIOLOGY

Mumps is an enveloped negative-sense RNA virus belonging to the Paramyxovirus family. In the United States between 2001 and 2005, only 200–300 cases of mumps were diagnosed annually. Between January and May, 2006, however, there were more than 2,500 outbreaks in 11 states. Unvaccinated individuals are particularly at risk for infection, though the majority of outbreak cases have occurred among those who have been vaccinated and have not achieved immunity.

Current recommendations are that children receive a first dose of MMR vaccine at ages 12 to 15 months and a second dose at ages 4 to 6 years. Two doses of MMR vaccine are also recommended for students attending colleges and other post–high school institutions and who do not have proof of two prior doses or other evidence of immunity.

CLINICAL FEATURES

Patients with mumps commonly present with painful, bilateral parotid swelling (Figure 11.1). They may also have fevers, dry mucous membranes, dysphagia, and trismus (Table 11.1). On questioning, the patient may describe prodromal symptoms including malaise, fevers, and a sore throat. Milking of saliva along Stenson's duct should reveal clear saliva (purulent saliva suggests a bacterial etiology).

Orchitis occurs in 25% of postpubertal males with mumps and is rare in prepubescent males, while oophoritis occurs in 5% of postpubertal females with mumps and is characterized by pelvic pain and tenderness. Mastitis may also occur.

DIFFERENTIAL DIAGNOSIS

Other etiologies of viral parotitis include Epstein-Barr virus (EBV), coxsackievirus, cytomegalovirus, influenza, and parainfluenza. Human immunodeficiency virus (HIV) infection can also be associated with a parotitis, though more commonly presents with isolated benign lymphoepithelial cysts.

Acute suppurative parotitis may present similarly. *Staphylococcus* species, *Streptococcus* species, *Escherichia coli*, *Haemophilus influenzae*, and anaerobes are likely agents. For these bacterial causes, antibiotics such as amoxicillin-clavulanate or ampicillin-sulbactam are first-line agents. A salivary gland stone blocking the duct may or may not be present.

Noninfectious etiologies of bilateral parotid enlargement include various autoimmune diseases, such as Sjögren's syndrome, sarcoidosis, and chronic self-purging, such as in bulimia. Alcoholism may produce bilateral parotid enlargement. Temporal mandibular joint syndrome or isolated bruxism may produce symptoms of bilateral pain that can be mistaken for mumps.

LABORATORY AND RADIOGRAPHIC FINDINGS

Diagnosis is made by clinical examination. Laboratory studies can also be submitted for analysis of antibodies to the mumps virus to demonstrate exposure.

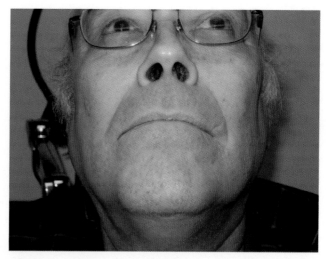

Figure 11.1 Mumps.

Table 11.1 Clinical Features: Mumps

Organism	Mumps virus
Signs and Symptoms	• Bilateral parotid gland swelling • Fever • Decreased appetite • Dry mucosal membranes • Trismus • Clear saliva from Stenson's • Orchitis, oophoritis, or mastitis
Laboratory and Radiographic Findings	• May have elevated leukocyte count • Imaging is usually not indicated unless a discrete lesion is being ruled out
Treatment	Supportive: • Pain medication • Antipyretics • Warm compresses • Parotid gland massage • Steroids can be considered

TREATMENT AND PROPHYLAXIS

Treatment of mumps infection is supportive. Patients may benefit from pain medication, antipyretics, massage of the parotid glands, and warm compresses. If the viral etiology is unclear and bacterial infection is suspected, antibiotics may also be prescribed. Steroids may help to decrease inflammation. Resolution occurs over a few weeks.

COMPLICATIONS AND ADMISSION CRITERIA

A variety of complications have been associated with mumps infection. These include sensorineural hearing loss, meningoencephalitis, and orchitis. Most patients with mumps infection do not require hospitalization, as supportive therapy is usually adequate. Patients with evidence of CNS involvement should be admitted for observation and treatment.

INFECTION CONTROL

The best prevention is vaccination. See Epidemiology above for current recommendations.

Control of outbreaks is indicated to limit the spread of disease. Perinatal transmission has also been noted, and an infected infant should be isolated from other infants.

Universal precautions should be observed. There are no additional isolation or contact precautions required.

PEARLS AND PITFALLS

1. Patients without vaccination are at higher relative risk.
2. Other causes of bilateral parotid swelling should also be considered.
3. Treatment is symptomatic.

REFERENCES

Fairbanks DNF. Pocket guide to antimicrobial therapy in otolaryngology – head and neck surgery, 12th ed. Washington, DC: American Academy of Otolaryngology, 2005.

Gurney TA, Murr AH. Otolaryngologic manifestations of human immunodeficiency virus infection. Otolaryngol Clin North Am 2003;36(4):607–24.

MMWR. Dispatch – mumps epidemic – Iowa. MMWR 2006;55(13):366–8.

MMWR. Notice to readers: updated recommendations of the Advisory Committee on Immunization Practices (ACIP) for the control and elimination of mumps. MMWR 2006 Jun 9;55(22):629–30.

12. Peritonitis

Ramin Jamshidi and William Schecter

INTRODUCTION

The tremendous complexity of the abdomen makes diagnosis and treatment of intraperitoneal disease one of the greatest challenges in clinical medicine. Many intra-abdominal processes prompt urgent evaluation and some of these require immediate intervention. These conditions manifest via peritonitis, which is inflammation or infection of the lining of the abdominal cavity. Peritonitis is classified as primary, secondary, or tertiary on the basis of its underlying pathophysiology; the distinction is useful when considering relevant microbiology and treatment.

Primary peritonitis occurs when bacteria seed the peritoneum hematogenously, via indwelling catheters, or by translocation across intestinal walls. Spontaneous bacterial peritonitis (SBP) and tuberculous peritonitis are examples of this process.

Secondary peritonitis is caused by inflammation and/or infection arising in abdominal organs as occurs with hollow viscus perforation, biliary tract disease, bowel ischemia, pancreatitis, and pelvic inflammatory disease. The process is generally polymicrobial, but the specific pathogens vary based on the source of infection.

Tertiary peritonitis refers to recurrent or persistent intra-abdominal infection after apparent definitive intervention with antibiotics and drainage.

EPIDEMIOLOGY

The single most common chief complaint for United States emergency department visits is abdominal pain. Although many such patients are suffering from self-limited disease, some require definitive intervention and an error or delay in diagnosis can be disastrous.

The most common cause of primary peritonitis is catheter-related peritonitis, due to peritoneal dialysis (Tenckhoff) catheters or peritoneovenous shunts. These chronically indwelling devices generate peritonitis at a rate of 1.3–1.4 episodes per patient per year. Usually a single organism is responsible, with gram-positive cocci in two thirds and gram-negative bacilli in the rest. Fungal infections occur infrequently and are due to *Candida* species in 80% of such cases.

The most common cause of secondary peritonitis is appendicitis. Lifetime risk of appendicitis in the United States is estimated to be 6–7%. Incidence is slightly lower in nonindustrialized nations with higher-fiber diets and less use of refined carbohydrates. Although the peak incidence is in the second and third decades of life, appendicitis can occur at any age.

Diverticulitis is another common cause of secondary peritonitis in the United States; incidence is considerably lower in countries with high-fiber diets. One-third of Americans older than age 45, one-half older than age 70, and two-thirds older than age 85 have colonic diverticula. Ten percent to 25% of these patients develop complications related to their diverticula.

Peptic ulcers are mucosal erosions of the stomach or duodenum that are estimated to affect roughly one in ten people worldwide. In the United States, it has been estimated that at any given time 2% of the general population has symptomatic peptic ulcer disease. *Helicobacter pylori* infection (30% prevalence in the United States), alcoholism, and use of nonsteroidal anti-inflammatory agents are the most common causes of the condition. Between 5% and 10% of patients suffer an ulcer perforation, and this is fatal in as many as 10%.

CLINICAL FEATURES

Visceral pain is often poorly localized or referred to a site not actually involved in the inflammatory process (Table 12.1). This is explained by the embryologic migration of nerves and the origin of the gut as a midline structure with symmetric visceral innervation.

Spontaneous bacterial peritonitis is a primary peritonitis (Table 12.2): Disease of the abdominal lining and its contained fluid is the central process. The presence of ascites is a necessary condition for developing such an infection, so this is

Table 12.1 Patterns of Referred Abdominal Pain

Structure	Innervation	Pain
Foregut	T5–T9 roots	Supraumbilical or epigastric
Midgut	T8–T11 roots	Periumbilical
Hindgut	T11–L1 roots	Infraumbilical or pelvic
Diaphragm	Phrenic nerve	Ipsilateral scapula or shoulder

Table 12.2 Clinical Features: Primary Peritonitis

Pathogenesis	Bacterial translocation across bowel or invasion along catheter
Organisms	Catheter-related: • *Streptococcus* sp. and *Staphylococcus* sp. (66%) • Gram-negative rods (33%) Spontaneous: • *Escherichia coli* (50%) • *Streptococcus* sp. (15–20%) • *Klebsiella* (10%)
Signs and Symptoms	Nonspecific: • Abdominal pain (<50%) • Pyrexia (80%) • Nausea • Catheter-site cellulitis • Encephalopathy
Laboratory Findings	• Leukocytosis • WBCs and organisms on paracentesis

WBC, white blood cell.

Table 12.3 Clinical Features: Peptic Ulcer Perforation

Pathogenesis	Chronic gastritis from alcohol, NSAID use, or H. pylori leading to mucosal erosion
Organisms	• *Helicobacter pylori* Peritoneal contamination by • *Streptococcus* sp. • *Lactobacillus* • *Candida*
Signs and Symptoms	Epigastric/upper abdominal pain: • history of prior episodes • acute onset • unrelenting
Laboratory and Radiographic Findings	• Leukocytosis • Subdiaphragmatic air on CXR
Treatment	• Antibiotics (see Treatment section) • Operative closure of perforation • Expectant management if perforation is small and contained

CXR, chest x-ray.

almost exclusively a disease of patients with liver disease or nephrotic syndrome. A deficiency in the reticuloendothelial system of patients with liver disease facilitates this process. Presentation of peritonitis can be subtle, with abdominal pain absent in more than half of patients with proven SBP. Fever, worsening renal function, nausea, or encephalopathy may be the only presenting symptoms. In-hospital mortality for SBP in cirrhotic patients is approximately 25–50% and recurrence rates are greater than 60% in 12 months.

Secondary peritonitis has a more distinct clinical presentation, almost always associated with abdominal pain and tenderness, and often with a history of acute onset. Any process that leads to intraperitoneal contamination or abscess formation can secondarily cause peritonitis. The following discussion highlights the most common etiologies of secondary peritonitis: peptic ulcers, appendicitis, diverticulitis, hepatic and splenic abscesses, and postoperative anastomotic leaks.

Viscus Perforation

Peptic ulcers are mucosal erosions of the stomach and duodenum. They are most commonly related to alcoholism, *H. pylori* infection, or anti-inflammatory medications. If these ulcers progress through the submucosa they can perforate freely into the peritoneum (Table 12.3). A less likely cause of gastric perforation is an advanced neoplasm. The spillage of acidic gastric contents, bacteria, and fungi into the peritoneum causes dramatic pain and can incite a septic cascade.

The appendix is a blind-ended tubular accessory of the cecum that does not have any known physiologic function in humans. When its lumen is obstructed (e.g., by a fecalith), continued mucosal secretion results in increased intraluminal pressure. Progressive increase in this pressure eventually impedes venous outflow and thus causes congestive ischemia with necrosis and possibly perforation. The typical chronology of symptoms and signs are pain, anorexia, tenderness, fever, and leukocytosis (Table 12.4). Essentially all patients with appendicitis complain of abdominal pain, 75% in the

Table 12.4 Clinical Features: Appendicitis

Pathogenesis	Obstruction by fecalith or swollen lymphatics causing venous congestion leading to ischemia
Organisms	• *Bacteroides fragilis* • *Escherichia coli* • *Enterococcus* (average of 10 organisms isolated)
Signs and Symptoms	• Umbilical/right lower abdominal pain • Anorexia (80%) • Nausea (80% – usually without emesis) • Fever
Laboratory and Radiographic Findings	• Modest leukocytosis (>10,000) • Appendix dilation and wall thickening • Stranding of periappendiceal fat
Treatment	• Antibiotics (see Treatment section) • Appendectomy • Percutaneous drainage of abscess

right lower quadrant, 15% periumbilically, and 10% diffusely. With timely treatment, most cases of appendicitis are benign, but perforation occurs in about 25% of patients, and 10% will develop abscesses.

Impaction of stool into a colonic diverticulum leads to inflammation and infection, defined as diverticulitis (Table 12.5). At the time of presentation the process may have progressed to localized microperforation or gross perforation with significant leakage of stool into the peritoneal cavity. Diverticula are most common in the sigmoid and descending segments so symptoms are usually lower abdominal in location. Bowel habits may be altered, but not uniformly or consistently: painful defecation, constipation, loose stools, dysuria, or urinary retention may occur.

Table 12.5 Clinical Features: Diverticulitis

Pathogenesis	Stool impaction in dilated portion of colonic wall
Organisms	• *Bacteroides fragilis* • *Escherichia coli* • *Enterococcus*
Signs and Symptoms	• Left lower abdominal pain (>90%) • Dysuria • Loose bowel movements or constipation • Fever (80%)
Laboratory and Radiographic Findings	• Leukocytosis • Diverticulosis • Free air or pericolonic air pocket • Localized colonic wall thickening/inflammation
Treatment	• Antibiotics • Bowel rest • Percutaneous drainage of abscess • Partial colectomy if recurrent or complicated

Anastomotic Leaks

Patients who have undergone resections or diversions of the enteric tract will have anastomoses that are prone to failed healing and leakage. Leakage of enteric contents into the abdomen will generate peritonitis and a clinical syndrome of pain, tenderness, anorexia, and possibly fever and chills. Such anastomotic leaks can manifest within the first days after operation or up to 3 weeks later. Typical timing is between 2 days and 1 week after operation, with a risk of 2–16% based on the type of operation. Anastomotic leaks are more common in patients who are malnourished or immunosuppressed (including chronic steroid users) and also in operations conducted in the setting of active infection.

Solid Organ Abscesses

Liver abscesses are classified as amebic, pyogenic, or hydatid, and are uncommon in North America (Table 12.6). Worldwide, amebic abscesses are the most common, but the pyogenic variety is more common in the United States.

Patients with hepatic abscesses do not have diffuse abdominal symptoms. Instead, the majority present with right upper quadrant tenderness (70%), fever (>80%), and leukocytosis (75%). With jaundice in approximately 33% and a positive Murphy's sign in approximately 20%, imaging is required to differentiate this condition from cholangitis. Overall mortality can be as high as 25% and is increased in patients with malignancy, low albumin (<2.5g/dL), and more abscess foci.

Peripancreatic abscesses are a subacute complication of acute pancreatitis (Table 12.7). Necrosis of a portion of the gland leaves dying tissue and profound regional inflammation, which may lead to infection and abscess formation. The onset is variable, from days to weeks after the initial onset of pancreatitis. The symptoms are similar to those of pancreatitis: nausea, vomiting, epigastric pain, and tenderness. Therefore, progression or nonresolution of pancreatitis (e.g., persistent pain with development of fever or leukocytosis) requires computed tomographic (CT) reevaluation to rule out pancreatic abscess formation. It is important to note that a necrotic gland does not necessarily indicate infection. When infection is present, *E. coli* and *Enterococcus* are generally involved (and *Staphylococcus*, *Pseudomonas*, and *Candida* to a lesser extent); anaerobes are not as prevalent as in other parts of the gastrointestinal (GI) tract. Peripancreatic infections carry serious morbidity and increased mortality; they predispose to pancreatic fistulae and hemorrhage from erosion of the gastroduodenal artery.

Splenic abscesses are the least common solid organ abscesses and are associated with high mortality rates (Table 12.8). Generally these are caused by direct extension or septic embolization, but up to 25% are cryptogenic. More than

Table 12.6 Clinical Features: Hepatic Abscess

	Pyogenic	Hydatid	Amebic
Pathogenesis	Biliary obstruction or GI infection which spreads via portal (15–30% cryptogenic)	Zoonotic infection harbored by rodents, contracted by exposure to feces	Environmentally acquired; invades liver from colon via portal system
Microbes	60% polymicrobial, 50% gram-negative enteric organisms: • *Escherichia coli* • *Klebsiella pneumoniae* (these two by far most common) • *Bacteroides* sp. • *Enterobacter* Sterile in 15%	• *Echinococcus granulosus* • *Echinococcus multilocularis* • *Echinococcus vogelii*	• *Entamoeba histolytica*
Laboratory and Radiographic Findings	• Majority are right lobed and solitary	• Eosinophilia (25%) • Hemagglutination and ELISA (80%) • Daughter cysts on CT	• Almost uniformly right lobed and solitary
Treatment	• Percutaneous/surgical drainage	• Pericystectomy • Albendazole 400 mg PO bid	• Metronidazole 500 mg PO tid

CT, computed tomography; ELISA, enzyme-linked immunosorbent assay.

Table 12.7 Clinical Features: Peripancreatic Abscess

Pathogenesis	Infection of inflamed or necrotic pancreas
Organisms	• Enterobacteriaceae • *Enterococcus* sp. • *Staphylococcus* sp. • *Candida* sp.
Signs and Symptoms	• Encephalopathy • Coagulopathy • Loss of glycemic control • Cerebral edema • Sepsis
Laboratory and Radiographic Findings	• Leukocytosis and fever • Fluid collection along pancreas
Treatment	• Imipenem-cilastatin 500 mg IV q6h • Open drainage and necrosectomy

Table 12.8 Clinical Features: Splenic Abscess

Pathogenesis	Direct extension or regional infection Hematogenous seeding (septic embolization)
Organisms	• Staphylococci and streptococci (hematogenous) • Polymicrobial as with viscus perforation (see above)
Signs and Symptoms	• Encephalopathy • Coagulopathy • Loss of glycemic control • Cerebral edema • Sepsis
Laboratory and Radiologic Findings	• Elevated AST or ALT (10^2–10^3 units/L) • PT >5 s above normal or INR >1.5
Treatment	• Nafcillin 2gm IV q4hr • Vancomycin 1gm IV q12hr • As for secondary peritonitis (see above)

INR, international normalized ratio; PT, prothrombin time.

90% will be accompanied by fever, 75% by left upper quadrant pain, and 66% by leukocytosis. Causative organisms are aerobes in more than 80% of cases, consistent with the known mechanism of septic embolization. Half of the cases are solitary abscesses and half are multiple.

DIFFERENTIAL DIAGNOSIS

Abdominal pain is a complaint relevant to a wide spectrum of disease processes. Work-up of peritonitis requires consideration of a complex differential diagnosis. Table 12.9 lists a number of potential causes with historical, exam, or diagnostic points that can help to identify them.

LABORATORY AND RADIOGRAPHIC FINDINGS

Paracentesis should be performed in patients with ascites and either abdominal pain or evidence of infection without an identifiable source. The fluid should be sent for cell count, Gram stain, and culture (and acid-fast stain as well if

Table 12.9 Differential Diagnosis of Abdominal Pain

Abdominal Trauma	History; abdominal wall ecchymosis
Adhesive Bowel Obstruction	Prior operations; lack of air in sigmoid/rectum on KUB; transition zone on CT
Cholecystitis	Gallbladder wall thickening on ultrasound
Constipation	Stool in colon on KUB; impaction on digital rectal
Ectopic Pregnancy	Low pelvic pain; elevated beta-HCG
Gastroesophageal Reflux	History; relief with antacids and repositioning
Gastritis	Alcoholism; NSAIDs; similar prior episodes
Hepatitis	Constitutional symptoms; history of exposure; ultrasound without evidence of cholecystitis
Hypercalcemia	Vague abdominal pain without tenderness; lab
Incarcerated Hernia	Palpable hernia; history of operation
Inflammatory Bowel Disease	Prior history; bloody stools; fistulae
Irritable Bowel Syndrome	Similar prior pain; normal labs and imaging
Ischemic Bowel	Acidosis; pain out of proportion to exam; vascular disease; bloody stools; bowel wall thickening on CT
Ketoacidosis	History of diabetes; hyperglycemia; ketosis
Lymphoma	Visceral or peripheral lymphadenopathy; LDH
Migraine Headache	History of migraine; abdominal CT normal
Omental Infarction	Clinically similar to appendicitis; CT diagnostic
Ovarian/Gonadal Torsion	Abdominal pain is referred; primary pain pelvic; ultrasound is diagnostic
Pancreatitis	Amylase or lipase elevation; gland inflammation without abscess on CT
Pelvic Inflammatory Disease	Tenderness on pelvic exam; normal gynecologic ultrasound
Pneumonia	Cough or URI symptoms; chest imaging
Porphyria	Elevated porphyrin levels
Pyelonephritis	Costovertebral tenderness; urinalysis findings
Sickle Cell Crisis	Sickle disease; dehydration
Tubo-ovarian Abscess	Pelvic ultrasound is diagnostic
Typhlitis	Neutropenia; normal appendix but cecal inflammation on CT
Uremia	Vague, diffuse pain with nausea; azotemia
Urolithiasis	Colicky flank pain; microscopic or gross hematuria
Zoster	Superficial pain; dermatomal distribution

HCG, human chorionic gonadotropin; KUB, kidney, ureter, and bladder radiograph; LDH, lactate dehydrogenase; NSAID, nonsteroidal anti-inflammatory drug; URI, upper respiratory infection.

Table 12.10 Imaging for Acute Abdominal Pain

Modality	Benefits	Limitations
KUB	Rapid, safe, portable Demonstrates bowel obstruction, free air, or constipation	Limited sensitivity for most conditions and may delay ordering other imaging studies
CT	Cross-sectional anatomy Casts "widest net" for abdominal findings	Potential contrast nephropathy Requires patient transport
US	Safe and portable Most sensitive for biliary anatomy or urogenital abnormalities	Availability and quality dependent on technologist Not useful for general abdominal survey

US, ultrasound.

Table 12.11 Antibiotics for Primary Peritonitis

Spontaneous Bacterial Peritonitis	ceftriaxone 2 g IV q24h *or* piperacillin-tazobactam 4.5 g IV q8h *or* ertapenem 1 g IV q24h
Catheter-Related Peritonitis	ceftriaxone 2 g IV q24h *plus* vancomycin 1 g IV q24h
Prophylaxis	ciprofloxacin 750 mg PO every week *or* trimethoprim-sulfamethoxazole 160/800 mg PO 5 days/week

tuberculous peritonitis is a consideration). A large-volume spun specimen should undergo cytologic testing if malignancy is a possibility. Presence of greater than 500 white blood cells/mL or 250 neutrophils/mL is diagnostic of peritonitis. Gram stain and culture are mandatory, though the stain may not reveal the organism. If a single organism is cultured, SBP is the most likely cause. Conversely, multiple organisms indicate secondary peritonitis, and the underlying process must be identified.

When seeking the source of abdominal pain, imaging studies are useful adjuncts and are sometimes critical (Table 12.10). The principal modalities are computed tomography and ultrasonography. However, plain radiography can be an useful initial study to evaluate bowel distension, presence of free air, and stool distribution.

CT with intravenous contrast carries a risk of contrast-induced nephropathy, which can occur in as many as 5% of patients with normal renal function. All patients should be well hydrated, and those with renal insufficiency should receive pretreatment with *N*-acetylcysteine and/or sodium bicarbonate. If there is any concern for bowel leakage, water-soluble oral contrast should be given to best distend and evaluate the bowel. Only water or a water-soluble contrast agent should be used (rather than barium) to avoid causing barium peritonitis. Rectal contrast is often neglected, but is important in the evaluation of lower GI structures such as colonic diverticula and the appendix. Discussing the clinical suspicions with the radiologist will optimize both technique and interpretation.

TREATMENT AND PROPHYLAXIS

Management of peritonitis depends on its etiology (Table 12.11). Therapy for SBP consists of antibiotics and supportive care. Standard treatment is 2 weeks of intravenous therapy. Duration may be shortened to 5 days in patients who are clinically well with sterile peritoneal fluid cultures and less than 250 neutrophils on repeat paracentesis. Recurrences are frequent, affecting more than 40% of patients within 6 months and nearly 70% within a year of the index episode. On this basis, prophylaxis is recommended with ciprofloxacin or trimethoprim-sulfamethoxazole; this decreases reinfection rates but does not affect overall survival.

Catheter-related peritonitis should be treated with intravenous or intraperitoneal antibiotics with a third-generation cephalosporin or vancomycin for 10–14 days. Broad coverage is appropriate until cultures allow tailoring of the regimen. Repeated bouts of peritonitis with a single organism may warrant removal of the catheter with replacement after a "line holiday."

Secondary peritonitis also necessitates antibiotic therapy (Table 12.12), but this is usually combined with a definitive intervention to remove the infected fluid/tissue and address its source either by percutaneous catheter drainage or operative exploration. Antibiotics should be initiated immediately and surgical consultation obtained.

If the intraperitoneal contamination is small and contained, antibiotics alone may be used. This approach is often combined with percutaneous catheter placement to drain the infected fluid collection. However, with diffuse infection or gross anastomotic leaks, surgery is almost always required to lavage the abdomen and achieve source control.

When definitive operations are performed, antibiotics are not indicated beyond 24–72 hours postoperatively unless an ongoing infection is identified. In patients who undergo catheter drainage, antibiotics are often continued for a predetermined period (5 days to 2 weeks) or as long as pus is draining, which is based on historical practice patterns rather than clinical evidence. Antibiotic prophylaxis has no role in the management of secondary peritonitis.

INFECTION CONTROL

Peritonitis is not a communicable disease, so special precautions are not required for protection of either the patient or others. Dressings and caps on peritoneal dialysis catheters should be managed in sterile fashion. Otherwise, standard precautions for patient contact are sufficient.

PEARLS AND PITFALLS

1. Integrate all available information when evaluating abdominal pain, as reliance on only lab studies or radiographs may delay accurate diagnosis and appropriate treatment.
2. A history of shifting pain suggests a surgical cause of the acute abdomen.
3. An unremarkable abdominal exam and normal laboratory studies do not rule out peritonitis in an elderly patient with abdominal pain.

Table 12.12 Antibiotics for Secondary Peritonitis

	Mild or Community-Acquired	Severe
Primary Treatment	piperacillin-tazobactam 4.5 g IV q8h *or* ampicillin-sulbactam 3 g IV q6h *or* ticarcillin-clavulanate 3.1 g IV q6h *or* ertapenem 1 g IV q24h	imipenem-cilastatin 750 mg IV q8h *or* meropenem 1 g IV q8h *or* ampicillin 500 mg IV q6h plus ciprofloxacin 400 mg IV q12h plus anti-anaerobe (clindamycin 600 mg IV q8h or metronidazole 500 mg IV q8h)
Penicillin-Allergic	ciprofloxacin 400 mg IV q12h plus anti-anaerobe (clindamycin 600 mg IV q8h or metronidazole 500 mg IV q8h)	aztreonam 1 g IV q12h plus ciprofloxacin 400 mg IV q12h plus anti-anaerobe (clindamycin 600 mg IV q8h or metronidazole 500 mg IV q8h)
Children	As above, but weight-based dosing and no fluoroquinolones	As above, but weight-based dosing and no fluoroquinolones

4. Do not use barium for radiographic contrast if visceral perforation is suspected. Water-soluble contrast should be substituted to avoid barium peritonitis.
5. Peritonitis is a process that evolves, so serial abdominal examination is essential.
6. Appendicitis can present in any fashion and should always be on the differential diagnosis of abdominal pain.

REFERENCES

Loutit J. Intra-abdominal infections. In: Wilson WR, Sande MA, eds. Current diagnosis & treatment in infectious diseases. New York: McGraw-Hill, 2001:164–76.

Nathens AB, Curtis JR, Beale RJ, et al. Management of the critically ill patient with severe acute pancreatitis. Crit Care Med 2004;32(12):2524–36.

Ng KK, Lee TY, Wan YL, et al. Splenic abscess: diagnosis and management. Hepatogastroenterology 2002;49(44):567–71.

Ordonez CA, Puyana JC. Management of peritonitis in the critically ill patient. Surg Clin North Am 2006;86(6):1323–49.

Schecter WP. Peritoneum and acute abdomen. In: Norton JA, Bollinger RR, Chang AE, et al., eds. Surgery: basic science and clinical evidence. New York: Springer, 2001.

Soybel DI. Acute abdominal pain. In: Souba WW, Fink MP, Jurkokvich GJ, eds. ACS surgery principles & practice. New York: American College of Surgeons, 2006.

13. Viral Hepatitis

Ramin Jamshidi and Francis Yao

Outline Introduction
Epidemiology
Clinical Features
Differential Diagnosis
Laboratory and Radiographic Findings
Treatment and Prophylaxis
Management and Admission Criteria
Infection Control
Pearls and Pitfalls
References
Additional Readings

INTRODUCTION

A number of viruses have been found to primarily infect hepatocytes, though not all cause clinically relevant disease. The classically recognized hepatotropic viruses are the hepatitis A, B, C, D, E, and G viruses. Of clinically apparent acute and chronic hepatitis, 10% to 20% is cryptogenic in nature and is thought to be caused by as yet unidentified viruses.

EPIDEMIOLOGY

Hepatitis viruses A and E are transmitted via the fecal-oral route, whereas B, C, and D are spread primarily via contact with infected blood or other body fluid. Hepatitis G is transferred by either route, but is not proven to cause clinical disease. Fecal-oral transmission of the A and E viruses is responsible for most acute outbreaks, whereas B and C constitute a major chronic public health burden.

Hepatitis A virus (HAV) infection accounts for approximately 25,000 cases of acute hepatitis annually in the United States, with as many as 40% of the urban population having serologic evidence of past infection. Outbreaks often affect clusters of persons exposed to a single source, such as a food handler or contaminated central water supply.

Persons infected with hepatitis B virus (HBV) carry the virus in all bodily fluids (blood, breast milk, saliva, semen, and urine). HBV can cause both acute and chronic hepatitis, the latter conferring risk of cirrhosis and hepatocellular carcinoma. It is estimated that 200 million people worldwide are chronically infected with HBV. In the United States, the prevalence is lower, though 200,000 to 300,000 new infections occur yearly.

Hepatitis C virus (HCV) can also cause both acute and chronic hepatitis. It is estimated that at least 4 million people in the United States have chronic HCV infection. It is currently the leading cause of chronic liver disease and the most common indication for liver transplantation. The highest prevalence of HCV is observed among hemophiliacs, injection drug users, hemodialysis recipients, and Vietnam veterans. Prior to screening of all blood products for HCV, the risk of transmission of HCV by transfusion was 1 in 10 transfusions, but the current estimated risk is 1 in 400,000. The rate of seroconversion from a needle-stick injury from a seropositive source ranges from 1% to 7% in various studies. (See Chapter 56, Blood or Body Fluid Exposure Management and Postexposure Prophylaxis for Hepatitis B and HIV.) Sexual and maternal-fetal transmission rates are lower than for HBV.

Hepatitis D virus (HDV) is transmitted parenterally and is dependent on HBV for survival. It has no replication machinery of its own and utilizes that of HBV. HDV infects the liver either simultaneously with HBV (co-infection) or in a person chronically infected with the B virus (superinfection). Worldwide, prevalence of HDV has been decreasing since the 1980s.

Hepatitis E virus (HEV) was named for its enteric transmission. Primary endemic regions are North Africa, Asia, Central America, and India. Outbreaks tend to occur after rainy seasons, when runoff from rainwater has been contaminated by feces. It is exceedingly rare in the United States but may be observed in recent travelers or immigrants. The mortality rate of acute HEV infection is 1–2%, but approaches 10–30% in pregnant women, with the worst outcomes in the third trimester.

Hepatitis G virus (HGV) is transmissible by enteral or parenteral routes, but it does not cause clinically significant liver disease. It is fairly prevalent, detected in 50% of IV drug users, 30% of patients on hemodialysis, 20% of hemophiliacs, and 15% of patients with chronic HBV or HCV infections.

In immunocompromised persons, cytomegalovirus (CMV), Epstein-Barr virus (EBV), or other herpesviridae may cause hepatitis. Other hepatotropic viruses are being investigated, though little clinical disease is attributable to them. These include dengue virus, TT virus, SEN virus, and GB virus (the latter three were named for the patients from whom they were isolated).

CLINICAL FEATURES
Acute Hepatitis

There are three phases of acute infection: prodrome, jaundice, and convalescence. The *prodrome* follows an incubation period that varies according to the causative hepatitis virus and consists of vague flulike symptoms: malaise, fatigability, myalgias, pharyngitis, anorexia, nausea, and pyrexia (Table 13.1).

Table 13.1 Clinical Features: Acute Hepatitis

Organisms	• Hepatitis A, E viruses • Hepatitis B, C, D viruses (less common) • Drugs and toxins
Incubation Period	Usually 1–4 weeks, may be up to months
Signs and Symptoms	Prodrome: • Vague "flulike" symptoms: fever, malaise, fatigability, myalgias, pharyngitis, anorexia, nausea Icteric phase: • Jaundice • Dark urine • Acholic stools • Pruritis Convalescence: • Clinical improvement • Serologic changes
Laboratory and Radiologic Findings	• Mild neutropenia or lymphocytosis • Elevated AST and ALT (100s – 1000s units/L) • Hyperbilirubinemia (predominantly indirect) • Virus-dependent serology (see below) • No biliary dilation on ultrasound
Treatment	• Supportive – symptom management • Interferon alpha for HCV, maybe for HBV • Careful hygiene to prevent spread

Table 13.2 Clinical Features: Fulminant Hepatic Failure

Organisms	• Hepatitis A, D, B are most common viral etiologies • Drugs and toxins are most common etiology overall
Incubation Period	Usually 1–4 weeks, may be up to months
Signs and Symptoms	• Encephalopathy • Coagulopathy • Loss of glycemic control • Cerebral edema • Sepsis
Laboratory Findings	• Elevated AST and ALT (1000s – 10,000s units/L) • PT >5 s above normal or INR >1.5
Treatment	• ICU admission and supportive care • Hemodynamic support • Monitor coagulopathy • Intracranial pressure monitoring • N-Acetylcysteine for acetaminophen overdose • Consider immediate liver transplantation

INR, international normalized ratio; PT, prothrombin time.

After the 2–4 weeks of prodrome, liver enzyme abnormalities develop and may be associated with hyperbilirubinemia or jaundice. During this *icteric phase*, patients may also present with dark urine, light-colored stools, and pruritis. In immunocompetent individuals, this will last about a month. *Convalescence* involves gradual clinical improvement and serologic changes (discussed below). Uncomplicated courses of acute HAV and HEV infection tend to present and resolve slightly more rapidly than B, C, and D; resolution of symptoms is generally over by 2–3 months for A and E, and 3–4 months for other serotypes.

Fulminant Hepatic Failure

Fulminant hepatic failure is a life-threatening condition, which complicates about 1% of all acute hepatitis. This devastating condition is defined by the presence of hepatic encephalopathy within 8 weeks after the onset of jaundice in a patient with no preexisting liver disease. It is associated with other clinical signs of liver failure including severe coagulopathy and perturbation of glycemic control (Table 13.2). Without liver transplantation, the mortality rate in patients with fulminant liver failure is from 50% to 80%. Death can occur within days of onset of encephalopathy and is most commonly due to intracranial hypertension with cerebral edema or sepsis.

Management of fulminant hepatic failure relies on prompt diagnosis and requires intensive care unit (ICU) admission, consultation with a gastroenterologist, and early referral to a liver transplant center.

Chronic Hepatitis

Of the hepatotropic viruses, only B, C, and D cause chronic infection. The principal long-term sequelae of chronic hepatitis are cirrhosis and hepatocellular carcinoma.

Cirrhosis is a complex entity that can lead to portosystemic hypertension with varix formation, ascites that may be complicated by spontaneous bacterial peritonitis, decreased protein synthesis, and hepatic encephalopathy. Chronic hepatitis predisposes to hepatocellular carcinoma, a primary malignancy of the liver that can progress in an indolent manner. By the time patients experience pain or recognize increasing abdominal girth, the tumors have typically grown quite large.

Clinical Course by Virus

HAV

HAV has an average incubation period of 30 days, is shed in the feces for 1–2 weeks before clinical illness arises, and continues to be infectious during the first week of symptoms. This infection often runs a mild course and the illness is typically subclinical in children, who can spread disease to family members. Complete clinical and laboratory recovery usually occurs by 9 weeks (Figure 13.1). Although HAV does not cause

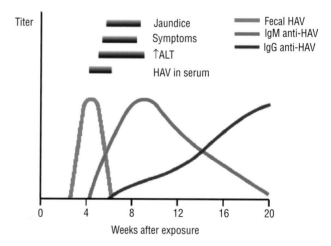

Figure 13.1 Chronology of HAV disease. Reprinted with permission of The McGraw-Hill Companies from *Current Medical Diagnosis & Treatment*, 2007.

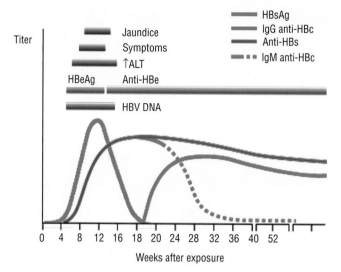

Figure 13.2 Chronology of HBV disease. Reprinted with permission of The McGraw-Hill Companies from *Current Medical Diagnosis & Treatment*, 2007.

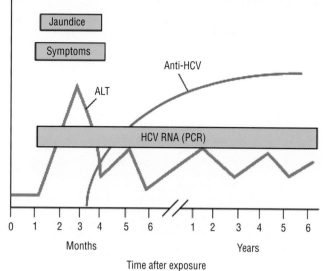

Figure 13.3 Chronology of HCV disease. Reprinted with permission of The McGraw-Hill Companies from *Current Medical Diagnosis & Treatment*, 2007.

chronic liver disease, a rare entity known as relapsing hepatitis A has been described, in which patients experience one or two relapses within the first 6 months after the index illness. Fulminant hepatic failure occurs in 1% of cases. The overall fatality rate for acute hepatitis A is 0.1%, but it is significantly greater in the elderly and patients with preexisting chronic hepatitis B or C.

HBV

HBV has a relatively long incubation period ranging from 6 weeks to 6 months, with an average of 12–14 weeks (Figure 13.2). Manifestation of acute hepatitis B is often insidious, and the majority of cases are minimally symptomatic. In 5–10% of patients with acute hepatitis B, a syndrome resembling serum sickness develops, with arthralgias, rash, angioedema, and rarely, proteinuria and hematuria. Fulminant liver failure occurs in less than 1% of patients. In endemic areas, most cases of HBV infection occur as a result of vertical transmission from infected mother to child at the time of delivery. For the HBV-infected neonate, the risk of developing chronic hepatitis B is greater than 90%, largely because of the lack of immune maturity. In contrast, immunocompetent adults who acquire acute HBV infection develop a chronic infection in only 3–8% of cases.

Among patients with chronic HBV infection, some have persistently normal liver enzymes with undetectable or very low levels of HBV DNA and negative hepatitis B e antigen (HBeAg). These patients are classified "inactive carriers" and have good long-term prognoses. Other patients with chronic hepatitis B have active viral replication based on HBV DNA and are at risk for progressive disease and development of cirrhosis. Patients with chronic HBV infection are at risk for developing hepatocellular carcinoma even in the absence of cirrhosis.

HCV

The typical incubation period for HCV infection is 6–7 weeks, after which a mild illness may follow, but acute hepatitis C is asymptomatic in 85% of cases (Figure 13.3). Fulminant hepatic failure is rarely associated with HCV, but 85% of patients acutely infected with HCV will develop chronic hepatitis, and 25–35% of those with chronic hepatitis C will develop cirrhosis after an average duration of about 20 years. In contrast to HBV, HCV-associated cirrhosis always precedes the development of HCV-associated hepatocellular carcinoma. The annual risk for carcinoma is 1–4% for patients with HCV-cirrhosis. HCV is implicated in many extrahepatic conditions, including cryoglobulinemia, which may manifest as neuropathy, glomerulonephritis, and arthropathy.

HDV

When acute HDV infection is synchronous with acute HBV ("co-infection"), the nature and severity of illness are similar to isolated acute HBV infection. In acute co-infection, spontaneous clearance of HBV and HDV occurs in 80–95% of cases. "Superinfection" occurs when patients with chronic hepatitis B are acutely infected by HDV. Superinfection is more likely to cause fulminant hepatitis (in 2 – 20% of cases, 10 times the rate for isolated HBV infection).

HEV

HEV is similar to HAV, in that infection manifests only as acute hepatitis and typically has a milder course in children. The virus has a long incubation period of 2–10 weeks, after which a transient macular skin rash may be observed. HEV infection generally lasts 1–4 weeks and is self-limited, though associated cholestasis may persist for 2–6 months.

DIFFERENTIAL DIAGNOSIS

The prodrome of acute viral hepatitis is nonspecific and can be difficult to distinguish from other viral syndromes. A clinical history of bodily fluid exposure or food- or water- related infection may support the diagnosis of acute viral hepatitis. Right upper quadrant pain and tenderness are often present in a patient with acute viral hepatitis, prompting consideration of acute cholecystitis and choledocholithiasis.

Nonmicrobial etiologies of acute hepatitis include autoimmune hepatitis, drugs, and toxins (Table 13.3). Acute acetaminophen overdose is the most common cause of acute liver failure in this country. Although greater than 140 mg/kg

Table 13.3 Some Common Hepatotoxic Medications

Injury Pattern	Hepatocellular	Cholestatic	Mixed
Lab Abnormality	ALT elevation	ALP and bilirubin elevation	ALP and ALT elevation
Medications or Classes	Acetaminophen Amiodarone Antiretrovirals Kava kava Ketoconazole SSRIs Statins Isoniazid (INH) Rifampin	Amoxicillin-clavulanate Anabolic steroids Clopidogrel Estrogens Macrolides Phenothiazines TCAs Rifampin	Amitriptyline Carba-mazepine Clindamycin Phenytoin Sulfonamides Trazodone Verapamil

ALP, alkaline phosphatase; ALT, alanine aminotransferase; SSRI, selective serotonin reuptake inhibitor; TCA, tricyclic antidepressant.

Table 13.4 HBV Serologic Tests and Interpretations

HBsAg (surface antigen)	*Currently* infected with HBV, (acute or chronic)

HBcAb (core antibody)
  IgG
  IgM
	
	Past exposure or false positive test
	Very recent *acute* HBV infection

HBsAb (surface antibody)	*Past* infection with resolution and *immunity*, or vaccination
Markers of viral replication (**Do these tests only if HBsAg+**)	
HBeAg (+)	
HBV-DNA (+)	

Table 13.5 Hepatitis B Viral Serology

	sAg	sAb	cAb	eAg	eAb
Vaccinated	−	+	−	−	−
Acutely Infected	+	+/−	IgM	+	−
Chronically Infected with Active Replication	+	−	IgG	+	−
Chronically Infected with Low Replication	+	−	IgG	−	+
Recovery from Infection	−	+	IgG	−	+/−
False Positive Versus Remote Prior Infection	−	−	IgG	−	−

(approximately 10 g in adults) is usually required to cause acute liver failure, patients with chronic liver disease may tip into failure with doses of only 3 g per day over days or weeks.

LABORATORY AND RADIOGRAPHIC FINDINGS

The basic liver panel includes alanine aminotransferase (ALT), aspartate aminotransferase (AST), total bilirubin, and alkaline phosphatase (ALP). The ALT or AST level in acute viral hepatitis generally ranges from several hundred to a few thousand units/liter. In drug-induced hepatitis, the peak ALT or AST levels may be even higher, sometimes exceeding 10,000. In acute alcoholic hepatitis, the ALT or AST level rarely exceeds 500, and the AST/ALT ratio is typically >2. Prothrombin time (PT) with international normalized ratio (INR) is the most important laboratory indicator for hepatic dysfunction, whereas the peak level of AST or ALT is of no proven prognostic significance.

The complete blood count (CBC) in viral hepatitis usually reveals a mild degree of neutropenia initially, followed by a mild lymphocytosis. Acute infections may cause reactive thrombocytosis, but many patients with cirrhosis have a low platelet count of less than 120×10^3/mL.

Once the diagnosis of acute viral hepatitis is suspected, specific serologic assays should be obtained to determine the etiology. The HAV IgM antibody becomes detectable about 4 weeks after acute HAV exposure. IgM titer peaks during the first week of clinical illness and disappears by 3–6 months, though it may be present for up to a year. HAV IgG becomes detectable about 2 weeks after the IgM and confers long-term immunity. Thus, a positive IgM antibody is a marker of acute infection, whereas positive IgG reflects prior exposure and ongoing immunity.

HBV has more intricate structural characteristics, which allows for multiple serologic assays to determine the nature of infection (Tables 13.4 and 13.5). Presence of surface antigen (HBsAg) indicates active infection (acute or chronic), whereas antibody against the surface antigen (HBsAb) indicates immunity due to either past infection or vaccination. HBV core antibody IgM can be detected in acute infection, whereas a positive HBV core IgG test reflects previous exposure. HBeAg and HBV DNA are markers of viral replication. They are useful in the evaluation of patients with chronic hepatitis B.

Pre-core mutants are common in the Mediterranean and Far East, unable to make HBeAg but detectable HBV DNA.

The presence of HCV antibody usually reflects active infection in association with circulating HCV RNA in the blood and does not confer immunity. Spontaneous clearance of HCV infection occurs in only 15–20% of patients following acute infection; the remaining patients develop chronic HCV infection. Spontaneous clearance of HCV infection, however, confers no protection against reinfection. Serologic conversion or appearance of HCV antibody may take 20–150 days (mean 50 days) after acute exposure. Consequently, a negative HCV antibody test during acute hepatitis does not exclude HCV infection. If acute hepatitis C is suspected, reverse transcriptase polymerase chain reaction (RT-PCR) assay should be used to determine the presence of HCV RNA, which becomes detectable 7–21 days after acute exposure.

Hepatitis D virus IgM antibody indicates acute infection and IgG reflects prior exposure and chronic immunity. HDV antigen (HDV Ag) testing is available in the research setting, but no commercial assays exist.

In the immunocompromised patient presenting with acute hepatitis, serologic testing for cytomegalovirus (serum antigen) and Epstein-Barr virus (monospot test) should also be included.

Ultrasound or computed tomography of the abdomen may be helpful in excluding biliary obstruction or gallbladder abnormalities, but their role in evaluating acute hepatitis is generally limited. It is important to remember that gallbladder wall thickening and pericholecystic fluid are nonspecific findings in some cirrhotic patients. Liver biopsy is not routinely performed in acute viral hepatitis, because the diagnosis can usually be determined by serologic testing and the results of the liver biopsy rarely change management.

TREATMENT AND PROPHYLAXIS

The mainstay of treatment of acute viral hepatitis has traditionally been supportive care for the symptomatic patient. However, it has recently been shown that interferon-alpha treatment of acute HCV infection can prevent the development of chronic hepatitis in some patients. In adults with acute HBV infection, the risk for developing chronic hepatitis B is only about 5%. Whether antiviral therapy using interferon-alpha or nucleic acid analogues is beneficial in acute HBV infection remains to be demonstrated. Primary prophylaxis is the key to prevention, and safe and effective vaccines are now available to prevent viral hepatitis A and B.

Inactivated HAV particles have been manufactured into two commercially available vaccines. A single dose provides 85% immunity for an average of 10 years, but a booster dose at 6–12 months increases efficacy to 94%. In recent years this vaccine has been recommended by the Centers for Disease Control and Prevention for children over 12 months. However, most older children and adults remain unvaccinated, so travelers to developing nations are advised to receive it before their trip. Household contacts of patients with hepatitis A should be treated with a dose of immune globulin to confer passive humoral immunity. This will prevent or attenuate disease in 85% of patients if received either preexposure, or postexposure during the 2- to 6-week incubation phase. However, immune globulin does not incite antibody production, and protection lasts only a few months.

HBV vaccine consists of recombinant surface antigen and confers humoral immunity for subsequent exposure to intact virus. The HBV vaccine series consists of three doses over a period of 6 months (at 0, 1, and 6 months) and produces lasting immunity in >90% of patients. Immunity lasts 10 years, at which point a booster dose is recommended. Hepatitis B immune globulin (HBIg) can attenuate disease severity and, in some cases, offers complete protection against infection as long as it is given within 7 days of exposure.

HDV immunity can be provided by immunization to HBV because HDV is completely dependent on the presence HBV for viral replication. No immunizations are currently available for hepatitis C, E, or G viruses.

A recombinant vaccine for HEV has been developed and results of phase II clinical testing were reported in 2007. While the agent appeared to be safe and effective in the prevention of clinically overt HEV infection, questions remain about lasting immunity and induction of chronic carrier states.

With acetaminophen toxicity of less than 24 hours, N-acetylcysteine should be given to reduce severity of hepatic injury. The standard regimen is an initial oral dose of 140 mg/kg followed by 17 oral doses of 70 mg/kg every 4 hours. There is evidence that shorter regimens of fewer doses are effective, and these protocols are in use in Canada and Europe. There is also an intravenous formulation of N-acetylcysteine available.

MANAGEMENT AND ADMISSION CRITERIA

Patients with acute hepatitis but without coagulopathy, severe electrolyte derangement, or signs of dehydration can be managed in the outpatient setting with close follow-up. Severe vomiting, diarrhea, or anorexia are indications for inpatient hydration and nutritional support. Elderly patients, those with comorbid medical conditions, and immunocompromised individuals should also be considered for hospitalization because of their diminished functional reserve and greater mortality risk. The presence of coagulopathy (PT 5 s above normal or INR > 1.5) is an indication for admission to monitor for signs of fulminant liver failure (progression of coagulopathy or onset of hepatic encephalopathy) necessitating ICU care to and referral to a liver transplant center.

All clusters or community outbreaks of viral hepatitis are reportable to the department of public health.

INFECTION CONTROL

Patients with suspected hepatitis should be treated with strict universal precautions. Those with acute hepatitis should be under contact precautions and be instructed to thoroughly wash their hands, especially following bowel movements.

PEARLS AND PITFALLS

1. Acute hepatitis can result from hepatotropic viruses A through E, but only B, C, and D cause chronic liver disease.
2. The most serious consequence of acute hepatitis is fulminant hepatic failure, defined as development of hepatic encephalopathy within 8 weeks from the onset of jaundice in a patient with no preexisting liver disease.
3. Hepatic encephalopathy or coagulopathy in a patient with acute viral hepatitis is an ominous sign and should prompt inpatient admission.
4. Fulminant liver failure necessitates admission to the intensive care unit and immediate referral to a liver transplant center. Clinical condition may deteriorate precipitously and death can occur within days of presentation.
5. In any patient with acute nonviral hepatitis, have a high level of suspicion for ingestion of hepatotoxic drugs. Serum acetaminophen level should be checked in any patient with unexplained elevated liver enzymes.
6. Acetaminophen overdose is the most common cause of acute liver failure in the United States. It is treated with N-acetylcysteine.
7. Acute viral hepatitis can cause cholestasis and abdominal pain. Ultrasound can help rule out the more common primary biliary cause of these symptoms.

REFERENCES

Dienstag JL, McHutchison JG. American gastroenterological association technical review on the management of hepatitis C. Gastroenterology 2006;130(1):231–64.

Fox RK, Wright TL. Viral hepatitis. In: Friedman S, ed. Current diagnosis & treatment in gastroenterology, 2nd ed. New York: McGraw-Hill, 2003.

Ganem D, Prince A. Hepatitis B virus infection – natural history and clinical consequences. N Engl J Med 2004;350(11):1118–29.

Menon KVN. Non-a to e hepatitis. Curr Opin Infect Dis 2002;15:529–34.

Navarro VJ, Senior JR. Drug-related hepatotoxicity. N Engl J Med 2006;354(7):731–9.

Pawlotsky JM. Molecular diagnosis of viral hepatitis. Gastroenterology 2002;122(6):1554–68.

Roberts SE, Goldacre MJ, Yeates D. Trends in mortality after hospital admission for liver cirrhosis in an English population. Gut 2005;54(11):1615–21.

Sookian S. Liver disease during pregnancy: acute viral hepatitis. Ann Hepatol 2006;5(3):231–6.

ADDITIONAL READINGS

Davern TJ. Fulminant hepatic failure. In: TM Bayless, AM Diehl eds. Advanced therapy in gastroenterology and liver disease, 5th ed. Ontario: BC Decker, 2006:629–37.

Pratt DS, Kaplan MM. Evaluation of abnormal liver-enzyme results in asymptomatic patients. N Engl J Med 2000;342(17): 1266–71.

14. Infectious Biliary Diseases: Cholecystitis and Cholangitis

Lan Vu and Hobart Harris

ACUTE CALCULOUS CHOLECYSTITIS

Epidemiology

The prevalence of gallstones in the general population is approximately 10–15%, and is higher in people with the following risk factors: female gender, multiparity, obesity, recent pregnancy, and hemolytic diseases (e.g., sickle cell disease). Of people with gallstones, 10–20% will develop complications such as biliary colic, cholecystitis, cholangitis, or gallstone pancreatitis.

Acute calculous cholecystitis is defined by sustained obstruction of the cystic duct or neck of the gallbladder with gallstones or sludge. In contrast, biliary colic is pain secondary to transient obstruction of the gallbladder. Acute cholecystitis is primarily a localized acute inflammatory process caused by gallbladder obstruction and subsequent distension, but is clinically managed as an infection. The pathophysiologic role of bacteria cultured from bile remains unknown.

Clinical Features

Although most patients with acute cholecystitis present with right upper quadrant tenderness, few actually present with the classic triad of fever, right upper quadrant pain, and leukocytosis. The pain of acute cholecystitis may radiate to the back and the right shoulder due to secondary irritation of the diaphragm. Acute cholecystitis can be distinguished from biliary colic by constant pain in the right upper quadrant and the presence of Murphy's sign, defined as inspiration limited by pain on palpation of the right upper quadrant. The presence of fever and leukocytosis in the setting of right upper quadrant pain is specific, but not sensitive for acute cholecystitis. Recent studies indicate that the presence of Murphy's sign has high sensitivity (97.2%) and positive predictive value (70%). Other less sensitive physical findings include a palpable gallbladder, jaundice, rebound tenderness, and guarding. Abnormal laboratory findings, which include elevated liver enzymes, hyperbilirubinemia, and elevated alkaline phosphatase levels, are nonspecific for acute cholecystitis, but can direct the work-up

for other disease processes. In particular, hyperbilirubinemia and elevated alkaline phosphatase levels may suggest choledocholithiasis or Mirizzi's syndrome, in which the common hepatic duct is obstructed by a stone impacted in the cystic duct or Hartmann's pouch (Table 14.1).

Differential Diagnosis

The differential diagnosis of upper abdominal pain includes gastrointestinal, cardiac, and pulmonary diseases.

Key features that may help to distinguish acute cholecystitis from biliary colic are:

- constant right upper quadrant pain, lasting >4–6 hours
- positive Murphy's sign (sonographic finding is more reliable than physical exam)
- leukocytosis and fever

Other conditions to consider are:

Gastrointestinal:

- hepatitis
- acute cholangitis
- biliary colic
- perforated ulcer disease
- dyspepsia
- appendicitis
- diverticulitis
- acute pancreatitis
- Fitz-Hugh–Curtis syndrome (perihepatitis caused by gonococcal infection)
- subhepatic or intra-abdominal abscess
- black widow spider envenomation

Urological:

- pyelonephritis
- nephrolithiasis
- renal infarct

Table 14.1 Clinical Features: Acute Cholecystitis

Signs and Symptoms	• Triad of fever, RUQ pain, leukocytosis (present in only 24% of cases) • Nausea/vomiting and postprandial RUQ pain (often following fatty meal) • Predisposition: female gender, multiparity, obesity, recent pregnancy, sickle cell disease • Majority of patients have gallbladder-associated symptoms prior to the development of acute cholecystitis • Diaphragmatic irritation may lead to right shoulder pain • Murphy's sign (inspiratory arrest during deep palpation over the gallbladder) highly sensitive (97.2%) but less specific (48.3%) • Palpable gallbladder is less frequent physical finding; represents body's effort to wall off the inflamed gallbladder • Rebound tenderness and guarding are less commonly found and indicate peritonitis
Laboratory and Radiographic Findings	• Elevated WBC, variable elevation of alkaline phosphatase, bilirubin, and transaminases • Hyperbilirubinemia and elevated alkaline phosphatase may suggest common bile duct stones or Mirizzi's syndrome • US: gallstones, edema or pericholecystic fluid, sonographic Murphy's sign; sensitivity >92–95% • Biliary scintigraphy: more expensive, but slightly more sensitive; sensitivity >97% • CT scan has minimal role except to exclude other diagnoses • Biliary scintigraphy is less specific in acalculous cholecystitis, and ultrasonography plays a larger role in diagnosis as does percutaneous cholecystostomy

CT, computed tomography; RUQ, right upper quadrant; US, ultrasound; WBC, white blood (cell) count.

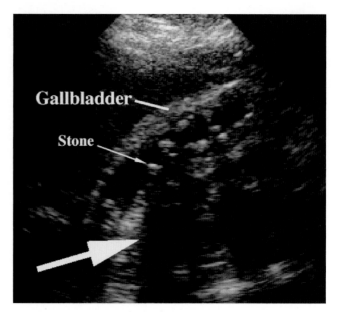

Figure 14.1 Sonographic findings of acute cholecystitis.

of 92%. Biliary scintigraphy, otherwise known as hydroxy-iminodiacetic acid (HIDA) scan, is a nuclear medicine study used to detect cystic duct obstruction associated with acute cholecystitis; sensitivity of this study is increased with the use of morphine, as it increases sphincter of Oddi pressure, causing a more favorable pressure gradient for the radioactive tracer to enter the cystic duct). When the diagnosis of acute cholecystitis is in question after sonographic evaluation, especially in the obtunded patient who cannot report pain on palpation, HIDA scan should be obtained.

Computed tomography (CT) scan can detect approximately 30% of gallstones. Common findings include gallbladder distension, gallbladder wall thickening, and pericholecystic inflammation and fluid; the last is the most specific finding.

Cardiac:

• acute coronary syndrome
• myocarditis
• pericarditis

Pulmonary:

• right lower lobe pneumonia
• pulmonary emboli
• empyema (other inflammatory pleural effusions)
• pulmonary infarction

Laboratory and Radiographic Findings

Sonography is the preferred initial test to evaluate gallstones and gallbladder pathology due to its high sensitivity for diagnosing acute calculous cholecystitis and accessibility in the acute care setting. Sonographic findings may include the presence of gallstones impacted in the gallbladder neck or cystic duct, positive sonographic Murphy's sign (pain when the gallbladder is palpated by the ultrasound probe), gallbladder distension, gallbladder wall thickening, and pericholecystic fluid (Figure 14.1). The presence of both gallstones and a sonographic Murphy's sign has a positive predictive value

Treatment

Once the diagnosis of acute calculous cholecystitis has been made, the patient should be admitted and evaluated for surgical intervention. A resuscitation phase involves fasting, intravenous hydration, and administration of analgesics and broad-spectrum antibiotics (Table 14.2). Acute calculous cholecystitis is mostly an acute inflammatory process that may lead to local or systemic infection. *Escherichia coli* and *Klebsiella* species are the most common organisms recovered from an acutely inflamed gallbladder; less common species include *Enterobacter* and *Proteus*. Standard current treatment is a third- or fourth-generation cephalosporin, or a ureidopenicillin with a beta lactamase inhibitor such as piperacillin-tazobactam. In addition, fluoroquinolones have been shown to have efficacy equivalent to that of third-generation cephalosporins in the treatment of both bacterial cholecystitis and cholangitis. Initial antibiotic therapy should be based on local or institutional bacterial resistance patterns of common gastrointestinal flora. There has historically been controversy on the use of opioids for acute calculous cholecystitis because they are thought to induce spasm of the sphincter of Oddi and potentially worsen obstruction; there is no clinical evidence, however, to support this phenomenon, and administration of opioid analgesia is standard.

Table 14.2 Therapeutic Recommendations for Acute Cholecystitis

1. Resuscitation	
Intravenous fluids Fasting Analgesics	
Antibiotic Therapy	
Often inflammatory and noninfectious, but treated as an infection Bile cultures frequently polymicrobial: *Escherichia coli* *Klebsiella* species *Enterobacter* species *Enterococcus*	**Recommended:** **Penicillins*:** ampicillin-sulbactam 3.0 g IV q6h piperacillin-tazobactam 3.375 g IV q6h or 4.5 g IV q8h ticarcillin-clavulanate 3.1 g IV q6h **Cephalosporins*:** third-generation: cefotaxime 2 g q6h or ceftriaxone 1 g IV qd fourth-generation: cefepime 1–2 g IV q12h **Alternative therapy:** **Fluoroquinolones:** ciprofloxacin 400 mg q12h or levofloxacin 500 mg IV qd
2. Intervention	
Cholecystectomy	Definitive therapy Laparoscopic cholecystectomy recommended within 72 hours of presentation Common bile duct exploration may be indicated in patients with persistent hyperbilirubinemia and elevated alkaline phosphatase
Percutaneous cholecystostomy	Recommended for high surgical risk patients Followed by elective cholecystectomy when patient is clinically stable
ERCP	Indicated for patients with persistent hyperbilirubinemia May be done prior to or after cholecystectomy, if common bile duct exploration is not done at the time of surgery

*Doses are based on patients with creatinine clearance greater than 60 mL/min and need to be adjusted for patients with renal impairment.
Escherichia coli and *Klebsiella* species are the most common Enterobacteriaceae; less common species include *Enterobacter* and *Proteus*. Pathogenicity is unclear for organisms cultured in bile from inflamed gallbladder unless they are also recovered in blood.
Anaerobes are less likely pathogens of cholecystitis unless a biliary-enteric anastomosis or fistula is present; in these cases, the most common are *Clostridium* species and *Bacteroides* species.

Definitive therapy for acute calculous cholecystitis is cholecystectomy. Acute cholecystitis was initially considered a relative contraindication for laparoscopic cholecystectomy because of the theoretical risk of higher rates of postoperative complications and conversion to laparotomy. Prospective trials have since shown that there is no difference in outcomes for patients randomized to early laparoscopic cholecystectomy (defined as within 72–96 hours of presentation) compared to those who underwent interval cholecystectomy (6–12 weeks after acute attack). In the early phase of acute inflammation, edematous adhesions are easily separated, whereas later fibrosis can make laparoscopic dissection more difficult. Early intervention also leads to fewer workdays lost and shorter overall hospital stays. The cumulative morbidity of laparoscopic cholecystectomy in the literature is approximately 7%, which is similar to open cholecystectomy, and includes biliary complications such as retained common bile duct stones, a bile leak or fistula, bile duct injury, split and lost gallstones potentially causing intraabdominal abscesses, cholangitis, and pancreatitis; and nonbiliary complications, such as wound infections, bleeding, cardiopulmonary complications, deep vein thrombosis, pulmonary embolism, and bowel perforation due to trocar placement.

Persistent hyperbilirubinemia and elevated alkaline phosphatase levels during resuscitation may indicate choledocholithiasis. Treatment options include intraoperative cholangiogram and common bile duct exploration, and preoperative or postoperative endoscopic retrograde cholangiopancreatography (ERCP) with stone retrieval and/or sphincterotomy.

Critically ill patients or those at high risk for surgical complications can be managed successfully with percutaneous cholecystostomy drainage (placement of a catheter into gallbladder). Clinical improvement occurs within 24 hours in 81–95% of patients. Ultrasound-guided cholecystostomy can now be done percutaneously by interventional radiologists. Laparoscopic cholecystectomy after cholecystostomy can be safely performed early, within 96 hours after resolution of toxemia, or 8 weeks later on an elective basis. For a minority of patients who remain a high surgical risk because of cardiac, pulmonary, or other system failure, percutaneous cholecystostomy along with percutaneous calculus extraction can be performed, with subsequent removal of the biliary drainage catheter after 6 weeks.

Complications and Admission Criteria

Approximately 15–20% of patients with acute calculous cholecystitis deteriorate clinically despite antibiotics and resuscitation, and require emergent cholecystectomy. The risks of conversion to open laparotomy, operative complications, and mortality are higher in this subset of patients. Complications include gangrenous cholecystitis, gallbladder perforation and peritonitis, gallbladder abscess, gallstone ileus, and emphysematous cholecystitis. Gangrenous cholecystitis is the most common complication of cholecystitis, particularly in older patients, diabetics, or those who delay care. The presence of sepsis is suggestive of gangrene, but gangrene may not be suspected preoperatively. Perforation of the gallbladder usually occurs secondary to gangrene and may cause a pericholecystic abscess. Less commonly, perforation occurs directly into the peritoneum, leading to generalized peritonitis. A cholecystoenteric fistula may result from erosion of the gallbladder directly into the duodenum, jejunum, or transverse colon. Fistula formation is more often due to longstanding pressure necrosis from stones than to acute cholecystitis. Passage of a gallstone through a cholecystoenteric fistula may lead to the development of mechanical bowel obstruction, usually in the terminal ileum (gallstone ileus). Emphysematous cholecystitis is caused by secondary infection of the gallbladder wall with gas-forming organisms (such as *Clostridium perfringens*).

Factors associated with the development of gangrenous cholecystitis include:

- male gender
- advanced age
- coexisting cardiovascular disease
- diabetes mellitus
- persistent leukocytosis of >15,000/mm^3 for 24–48 hours

Emergent cholecystectomy is required for all of these complications except gallstone ileus, in which the primary surgical goal is to alleviate the obstruction; cholecystoenteric fistulas will usually close spontaneously and subsequent elective cholecystectomy can be done.

Special Considerations

ACUTE CHOLECYSTITIS IN PREGNANCY

Although uncommon in pregnancy, gallstone disease is an important consideration in pregnant women who present with abdominal pain because of the high potential for maternal and fetal morbidity. Pregnant patients with cholecystitis may present with atypical abdominal pain depending on the gestational age of the fetus. Right upper quadrant ultrasound is the ideal diagnostic imaging study to evaluate the gallbladder. Rarely, CT scan may be indicated to evaluate other possible causes of abdominal pain, such as appendicitis, though teratogenicity is a concern and the risks and benefits for the mother and fetus must be considered carefully (see Chapter 53, Fever in Pregnancy, for a full discussion of fetal exposure to diagnostic imaging).

Obstetric and surgical consultants should be contacted early when acute cholecystitis is suspected for specific guidance on further management, such as fetal monitoring, the use of tocolytics and nonteratogenic antibiotics, and discussion of possible surgical intervention. Recent reviews show that laparoscopic cholecystectomy can be performed safely in pregnant women who have refractory biliary symptoms after nonoperative management.

ACUTE ACALCULOUS CHOLECYSTITIS

Acute acalculous cholecystitis accounts for 10–15% of cases of acute cholecystitis and occurs in severely ill patients, such as those with severe trauma or burns, major surgery, long-term fasting, total parenteral nutrition, sepsis, diabetes mellitus, atherosclerotic disease, systemic vasculitis, acute renal failure, and acquired immunodeficiency syndrome (AIDS). Acute acalculous cholecystitis is usually a disease of hospitalized patients. The pathophysiology includes gallbladder ischemia, bile stasis or sludge, and local or systemic infection. Presenting symptoms are often vague and nonspecific, and diagnosis is especially difficult in noncommunicative patients. Diagnostic imaging is similar to that previously described, but has a lower sensitivity for acute acalculous cholecystitis than for acute calculous cholecystitis. Delayed diagnosis and comorbidities contribute to the higher mortality rate of acute acalculous cholecystitis, reported between 10% and 50%, compared to <0.5% in patients with acute calculous cholecystitis.

ACUTE BACTERIAL CHOLANGITIS

Epidemiology

Acute cholangitis is a bacterial infection of the biliary tract superimposed on biliary obstruction. The incidence and mortality is higher in the elderly population because of comorbidities and delayed diagnosis. However, early intervention has lowered mortality to 0.4–7.0% overall, and current management usually involves a multidisciplinary team of internists, interventional radiologists, gastroenterologists, and surgeons.

The most common cause of cholangitis in the United States is choledocholithiasis secondary to cholelithiasis. Approximately 6–9% of patients with symptomatic gallstone disease in the United States will develop acute cholangitis. In contrast, primary bile duct stones are endemic in Hong Kong and Southeast Asia and the incidence of cholangitis is much higher. Other less common causes of cholangitis include primary malignancies of the bile duct, pancreas, and gallbladder, metastatic disease, benign strictures from bile duct reconstruction and biliary interventions, and sclerosing cholangitis. Common bile duct stones usually lead to incomplete biliary obstruction and subsequent ascending infection, whereas malignant obstruction is often complete and infection occurs as a result of translocation of bacteria via the portal system or due to biliary intervention with incomplete drainage. Bile stasis and increased intraluminal pressure in an obstructed biliary system allows for bacterial multiplication and translocation. Translocation occurs at the level of the bile canaliculi; and venous sinusoids, where bile and portal blood are in close proximity.

Clinical Features

Acute cholangitis can be a diagnostic challenge (Table 14.3), and the clinical presentation can range from isolated fever, especially in the elderly, to florid sepsis. The complete Charcot's triad, defined as fever, right upper quadrant pain, and jaundice, rarely occurs in patients with cholangitis. Reynolds' pentad, which includes the additional symptoms of hypotension and altered mental status, occurs in only 10–30% of patients. Laboratory findings that distinguish cholangitis from acute calculous cholecystitis are hyperbilirubinemia and elevated alkaline phosphatase. Risk factors predicting overall poor prognosis include acute renal failure, age older than 50 years, female gender, cirrhosis, cholangitis associated with liver abscess, high malignant biliary stricture, and a history of transhepatic cholangiography.

Table 14.3 Clinical Features: Acute Bacterial Cholangitis

Signs and Symptoms	• Diagnostic challenge: spectrum of presentation ranges from fever to sepsis • Charcot's triad: fever, RUQ pain, and jaundice (rarely present simultaneously) • Reynolds' pentad: Charcot's triad plus hypotension and altered mental status present in 10–30% of patients • 6–9% of patients had previous history of symptomatic gallbladder disease
Laboratory and Radiographic Findings	• Elevated WBC, alkaline phosphatase, and direct bilirubin; variable elevation in LFT (may indicate the development of hepatic abscesses) • Ultrasonography as first radiographic study; very sensitive for gallstones, but poor imaging of distal common bile duct • Normal US does not rule out cholangitis • MRCP excellent imaging of biliary anatomy • ERCP is both diagnostic and therapeutic

LFT, liver function test; MRCP, magnetic resonance cholangiopancreatography; RUQ, right upper quadrant; US, ultrasound; WBC, white blood (cell) count.

Laboratory and Radiographic Findings

The diagnosis of acute cholangitis is usually made based on clinical presentation, but imaging studies can evaluate the cause of the obstruction, the degree of biliary dilation, and the presence of other complications, including hepatic abscess. Ultrasonography and CT scan of the abdomen and pelvis are the most common initial studies obtained in the acute setting. Ultrasound has a high sensitivity for gallstones and can detect biliary dilation, but cannot evaluate the distal common bile duct very well. Importantly, a normal ultrasound of the right upper quadrant does not rule out acute cholangitis. CT scan has been reported to be superior to ultrasound in detecting choledocholithiasis, especially calcified stones, and at specifying the level of obstruction. CT scan also has the advantage of imaging the entire abdomen and evaluating for mass lesions that may be the cause of the obstruction. Magnetic resonance cholangiopancreatography (MRCP), an alternative to the more invasive ERCP, is accurate in defining the biliary anatomy in cases of malignancies or sclerosing cholangitis, but is generally not helpful in the setting of acute cholangitis. ERCP is potentially both diagnostic and therapeutic, but because of the risk of complications, it should be reserved for patients in whom intervention is likely.

Treatment

Patients diagnosed with acute cholangitis require resuscitation with intravenous fluids, antibiotics, and subsequent biliary decompression (Table 14.4). Patients can deteriorate quickly in the setting of acute cholangitis and must be monitored closely for the first 24–48 hours. Of patients with cholangitis, 50% will present with septicemia and 20–30% will have positive blood cultures. Blood cultures should be sent in all patients. Initial antibiotic therapy should be broad, though may be tailored to suspected etiology. Bile specimens from patients with presumed choledocholithiasis will usually grow gram-negative rods, such as *Escherichia coli*, *Klebsiella*, *Proteus*, and *Pseudomonas*, whereas cultures from patients who have undergone previous biliary interventions or reconstruction may grow nosocomial organisms, such as *Pseudomonas*, *Enterobacter*, *Bacteroides*, *Enterococcus*, and yeast (i.e., *Candida*), which are more resistant to the conventional antibiotic therapy. Antibiotic recommendations are similar to those for acute cholecystitis and should be based on the cause of obstruction and the patient's prior history of biliary instrumentation. Monotherapy with a fluoroquinolone or third-generation cephalosporin is usually sufficient in uncomplicated cases. However, when there is concern for anaerobic infections (history of biliary reconstruction and instrumentation) and/or penicillin resistance, the addition of metronidazole or the use of piperacillin-tazobactam may be required for adequate coverage.

Biliary decompression is the key to the treatment of acute cholangitis and can occur spontaneously or require mechanical decompression. Approximately 10–15% of patients, despite supportive measures, will not respond to medical therapy alone and will require urgent biliary decompression within 12 to 24 hours of presentation. Nonoperative biliary drainage modalities have greatly reduced mortality as compared to surgical decompression of the biliary tract. Endoscopic decompression consists of cholangiography for diagnosis and stone extraction with optional sphincterotomy or stent placement

Table 14.4 Therapeutic Recommendations for Acute Bacterial Cholangitis

1. Resuscitation	
Intravenous fluids Fasting	
Antibiotic Therapy	Similar to therapy for acute cholecystitis

Frequently polymicrobial
Stone disease:
  Escherichia coli,
  Klebsiella,
  Proteus, and
  Pseudomonas
Previous biliary
  interventions:
Concern for more resistant
  bacteria:
  Pseudomonas,
  Enterobacter,
  Bacteroides,
  Enterococcus, and
  fungus (i.e., *Candida*).
	Recommended:
	Penicillins*:
	ampicillin-sulbactam 3.0 g IV q6h
	piperacillin-tazobactam 3.375 g IV q6h
	  or 4.5 g IV q8h
	ticarcillin-clavulanate 3.1 g IV q6h
	Cephalosporins*:
	third-generation: cefotaxime 2 g q6h
	  or ceftriaxone 1 g IV qd
	fourth-generation: cefepime 2 g IV q12h
	Alternative therapy:
	Fluoroquinolones:
	ciprofloxacin 400 mg q12h or levofloxacin
	  500 mg IV qd
	Addition of metronidazole (500 mg IV/PO
	  tid) with concern for anaerobes.

2. Intervention	
Biliary Decompression	
Endoscopic drainage	Includes ERCP with stone extraction and sphincterotomy or stent placement
Transhepatic drainage	Indicated for patients whose biliary system is not endoscopically accessible
Surgical drainage	Indicated for patients who fail other modalities Higher mortality rates

Interval Cholecystectomy	Recommended for patients with gallstones
	  because of the 20–25% incidence of
	  recurrent biliary symptoms
	Done electively when cholangitis has
	  resolved

*Doses are based on patients with creatinine clearance greater than 60 mL/min and need to be adjusted for patients with renal impairment.

(Figure 14.2). The emphasis should be on decompression and not definitive treatment for critically ill patients. Surgical decompression becomes necessary when nonoperative drainage has failed. However, prognosis can be poor, especially in patients with comorbid conditions. Interval cholecystectomy is recommended after resolution of cholangitis because of the high incidence of recurrent biliary symptoms, approximately 20–25% within 2 years.

Special Considerations

PARASITIC CHOLANGITIS

Helminthic biliary infections are most prevalent in tropical countries where parasites are endemic are the second most common cause of cholangitis worldwide. However, with increasing migration and tourism, the incidence in developed countries has increased. Biliary parasites cause damage to the bile ducts by a number of mechanisms:

- irritating composition of the parasite, parasitic secretions, or eggs
- physical obstruction of the bile ducts
- induction of biliary stone formation

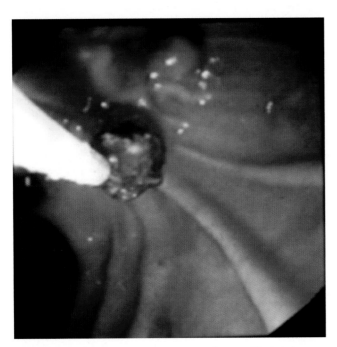

Figure 14.2 Endoscopic drainage and extraction of common bile duct stone.

- introduction of bacteria into the biliary system during migration from the duodenum
- Supervening bacterial infection on any of the above.

Common biliary parasites include the nematode *Ascaris lumbricoides* and the hermaphroditic trematodes *Clonorchis sinensis*, *Opisthorchis viverrini* and *felineus*, *Dicrocoelium dendriticum*, and *Fasciola hepatica* and *gigantica*. Infection is transmitted by ingestion of human feces, raw fish, and freshwater plants. Cholangitis is a complication of biliary fluke infections. Patients with biliary ascariasis will also present with intestinal ascariasis, including symptoms of vomiting, intestinal colic, and/or palpable mass of intestinal worms. *Clonorchis* can cause a chronic infection and may be associated with recurrent pyogenic cholangitis secondary to intrahepatic biliary stone formation. The chronic irritation and inflammation in the bile ducts carries an associated risk of biliary tract malig-

Table 14.5 Medical Therapy of Parasitic Biliary Diseases*

Parasite	Drug	Adult and Pediatric Dose
Ascaris	pyrantel pamoate *or* mebendazole *or* piperazine citrate	Single dose of 1 mg/kg (max 1 g) 100 mg PO bid for 3 days 75 mg/kg (max 3–5 g/day) PO for 2 days
Clonorchis sinensis	praziquantel *or* abendazole	25 mg/kg PO tid for 2 days ≥ 60 kg: 400 mg PO q12h for 1 day < 60 kg: 15 mg/kg PO q12h for 1 day
Fasciola hepatica	triclabendazole *or* bithionol	Single dose 10 mg/kg PO, may be repeated after 2 weeks or 6 months (severe cases: 20 mg/kg PO divided into two doses, 12 hours apart) 30–50 mg/kg on alternate days, 10–15 days

*References include World Health Organization and Center for Disease Control and Prevention.

nancies. *Fasciola* is distinguished from the other biliary parasites by its ability to migrate through the duodenal wall into the peritoneal cavity and penetrate the liver. Biliary obstruction in parasitic infection results from the presence of adult flukes and stone formation. The clinical presentation is similar to that of bacterial infection. Diagnosis of parasitic cholangitis is based primarily on identification of eggs in feces and endoscopic evaluation.

Key features that may help distinguish parasitic from bacterial cholangitis are:

- travel to endemic area within the past year
- associated gastrointestinal symptoms
- eosinophilia
- demonstration of eggs in feces or duodenal contents

TREATMENT OF PARASITIC CHOLANGITIS

Treatment modalities include anthelmintic therapy, endoscopy, and surgery (Table 14.5). As with other causes

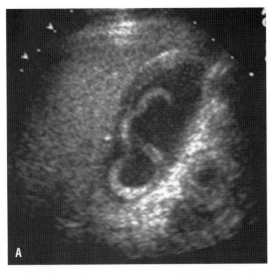
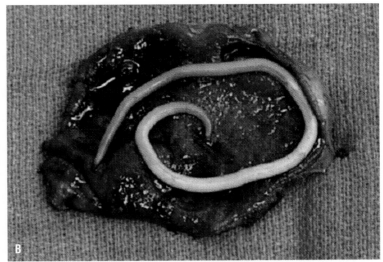

Figure 14.3 Presence of *Ascaris* in the gallbladder (A) by ultrasound and (B) at the time of surgery.

of cholangitis, operative drainage has a higher mortality rate than endoscopic (parasite and stone) extraction with sphincterotomy. Patients with associated acute or chronic cholecystitis from parasite migration into the gallbladder will require cholecystectomy (Figure 14.3).

PEARLS AND PITFALLS

1. Acute cholecystitis is often an inflammatory process without infection. When infection occurs, it is usually polymicrobial.
2. Patients with acute cholecystitis require hospitalization, and the definitive treatment is cholecystectomy (may be required emergently, e.g., emphysematous cholecystitis).
3. Over 90% of patients with acute cholecystitis have calculous cholecystitis. Acalculous cholecystitis has different epidemiology and pathophysiology, and is usually a disease of hospitalized patients.
4. Acute cholangitis can present with isolated fever or with florid sepsis.
5. Normal ultrasonography does not rule out cholangitis.
6. Early decompression of biliary system is indicated for acute cholangitis that does not respond to conservative measures.
7. Consider parasitic cholangitis in patients who have traveled to endemic areas.

REFERENCES

Akyurek M, Salman B, Yuksel O, et al. Management of acute calculous cholecystitis in high-risk patients: percutaneous cholecystostomy followed by early laparoscopic cholecystectomy. Surg Laparosc Endosc Percutan Tech 2005;15(6):315–20.

Bornman PC, Van Beljon JI, Krige JEJ. Management of cholangitis. J Hepatobiliary Pancreat Surg 2003;10:406–14.

Fagan SP, Awad SS, Rahwan K, et al. Prognostic factors for the development of gangrenous cholecystitis. Am J Surg 2003;186:481–5.

Gigot JF, Leese T, Bereme T, et al. Acute cholangitis. Multivariate analysis of risk factors. Ann Surg 1989;209:435–8.

Glasgow RE, Visser BC, Harris HW, et al. Changing management of gallstone disease during pregnancy. Surg Endosc 1998;12:241–6.

Gruber PJ, Silverman RA, Gottesfeld S, et al. Presence of fever and leukocytosis in acute cholecystitis. Ann Emerg Med 1996;28:273–7.

Lai EC, Mok FP, Tan ES, et al. Endoscopic biliary drainage for severe acute cholangitis. N Engl J Med 1992;326:1582–6.

Lai PBS, Kwong KH, Leung KL, et al. Randomized trial of early versus delayed laparoscopic cholecystectomy for acute cholecystitis. Br J Surg 1998;85:764–7.

Lo CM, Liu CI, Fan ST, et al. Prospective randomized study of early versus delayed laparoscopic cholecystectomy for acute cholecystitis. Ann Surg 1998;227:461–7.

Lowe SA. Diagnostic radiography in pregnancy: risks and reality. Aust N Z J Obstet Gynaecol 2004;44:191–6.

Osman M, Laustern SB, El-Sefi T, et al. Biliary parasites. Dig Surg 1998;15:287–96.

Poon RT, Liu CL, Lo CM, et al. Management of gallstone cholangitis in the era of laparoscopic cholecystectomy. Arch Surg 2001;136:11–6.

Singer AJ, McCracken G, Henry MC, et al. Correlation among clinical, laboratory, and hepatobiliary scanning findings in patients with suspected acute cholecystitis. Ann Emerg Med 1996;28:267–72.

Sung JJ, Lyon DJ, Suen R, et al. Intravenous ciprofloxacin as treatment for patients with acute suppurative cholangitis: a randomized, controlled clinical trial. J Antimicrob Chemother 1995;35:855–64.

Yusoff IF, Barkun JS, Barkun AN. Diagnosis and management of cholecystitis and cholangitis. Gastroenterol Clin North Am 2003; 32:1145–68.

ADDITIONAL READINGS

IDSA Guidelines. Clin Infect Dis 2003 October 15;37:997.

Indar AA, Beckingham IJ. Acute cholecystitis. BMJ 2002; 325:639–43.

Lillemoe KD. Surgical treatment of biliary tract infections. Am Surg 2000 Feb;66(2):138–44.

Mazuski JE, Sawyer RG, Nathans AB, et al. The Surgical Infection Society guidelines on antimicrobial therapy for intra-abdominal infections: an executive summary. Surg Infect 2002;3(3).

Solomkin JS, Mazuski JE, Baron EJ, et al. Guidelines for the selection of anti-infective agents for complicated intra-abdominal infections. Clin Infect Dis 2003 Oct 15;37:997–1005.

Westphal JF, Brogard JM. Biliary tract infections: a guide to treatment. Drugs 1999 Jan;57(1):81–91.

15. Acute Infectious Diarrhea

Kimberly Schertzer and Gus M. Garmel

INTRODUCTION

Acute diarrhea, defined as the presence of three or more loose stools per day for less than 2 weeks, is usually self-limited and infectious in etiology. In contrast, chronic diarrhea has a duration of more than 3–4 weeks, is less likely to resolve spontaneously, and is more likely to be mechanical in origin. In general, the pathophysiology of diarrhea is osmotic, secretory, inflammatory, or mechanical. *Osmotic diarrhea* is the result of poorly absorbed molecules, such as lactulose, that draw water into the intestinal lumen. *Inflammatory diarrhea* occurs when inflammation of the bowel mucosa causes decreased fluid resorption. *Secretory diarrhea* occurs when there is an increased amount of fluid secreted into the bowel lumen, usually secondary to the effects of bacterial enterotoxin or other secretagogues on the mucosa. *Mechanical diarrhea* occurs with increased gut motility and is often seen in irritable bowel disease or following surgery. Acute infectious diarrhea is generally inflammatory, secretory, or a combination of both.

EPIDEMIOLOGY

Infectious diarrhea is among the leading causes of adult mortality worldwide and is the single leading cause of childhood mortality, resulting in the deaths of 1.6 to 2.5 million children every year. In the United States, as many as 375 million episodes of diarrheal illness are estimated to occur annually. Diarrheal illness is responsible for approximately 5% of U.S. emergency department (ED) visits, as well as 900,000 hospitalizations and 6000 deaths each year.

CLINICAL FEATURES

Inflammatory diarrhea tends to cause frequent, small, bloody bowel movements and is generally associated with fevers, significant abdominal pain, and tenesmus, defined as the frequent urge to have a bowel movement. Large numbers of fecal leukocytes are identified in most cases of inflammatory diarrhea (Table 15.1).

Noninflammatory diarrhea tends to be watery, nonbloody, and large volume, often exceeding a liter per day. Though it is generally milder in its course, significant fluid and electrolyte imbalances may occur. Associated nausea, vomiting, and mild abdominal cramping are common, although fever is generally absent. Fecal leukocytes are uncommon.

DIFFERENTIAL DIAGNOSIS

Although medications and mechanical factors may cause acute diarrhea, its origin is usually infectious. Viral etiologies are most common (50–70%), followed by bacterial (15–20%) and parasitic (10–15%).

Viruses Causing Acute Diarrhea

Viral diarrhea most commonly occurs during winter months as a result of family and community outbreaks of noroviruses or rotavirus. Other pathogens include astrovirus, calicivirus, enterovirus, and adenovirus. Incubation periods range from 1 to 3 days, and the resulting illnesses are generally mild and self-limited (less than 4 days). Viral diarrhea is characterized by an abrupt onset of abdominal cramps and nausea, followed

Table 15.1 Clinical Features: Acute Infectious Diarrhea

	Pathogen	Signs and Symptoms
Inflammatory	*Campylobacter jejuni* *Clostridium difficile* Enterohemorrhagic and enteroinvasive *Escherichia coli* *Shigella* Non-typhi *Salmonella* *Entamoeba histolytica*	Bloody Associated with fever, abdominal pain, and tenesmus Frequent, small-volume stool Fecal leukocytes
Noninflammatory	Rotavirus Norwalk virus Adenovirus *Giardia lamblia* *Cryptosporidium parvum* *Vibrio cholerae* Enterotoxigenic *E. coli*	Nonbloody Nausea, vomiting, mild abdominal pain Watery, large-volume stool

Table 15.2 Infectious Viral Diarrhea

Pathogen	Key Features	Diagnosis	Treatment
Norovirus and Norwalk-like Virus	• Frequent cause of community and cruise ship outbreaks	Clinical suspicion	Supportive
Rotavirus	• Frequently affects children • Peak incidence 3–35 months of age	Stool enzyme immunoassay and serum antibody tests	Supportive
Astrovirus	• Frequent cause of U.S. epidemics • Milder clinical symptoms	Electron microscopy (seldom used)	Supportive

by diarrhea with or without vomiting. Fever occurs in approximately half the cases, often accompanied by headache, myalgias, and symptoms of upper respiratory infection (Table 15.2).

NOROVIRUSES

In the United States, noroviruses are the most common cause of gastroenteritis. Two noroviruses, Norwalk and Norwalk-like virus, are frequently implicated in community outbreaks. Of the 13.8 million cases of foodborne illness reported in the United States annually, 9.2 million are due to noroviruses. The mode of transmission is predominantly foodborne (37%), followed by person-to-person contact (20%), oysters (10%), and contaminated water (6%).

ROTAVIRUS

Worldwide, rotavirus is the most common cause of severe diarrheal disease in young children and infants. It is thought to be responsible for as many as 20% of the deaths attributed to diarrhea. Rotavirus has a peak incidence between 3 months and 35 months of age, though adults may acquire it from their children. It has been implicated in 10% of cases of traveler's diarrhea. Prior illness exposure seems to afford some protection against severe recurrences. Diagnostic stool enzyme immunoassay and serum antibody tests exist, although they are not generally recommended.

ASTROVIRUS

Astrovirus is associated with 2–9% of cases of diarrhea globally. In general, symptoms are similar but milder than those associated with rotavirus, with less nausea, fever, and vomiting. Astrovirus is a frequent cause of U.S. day care and hospital epidemics.

Bacteria Causing Acute Diarrhea (Table 15.3)

CAMPYLOBACTER

Campylobacter now represents the most common cause of bacterial diarrhea in developed countries. It accounts for approximately 2.4 million annual cases in the United States, nearly all due to *Campylobacter jejuni*. The incidence of *Campylobacter*-related diarrhea peaks in late summer and early fall. Spread is most frequently via undercooked poul-

try, although dogs, cats, and birds have also been identified as reservoirs; person-to-person spread is rare. *Campylobacter* often causes an ileocolitis, which may produce either a watery or hemorrhagic diarrhea. Of patients with *Campylobacter*, more than 50% will have gross or occult blood in their stool. Symptoms include fever, abdominal pain, nausea, and malaise, which may be mistaken for appendicitis or irritable bowel syndrome. The frequency of diarrhea may be dramatic; approximately 20% of individuals with *Campylobacter* diarrhea will have more than 15 bowel movements daily. Symptoms generally resolve within a week even without antibiotics, although they may persist for 1–3 weeks in up to 20% of patients.

Complications of *Campylobacter* infection vary according to the age and characteristics of the affected host (Table 15.4). Preceding infection with *Campylobacter* has been identified in as many as 20–40% of patients with Guillain-Barré.

SALMONELLA

Salmonella accounts for an estimated 1.4 million cases of diarrhea in the United States yearly. It occurs most frequently in the summer and fall months and is commonly implicated in epidemics. The most common serotypes in the United States are *Salmonella enteritidis* and *Salmonella typhimurium*. Transmission is generally foodborne from contaminated poultry, meats, eggs, and milk, though other vectors, such as household pets (especially turtles or lizards), have been identified. Symptoms of *Salmonella* infection include nausea, vomiting, abdominal discomfort (frequently mimicking appendicitis), and occasionally bloody diarrhea. The bacteria usually invade small intestine epithelium, although colonic invasion also occurs. Symptoms generally last from 2 to 24 days. The most at-risk individuals for salmonellosis are the elderly and children less than 1 year of age. Normal gastric activity effectively kills more than 99.9% of gram-negative bacteria, including *Salmonella*, and patients with raised gastric pH levels, either through gastrectomy or pharmacologic therapy, are at increased risk of *Salmonella* infection.

Salmonellosis has a high rate of complications, including microabscess formation, toxic megacolon, and a notable 2–4% rate of bacteremia. Risk factors for the development of these complications include hemolytic or sickle cell anemias, malignancy, steroid use, chemo- or radiation therapy, and acquired immunodeficiency syndrome (AIDS). The elderly are less likely to present with classic symptoms of *Salmonella* gastroenteritis, and they are at greater risk of developing invasive disease.

SHIGELLA

Shigella infections account for 10–20% of bacterial diarrhea in the United States. *Shigella sonnei* accounts for 75% of *Shigella* isolates, and only the *Shigella dysenteriae* strain produces the shiga toxin responsible for serious complications. The inoculum needed to cause infection is extremely small (as low as 200 organisms), and transmission of infection is predominately person-to-person or from contaminated food and water supplies. *Shigella* outbreaks are common in nursing facilities, day care centers, and other institutions. Homosexual men are at increased risk for infection with *Shigella flexneri*.

Shigella infections generally begin with fever, fatigue, anorexia, and malaise. This is followed by watery diarrhea that may progress to dysentery, defined as inflammation of

Table 15.3 Infectious Bacterial Diarrhea

Pathogen	Epidemiologic Settings or Modes of Transmission	Key Features	Diagnosis	Treatment (see Table 15.9)
Campylobacter	• Community acquired • Foodborne	• Frequently from undercooked poultry • Causes an ileocolitis that may produce watery or hemorrhagic diarrhea • May be related to development of Guillain-Barré	• Fecal leukocytes • Stool culture on antibiotic medium	• Supportive • Antibiotics if immunocompromised, high fever, bloody stools, or duration >1 week
Salmonella	• Community acquired • Foodborne	• Foodborne from contaminated poultry, meats, eggs, and milk, and pets • Symptoms may mimic appendicitis • May cause microabscess formation or asymptomatic carrier state	• Stool culture on special agar	• Supportive • Antibiotics for high-risk patients only*
Shigella	• Community acquired • Person-to-person spread	• Causes colonic involvement and mucosal breakdown • Malaise and anorexia are common	• Stool culture	• Antibiotics
E. coli shiga-toxin producing (*E. coli* 0157:H7)	• Sporadic infection • Community outbreaks • Foodborne (undercooked hamburger, contaminated produce)	• Most patients are afebrile (may report fever at home) • Presents with severe abdominal pain and tenderness • Often mistaken for other abdominal illnesses	• Stool culture on sorbitol-MacConkey's agar	• Supportive • Avoid antibiotics as they predispose to HUS-TTP
Clostridium difficile	• Antibiotic use • Nosocomial spread	• Overgrowth of bacteria producing enterotoxins • Highly contagious among hospitalized patients	• Anaerobic stool culture	• Antibiotics • Avoid antimotility agents
Yersinia enterocolitica	• Community acquired • Domestic animals • Foodborne	• Most commonly affects children under 10 years • Found in lakes, streams • Most common sign is diffuse, vague abdominal discomfort	• Stool culture on *Yersinia*-selective agar	• Supportive • Antibiotics if enteritis or arthritis present
Vibrio cholerae	• Seafood • Foreign travel	• Acute onset of profound, watery diarrhea • Significant dehydration may occur	• Stool culture	• Supportive • Antibiotics

*High-risk patients include immunosuppressed patients, patients at extremes of age, pregnant patients, or those with cardiac disorders or prosthetic implants.

Table 15.4 Complications of *Campylobacter* Infection

Population	Complication
Children and Young Adults	• Appendicitis • Mesenteric adenitis • Toxic megacolon • Pseudomembranous colitis • Cholecystitis
Adults (Otherwise Healthy)	• Reactive arthritis
Adults with Liver Disease	• Spontaneous bacterial peritonitis
Infrequent Complications	• Hemolytic anemia • Carditis • Encephalopathy • Guillain-Barré syndrome

the intestine associated with bloody stool and pain. Frequent bowel movements are common, and patients may have up to 100 per day in severe cases. Duration of illness ranges from a few days to 1 week. Significant complications include colonic hemorrhage, HUS-TTP (hemolytic uremic syndrome–thrombotic thrombocytopenic purpura), bacteremia, generalized seizures or encephalopathy, and reactive arthritis.

ENTEROINVASIVE *E. COLI* (EIEC)

Similar to *Shigella* infection, though without toxin production, EIEC is marked by fever, predominantly watery diarrhea, and tenesmus. Spread is person-to-person, foodborne or waterborne.

ENTEROAGGREGATIVE *E. COLI* (EAEC)

Responsible for several outbreaks in the United States and industrialized nations, EAEC is also known to cause a persistent chronic diarrhea in children and is an increasingly important pathogen affecting travelers. In some regions of Latin America, it is the second most common bacterial cause of traveler's diarrhea. Transmission is likely foodborne, although exposure does not always result in diarrhea. Symptoms may include watery diarrhea with or without blood or mucus, abdominal pain, nausea, vomiting, fever, and borborygmi. The incubation period ranges from 8 to 18 hours, and duration of symptoms is highly variable, often lasting weeks.

SHIGA-TOXIN-PRODUCING *ESCHERICHIA COLI* (STEC, ALSO KNOWN AS ENTEROHEMORRHAGIC *E. COLI* OR EHEC)

E. coli 0157:H7 differs from other forms of *E. coli* in that it produces shiga toxins 1 and 2. These toxins inhibit protein synthesis and cause cell injury and cell death. Most infections occur in the summer and fall months. After an incubation period of 3–4 days, *E. coli* 0157:H7 causes an initially non-bloody diarrhea that may be followed by a bloody diarrhea after 1–3 days. Prediarrheal signs include fever, abdominal pain, irritability, fatigue, headache, myalgias, and confusion. There may be severe abdominal pain, pain on defecation, and abdominal tenderness on exam. Patients are generally afebrile on presentation, though they may report a history of fever at symptom onset. STEC infection in children may be mistaken for intussusception, inflammatory colitis, or appendicitis, and in adults, for diverticulitis, cancer, hemorrhoids, ischemic colitis, or bowel infarction.

A minority of cases of *E. coli* 0157:H7 infection will be complicated by the hemolysis and acute renal failure of HUS, and *E. coli* 0157:H7 is the most common cause of HUS in the world. There is no correlation between the severity of diarrheal symptoms and the development of HUS, though children younger than 5 years and the elderly are at increased risk of this complication.

The spread of *E. coli* 0157:H7 is primarily foodborne, waterborne, or person-to-person. Outbreaks have been reported in day care centers. Detection is by culture on a sorbitol-MacConkey's agar, which may not be included in the standard stool culture orders at all hospitals. Treatment is primarily supportive, consisting of rehydration and time, though patients with HUS often require temporary dialysis. Antibiotics and antimotility agents are contraindicated, as they may increase the likelihood of HUS. Additionally, narcotics and nonsteroidal anti-inflammatory agents are not recommended. All cases of *E. coli* 0157:H7 require involvement of the health department.

CLOSTRIDIUM DIFFICILE

This anaerobic, spore-forming bacillus is a common cause of acute diarrhea among hospitalized patients. Following a disturbance of normal colonic flora, usually due to antibiotics, *C. difficile* enterotoxins A and B interact to cause colitis and pseudomembranes. Nearly all antibiotics have been implicated in the development of *C. difficile* colitis, but the most frequent offenders are clindamycin, cephalosporins, amoxicillin, and ampicillin. Administration of antibiotics within the previous 3 months may contribute to the development of *C. difficile* diarrhea. The incubation period is unknown. Initial symptoms include a profuse, watery diarrhea, which may progress to bloody diarrhea. This may be accompanied by fever, abdominal cramping, and leukocytosis. Risk factors for symptomatic infection include older age, comorbid illness, elevated gastric

pH, presence of a nasogastric (NG) tube, duration of antibiotic use, recent intensive care unit (ICU) stay, and overall length of hospitalization.

The diagnosis of *C. difficile* is made by detection of the specific toxin through one of several laboratory tests. Although *C. difficile* diarrhea resolves without treatment in 20% of cases, most clinicians administer oral metronidazole (first line) or oral vancomycin in addition to stopping any potentially responsible antibiotic. The rates of relapse approach 20%. Antimotility agents should be avoided, as they increase the risk of toxic megacolon.

YERSINIA ENTEROCOLITICA

More common in winter months, *Yersinia* most frequently affects children under 10 years of age. It is found in streams, lake water, and contaminated milk and is transmitted by animals (including dogs, cats, and farm animals). The most common symptom is diffuse, poorly localized abdominal pain, which occurs in up to 84% of cases and may be mistaken for appendicitis. In addition, patients may present with hemorrhagic diarrhea, nausea, vomiting, and arthritis. Laboratory work-up may demonstrate a leukocytosis, elevated ESR, and occult positive stool. Diagnosis is made with stool cultures on *Yersinia*-selective agar.

VIBRIO CHOLERAE AND NONCHOLERA VIBRIOS

Vibrio cholerae is rarely seen in the United States, with only 61 cases reported over the past 5 years. Most cases occur in individuals returning from travel abroad, or among those ingesting shellfish from the Gulf Coast. *Vibrio cholerae* produces a profuse, "rice water" diarrhea that is severe, acute in onset, and accompanied by significant dehydration. This diarrhea generally lasts 2–3 days. Noncholera *Vibrio* strains, such as *Vibrio parahemolyticus*, are seen more frequently in the United States as a result of contaminated shellfish.

Parasites Causing Acute Diarrhea

In general, parasitic disease tends to be travel-related. Spread is person-to-person or through contact with contaminated food or water. Common offending parasites include *Giardia lamblia*, *Cryptosporidium*, *Isospora belli*, *Cyclospora*, and *Entamoeba histolytica* (Table 15.5). In the United States, the most common causes of chronic infectious diarrhea both among immunocompetent and immunocompromised hosts are *Giardia* and *Cryptosporidium*.

GIARDIA LAMBLIA

Acquisition of *Giardia lamblia* is usually by drinking contaminated lake or stream water. However, spread can also be person-to-person, and *Giardia* is a frequent cause of outbreaks in day care centers and nursing homes. Although some carriers may be asymptomatic, most develop a chronic, watery diarrhea often associated with mucus. Nausea, abdominal pain, significant flatulence, weight loss, and steatorrhea are common.

CRYPTOSPORIDIUM

Cryptosporidium causes an acute, watery diarrhea that resolves spontaneously in 2–3 days in immunocompetent adults. However, it is a common cause of chronic diarrhea (4–6 weeks) in AIDS patients and immunocompetent children. *Cryptosporidium*-related diarrhea is thought to occur as frequently as *Giardia* infection in children. Symptoms of infection

Table 15.5 Infectious Parasitic Diarrhea

Pathogen	Key Features	Diagnosis	Treatment
Giardia lamblia	• Watery diarrhea, steatorrhea, flatulence • Acquired from contaminated water and community outbreaks	• Stool ova and parasite testing	• Metronidazole or tinidazole
Cryptosporidium	• Long-term intestinal damage may occur • Fatigue, flatulence and abdominal discomfort common	• Acid-fast smear of stool samples	• Supportive if immunocompetent • Nitazoxinide in children and in HIV-positive adults
Isospora	• Malaise, headache and vomiting common • Causes direct cell damage	• No direct test available • Peripheral eosinophilia seen on CBC	• Supportive • Trimethoprim-sulfamethoxazole
Cyclospora cayetanensis	• Causes a watery diarrhea with muscle aches and nausea • Often relapsing episodes • Travel to endemic area is common	• Modified acid-fast smear	• Trimethoprim-sulfamethoxazole
Entamoeba histolytica	• Secretion of toxins causes intestinal ulceration • Complications include liver abscess	• Direct identification of cysts in stool • Serological studies in long-standing infection	• Metronidazole

CBC, complete blood count; HIV, human immunodeficiency virus.

include afebrile diarrhea, fatigue, flatulence, and abdominal pain. *Cryptosporidium* transmission is primarily via water, and outbreaks have occurred from contaminated city water supplies. It is also spread through contact with livestock and person-to-person, and has been implicated in day care center outbreaks. Diagnosis is made with a modified acid-fast smear of stool samples.

ISOSPORA

Isospora spread is usually through contaminated water. Predominantly affecting immunocompromised patients, *Isospora* outbreaks have occurred in day care centers and institutions. Symptoms include watery diarrhea, steatorrhea, headache, fever, malaise, abdominal pain, and vomiting. *Isospora* is difficult to distinguish clinically from *Giardia* infection.

CYCLOSPORA CAYETANENSIS

Travel to an endemic area usually precedes *Cyclospora* infection, which results in a chronic, watery, relapsing diarrhea even in immunocompetent patients. *Cyclospora* causes a prolonged watery diarrhea, typically preceded by a 1-day prodrome of malaise and fever, lasting for several weeks. Symptoms include abdominal cramping, nausea, and muscle aches. Disease is primarily transmitted via contaminated food or water. Diagnosis is by modified acid-fast smear of stool.

ENTAMOEBA HISTOLYTICA

Entamoeba infection has been implicated in outbreaks in day care centers and institutions. Spread is generally through contaminated water or food. Clinical disease may be asymptomatic, but more commonly manifests as severe bloody diarrhea. In addition, patients may experience abdominal cramping and malaise. Rare complications include the development of liver abscesses.

LABORATORY AND RADIOGRAPHIC FINDINGS

Viruses are the most common causes of acute diarrhea. Most of these are self-limited, requiring only symptomatic treatment.

Table 15.6 Indications for Stool Culturing in the Acute Care Setting

• Bloody diarrhea
• Fever of 38.5°C (101.3°F) or higher
• History
• Recent travel
• Anal intercourse
• High-risk employment (food handler, day care worker, nursing facility worker)
• Immunocompromised status
• Toxic appearance
• Signs of significant dehydration
• Extremes of age (<1 year or >65 years)
• Severe diarrheal disease
• Presence of six or more stools in 24 hours
• Diarrhea lasting longer than 48 hours

Based on Ilnyckyj A. Clinical evaluation and management of acute infectious diarrhea in adults. Gastroenterol Clin North Am 2001 Sep;30(3):599–609.

As a result, laboratory work-up is indicated only for specific concerning elements in the history or physical examination.

It is prudent to check serum electrolytes in a patient experiencing profuse diarrhea. In addition, if bloody diarrhea is present, a complete blood count assists in quantifying the amount of blood lost. Bandemia in a toxic-appearing patient suggests an invasive pathogen. Fecal leukocytes indicate colonic inflammation and are neither very sensitive nor specific for acute bacterial infection, though in conjunction with a suggestive clinical history may increase the likelihood of this etiology.

Bacterial stool cultures have limited utility in most patient populations, though they are frequently ordered. Their overall yield is low, with a positive rate reported as low as 1.5–1.6%. Table 15.6 provides a list of indications for obtaining stool cultures in the acute care setting.

Patients with a history of hospitalization or antibiotic use within the previous three months should have their stool tested for *C. difficile* toxin. The presentation of *C. difficile*

Table 15.7 Indications for Ova and Parasite Testing in the Acute Care Setting

- History of recent travel to mountain regions
- Exposure to groups of infants with diarrhea
- History of homosexual activity
- AIDS
- Chronic diarrhea without previous diagnosis or prior testing

diarrhea or colitis may be delayed for several months after the initial infection with this pathogen.

There is no indication to test for ova and parasites in most immunocompetent patients, although testing for parasites is indicated in patients with the risk factors described in Table 15.7.

TREATMENT AND PROPHYLAXIS

Fluid Replacement

Dehydrated patients often describe symptoms of dizziness, lightheadedness, and thirst. Clinical signs of dehydration include hypotension, tachycardia, delayed capillary refill, and decreased urine output. Mild to moderate dehydration generally responds well to oral rehydration, and patients should be encouraged to drink fluids containing some glucose. Milk or milk products should be avoided, because a temporary lactase deficiency is often associated with diarrhea.

Severe dehydration requires parenteral fluid resuscitation. Lactated Ringer's is the crystalloid of choice, because it contains both glucose and potassium. One study recommends that the patient's estimated fluid deficit be determined, with 50% replaced in the first hour of treatment. The remainder should be replaced in the subsequent 3 hours, with close observation for signs of hyponatremia (irritability, restlessness, altered mental status or weakness).

Dietary Therapy

Many clinicians continue to recommend the gradual introduction of a limited diet of bananas, rice, applesauce, and toast (BRAT diet), although there is no scientific support for this practice. It is prudent to recommend avoiding caffeine, which increases gastrointestinal motility, and sorbitol, which increases osmotic loads. Adults should gradually increase their intake of sodium (soups, crackers), potassium (fruit juice, bananas), and carbohydrates (crackers, rice, bread, pasta), without spices or sauces.

Probiotics

Probiotics are nonpathogenic bacteria that eliminate or reduce the effects of pathogenic bacteria. Although there are numerous agents, the most information is available for lactobacilli and bifidobacteria. Probiotics may decrease the duration of acute diarrhea by 1 day and the number of stools by 1.5 per day.

Antimotility Agents

Antimotility agents (loperamide) slow intraluminal fluid transport and increase intestinal absorption of fluid, decreasing the number of watery stools. They are not recommended in children under 5 years of age or in patients with high fever, hemorrhagic diarrhea, or immunocompromised status, as they can delay pathogen clearance and increase tissue invasion. In cases of *C. difficile* and *Shigella*, they increase the risk of toxic megacolon, and in cases of *E. coli* 0157:H7, they increase the development of HUS-TTP.

Bismuth Subsalicylate

Bismuth subsalicylate has both an antisecretory effect and antibacterial activity. It may have anti-inflammatory properties as well. It has been shown to reduce the frequency of stools in children and decrease the duration of diarrhea by hours in adults. Despite this, current pediatric guidelines do not encourage its use in children, as it contains aspirin, which may increase the likelihood of Reye's syndrome.

Antimicrobial Therapy for Bacterial Diarrhea

The use of antibiotics in acute diarrhea is limited by the fact that more than half the etiologies are viral in origin. There are increasing concerns about antibiotic resistance and adverse effects of the drugs themselves. In addition, antibiotics may increase the complication rates of certain infections. (See Table 15.8.)

Antibiotics are not indicated for EHEC infection because they offer no improvement in outcome and are associated with an increased incidence of hemolytic-uremic syndrome. Some experts recommend *against* starting empiric antibiotics until the *absence* of an *E. coli* 0157:H7 infection is confirmed by culture. Although no specific clinical trials have explored the use of antibiotics for EIEC, antibiotics are nevertheless recommended, and treatment with antibiotics significantly decreases the duration of illness in enteroaggregative *E. coli* (EAEC). The choice of antibiotics is influenced by resistance patterns; quinolones, azithromycin, or piperacillin are current recommendations as possible therapeutic agents.

Antibiotics are usually not recommended for *Salmonella* infections because they do not reduce symptoms and may prolong the carrier state. However, as up to 4% of these patients will have concomitant bacteremia, antibiotics should be prescribed to anyone who is immunosuppressed, at the extremes of age, pregnant, or has a cardiac disorder, prosthetic implant, or severe diarrhea.

Except in high-risk individuals, such as pregnant women and the immunocompromised, antibiotics are not recommended for *Campylobacter* infection because they offer no

Table 15.8 Role of Antibiotics for Various Pathogens

Pathogens for Which Antibiotics May Be Beneficial
- *Shigella*
- *Vibrio*
- *Clostridium difficile*
- Enteroinvasive *E. coli* (EIEC)
- Enteroaggregative *E. coli* (EAEC)

Pathogens for Which Antibiotics Are Not Generally Recommended
- *Campylobacter* *
- Enterohemorrhagic *E. coli* (EHEC)*,‡
- *Salmonella*†
- *E. coli* 0157:H7‡

*Offers no benefit.
†Prolongs fecal shedding.
‡Increases risk of relapse or other complications.

Table 15.9 Antibiotic Therapy for Acute Bacterial Diarrhea

Pathogen	Therapy Recommendation
Campylobacter	Antibiotics only for severe disease or immunocompromised patients azithromycin 500 mg PO qd × 3 days *or* ciprofloxacin 500 mg PO bid (regional resistance to quinolones exists)
Salmonella	Antibiotics only for severe disease or immunocompromised patients ciprofloxacin, 500 mg PO bid × 5–7 days *or* azithromycin 1 g PO once, then 500 mg PO qd × 6 days
Shigella	Adults: ciprofloxacin or levofloxacin, 500 mg PO bid × 3 days *or* TMP-SMX DS PO bid × 3 days Children: TMP-SMX 5/25 mg per kg PO qd × 3 days Treat immunocompromised children and adults for 7–10 days
E. coli shiga-toxin producing (*E. coli* 0157:H7)	NO TREATMENT. Increased risk of HUS-TTP with antimicrobial and antimotility treatment.
Clostridium difficile	metronidazole 500 mg PO tid or 250 mg qid × 10–14 days Severe disease: vancomycin 125 mg PO qid × 10–14 days
Yersinia enterocolitica	Antibiotics only for severe disease or immunocompromised patients doxycycline 100 mg IV q 12h plus gentamicin or tobramycin 5 mg/kg q24h
Vibrio cholerae	ciprofloxacin 1g PO × 1 dose Children or pregnant adults: TMP-SMX DS PO bid × 2 days
Vibrio parahemolyticus	Generally supportive therapy is best. Doxycycline 200 mg PO/IV bid × 3 days, then 100–200 mg PO bid × 14 days. May consider fluoroquinolones or parenteral third-generation cephalosporins depending on organism sensitivity
EIEC (Enteroinvasive *E. coli*)	Generally supportive therapy is best May treat severe disease with ciprofloxacin 500 mg PO bid × 3–5 days *or* TMP-SMX DS PO bid × 3–5 days
EAEC (Enteroaggregative *E. coli*)	Generally supportive therapy is best May treat severe disease with ciprofloxacin 500 mg PO bid × 3–5 days *or* TMP-SMX DS PO bid × 3–5 days
EHEC (Enterohemorrhagic *E. coli*)	Antibiotics not recommended

Adapted from Gilbert DN, Moellering RC, Eliopoulos GM, Sande MA. Sanford guide to antimicrobial therapy 2006, 36th ed. Sperryville, VA: Antimicrobial Therapy, 2006.
DS, double strength.

benefit. Antibiotics do not alter the course of *Yersinia* infection, though a fluoroquinolone or trimethoprim-sulfamethoxazole (TMP-SMX) is recommended for severe enteritis and complications such as mesenteric adenitis, arthritis, and erythema nodosum. Treatment with antibiotics decreases mortality and shortens the duration of illness for all patients with *Shigella*. *Vibrio* cholera treatment is with oral ciprofloxacin. (See Table 15.9.)

Antimicrobial Therapy for Parasitic Diarrhea

Diarrheal illness due to parasites is generally related to travel. Parasitic infection often results in longer periods of diarrhea than viral or bacterial etiologies. Once identified, parasitic organisms typically respond to directed antibiotic therapy, although treatment in immunocompromised hosts is more difficult. (See Table 15.10.)

COMPLICATIONS AND ADMISSION CRITERIA

Most of the morbidity and mortality associated with acute diarrhea is the result of either dehydration or electrolyte imbalances. It is rare that the infectious nature of acute diarrhea causes problems, unless the patient is significantly immunocompromised. Patients with signs of severe

Table 15.10 Therapy for Acute Parasitic Diarrhea

Pathogen	Therapy Recommendation
Giardia	Antibiotic resistance is rare metronidazole 500–750 mg PO tid × 5 days
Cryptosporidium	Antibiotics only for severe disease or immunocompromised patients Nitazoxanide recommended for HIV-positive adults and immunocompetent children.
Isospora	Immunocompetent adults: TMP-SMX DS PO bid × 10 days Adults with AIDS: TMP-SMX DS PO q6hr × 10 days then q12h × 3 weeks
Cyclospora	Immunocompetent adults: TMP-SMX DS PO bid × 10 days Adults with AIDS: TMP-SMX DS PO qid × 10 days then q12h × 3 weeks
Entamoeba	metronidazole 500–750 mg PO tid × 10 days

dehydration (specifically hypotension or orthostasis) after fluid administration, those unable to maintain a reasonable hydration status, and those with significant metabolic abnormalities due to electrolyte disturbances warrant admission for IV fluid resuscitation and correction of electrolyte abnormalities. Immunocompromised individuals and those at the extremes of age warrant special consideration for possible admission, as do individuals with poor social circumstances.

INFECTION CONTROL

In general, good hand-washing and hygiene techniques are recommended to control the spread of infection in patients with acute diarrhea. Isolation, especially in cases of patients hospitalized with *C. difficile* or rotavirus, is also recommended to decrease disease transmission. Cases of salmonellosis, shigellosis, and STEC infection should be reported to the Department of Public Health (Table 15.11). Food handlers and individuals who work with infants and/or the elderly should be kept from work until their diarrhea has resolved.

Table 15.11 Diarrheal Illnesses Requiring Health Department Notification (National Standards)

- Cholera
- Cryptosporidiosis
- Cyclosporiasis
- Giardiasis
- Hemolytic uremic syndrome, postdiarrheal
- Salmonellosis
- Shiga toxin-producing *Escherichia coli* (STEC)
- Shigellosis
- Tuberculosis

Based on the 2006 Nationally Notifiable Disease list produced by the Centers for Disease Control and Prevention (available at http://www.cdc.gov/epo/dphsi/phs/infdis2006.htm)

PEARLS AND PITFALLS

1. Important historical features that should prompt diagnostic testing in the acute care setting include high-risk sexual behavior, antibiotic use or hospitalization in the preceding 3 months, high-risk employment (e.g., food handlers, day care workers), and travel abroad or to mountainous regions.
2. Stool cultures are overutilized. They are seldom indicated in cases of acute nonbloody diarrhea, though they should be sent on all patients with chronic diarrhea.
3. Cultures for ova and parasites are indicated in select patients only, including patients with AIDS, patients with recent mountain travel, patients with a history of homosexual activity, and patients with exposure to groups of young children.
4. Rehydration and electrolyte management constitute the primary treatment of patients with both acute and chronic diarrhea.

REFERENCES

Banks JB, Sullo EJ, Carter L. Clinical inquiries. What is the best way to evaluate and manage diarrhea in the febrile infant? [comment]. J Fam Pract 2004;53(12):996–9.

Beaugerie L, Petit J-C. Microbial-gut interactions in health and disease. Antibiotic-associated diarrhoea. Best Pract Res Clin Gastroenterol 2004;18(2):337–52.

Casburn-Jones AC, Farthing MJG. Management of infectious diarrhoea. Gut 2004;53(2):296–305.

Dennehy PH. Rotavirus vaccines: an update. Curr Opin Pediatr 2005;17(1):88–92.

Elmer GW, McFarland LV. Biotherapeutic agents in the treatment of infectious diarrhea. Gastroenterol Clin North Am 2001;30(3):837–54.

Gendrel D, Treluyer JM, Richard-Lenoble D. Parasitic diarrhea in normal and malnourished children. Fundam Clin Pharmacol 2003;17(2):189–97.

Goldsweig CD, Pacheco PA. Infectious colitis excluding *E. coli* O157:H7 and *C. difficile*. Gastroenterol Clin North Am 2001;30(3):709–33.

Goodgame RW. Viral causes of diarrhea. Gastroenterol Clin North Am 2001;30(3):779–95.

Gore JI Surawicz C. Severe acute diarrhea. Gastroenterol Clin North Am 2003;32(4):1249–67.

Huang DB, Okhuysen PC, Jiang ZD, et al. Enteroaggregative *Escherichia coli*: an emerging enteric pathogen. Am J Gastroenterol 2004;99(2):383–9.

Ilnyckyj A. Clinical evaluation and management of acute infectious diarrhea in adults. Gastroenterol Clin North Am 2001;30(3):599–609.

Kosek M, Bern C, Guerrant RL The global burden of diarrhoeal disease, as estimated from studies published between 1992 and 2000. Bull World Health Organization 2003;81(3):197–204.

Kyne L, Farrell RJ, Kelly CP. *Clostridium difficile*. Gastroenterol Clin North Am 2001;30(3):753–77.

Lee SD, Surawicz CM. Infectious causes of chronic diarrhea. Gastroenterol Clin North Am 2001;30(3):679–92.

Mack DR. Probiotics-mixed messages [comment]. Can Fam Physician 2005;51:1455–7, 1462.

Nataro JP, Sears CL. Infectious causes of persistent diarrhea. Pediatr Infect Dis J 2001;20(2):195–6.

Ramaswamy K, Jacobson K. Infectious diarrhea in children. Gastroenterol Clin North Am 2001;30(3):611–24.

Ramzan NN. Traveler's diarrhea. Gastroenterol Clin North Am 2001;30(3):665–78.

Sellin JH. The pathophysiology of diarrhea. Clin Transplantation 2001;15 Suppl 4:2–10.

Seupaul R. Diarrhea. In: Mahadevan S, Garmel G, eds, An introduction to clinical emergency medicine: guide for practitioners in the emergency department. Cambridge, UK: Cambridge University Press, 2005:233–9.

Slotwiner-Nie PK, Brandt LJ. Infectious diarrhea in the elderly. Gastroenterol Clin North Am 2001;30(3):625–35.

Starr J. *Clostridium difficile* associated diarrhoea: diagnosis and treatment. BMJ 2005;331(7515):498–501.

Steffen R, Gyr K. Diet in the treatment of diarrhea: from tradition to evidence [comment]. Clin Infect Dis 2004;39(4):472–3.

Sullivan A, Nord CE. Probiotics and gastrointestinal diseases. J Intern Med 2005;257(1):78–92.

Tarr PI, Gordon CA, Chandler WL. Shiga-toxin-producing *Escherichia coli* and haemolytic uraemic syndrome. Lancet 2005;365(9464):1073–86.

Tarr PI, Neill MA, *Escherichia coli* O157:H7. Gastroenterol Clin North Am 2001;30(3):735–51.

The Sanford guide to antimicrobial therapy, 36th ed. DN Gilbert et al., eds. Sperryville, VA: Antimicrobial Therapy, 2006.

Thielman NM, Guerrant RL. Clinical practice. Acute infectious diarrhea [comment]. N Engl J Med 2004;350(1):38–47.

Wilhelmi I, Roman E, Sanchez-Fauquier A. Viruses causing gastroenteritis. Clin Microbiol Infect 2003;9(4):247–62.

Yates J. Traveler's diarrhea. Am Fam Physician 2005; 71(11):2095–100.

ADDITIONAL READINGS

Gore JI, Surawicz C. Severe acute diarrhea. Gastroenterol Clin North Am 2003 Dec;32(4):1249–67.

Ilnyckyj A. Clinical evaluation and management of acute infectious diarrhea in adults. Gastroenterol Clin North Am 2001 Sep;30(3):599–609.

Talan D, Moran GJ, Newdow M, et al. EMERGEncy ID NET Study Group. Etiology of bloody diarrhea among patients presenting to United States emergency departments: prevalence of *Escherichia coli* O157:H7 and other enteropathogens. Clin Infect Dis 2001 Feb 15; 32(4):573–80.

Thielman NM, Guerrant RL. Clinical practice. Acute infectious diarrhea. N Engl J Med 2004 Jan 1;350(1):38–47.

16. Diarrhea in HIV-Infected Patients

George Beatty

INTRODUCTION

A useful initial approach to evaluating diarrhea in an individual infected with human immunodeficiency virus (HIV) is to distinguish acute from chronic diarrhea, and small from large bowel involvement. In addition, particular consideration should be given to the stage of HIV disease, current medications, and sexual history, as these factors help determine likely pathogens. Finally, evaluating the degree of systemic illness is essential to assessing the need for hospital admission.

Initial Approach

Acute diarrhea is defined as the presence of three or more loose or watery stools per day for less than 2 weeks. Diarrhea is defined as persistent if it has been present between 2 and 4 weeks and is considered chronic when present for 4 weeks or more. Pathogens infecting the small bowel affect the secretory and nutritional absorption functions of the gastrointestinal (GI) tract and typically present with large volumes of watery stool, often accompanied by cramps, bloating, and abdominal gas (Table 16.1). Severe or prolonged diarrhea may result in dehydration, malnutrition, and weight loss. Large bowel involvement primarily affects water resorptive capacity and typically causes frequent, small-volume diarrhea that may be bloody or mucoid and is often accompanied by pain.

EPIDEMIOLOGY

Overall, up to 40% of patients with HIV infection report at least one episode of diarrhea in any given month, and approximately one quarter of patients experience chronic diarrhea at some point. The prevalence of diarrhea increases with decreasing CD4 T-cell counts. More than 50% of patients with a CD4 count below 50 will experience at least one episode of diarrhea each year, and in some areas this number will approach 100%. Approximately one half of patients hospitalized with complications of HIV infection report diarrhea. Diarrhea has been shown to be an independent predictor of death in this population.

ASSOCIATED CLINICAL FEATURES

In general, diarrheal symptoms are nonspecific in HIV-infected patients, as they are in the HIV-negative host. Patients with bacterial diarrhea will often, though not invariably, present with associated crampy abdominal pain. The lack of associated abdominal pain or other symptoms should suggest viral acute gastroenteritis or medication side effects. In patients with the large volume, watery diarrhea characteristic of small bowel infections, volume loss may result in dizziness, syncope, pallor, electrolyte imbalances (hypokalemia, hyponatremia), and acute renal insufficiency. Signs of invasive or systemic involvement include the presence of fever, severe abdominal cramps, and bloody stools. Patients with long-standing chronic diarrhea may exhibit obvious wasting or malnutrition, but these may also result from advanced HIV infection.

Table 16.1 Small Versus Large Bowel Diarrhea

	Common Pathogens	Symptoms
Small Bowel	• *Salmonella** • *Escherichia coli* • Viral (e.g., rotavirus) • *Giardia* • MAC • *Cryptosporidium** • *Microsporidium** • Malabsorption	• Large volume • Watery stool • Upper abdominal cramps • Bloating • Gas • Weight loss • Malnutrition • Dehydration
Large Bowel	• *Yersinia* • *Campylobacter** • *Shigella* • *Clostridium difficile* • CMV • Enteroinvasive *E. coli* • *Entamoeba histolytica* • Gonorrhea	• Small volumes • Frequent bowel movements • Mucoid or bloody stool • Tenesmus • Lower abdominal cramps

*May involve both small and large bowel, but typically presents as listed.
CMV, cytomegalovirus; MAC, *Mycobacterium avium* complex.

DIFFERENTIAL DIAGNOSIS

Diarrhea in HIV-infected patients poses a diagnostic dilemma in the acute care setting, as these patients are susceptible to all of the infections associated with diarrhea in the normal host, as well as a multitude of opportunistic infections and medication side effects. Some pathogens are unique to HIV disease, and others that cause mild or self-limiting disease in immunocompetent hosts may cause severe and prolonged disease in the setting of advanced HIV infection.

A careful history may provide important diagnostic clues as to the possible etiology of diarrhea (see Table 16.2). The patient's most recent and nadir CD4 T-cell count, history of opportunistic infections, currently prescribed antiretroviral regimen, and prophylactic antibiotics all help determine the pathogens to which the patient is susceptible.

The duration, frequency, volume, and character of the diarrhea, as well as associated symptoms such as weight loss, fever, and abdominal pain, will also help narrow the differential. For example, several weeks of voluminous watery diarrhea with cramps, bloating, and nausea in a patient with low CD4 counts would suggest small bowel infection with *Cryptosporidium, Microsporidium, Isospora belli*, or *Giardia* organisms.

Similarly, a recent onset of small-volume diarrhea with hematochezia and tenesmus would raise suspicion for *Shigella* or *Campylobacter* infection of the large bowel, whereas a longer duration of these symptoms would suggest colitis from cytomegalovirus (CMV), herpes, or *Clostridium difficile*.

In addition, a complete list of current medications should be obtained, and particular attention given to antiretroviral medications, any recent changes in medications, recent antibiotic use, over-the-counter (OTC) medications, and medications that decrease gastric acidity (H2 antagonists and proton pump inhibitors). The last have been shown to increase the risk of *C. difficile*. Finally, an explicit sexual history should be taken, as anal-oral contact increases the risk of certain pathogens.

As with all cases of diarrhea, a complete history should include information about recent travel, dietary changes, pets, water sources, sick contacts (especially children), comorbid conditions, and family history of chronic diarrhea or irritable bowel disease. If the patient is employed in a food-handling or child care industry, health department notification may be required.

Physical examination should focus on the abdominal exam, noting tenderness, quality of bowel sounds, stool color and guaiac, and any hepatosplenomegaly or masses. The presence of fever and signs of dehydration, such as dry mucous membranes and tachycardia, should be noted.

In patients with relatively intact immune function, as measured by a current CD4 count greater than 200 cells/mm^3, viral gastroenteritis and medication side effects account for a majority of cases of acute diarrhea. With decreasing CD4 counts, other pathogens increasingly predominate, and the prevalence of persistent and chronic diarrhea increases several fold. It is important to remember that all chronic diarrhea begins acutely (Tables 16.3 and 16.4).

CD4 Count and Risk of Diarrhea-Causing Opportunistic Infections

Stratifying patients on the basis of their most recent CD4 count provides a useful way to identify which patients are at risk

Table 16.2 Key Components of History and Examination

History
- HIV status: current CD4 T-cell count, antiretroviral treatment, and history of opportunistic infections
- Duration of symptoms, frequency, characteristics of stool, amount, weight loss
- Medications: including OTCs, recent change in meds, HIV meds, use of proton pump inhibitors or H2 blockers
- Recent antibiotic use or hospitalization
- Abdominal symptoms or constitutional symptoms
- Travel, food habits, sexual activity
- Pets
- Water source
- Sick contacts, children, day care
- Comorbidities (e.g., diabetes, pancreatitis)
- Family history of bowel disease (e.g., irritable bowel disease)
- Employment (e.g., food service employee)

Physical Examination
- Vital signs, fever, weight
- signs of dehydration, orthostatic hypotension, tachycardia, dry mucous membranes
- Abdominal exam, tenderness, hepatosplenomegaly
- Skin evidence of rash or Kaposi's sarcoma
- Signs of systemic illness

for infections unique to HIV and at increased risk of complications from more common pathogens.

In addition to the common etiologies of diarrhea in the normal host, HIV-infected patients are at higher risk of the following pathologies, based on CD4 count:

CD4 greater than 200:

- HIV medication associated diarrhea
- self-limiting bacterial acute gastroenteritis (AGE)
- Viral acute gastroenteritis
- *Giardia*
- *Entamoeba histolytica*
- self-limiting *Cryptosporidium*
- tuberculosis
- small bowel overgrowth

CD4 50–200:

- all of the above
- invasive/systemic *Salmonella*
- invasive bacterial enteritis
- *C. difficile*

CD4 less than 50:

- all of the above
- *Mycobacterium avium* complex
- chronic and severe *Cryptosporidium* and *Microsporidium*
- HIV enteropathy
- CMV colitis

Patients with HIV are often at risk for additional infections because of overlapping risk factors for sexually transmitted infections. Proctitis due to gonorrhea and *Chlamydia* may be mistaken for colitis. Infections causing enteritis that may be transmitted via a fecal-oral route include *Salmonella, Shigella, Campylobacter jejuni*, hepatitis A, *Yersinia, Giardia lamblia, Entamoeba histolytica, Cryptosporidium,* and herpes simplex.

Table 16.3 Causes of Acute Diarrhea in HIV*

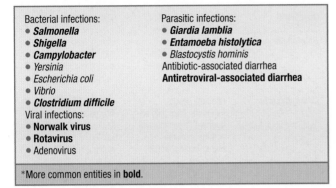

Bacterial infections:	Parasitic infections:
• **Salmonella**	• **Giardia lamblia**
• **Shigella**	• **Entamoeba histolytica**
• **Campylobacter**	• Blastocystis hominis
• Yersinia	Antibiotic-associated diarrhea
• Escherichia coli	**Antiretroviral-associated diarrhea**
• Vibrio	
• **Clostridium difficile**	
Viral infections:	
• **Norwalk virus**	
• **Rotavirus**	
• Adenovirus	

*More common entities in **bold**.

Table 16.4 Causes of Persistent and Chronic Diarrhea in HIV*

Bacterial and mycobacterial infections:	Viral infections:
• Escherichia coli	• Cytomegalovirus
• Salmonella	• Herpes
• Shigella	• HIV (AIDS enteropathy)
• Campylobacter jejuni	Other causes:
• **Clostridium difficile**	• Kaposi's sarcoma
• TB	• Lymphomas
• **MAC**	• Malabsorption
Parasitic infections:	• **Medication side effects**
• **Cryptosporidium**	• Small bowel overgrowth
• **Microsporidium**	• Functional disorders
• Isospora belli	• Irritable bowel syndrome
• **Giardia lamblia**	• Pancreatic insufficiency (MAC,
• Cyclospora	CMV, pentamidine, didanosine)
• **Entamoeba histolytica**	

*More common entities in **bold**.
TB, tuberculosis.

Associated symptoms such as long-standing fever and night sweats may suggest underlying mycobacterial disease, such as MAC or TB. Profound dehydration in a patient with less than 200 CD4 T-cells may suggest cryptosporidial infection. Patients with CMV colitis may experience odynophagia or visual field defects from concomitant esophageal and retinal CMV infection.

Additional focused exam may be useful depending on the clinical scenario. A patient with CD4 less than 50 and symptoms referable to colitis should have a retinal exam for CMV. The presence of a violaceous nodular rash consistent with Kaposi's sarcoma or the presence of the white patchy mucosal lesions of oral or vaginal candidiasis suggests a CD4 count less than 200 in a patient whose stage of HIV disease is unknown.

Because patients with HIV may receive multiple antibiotics, higher rates of both small bowel overgrowth and *C. difficile* are reported. The prevalence of small bowel overgrowth in HIV-infected patients may be greater than 30%. Small bowel overgrowth is characterized by excess growth of mostly gram-negative enteric flora, resulting in chronic diarrhea and malabsorption, culminating in malnutrition and vitamin deficiencies.

Finally, HIV itself infects the gut wall and can cause a chronic diarrheal illness associated with malabsorption and weight loss. This so-called "HIV enteropathy" remains poorly defined and is generally seen in very advanced HIV disease (CD4 <100). It is a diagnosis of exclusion.

Table 16.5 Commonly Used HIV Medications That Can Cause Diarrhea

HIV Protease Inhibitors:	HIV Nucleoside Reverse Transcriptase Inhibitors:
• amprenavir (Agenerase)	• abacavir (Ziagen)
• darunavir (Prezista)	• didanosine (Videx)
• fosamprenavir (Lexiva)	• stavudine (Zerit)
• lopinavir (Kaletra)	• tenofovir (Viread)
• nelfinavir (Viracept)	**Antibiotics:**
• ritonavir (Norvir)	• clindamycin
• saquinavir (Fortovase)	• TMP-SMX
• tipranavir (Aptivus)	

TMP-SMX, trimethoprim-sulfamethoxazole.

Noninfectious Causes of Diarrhea

The most common noninfectious causes of diarrhea in HIV-infected patients are medication side effects, particularly protease inhibitors, which are the backbone of many antiretroviral regimens. Patients will report a temporal association with initiation of the medication and will generally report moderate-to low-volume watery diarrhea or loose stools, possibly with abdominal bloating, gas, and discomfort (Table 16.5). Abdominal cramps, fever, bloody stool, and dehydration are absent. The diarrhea may wane after 4–6 weeks on the medication but will often persist, particularly with nelfinavir, ritonavir, and lopinavir.

Other noninfectious causes include infiltrative diseases such as gastrointestinal Kaposi's sarcoma and non-Hodgkin's lymphoma. Up to 15% of patients with visceral Kaposi's sarcoma will not have skin involvement.

LABORATORY FINDINGS

Because of the broad range of possible enteric pathogens requiring distinct treatments, particularly in patients with advanced HIV disease, microbiologic diagnosis should always be pursued. Depending on the clinical scenario, the following investigations may be appropriate:

- stool culture and sensitivity (specify cultures for *E. coli* 0157, *Vibrio*, and *Yersinia* if diarrhea is bloody or patient systemically ill)
- stool ova and parasite exam × 3 (order *Cryptosporidium/Microsporidium* separately if CD4 is less than 200)
- *Giardia* antigen test
- *C. difficile* toxin assay
- stool for leukocytes, occult blood, fecal fat
- serum electrolytes Na and K looking for an osmotic gap

Although certain pathogens will require upper or lower endoscopy with mucosal aspirate cultures and/or biopsy for diagnosis, it is reasonable to initiate a stepwise approach in the acute care setting. Initial evaluation should include stool culture and sensitivity and exam for ova and parasites (O&P). Because of the relatively low sensitivity of only one O&P exam (~50%), patients should have follow up O&P exam on a second and third stool sample. If the CD4 count is less than 200, exams for *Microsporidium* and *Cryptosporidium* should also be specifically requested with the O&P exam. A history of recent antibiotic therapy or hospital admission should prompt stool collection for *C. difficile* toxin assay, though this study should be considered in all patients, as there is an increasing prevalence of community-acquired *C. difficile* diarrhea in individuals with no known risk factors. Fecal leukocytes may support a diagnosis of bacterial gastroenteritis, but their absence does not rule out infection in an HIV-infected patient, and this is generally not a useful test in this population. All febrile patients should receive blood cultures to rule out bacteremia from *Salmonella* or other enteric bacteria, and separate mycobacterial blood culture should be sent in febrile patients with CD4 less than 100 to rule out MAC.

Additional Work-Up

Patients with persistent or chronic diarrhea in whom this initial work-up has not revealed a cause should be referred for endoscopic evaluation, and a noninfectious cause, such as medication side effect or irritable bowel syndrome, should be considered. Colonoscopy or sigmoidoscopy with mucosal biopsy is generally required for diagnosis of CMV colitis. Diagnosis of MAC is usually made by mycobacterial blood culture, though it may only appear in mucosal aspirate. Other diagnoses that may require upper or lower endoscopy with biopsy and/or microbiologic examination of mucosal aspirate include *Microsporidium* and *Cryptosporidium*. The diagnostic value of radiographic studies in evaluating diarrhea is very low compared with endoscopy. While radiography is generally not indicated, a plain film may show dilated bowel loops suggesting obstruction, free air suggesting perforation, or thumbprinting indicating mucosal edema. Computed tomography (CT) may also show signs of perforation, obstruction, or bowel wall inflammation.

TREATMENT

In patients with CD4 counts greater than 200, the majority of cases of acute diarrhea are self-limiting infections that can be managed conservatively with oral rehydration, symptomatic treatment, and dietary modifications, with early follow-up for results of stool studies. Patients with CD4 counts less than 200, febrile patients, patients with evidence of systemic involvement, and patients requiring admission for other reasons may be empirically treated with antimicrobials once appropriate specimens have been obtained. Patients who already have a microbiologic diagnosis should receive appropriate pathogen-directed therapy. (See Table 16.6.)

Empiric therapy should be directed at common gram-negative enteric pathogens, e.g., *Salmonella*, *Shigella*, *Yersinia*, *Campylobacter*. A quinolone, such as ciprofloxacin 500 mg bid or levofloxacin 500 mg qd × 5 days, is recommended. If clinical suspicion for a parasitic infection, such as *Giardia* or *Entamoeba histolytica*, is high, metronidazole 250–750 mg tid or tinidazole 2 gm daily can be substituted.

Patients presenting to the emergency department with persistent or chronic diarrhea despite treatment for enteric bacteria may be empirically treated with metronidazole or tinidazole for parasites, and to complete treatment for bacterial overgrowth, but if the stool O&P is negative and their symptoms are more consistent with an infectious cause than a medication side effect or irritable bowel syndrome (IBS), these patients should be referred for endoscopy. Both IBS and transient lactose intolerance can follow an acute bacterial gastroenteritis. Finally, local health departments may require notification of positive culture results for certain pathogens (e.g., *Shigella*, gonorrhea), and sexual partner notification may be warranted.

Table 16.6 Clinical Features and Treatment of HIV Associated Diarrhea

Organism	Clinical Features	Treatment
Salmonella	May be septic and invasive in low CD4. Usually food acquired.	ciprofloxacin 500–750 mg PO bid × 14 days, or ceftriaxone IV. If CD4 <200, treat 4–6 weeks.
Campylobacter	Possible sexual exposure. May also be invasive (bloody, fever) with bacteremia/extraintestinal in CD4 <200.	ciprofloxacin 500 mg PO bid × 3–5 days (2 weeks if bacteremic) *or* azithromycin 500 mg PO qd × 3–5 days (some quinolone resistance)
Shigella	Possible sexual exposure. May be bloody, with fever and upper GI symptoms	ciprofloxacin 500 mg PO bid × 3–5 days
Giardia	Gas, bloating, cramps, foul-smelling stools	metronidazole 250–500 mg tid × 7 days *or* tinidazole 2 gm × 1
Isospora	Watery, afebrile	TMP-SMX DS PO qid × 10 days
Entamoeba histolytica	Gas, bloating, cramps, foul-smelling stools, may be bloody	metronidazole 750 mg PO tid × 10 days *or* tinidazole 2 g PO qd × 3–5 days
MAC	Occurs exclusively in low CD4. Fever, weight loss, anemia, night sweats, hepatomegaly, elevated alkaline phosphatase	clarithromycin 500 mg PO bid plus ethambutol 20 mg/kg/day PO indefinitely, and antiretroviral therapy
Clostridium difficile	Previous antibiotics or hospitalization	metronidazole 500 mg PO tid × 10 days
Cryptosporidium	Large volumes, nausea/vomiting, cramps, electrolyte imbalance, acidosis in low CD4	**Immunocompetent**: nitazoxanide 500 mg PO bid × 3–5 days **CD4 < 100**: nitazoxanide 500 mg PO bid *or* paromomycin 1 g PO bid plus azithromycin 600 mg PO qd; plus antiretroviral therapy
Microsporidium	Watery stools, malabsorption. Fever uncommon.	albendazole 400–800 mg PO qh12 × 2–4 weeks
CMV	Occurs exclusively in CD4 <50. Colitis–lower abdominal pain, bright red blood per rectum. May coexist with retinitis. Requires biopsy for diagnosis.	ganciclovir 5 mg/kg IV bid and antiretroviral therapy

TMP-SMX DS, trimethoprim-sulfamethoxazole double strength.

Symptomatic Treatment

Dietary modification may assist in ameliorating diarrhea in all patients. Recommended foods include complex carbohydrates in the form of boiled starches and cereals, such as potatoes, noodles, rice, wheat, and oats, with salt, along with boiled vegetables and lean meats. Soups, crackers, yogurt, and bananas are often well-tolerated. Lactose-containing foods and high-fat foods should be avoided. For symptomatic treatment of patients with chronic diarrhea and in select afebrile patients with acute nonbloody diarrhea, anti-motility agents such as loperamide (4 mg initially, then 2 mg after each unformed stool) or diphenoxylate (4 mg qid) may be used. These agents can increase the risk of severe complications in patients with *C. difficile* and some other bacterial diarrheas, and should only be used after an initial work-up has been completed. Bulking agents such as psyllium are often beneficial. Patients with advanced HIV disease and infections such as cryptosporidium or MAC may experience severe chronic diarrhea causing dehydration, malnutrition, and weight loss. In these patients, a more aggressive attempt at slowing intestinal motility can include oral tincture of opium or subcutaneous administration of octreotide. In all patients with dehydration, oral rehydration solutions provide more effective rehydration than sports drinks such as Gatorade and are less likely to cause hypernatremia than high-sodium foods such as chicken soup. Intravenous (IV) rehydration is indicated for all patients with moderate to severe dehydration. Finally, although antiretroviral medications undoubtedly contribute to diarrhea in patients with infectious causes, many of these infections will prove incurable without sustained treatment of HIV and immune restoration. Antiretroviral medications should be discontinued only as a last resort and in consultation with the prescribing practitioner, as any changes may affect antiretroviral drug resistance patterns and future HIV treatment options.

COMPLICATIONS AND ADMISSION CRITERIA

Sepsis

HIV-infected patients with lower CD4 counts are at higher risk of *Salmonella* bacteremia and septicemia. Complications of *Salmonella* bacteremia in this population include septicemia, pyelonephritis, intra-abdominal abscesses, osteomyelitis, and septic arthritis. Patients with suspected or known *Salmonella* bacteremia should be admitted for treatment with an IV quinolone, further work-up, and observation. Patients with CD4 counts less than 200 and *Salmonella* bacteremia should be treated for 4–6 weeks and, if relapse occurs, should be maintained indefinitely on suppressive fluoroquinolone therapy, such as ciprofloxacin.

Dehydration and Electrolyte Imbalance

Patients with advanced HIV and opportunistic enteric infections (particularly *Cryptosporidium*) can have massive volume loss resulting in hemodynamic compromise, significant electrolyte imbalance (especially hypokalemia), and refractory acidosis from loss of bicarbonate. Such patients will require admission for aggressive IV rehydration, electrolyte repletion, antimotility agents, and correction of acidosis.

Malnutrition

Patients with low CD4 counts and chronic diarrhea from conditions such as MAC, *Microsporidium*, *Cryptosporidium*, or HIV enteropathy can develop nutritional, caloric, and vitamin deficiencies. In concert with the catabolic state often seen in advanced HIV, this can result in a state resembling starvation that, in its severe form, will require admission.

Other

Rarely, patients with extensive gastrointestinal Kaposi's sarcoma can experience gastrointestinal hemorrhage. Severe infectious colitis (e.g., *C. difficile*) or infiltrative processes (e.g., lymphoma) can cause perforation.

Admission Criteria

Admission to the hospital is recommended for patients with:

- CD4 less than 200 who have fever and/or signs or symptoms of systemic involvement
- known or suspected bacteremia
- CD4 less than 200 and known *Salmonella* infection
- severe dehydration, acidosis, or electrolyte imbalance

Admission to the hospital should be considered in:

- any patient with CD4 less than 200
- patients with hepatosplenomegaly

INFECTION CONTROL

Universal blood and bodily fluid precautions are sufficient infection control methods for most pathogens associated with diarrhea in HIV-infected patients. When caring for patients with known *C. difficile* infection, use soap and water for hand hygiene, as alcohol-based hand rubs may not be as effective against spore-forming bacteria. Place these patients in private rooms when available, and use gloves and dedicated equipment for all patient care.

PEARLS AND PITFALLS

1. Admit patients with CD4 less than 200 and fever or systemic symptoms.
2. Admit patients with severe dehydration, acidosis, electrolyte imbalance.
3. Chronic diarrhea in patients with CD4 greater than 200 is often due to HIV medications.
4. Ova and parasite exam should be sent on three different stools.
5. Remember *C. difficile*.
6. *Salmonella* is much more pathogenic and more likely to cause sepsis in patients with HIV.
7. In patients with CD4 greater than 200 consider viral and common bacterial causes, and medication side effects.
8. In patients with CD4 less than 200 consider *Cryptosporidium*, parasites, MAC.
9. In patients with severe dehydration, electrolyte disturbances, weight loss, and CD4 less than 200 consider *Cryptosporidium*.

REFERENCES

Angulo FJ, Swerdlow DL. Bacterial enteric infections in persons infected with human immunodeficiency virus. Clin Infect Dis 1995 Aug;21(Suppl 1):S84–93.

Asmuth DM, DeGirolami PC, Federman M, et al. Clinical features of microsporidiosis in patients with AIDS. Clin Infect Dis 1994 May;18(5):819–25.

Blanshard C, Francis N, Gazzard BG. Investigation of chronic diarrhoea in acquired immunodeficiency syndrome. A prospective study of 155 patients. Gut 1996 Dec;39(96):824–32.

Call SA, Heudebert G, Saag M, Wilcox CM. The changing etiology of chronic diarrhea in HIV-infected patients with CD4 cell counts less than 200 cells/mm^3. Am J Gastroenterol 2000 Nov;95(11):3142–6.

Chen XM, Keithly JS, Paya CV, LaRusso NF. Cryptosporidiosis. N Engl J Med 2002 May 30;346(22):1723–31.

Mayer HB, Wanke CA. Diagnostic strategies in HIV-infected patients with diarrhea. AIDS 1994 Dec;8(12):1639–48.

Sharpstone D, Gazzard B. Gastrointestinal manifestations of HIV infection. Lancet 1996 Aug 10;348(9024):379–83.

Sherman DS, Fish DN. Management of protease inhibitor-associated diarrhea. Clin Infect Dis 2000 Jun;30(6):908–14.

ADDITIONAL READINGS

Cohen J, West AB, Bini EJ. Infectious diarrhea in human immunodeficiency virus. Gastroenterol Clin North Am 2001 Sep;30(3):637–64.

Kearney DJ, Steuerwald M, Koch J, Cello JP. A prospective study of endoscopy in HIV-associated diarrhea. Am J Gastroenterol 1999 Mar;94(3):596–602.

Morpeth SC, Thielman NM. Diarrhea in patients with AIDS. Curr Treat Options Gastroenterol 2006 Feb;9(1):23–37.

Sanchez TH, Brooks JT, Sullivan PS, et al. Bacterial diarrhea in persons with HIV infection, United States, 1992–2002. Clin Infect Dis 2005 Dec 1;41(11):1621–7.

Weber R, Ledergerber B, Zbinden R, et al. Enteric infections and diarrhea in human immunodeficiency virus-infected persons: prospective community-based cohort study. Swiss HIV Cohort Study. Arch Intern Med 1999 Jul 12;159(13):1473–80.

17. Ulcerative Sexually Transmitted Diseases

Diane Birnbaumer

INTRODUCTION – AGENTS

Sexually transmitted infections can be divided into those that cause genital ulcers and those that do not. In North America, ulcerative sexually transmitted diseases are most commonly caused by herpes genitalis, syphilis, and, occasionally, chancroid; much rarer causes include lymphogranuloma venereum and granuloma inguinale. Definitive diagnostic tests often are not available in the acute care setting, and empiric treatment with close follow-up is often the best approach.

HERPES GENITALIS

Epidemiology

Genital herpes infection is caused by herpes simplex virus (HSV) types 1 and 2. This is by far the most common cause of ulcerating genital disease in North America: More than 50 million persons in the United States have the disease. Most U.S. cases are caused by HSV-2.

Clinical Features

Herpes genitalis can present with a broad range of symptoms. Serologic testing suggests that many infected patients are asymptomatic or have minimal symptoms. Those with an initial genital infection caused by HSV-1 tend to have milder symptoms than those infected with HSV-2. In addition, patients who already have antibodies to HSV-1 (e.g., those with a history of fever blisters) often have milder symptoms with initial HSV-2 genital infection. Symptomatic patients with genital infection caused by HSV-2 who have no prior HSV antibodies tend to present with the most severe disease. In all cases of genital herpes, recurrences may occur and are more common in patients infected with HSV-2.

Typically, patients presenting with genital herpes complain of multiple painful genital ulcers (Table 17.1). Some patients, particularly men, may note vesicles prior to developing ulcers (Figure 17.1). The ulcers are multiple, shallow, clean-based, and very painful. In severe cases, these ulcers may coalesce, particularly in women (Figure 17.2). In mild cases, the ulcers heal in several days to a week; in severe cases, the lesions may take up to 2 weeks to heal. Adenopathy, when present, is mild, bilateral, minimally tender, and nonfluctuant. Patients with severe initial infection may develop systemic symptoms such as fever and myalgias prior to appearance of the genital ulcers.

Patients with known herpes genitalis may present with a recurrence. Frequently these episodes are heralded by local tingling, dysesthesias, or itching that precede the vesicles and ulcers. Recurrences tend to last only several days. Recurrences are more common in patients infected with HSV-2.

Differential Diagnosis

All of the sexually transmitted diseases (STDs) that cause genital ulcers should be considered in patients presenting with this complaint:

Table 17.1 Clinical Features: Herpes Genitalis

Organisms	Herpes simplex virus type 1 and type 2
Incubation Period	Variable; may be weeks to years
Transmission	Direct contact
Signs and Symptoms	• Patients with initial primary infection may have systemic symptoms including fever and myalgias • Vesicles may be noted prior to ulcers • Multiple painful genital ulcers are noted; in initial infection these lesions may coalesce, particularly in women • Shotty bilateral adenopathy may develop
Laboratory Findings	• Serology may be positive for HSV-1 or HSV-2 • Viral cultures may be positive • PCR testing not currently FDA-approved

FDA, Food and Drug Administration; PCR, polymerase chain reaction.

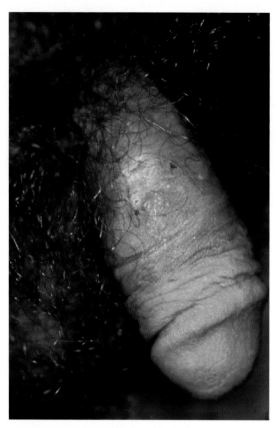

Figure 17.1 Genital herpes lesions on the penile shaft. Image courtesy of the Australasian Chapter on Sexual Health Medicine.

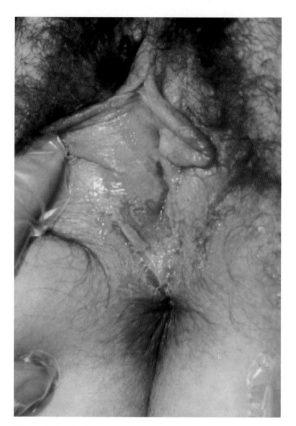

Figure 17.2 Coalescent primary herpes lesions on the vulvae. Image courtesy of the Australasian Chapter on Sexual Health Medicine.

- syphilis
- chancroid
- granuloma inguinale
- lymphogranuloma venereum
- scabies

Noninfectious conditions that can mimic genital herpes include Behçet's syndrome, trauma, contact dermatitis, erythema multiforme, Reiter's syndrome, psoriasis, fixed drug eruptions, Crohn's disease, and lichen planus.

Key features that may help distinguish herpes from other STDs are:

- systemic symptoms suggest primary genital herpes infection
- multiple painful genital ulcers with a clean base suggest herpes, but may also be seen in patients with chancroid
- recurrences are common and suggest herpes infection, but may also be seen in some other entities (e.g., Behçet's syndrome)

Laboratory Findings

Until relatively recently, viral culture was the only way to make the diagnosis of herpes genitalis. The sensitivity of culture is low, particularly in recurrences or when lesions have begun to heal, so a negative culture does not rule out the disease. Polymerase chain reaction testing is now available for testing genital lesions but has not been approved by the Food and Drug Administration (FDA).

Serologic testing is available that can diagnose the infection and determine the type of HSV involved. Some of these tests are available for point-of-care testing. False-negative results may occur in the early stages of infection. The presence of serum HSV-2 antibodies is considered diagnostic of anogenital infection.

Serologic testing is recommended in the following patients: (1) those with recurrent or atypical symptoms with negative HSV cultures, (2) those with a clinical diagnosis of herpes without laboratory confirmation, and (3) those with a partner with genital herpes.

Treatment and Prophylaxis

Primary and recurrent herpes infection can be treated with antiviral agents including acyclovir, famciclovir, and valacyclovir (Table 17.2). Severe cases (meningitis, severe local disease, urinary retention) require hospitalization and should be treated with intravenous acyclovir.

Patient having six or more recurrences per year can be placed on acyclovir, famciclovir, or valacyclovir for prophylaxis. Acyclovir has been proven safe for up to 7 years.

Complications and Admission Criteria

Viral meningitis may develop in 33% of women and 10% of men who have primary genital HSV infection. These patients usually present as their genital lesions are beginning to resolve. Patients have symptoms typical for viral meningitis, including headache, photophobia, neck pain and stiffness, and fever. Lumbar puncture usually shows a

Table 17.2 Treatment of HSV Infections

Patient Category	Therapy Recommendations
Adults: Mucocutaneous	**Genital HSV and proctitis – first clinical episode**: (all prescriptions for 7–10 days) acyclovir 400 mg PO tid *or* acyclovir 200 mg PO 5 × day *or* famciclovir 250 mg PO tid *or* valacyclovir 1 g PO bid
	Genital HSV and proctitis – episodic disease: (all for 5 days unless otherwise noted) acyclovir 400 mg PO tid *or* acyclovir 200 mg PO 5 × day *or* acyclovir 800 mg PO bid *or* famciclovir 125 mg PO bid *or* valacyclovir 500 mg PO bid × 3–5 days
	Genital HSV or proctitis – suppressive daily therapy for recurrent disease: acyclovir 400 mg PO bid *or* famciclovir 250 mg PO bid *or* valacyclovir 500 mg PO qd *or* valacyclovir 1 g PO qd
	Severe genital HSV or proctitis: acyclovir 5–10 mg/kg IV q8h × 5–7 days or until clinical resolution; suppressive therapy thereafter, if indicated
	Genital HSV in pregnancy: acyclovir per above regimen w/initial HSV or highly symptomatic recurrent HSV; give IV with life-threatening infection
Immunosuppressed	**Prophylaxis for acute immunosuppression in organ and bone marrow seropositives**: initiation – acyclovir 5 mg/kg IV q8h × 7 days follow-up – acyclovir 200–400 mg PO tid-5 × day × 1–3 months
	Episodic prescription for recurrent infection in HIV-infected patients: (all drugs for 5–10 days) acyclovir 200 mg PO 5 × day *or* acyclovir 400 mg PO tid *or* famciclovir 500 mg PO bid *or* valacyclovir 1 g PO bid
	Daily suppressive prescription in HIV-infected patients: acyclovir 400–800 mg PO bid-tid *or* valacyclovir 500 mg *or* famciclovir 500 mg bid
Antiviral Resistant Strains	foscarnet 40 mg/kg IV q8h until clinical resolution topical cidofovir gel 1% for genital or perirectal lesions qd × 5 days may be tried (local pharmacy must compound)

leukocytosis with lymphocytic predominance. These patients should be admitted for intravenous antiviral treatment.

Primary genital herpes may also be complicated by sacral radiculopathy syndrome, characterized by urinary retention and constipation. These symptoms usually resolve spontaneously, although the patients may temporarily need urinary catheterization to aid in voiding and should be admitted for initial management.

Congenital herpes infection is a very serious infection of newborn infants born to women with active herpes infection. Women of childbearing age with genital herpes must tell their obstetrician about their history of the infection whenever they become pregnant, so they can be followed closely for the signs of the infection as they near term.

Infection Control

Patients with active lesions are infectious and should refrain from sexual activity until the lesions resolve. Patients who have no evidence of active lesions, but who have a history of the disease or are serologically positive for HSV, may pass the infection on to sexual partners, even when asymptomatic. In the health care setting, universal precautions should be observed at all times.

Pearls and Pitfalls

1. Viral meningitis may develop in 33% of women and 10% of men who have primary genital HSV infection.
2. Visceral involvement and disseminated HSV can be life-threatening in HIV-infected patients. Encephalitis is a rare but life-threatening complication of HSV; presentation is often atypical.
3. HSV-1 is the leading cause of sporadic encephalitis in U.S. adults. Benign recurrent lymphocytic meningitis can follow recurrence of genital HSV by 5–7 days.
4. Severe recurrent genital and perirectal symptoms are commonly seen with acquired immunodeficiency syndrome (AIDS) especially in patients with low CD4 counts and high viral loads. HIV-infected patients, especially those with AIDS, need longer treatment and/or higher doses for episodic cutaneous HSV.
5. Between 15% and 65% of all cases of erythema multiforme, and over 70% of recurrent cases, have been associated with HSV.
6. Cutaneous HSV is worse in patients with abnormal skin, such as those with eczema or varicelliform eruption.

SYPHILIS

Epidemiology

Compared to herpes genitalis, syphilis is orders of magnitude less common; annually, the incidence ranges from 7000 to 25,000 cases. This infection is most commonly seen in patients of lower socioeconomic status or in those who abuse drugs, though cases in men who have sex with men without other risk factors have accounted for much of the recent increase in incidence.

Table 17.3 Clinical Features: Syphilis

Organism	*Treponema pallidum*
Incubation Period	• Primary: 3 weeks • Secondary: 7–14 weeks after inoculation • Tertiary: Months to years
Transmission	Syphilis may be spread by contact with the primary chancre, mucous patches in the mouth, the skin lesions of secondary syphilis, or genital condyloma lata.
Signs and Symptoms	• Primary: Usually painless chancre at site of inoculation • Secondary: Rash, usually truncal, may involve palms and soles. Generalized lymphadenopathy. Condyloma lata, mucous patches. May see alopecia. • Tertiary: Dementia, tabes dorsalis, alopecia, gummata.
Laboratory Findings	• Nontreponemal tests (RPR, VDRL): Positive suggests disease; may see false positives; should confirm with treponemal test; activity of test reflects disease activity • Treponemal tests (FTA, MHA-TP): Specific to spirochete; confirmatory test; usually positive for life; activity does not correlate with disease activity

FTA, fluorescent treponemal antibody absorbed; MHA-TP, microhemagglutination assay–*Treponema pallidum*; RPR, rapid plasma reagin; VDRL, venereal disease research laboratory.

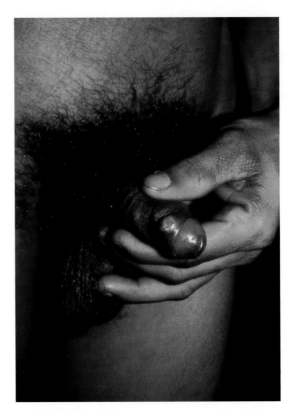

Figure 17.3 Primary syphilitic chancre on the penis. Image courtesy of the Australasian Chapter on Sexual Health Medicine.

Clinical Features

Caused by the spirochete *Treponema pallidum*, syphilis progresses through several stages if untreated (Table 17.3). The primary stage occurs 3 weeks after inoculation with the spirochete. A chancre, usually painless, develops at the site of inoculation (Figure 17.3); occasionally patients may develop multiple lesions, but rarely more than two lesions (Figure 17.4). After 3 weeks the lesion resolves, and the patient becomes asymptomatic.

Four to 10 weeks later the patient may develop symptoms of secondary syphilis. This stage is characterized by a rash, lymphadenopathy, and, occasionally, alopecia. The rash begins as a macular rash and rapidly becomes papulosquamous, occurring primarily on the torso (Figure 17.5); it may also involve the extremities and may involve the palms (Figure 17.6) and soles.

Lesions in the mouth are known as mucous patches and those on the genitalia are condyloma lata (Figure 17.7). All skin, mouth, and genital lesions are infectious. During this stage patients may develop generalized, mildly enlarged lymph nodes. Even untreated, this stage will resolve to latent disease.

Tertiary syphilis may develop decades after primary infection in up to 40% of untreated patients. In this stage, complications such as aortic root aneurysms, skin gummata, and central nervous system disease can cause severe morbidity.

Differential Diagnosis

All of the sexually transmitted diseases that cause genital ulcers should be considered in patients presenting with this complaint:

• herpes genitalis
• chancroid
• granuloma inguinale
• lymphogranuloma venereum

Conditions such as Behçet's syndrome, fixed drug eruptions, scabies, pyoderma gangrenosum, and trauma are also in the differential diagnosis.

Key features that may help to distinguish syphilis from other STDs are:

• patients typically have a single painless genital ulcer
• a truncal papulosquamous rash involving palms and soles
• condyloma lata and/or mucous patches

Laboratory Findings

Both nontreponemal and treponemal tests are available for diagnosing syphilis. Nontreponemal tests such as the rapid plasma reagin (RPR) and venereal disease research laboratory (VDRL) assay determine presence and activity of disease, but false positives may occur, and these tests may be falsely negative in early primary syphilis and long-standing latent disease. Because these tests are quantitative and correlate with disease activity, they can be used to monitor response to therapy. Positive nontreponemal tests should be confirmed with a treponemal test, such as the fluorescent treponemal antibody absorbed (FTA), the treponemal pallidum particle agglutination (TP-PA), or the microhemagglutination assay–*Treponema pallidum* (MHA-TP), which is rarely used anymore. These treponemal tests are specific for the treponeme, and the test is

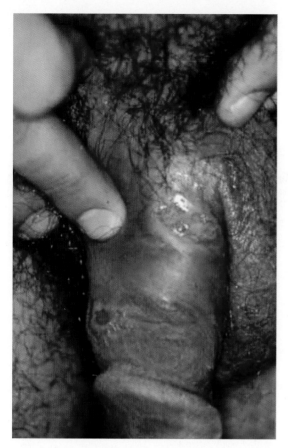

Figure 17.4 Two primary syphilitic lesions on the penile shaft. Image courtesy of the Australasian Chapter on Sexual Health Medicine.

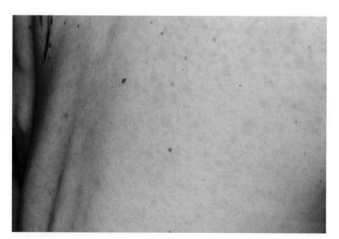

Figure 17.5 The rash of secondary syphilis. Image courtesy of the Australasian Chapter on Sexual Health Medicine.

usually positive for life. Treponemal tests results do not correlate well with disease activity and cannot be used to monitor response to treatment.

Treatment and Prophylaxis

Primary syphilis is treated with one dose of benzathine penicillin G (BPG), 2.4 million units intramuscularly. It is critical to use only benzathine penicillin G, not another formulation or a combination of types of penicillin.

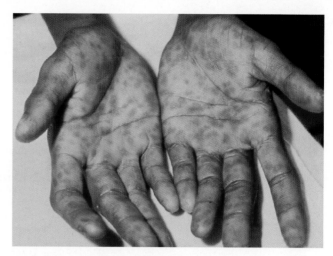

Figure 17.6 Palmar rash due to secondary syphilis. Image courtesy of the Australasian Chapter on Sexual Health Medicine.

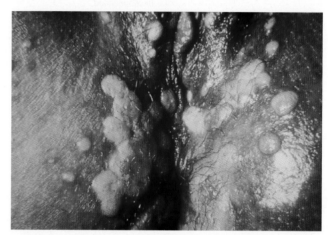

Figure 17.7 Condyloma lata of secondary syphilis. Image courtesy of the Australasian Chapter on Sexual Health Medicine.

Secondary and early latent syphilis are also treated with one dose of benzathine penicillin G, 2.4 million units intramuscularly. Patients with late latent syphilis should receive 1.2 million units intramuscularly once a week for 3 weeks.

Neurosyphilis is treated intravenously with aqueous crystalline penicillin G 18–24 million units daily, given as 3–4 million units intravenous (IV) every 4 hours for 10–14 days (Table 17.4).

Complications and Admission Criteria

Patients with primary and secondary syphilis are managed as outpatients. Neurosyphilis is usually managed in the inpatient setting. Patients infected with HIV may have a more aggressive syphilis infection, and their response to treatment must be monitored closely.

Infection Control

Syphilis may be spread by contact with the primary chancre, mucous patches in the mouth, the skin lesions of secondary syphilis, or genital condyloma lata. Universal precautions should be observed in the health care setting.

Table 17.4 Treatment of Syphilis

Patient Category	Therapy Recommendations
Primary and Secondary Syphilis	Benzathine penicillin G 2.4 million units IM × 1. PCN allergy (nonpregnant, preferred): doxycycline 100 mg PO bid × 14 days *or* tetracycline 500 mg PO qid × 14 days Requires well-documented close follow-up.
Latent syphilis	**Early latent (<1 year infection duration) (with normal CSF exam, if done):** benzathine penicillin G 2.4 million units IM × 1 **Late latent or latent of unknown duration (with normal CSF exam, if done):** benzathine penicillin G 2.4 mil units IM q wk × 3 weeks If any dose >2 days late, must recommence prescription from first dose **PCN allergy recommended:** doxycycline 100 mg PO bid × 4 wks *or* tetracycline 500 mg PO qid × 4 weeks
Neurosyphilis	Only penicillin is currently recommended; allergic persons should be desensitized and treated with penicillin. **Recommended:** aqueous crystalline penicillin G 18–24 million units/day IV, administer as 3–4 million units IV q4h × 10–14 days **Alternative:** procaine penicillin 2.4 million units IM qd, *plus* probenecid 500 mg PO qid × 10–14 days
Syphilis in HIV-Infected	Penicillin is the highly preferred regimen for all stages of syphilis in HIV-infected persons Primary, secondary, and early latent syphilis: use benzathine penicillin G as for non-HIV persons; some experts recommend three weekly doses (i.e., as for late latent syphilis) PCN-allergic HIV with primary, secondary, or early latent syphilis: can be treated as allergic HIV-negative person (although *not* the ideal) Late latent syphilis or syphilis of unknown duration requires a lumbar puncture to rule out neurosyphilis. All require PCN-based treatment. Desensitization required.
Syphilis in Pregnancy	Only penicillin is currently recommended. Treatment during pregnancy should be the penicillin regimen appropriate to the stage of syphilis diagnosed; desensitization required for PCN-allergic pregnant patients. Some experts recommend a second dose of benzathine penicillin G 2.4 million units IM 1 week after the initial dose for primary, secondary, or early latent syphilis in pregnancy.

CSF, cerebrospinal fluid; PCN, penicillin.

Pearls and Pitfalls

1. The rash of secondary syphilis may appear very similar to that of pityriasis rosea. Sexually active patients with a rash that looks like pityriasis rosea should be tested for syphilis.
2. Consider syphilis in *any* sexually active person with a generalized rash or genital ulcer.
3. Treatment of sex partners is key to control of syphilis.
4. Indications for a lumbar puncture in syphilis include neurologic or ophthalmologic signs or symptoms; other evidence of active tertiary syphilis; treatment failure; or HIV infection with latent syphilis or syphilis of unknown duration.
5. Treatment failure can occur with any regimen.
6. Treat high-risk persons before lab results are available because the patient may not return for results.
7. Advancement through stages may be more rapid in HIV-infected persons.
8. Syphilitic lesions usually resolve without treatment while latent infection persists.

CHANCROID

Epidemiology

This ulcerating sexually transmitted disease, caused by *Haemophilus ducreyi*, is uncommon in the United States but may occur in sporadic outbreaks.

Clinical Features

Patients complain of multiple painful genital ulcers within 1–2 weeks of primary infection (Table 17.5); these ulcers are very similar to those of herpes genitalis. Within a week, up to 40% of patients will develop an inguinal bubo, usually unilateral and frequently painful and fluctuant. These buboes may spontaneously rupture and cause a chronic draining sinus. The combination of painful genital ulcers and fluctuant inguinal lymphadenopathy should raise suspicion for this disease (Figure 17.8).

Patients with chancroid can transmit the infection until the ulcer heals. The ulcer heals with or without treatment, but

Table 17.5 Clinical Features: Chancroid

Organism	*Haemophilus ducreyi*
Incubation Period	3–5 days; may be as long as 14 days
Transmission	Direct contact with the lesion
Signs and Symptoms	● Multiple painful genital ulcers ● Painful, enlarged, fluctuant inguinal lymph node
Laboratory Findings	● Diagnosis usually made clinically ● Organism can be cultured, but requires special medium not usually available

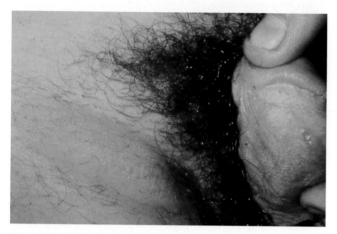

Figure 17.8 Ulcerative lesions on the penis from chancroid with accompanying fluctuant, tender, erythematous lymphadenitis (bubo). Image courtesy of the Australasian Chapter on Sexual Health Medicine.

treatment speeds healing. Chancroid infection increases risk of HIV infection and transmission.

Patients may develop chancroid of the eye or fingers, usually caused by autoinoculation.

Sites of infection include:

● genitalia: genital ulcer(s)
● inguinal lymph nodes: following small, missed genital ulcer or with genital ulcer
● conjunctivae: autoinoculation from genital source
● fingers: can follow autoinoculation or foreplay

Differential Diagnosis

All of the sexually transmitted diseases that cause genital ulcers should be considered in patients presenting with this complaint:

● syphilis
● chancroid
● granuloma inguinale
● lymphogranuloma venereum

Conditions such as Behçet's syndrome, fixed drug eruptions, scabies, pyoderma, and trauma are also in the differential diagnosis.

Key features that may help to distinguish chancroid from other STDs are:

● the presence of a painful, fluctuant inguinal lymph node
● multiple, painful genital ulcers; may look very similar to herpes genitalis

Laboratory Findings

The causative organism, *Haemophilus ducreyi*, is fastidious and requires special growth medium for culture. This medium is not commonly available in most microbiology labs, and the diagnosis is usually made clinically. The criteria for making this diagnosis are:

● The patient has one or more painful genital lesions.
● The patient has no evidence of *T. pallidum* infection by dark-field examination of ulcer exudates or by a serologic test for syphilis performed at least 7 days after the onset of ulcers.
● The clinical presentation, appearance of genital ulcers, and, if present, regional adenopathy are typical for chancroid.
● A test for HSV on the ulcer exudate is negative.

Treatment and Prophylaxis

Recommended treatment for chancroid consists of one of the following: azithromycin, ceftriaxone, ciprofloxacin, or erythromycin base (Table 17.6).

Buboes should not be incised and drained initally, even if they are very fluctuant. If the bubo appears at risk for spontaneous rupture, needle aspiration of the fluid may help relieve pressure. Buboes that do not respond to antibiotic therapy require incision and drainage.

Complications and Admission Criteria

The most serious complication of chancroid is scarring of the lymphatics of the groin caused by lymphadenitis. Early treatment usually prevents this complication; however, patients who present with advanced disease may develop this complication despite appropriate therapy.

Infection Control

This infection is acquired by direct contact with the genital ulcers characteristic of this disease. Universal precautions should be observed.

Pearls and Pitfalls

1. The genital ulcers of chancroid look very much like those seen in patients with herpes genitalis.
2. As chancroid is significantly more rare than herpes and tends to occur in sporadic outbreaks in the United States, cases of this infection can be missed.
3. The combination of painful genital ulcers and a suppurative lymph node suggests a high probability of chancroid. Any patient with painful genital ulcers and fluctuant inguinal lymphadenopathy should be evaluated for chancroid and empiric treatment prior to test results is usually indicated.
4. Up to 10% of patients are co-infected with syphilis; therefore patients with chancroid *must* also be treated for syphilis.

Table 17.6 Treatment of Chancroid Infections

Patient Category	Therapy Recommendations
Recommended Regimen	azithromycin 1 g PO × 1 *or* ceftriaxone 250 mg IM × 1 *or* ciprofloxacin 500 mg PO bid × 3 days *or* erythromycin base 500 mg PO qid × 7 days
Regimens in Pregnancy	ceftriaxone 250 mg IM × 1 *or* erythromycin base 500 mg PO qid × 7 days *or* azithromycin: safety and efficacy in pregnancy and lactation not established
Treatment in HIV Infection	• Some experts recommend the 7-day erythromycin regimen because of slow healing in this group of patients • Efficacy of azithromycin and ceftriaxone unknown in this group. Use only if follow-up is ensured.
Management of Fluctuant Buboes	• Incision and drainage is probably preferred treatment in those not adequately responding to antibiotics alone. • Bubo aspiration is simpler and safer than incision and drainage, but reaspiration is often needed; sinus tracts may form.
Other Management Considerations	• Follow-up: Examine all patients 3–7 days after initiation of treatment. If no clinical improvement: (1) Reassess diagnosis, (2) consider co-infection with another STD or HIV, (3) consider noncompliance, (4) consider antibiotic resistance. • Sex partners: all sex partners from 10 days prior to symptom onset up to the time of treatment should be examined and treated regardless of symptoms. • Candidates for longer treatment and close follow-up: HIV-infected persons; uncircumcised men.

5. Uncircumcised men may be at higher risk and make take longer to cure.
6. No immunity develops after infection.
7. Chancroid is more commonly diagnosed in men, especially if partners include commercial sex workers.

REFERENCES

ACOG. Practice bulletin: management of herpes in pregnancy. Clinical guidelines for obstetrician-gynecologists. Int J Gynaecol Obstet 2000;68:165–73.

Armstrong GL, Schillinger J, Markowitz L, et al. Incidence of herpes simplex type 2 infection in the United States. Am J Epidemiol 2001;153:912–20.

Augenbraum M. Treatment of latent and tertiary syphilis. Hosp Pract 2000;35(4):89–95.

Centers for Disease Control and Prevention (CDC). Brief report: a treatment failures in syphilis infections – San Francisco, California, 2002–2003. MMWR 2004;53(9):197–8.

Centers for Disease Control and Prevention (CDC). Sex CDC. Sexually transmitted diseases: treatment guidelines, 2006. MMWR 2006;55(RR-11).

Gene M, Ledger WJ. Syphilis in pregnancy. Sex Transm Infect 2000;76(2):73–9.

Kimberlin DW, Rouse DJ. Genital herpes. N Engl J Med 2004;350:1970–7.

Lukehart SA, Godornes C, Molini BJ, et al. Macrolide resistance in *Treponema pallidum* in the United States and Ireland. N Engl J Med 2004;351:154–8.

Singh AE, Romanowki B. Syphilis: review with emphasis on clinical, epidemiological, and some biologic features; Clin Microbiol Rev 1999;12(2):187–209.

Steiner I, Biran I. Herpes simplex encephalitis. Curr Treat Options Infect Dis 2002;4:491–9.

Whittington WL, Celum CL, Cent A, et al. Use of a glyco-protein G-based type-specific assay to detect antibodies to herpes simplex virus type among personnel attending sexually transmitted disease clinics. Sex Transm Dis 2001;28:99–104.

ADDITIONAL READINGS

Ernst AA, Marvez-Valls E, Martin DH. Incision and drainage versus aspiration of fluctuant buboes in the emergency department during an epidemic of chancroid. Sex Transm Dis 1995;22:217–20.

Lewis DA. Diagnostic tests for chancroid. Sex Transm Infect 2000;76:137–41.

Steen R, Dallabetta G, Genital ulcer disease control and HIV prevention. J Clin Virol 2004;29:143–51.

18. Nonulcerative Sexually Transmitted Diseases

Diane Birnbaumer

INTRODUCTION – AGENTS

Sexually transmitted diseases are best divided into two major groups: those that cause ulcerative lesions (see Chapter 17, Ulcerative Sexually Transmitted Diseases) and those that do not. Diseases that fall into this latter group include chlamydial infections, gonococcal infections, nongonococcal urethritis, and human papilloma virus (HPV). Although new tests make diagnosis easier, results are often not available during an acute care visit, and empiric treatment with appropriate follow-up is often the best approach.

CHLAMYDIA

Epidemiology

Chlamydia trachomatis, when sexually transmitted, most commonly causes urethritis in men and cervicitis in women. The incidence of this infection is 3 to 5 million cases annually, making it the most common sexually transmitted infection in the United States.

Clinical Features

In men, _C. trachomatis_ most commonly causes urethritis with dysuria and/or a clear urethral discharge (Table 18.1). Women, in contrast, are asymptomatic in 70–80% of cases, though rare complaints include dysuria, vaginal discharge, and spotting.

Differential Diagnosis

The differential diagnosis for _Chlamydia_ includes:

Urethritis:

- _Neisseria gonorrhoeae_
- _Mycoplasma genitalium_
- _Ureaplasma urealyticum_
- adenovirus
- herpes simplex virus
- _Trichomonas vaginalis_

Noninfectious causes such as Reiter's syndrome and contact dermatitis from topical preparations or latex condoms should also be considered in the differential diagnosis.

Cervicitis:

C. trachomatis and _N. gonorrhoeae_ are the most common causes of acute cervicitis. As mentioned above, noninfectious causes, including contact dermatitis from douches, scented tampons, vaginal creams, or latex condoms should also be considered.

GONORRHEA

Epidemiology

Gonorrhea is caused by the organism _Neisseria gonorrhoeae_. It is highly infectious and can disseminate beyond the genital tract to other parts of the body. The risk of transmission after a single sexual encounter with a person infected with gonorrhea is around 50%.

Table 18.1 Clinical Features: _Chlamydia_

Organism	Chlamydia trachomatis
Signs and Symptoms	**Men:** • Dysuria and/or clear urethral discharge **Women:** • Frequently asymptomatic
Laboratory Findings	• Male urethritis: Urine positive for leukocyte esterase; ≥10 WBC per hpf on examination of urine sediment; ≥5 WBC per hpf on Gram stain of the urine • Male urethritis: Urine/urethral swabs: nucleic acid amplification test (NAAT) positive for _Chlamydia_ • Female cervicitis: Urine/cervical swabs: NAATs positive for _Chlamydia_
hpf, high-power field; NAAT, nucleic acid amplification test; WBC, white blood cell.	

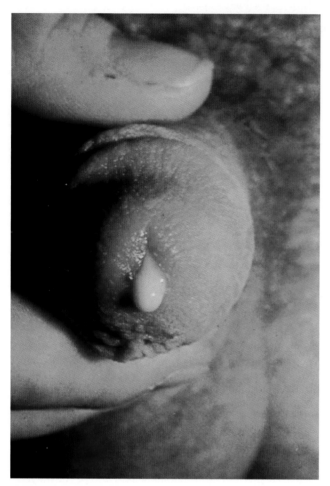

Figure 18.1 Purulent urethral discharge in a patient with gonorrhea. Image courtesy of the Australasian Chapter on Sexual Health Medicine.

Table 18.2 Clinical Features: Gonorrhea

Organism	*Neisseria gonorrhoeae*
Incubation period	Less than 1 week; may be as little as 2 days
Signs and Symptoms	**Ophthalmology**: May develop corneal ulceration, hyperopion, and endophthalmitis **Disseminated gonococcal infection**: Septic arthritis and skin lesions; rare cases of meningitis and endocarditis **Genitourinary**: **Men**: ● Dysuria and purulent urethral discharge **Women**: ● Cervicitis ● Often infection is asymptomatic ● Nonspecific symptoms such as a mild vaginal discharge or spotting, particularly after intercourse, may occur
Laboratory Findings	● Gram stain positive for gram-negative intracellular diplococci (urethral or conjunctival discharge). Negative Gram stain does not rule out the diagnosis, and other testing is needed. ● Male urethritis: Urine or urethral swabs: NAAT positive for gonorrhea ● Female cervicitis: Urine/cervical swabs: NAATs positive for gonorrhea; cervical swabs preferred specimen source in women

NAAT, nucleic acid amplification test.

Clinical Features

In men, gonorrhea most commonly causes urethritis characterized by a purulent urethral discharge (Figure 18.1) and dysuria. Women infected with gonorrhea often have cervicitis, which may present with a mild vaginal discharge, or spotting, particularly after intercourse (Table 18.2). Gonorrhea may also infect the rectum and pharynx, but patients are often asymptomatic when infection occurs in these areas.

Gonococcal conjunctivitis is a potentially sight-threatening infection. Patients present with a purulent eye discharge and chemosis and may develop corneal ulceration, hypopion, and endophthalmitis. Globe perforation may occur in neglected, inadequately treated, or advanced cases.

Gonorrhea disseminates in 0.5–3% of untreated patients. Patients with disseminated gonococcal infection most commonly develop septic arthritis and skin lesions; in rare cases, the infection may cause meningitis and endocarditis. The septic arthritis is usually mono- or oligoarticular, most frequently involving the knee. The skin lesions are commonly described as necrotic pustules on an erythematous base. They occur on the distal extremities and usually total fewer than 20 lesions.

Differential Diagnosis

The differential diagnosis includes:

● Conjunctivitis: Other causes including *Staphylococcus*, *Streptococcus*, and viruses should be considered.

● Gonococcal arthritis: As gonococcal arthritis is a true septic process, not a reactive arthritis, other bacterial causes including *Staphylococcus aureus* should also be considered. Trauma, rheumatologic conditions, and degenerative joint disease may also cause joint symptoms.

● Gonococcal skin lesions: Community-acquired methicillin-resistant *S. aureus* infection may cause skin lesions similar to those caused by *N. gonorrhoeae*.

Key features that may help to distinguish gonorrhea from other STDs are:

● presence of a purulent discharge, which may be copious in men with urethritis
● marked chemosis in patients with conjunctival infections
● a single septic knee joint in a sexually active patient should suggest disseminated gonococcal infection

Laboratory Findings

Gram stain may be useful in making the diagnosis in patients with conjunctivitis, or urethritis when there is exudate at the urethral meatus. In men, a Gram stain positive for gram-negative intracellular diplococci is more than 99% specific and 95% sensitive in making the diagnosis of gonorrhea; however, a negative Gram stain does not rule out the diagnosis and further testing is needed in these cases.

Nucleic acid amplification tests (NAATs) on urine, urethral swabs, or cervical swabs can be used to diagnose gonorrhea and *Chlamydia*. Urine testing in men has adequate sensitivity and specificity to make the diagnosis (95–97% sensitive,

Table 18.3 Treatment of *Chlamydia* Infections

Recommended regimen:
azithromycin 1 g PO single dose
or
doxycycline 100 mg PO bid × 7 days
Alternative regimens:
(all 7-day regimens)
erythromycin 500 mg PO qid
or
ofloxacin 300 mg PO bid
or
levofloxacin 500 mg PO qd
or
erythromycin ethylsuccinate 800 mg PO qid

Table 18.4 Treatment of Gonorrheal Infections

Uncomplicated Infections of Urethra, Cervix or Rectum	ceftriaxone 125 mg IM *or* cefixime 400 mg PO Plus treatment for *Chlamydia* unless ruled out by negative testing
Uncomplicated Pharyngeal Infection	ceftriaxone 125 mg IM single dose Plus treatment for *Chlamydia* unless ruled out by negative testing
Adult Conjunctivitis	Consider hospitalization Normal saline irrigation and ceftriaxone 1 g IM once
Disseminated Gonococcal Infection (see Chapter 4, Systemic Diseases Causing Fever and Rash)	Strongly consider hospitalization **Recommended regimen:** ceftriaxone 1 g IM or IV every 24 hours **Alternative regimens:** cefotaxime 1 g IV q8h *or* ceftizoxime 1 g IV q8h *or* spectinomycin* 2 g IM q12h Treatment should be continued for 24–48 hours after improvement, at which time therapy may be switched to one of the following regimens to complete at least 1 week of antimicrobial therapy. cefixime† 400 mg PO bid *or* cefixime 400 mg by suspension (200 mg/5 ml) bid *or* cefpodoxime 400 mg PO bid

Important note: Because of a high level of resistance, fluoroquinolones are no longer recommended to treat gonorrhea.
*Spectinomycin is currently not available in the United States.
†The tablet formulation of cefixime is currently not available in the United States.

>99% specific); in women, the sensitivity of NAAT is particularly dependent on the assay and urine collection method, and some institutions prefer endocervical swabs to diagnose gonorrhea (urine sensitivity 90–95%; cervical swab sensitivity 95–99%; specificity >99% for both).

There are only a few NAATs approved for the diagnosis of pharyngeal or rectal infection, and these often must be sent to a specific lab. When these tests are not available, pharyngeal or rectal swab should be sent for culture and sensitivity.

In all cases, NAATs cannot be used to determine organism antibiotic sensitivity, and are not a replacement for cultures if sensitivities are important to patient management or public health.

Testing for culture and sensitivity is recommended for any patient suspected of having disseminated gonococcal infection. Cultures from the symptomatic site (e.g., of arthrocentesis fluid or skin lesions), and blood are indicated. In addition, patients need cultures of the sites that are potential sources of dissemination; this includes the rectum and pharynx in both genders, and the urethra in men and cervix in women.

CHLAMYDIA AND GONORRHEA: TREATMENT

Chlamydia

Chlamydia is treated with a single dose of oral azithromycin; an alternative regimen is doxycycline for 7 days (Table 18.3). Although more expensive and with some documented treatment failures, the single dose of azithromycin can be given during the patient's index visit and ensures compliance with a complete therapeutic course.

Alternative treatment regimens include erythromycin, ofloxacin, levofloxacin, or erythromycin ethylsuccinate.

Gonorrhea

There are several single-dose regimens that can be used to treat uncomplicated gonorrheal infections of the urethra, cervix, or rectum (Table 18.4). Cefixime and ceftriaxone are options; the prevalence of quinolone-resistant *N. gonorrhoeae* (QRNG) is increasing rapidly in the United States, and fluoroquinolones are no longer recommended.

Pharyngeal gonorrhea should be treated with ceftriaxone.

Gonococcal conjunctivitis is treated with ceftriaxone. These patients should also undergo saline lavage of the infected eye.

Patients with disseminated gonorrhea should be admitted for initial therapy. The recommended regimen is ceftriaxone, 1 g intramuscularly (IM) or intravenously (IV) every 24 hours. Alternative regimens include cefotaxime, or ceftizoxime, or spectinomycin.

Until recently, patients treated for gonorrhea were also treated for *Chlamydia* because of the high rate of co-infection with both organisms. In institutions where NAAT results are immediately available, a negative *Chlamydia* NAAT result mitigates the need for additional treatment. If, however, results will not be available during the patient's acute care stay, patients should be treated presumptively for both infections.

CHLAMYDIA AND GONORRHEA: COMPLICATIONS AND ADMISSION CRITERIA

Chlamydia

Patients with *Chlamydia* infections rarely develop complications during the index infection. Women may go on to develop pelvic inflammatory disease (PID); criteria for admitting these patients are listed in the PID section below. Men may develop epididymitis and/or orchitis, but rarely require admission.

Gonorrhea

Disseminated gonococcal infection is the most common complication of untreated gonorrhea infections; these patients should usually be admitted as part of their initial treatment. Men may also develop epididymitis and/or orchitis; rarely, these patients are symptomatic enough to need hospitalization. Women with gonococcal PID may be very ill and require hospitalization.

NONGONOCOCCAL URETHRITIS
Epidemiology

While commonly caused by *Chlamydia* and gonorrhea, urethritis may also be caused by *Mycoplasma genitalium, Ureaplasma urealyticum, Trichomonas vaginalis*, HSV, and adenovirus. With a recent decrease in rates of infection with *C. trachomatis*, these organisms are becoming more frequently recognized as causes of nongonococcal urethritis (NGU) in men. These patients present with typical symptoms of urethritis and frequently return for care when initial treatment for *Chlamydia* and gonorrhea does not cure their symptoms.

Clinical Features

Patients commonly present with dysuria and/or a urethral discharge and may have been treated for urethritis already.

Differential Diagnosis

The differential diagnosis includes other infectious agents such as *Chlamydia* and gonorrhea, as well as Reiter's syndrome and local irritants.

Laboratory Findings

Patients with this infection often fail initial treatment for *Chlamydia* and gonorrhea and return with persistent symptoms. The diagnosis of NGU is made in patients who have negative *Chlamydia* and gonorrhea testing, and who meet criteria for urethritis.

Diagnostic criteria include:

- mucopurulent or purulent discharge
- Gram stain showing 5 or more WBCs per oil immersion field
- positive leukocyte esterase test on first-void urine or specimen that has at least 10 WBCs per high power field.

Treatment

Treatment is either azithromycin 1 g orally once or doxycycline 100 mg orally twice a day for 7 days (if this regimen was not used during an earlier visit). Alternative regimens include erythromycin base, or erythromycin ethylsuccinate, or ofloxacin, or levofloxacin for 7 days. Patients who have recurrent or persistent urethritis despite this treatment should receive metronidazole 2 g orally as a single dose, or tinidazole 2 g orally as a single dose, or azithromycin 1 g orally as a single dose (if not used for initial treatment).

Table 18.5 Clinical Features: Nongonococcal Urethritis

Organisms	• *Chlamydia trachomatis* • *Mycoplasma genitalium* • *Ureaplasma urealyticum* • *Trichomonas vaginalis* • HSV • adenovirus
Incubation period	Variable
Signs and Symptoms	Dysuria with or without urethral discharge
Laboratory Findings	(1) Mucopurulent or purulent discharge, (2) Gram stain showing ≥5 WBCs per oil immersion field, and (3) positive leukocyte esterase test on first-void urine or specimen that shows ≥10 WBCs per high-power field.
Treatment	**Recommended regimen:** azithromycin 1 g PO single dose *or* doxycycline 100 mg PO bid × 7 days **Alternative regimens:** erythromycin base 500 mg PO qid × 7 days *or* erythromycin ethylsuccinate 800 mg PO qid × 7 days *or* ofloxacin 300 mg PO bid × 7 days *or* levofloxacin 500 mg PO qd × 7 days **Treatment for persistent or recurrent NGU:** metronidazole 2 g PO single dose *or* tinidazole 2 g PO single dose *or* azithromycin 1 g PO single dose (if not used for initial treatment)

WBC, white blood cell.

Complications and Admission Criteria

Complications of this infection are rare.

PELVIC INFLAMMATORY DISEASE
Epidemiology

Nearly 1 million cases of PID are diagnosed annually in the United States. This infection of the upper female genital tract can be caused by several organisms, including *C. trachomatis, N. gonorrhoeae, Mycoplasma, Ureaplasma*, vaginal aerobes, and facultative anaerobes; in fact, infection caused by multiple organisms is common. PID can be a life-altering infection, as complications are common.

Clinical Features

This infection of the female upper genital tract causes a wide array of symptoms (Table 18.6). Patients may be asymptomatic, have mild symptoms such as pelvic pain and dyspareunia, or have severe illness characterized by peritoneal signs and systemic toxicity. Making the diagnosis of PID is

Table 18.6 Clinical Features: Pelvic Inflammatory Disease

Organisms	• *Chlamydia trachomatis* • *Neisseria gonorrhoeae* • *Mycoplasma* • *Ureaplasma* • Vaginal aerobes and facultative anaerobes
Incubation period	Days to years
Signs and Symptoms	• Severe cases: fever, abdominal pain, peritoneal signs, systemic toxicity • Mild cases: dyspareunia, pelvic pain, abdominal pain • May be asymptomatic
Laboratory Findings	• Laboratory testing may be misleadingly normal • Patients may have an elevated erythrocyte sedimentation rate, peripheral WBC count, or C-reactive protein
Treatment	**Outpatient Therapy** **Regimen A**: ceftriaxone 250 mg IM once *plus* doxycycline 100 mg PO bid × 14 days *with or without* metronidazole 500 mg PO bid × 14 days **Regimen B**: cefoxitin 2 g IM plus probenecid 1 g PO concurrently ×1 *plus* doxycycline 100 mg PO bid × 14 days *with or without* metronidazole 500 mg PO bid × 14 days **Inpatient Therapy** **Regimen A**: cefoxitin 2 g IV q6h (or cefotetan 2 g IV q12h) *plus* doxycycline 100 mg PO or IV q12h Continue until at least 48 hours after improvement Continue doxycycline for a 10- to 14-day course total **Regimen B**: clindamycin 900 mg IV q8h *plus* gentamicin 2 mg/kg load IV or IM Then 1.5 mg/kg IV or IM q8h Continue until at least 48 hours after improvement Continue doxycycline for 10–14 days total

Important note: Because of a high level of resistance, fluoroquinolones are no longer recommended to treat gonorrhea.
WBC, white blood cell.

often difficult. The "gold standard" is laparoscopy, but the diagnosis of PID is usually made clinically, based on the following criteria:

1. complaints of pelvic or lower abdominal pain, *and*
2. cervical motion tenderness, adnexal tenderness, or uterine tenderness.

The goal of using this low diagnostic threshold is to identify and treat the mild cases of PID in an attempt to prevent complications, such as chronic pelvic pain, infertility, and ectopic pregnancy.

Differential Diagnosis

Any condition that causes lower abdominal symptoms in women may mimic PID:

- ovarian cysts
- ovarian torsion
- ectopic pregnancy
- appendicitis
- tubo-ovarian abscess
- diverticulitis

Unfortunately, presentation of these conditions may appear clinically to be quite similar; often, further testing such as ultrasound or computed tomographic (CT) scanning may be necessary to make the diagnosis. In clinically unclear cases, laparoscopy may lead to a definitive diagnosis.

Laboratory Findings

Though the diagnosis is usually made clinically, and laparoscopy is the gold standard, there is limited evidence suggesting that greater than 5 WBCs on wet mount microscopy of endocervical swab in the setting of abdominal pain is highly predictive of PID.

Treatment

Because of a high level of fluoroquinolone resistance, these agents are no longer recommended to treat gonorrhea. Treatment choices are (1) ceftriaxone *plus* doxycycline with or without metronidazole, *or* (2) cefoxitin *plus* probenecid *plus* doxycycline with or without metronidazole.

Inpatient treatment consists of two possible regimens. The recommended regimen A is cefoxitin *or* cefotetan, *plus* doxycycline. Recommended inpatient regimen B is clindamycin *plus* gentamicin. Alternative regimens are (1) levofloxacin with or without metronidazole, or (2) ofloxacin with or without metronidazole, or (3) ampicillin-sulbactam *plus* doxycycline. Again, local susceptibility patterns must be confirmed prior to treating PID with quinolones. Please see Table 18.6 for specific doses.

Complications and Admission Criteria

Early complications of this infection are tubo-ovarian abscess and the right upper quadrant pain of perihepatitis (Fitz-Hugh–Curtis syndrome). Because of scarring of the upper genital tract, long-term complications include chronic pelvic pain, chronic dyspareunia, infertility, and an increased risk of ectopic pregnancy.

Criteria for admission in the setting of PID include:

- pregnancy
- failure to respond clinically to oral antimicrobials
- inability to complete or tolerate an outpatient oral regimen
- severe illness, nausea and vomiting, or high fever
- concomitant tubo-ovarian abscess

Table 18.7 Clinical Features: Human Papilloma Virus

Organism	Human papilloma virus
Incubation period	Variable – weeks to years
Signs and Symptoms	• Flat, papular, or pedunculated warts on the genitalia or around the anus • Patients often are asymptomatic
Laboratory Findings	• Pap smear with cytologic testing is the standard screening procedure, looking for cervical neoplasia • Tissue biopsy may be necessary • HPV DNA testing includes hybrid capture II and polymerase chain reaction testing; both are highly sensitive

Treatment	**Patient-Applied:**
	• Podofilox 0.5% solution or gel
	  Apply solution with a cotton swab or gel with a finger.
	  Apply to visible genital warts twice a day for 3 days, followed by 4 days of no therapy. This cycle may be repeated, as necessary, for up to four cycles.
	  The total wart area treated should not exceed 10 cm^2.
	  Total volume of podofilox should be limited to 0.5 mL per day.
	  Demonstrate the proper application technique and identify which warts should be treated.
	    The safety of podofilox during pregnancy has not been established.
	  or
	• Imiquimod 5% cream
	  Apply imiquimod cream once daily at bedtime, three times a week for up to 16 weeks.
	  The treatment area should be washed with soap and water 6–10 hours after the application.
	  The safety of imiquimod during pregnancy has not been established.
	Provider-Administered:
	• Cryotherapy
	  Liquid nitrogen or cryoprobe.
	  Repeat applications every 1–2 weeks.
	  or
	• Podophyllin resin 10%–25% in a compound tincture of benzoin
	  Apply a small amount to each wart and allow to air dry.
	  Treatment can be repeated weekly, if necessary.
	  To avoid the possibility of complications associated with systemic absorption and toxicity:
	  1. Application should be limited to <0.5 mL of podophyllin or an area of <10 cm^2 of warts per session, and
	  2. No open lesions or wounds should exist in the area to which treatment is administered. Some specialists suggest that the preparation should be thoroughly washed off 1–4 hours after application to reduce local irritation.
	  The safety of podophyllin during pregnancy has not been established.
	  or
	• Trichloroacetic acid or bichloroacetic acid 80–90%
	  Apply a small amount only to the warts and allow to dry, at which time a white "frosting" develops.
	  If an excess amount of acid is applied, the treated area should be powdered with talc, sodium bicarbonate (i.e., baking soda), or liquid soap preparations to remove unreacted acid.
	  This treatment can be repeated weekly, if necessary.
	  or
	• Surgical removal

• cases in which other surgical emergencies such as appendicitis cannot be excluded

HUMAN PAPILLOMA VIRUS

Epidemiology

Two hundred million Americans are infected with human papilloma virus (HPV), the virus that causes condyloma acuminata, or genital warts. Although some infections cause lesions, most are asymptomatic or unrecognized. The prevalence of HPV infection is 22–35% in women and 2–35% in men. More than 100 types of HPV exist and 30 to 40 of these can cause genital infection. Whereas types 6 and 11 are most commonly associated with genital warts, others are strongly associated with cervical neoplasia (types 16, 18, 31, 33, and 35).

Clinical Features

Most HPV infections are asymptomatic and self-limited. When HPV causes symptoms, patients complain of lesions on the genital mucosa (Table 18.7). These warts can be flat, papular, or pedunculated growths and are found on moist surfaces such as the vulvae, introitus, and cervix, perianally, and on the shaft of the penis. Women additionally may have cervical infection manifested by flat warts only seen on colposcopy.

Differential Diagnosis

Condyloma lata, a skin condition seen in secondary syphilis, and malignancy such as squamous cell carcinoma should be considered in the differential diagnosis.

Laboratory Findings

Anogenital lesions are often highly suggestive of HPV infection, and treatment is frequently based on a clinical diagnosis. As this is a sexually transmitted disease, evaluation for other sexually transmitted disease is often indicated. Syphilis testing, including dark-field examination, should be considered, as flat condyloma acuminata lesions may resemble those seen with the condyloma lata seen in secondary syphilis.

The most common way to diagnose HPV infection is through screening with routine Pap smears with cytologic testing. Cervical dysplasia or neoplasia should prompt further testing and tissue biopsy may be necessary. HPV DNA testing of cervical scrapings is available and includes HC II (hybrid capture II) and PCR (polymerase chain reaction) testing. Both tests are highly sensitive.

Treatment and Admission Criteria

HPV is treated topically with the goal of eradicating or reducing symptoms. There are many topical options available, and none has been demonstrated to be significantly superior to any other. Multiple treatment applications are required over weeks to months. These treatments may rarely cause local skin reactions and pain.

The two categories of treatments are immune response modifiers and cytotoxic agents. Immune response modifiers include imiquimod and interferon α, and cytotoxic agents include antiproliferative (podofilox, podophyllin, and 5-fluorouracil) and chemodestructive (salicylic acid, trichloroacetic acid [TCA] and bichloroacetic acid [BCA]) agents.

Surgical treatment may be necessary for extensive lesions or those unresponsive to topical medications. Advantages of surgical therapy include single-treatment regimens with decreased recurrence, although cryosurgery may require multiple sessions to eradicate the lesions.

Complications

The most concerning complication of HPV infection is cervical cancer, particularly its association with HPV serotypes 16, 18, 31, 33, and 35. Patients with anogenital HPV infection are also at increased risk of developing vaginal and anal carcinoma.

Prevention

In 2006, the FDA licensed an HPV vaccine for use in women aged 9–26 years. This vaccine is virtually 100% protective against four HPV types, which together are responsible for 70% of cases of cervical cancer and 90% of cases of anogenital warts. The full vaccination series requires three injections over a 6-month period.

Abstinence is the only way to eliminate the risk of transmission of sexually transmitted diseases, but safe sex practices dramatically decrease this risk. Education about barrier protection and safe sex practice is an essential addition to treatment.

INFECTION CONTROL

Universal precautions should be observed for all patients with sexually transmitted infections. No isolation is required.

PEARLS AND PITFALLS

1. Patients diagnosed with *Chlamydia* and gonorrhea should refrain from sexual activity during and for 7 days after completion of treatment; treat all partners from the period of 60 days prior to diagnosis.
2. Have a low threshold to treat patients presenting to the emergency department with symptoms suggestive of *Chlamydia* or gonorrhea. Deferring treatment until the patient has definitive test results may lead to undertreated disease and increased transmission.
3. Any sexually active patient who presents with a single septic joint should be evaluated for disseminated gonococcal infection.
4. Chemosis and purulent eye discharge suggest a gonococcal conjunctivitis. Consider sending a Gram stain and culture of the discharge and treat empirically if there is a high suspicion of the infection.
5. Patients who present for care who have been adequately treated for *Chlamydia* and gonorrhea but remain symptomatic should have diagnostic testing to ensure that the patient has urethritis and treated accordingly.
6. The Centers for Disease Control and Prevention recommend a low clinical threshold to diagnose and treat PID. Failure to do so may put the patient at risk for long-term complications from untreated PID, including chronic pelvic pain, chronic dyspareunia, infertility, and increased risk for ectopic pregnancy.
7. Patients with HPV infections should be referred to a primary care provider who can initiate or continue treatment and monitor the patient's response and follow Pap smears in women with the infection.
8. Testing for other sexually transmitted disease is indicated, particularly syphilis, which can also present with skin lesions.

REFERENCES

Centers for Disease Control and Prevention (CDC). Screening tests to detect *Chlamydia trachomatis* and *Neisseria gonorrhoeae* infections, 2002. MMWR 2002;51(RR-15).

Centers for Disease Control and Prevention (CDC). Increased in fluoroquinolone-resistant Neisseria gonorrhoeae among men who have sex with men – United States, 2003 and revised recommendations for gonorrhea treatment, 2004. MMWR 2004;53(16):335–8.

Centers for Disease Control and Prevention (CDC). Sexually transmitted diseases: treatment guidelines, 2006. MMWR 2006;55(RR-11).

Lau C-Y, Qureshi AK; Azithromycin versus doxycycline for genital chlamydial infections: a meta-analysis of randomized clinical trials. Sex Transm Dis 2002;29(9):497–502.

Mehta SD, Rothman RE, Kelen GD, et al. Clinical aspects of diagnosis of gonorrhea and *Chlamydia* infection in an acute care setting. Clin Infect Dis 2001;32:655–9.

Mehta SD, Rothman RE, Kelen GD, et al. Unsuspected gonorrhea and chlamydia in patients of an urban adult emergency department: a critical population for STD control intervention. Sex Transm Dis 2001;28:33–9.

Rousseau MC, Pereira JS, Prade JC, et al. Cervical coinfection with human papillomavirus (HPV) types as a predictor of acquisition and persistence of HPV infection. J Infect Dis 2001;184:1508–17.

Westrom L. Consequences of pelvic inflammatory disease. New York: Raven Press, 1992:100–10.

Whittington WL, Celum CL, Cent A, et al. Use of a glycoprotein G-based type-specific assay to detect antibodies to herpes simplex virus type among personnel attending sexually transmitted disease clinics. Sex Transm Dis 2001;28:99–104.

19. Vulvovaginitis

Diane Birnbaumer

INTRODUCTION

Vulvovaginitis prompts more than 10 million physician visits annually in the United States. Most cases are caused by infectious agents, including *Gardnerella vaginalis*, *Trichomonas vaginalis*, and *Candida* species.

Diagnosis of a specific causative organism in patients with vulvovaginitis can be difficult. Although signs, symptoms, and laboratory testing may suggest an organism, significant overlap exists in the specificity and sensitivity of these diagnostic tools, and empiric treatment may be the best approach.

BACTERIAL VAGINOSIS

Epidemiology

Bacterial vaginosis is caused by *Gardnerella vaginalis*, an anaerobic bacillus. Infection occurs when this organism replaces the usual *Lactobacillus* species found in vaginal flora. Although infection is associated with multiple sexual partners, women who are not sexually active may acquire this infection; as such, it should not be considered a sexually transmitted disease. This organism is found in up to 40% of asymptomatic women, and men may harbor the organism asymptomatically in the urethra, posing a potential infectious source.

Clinical Features

Symptomatic patients present complaining of a foul or fishy vaginal odor and may have a vaginal discharge (Table 19.1). Only a minority of patients with this infection complain of pruritis. On examination, the vaginal mucosa is not usually inflamed, but there is frequently a thin, homogeneous, gray-white vaginal discharge that may be fishy or foul smelling.

Laboratory Findings

A vaginal swab should be obtained for Gram stain and/or wet preparation. To increase diagnostic accuracy, vaginal fluid should be pH tested.

The Centers for Disease Control and Prevention diagnostic criteria for bacterial vaginosis are:

- homogenous, white, inflammatory discharge that smoothly coats the vaginal walls
- vaginal fluid pH greater than 4.5
- fishy odor of vaginal discharge before or after the addition of 10% KOH (a positive amine odor test or "whiff" test)

Treatment

Bacterial vaginosis can be treated with oral or topical metronidazole or clindamycin (Table 19.2). Patients taking metronidazole should be instructed to refrain from consuming alcohol until at least 24 hours after taking the last dose of the medication.

Treatment is not recommended for nonpregnant, asymptomatic women. All pregnant women who meet diagnostic criteria for bacterial vaginosis (BV) and are symptomatic *or* at risk for preterm delivery should be treated. Treatment of asymptomatic pregnant women with bacterial vaginosis and no other risk factors for preterm delivery is controversial; consider an obstetreics consult.

Table 19.1 Clinical Features: Bacterial Vaginosis

Organism	*Gardnerella vaginalis*
Signs and Symptoms	• Foul or fishy vaginal odor • Vaginal discharge; usually thin, gray-white in color
Laboratory Findings	• Gram stain or wet mount positive for clue cells • Vaginal fluid pH >4.5 • May see WBCs on wet mount
WBC, white blood cell.	

Table 19.2 Treatment of Bacterial Vaginosis

Patient Category	Therapy Recommendations

Adults:
Nonpregnant Patient
	Recommended regimens:
	metronidazole 500 mg orally bid × 7 days
	or
	metronidazole gel 0.75%, one applicator
	  intravaginally bid × 5 days
	or
	clindamycin cream 2%, one applicator
	  intravaginally at bedtime × 7 days
	Alternative regimens:
	clindamycin 300 mg orally bid × 7 days
	or
	clindamycin ovules 100 g intravaginally once at
	  bedtime ×3 days

Adults:
Pregnant Patient
	metronidazole 500 mg orally bid × 7 days
	or
	metronidazole 250 mg orally three times
	  a day × 7 days
	or
	clindamycin 300 mg orally bid × 7 days
	Use clindamycin only during the first half of
	  pregnancy because of risk of adverse events
	  in fetus

Patients taking metronidazole should be instructed to refrain from consuming alcohol until at least 24 hours after taking the last dose of the medication. Treatment of nonpregnant, asymptomatic women with BV is not recommended.

Complications and Admission Criteria

Complications are rare in nonpregnant women. However, bacterial vaginosis during pregnancy is associated with increased risk of adverse pregnancy outcomes, particularly premature birth in women with risk factors for preterm delivery.

Infection Control

Treatment of sexual partners does not affect the patient's response to treatment or risk of relapse; therefore the treatment of sexual partners is not recommended. As this infection may occur in women who are not sexually active, abstinence does not mitigate the risk of infection.

TRICHOMONIASIS

Epidemiology

Trichomonas causes 2–3 million infections annually and is commonly co-transmitted with other sexually transmitted diseases. Caused by the flagellated protozoan *Trichomonas vaginalis*, this infection is found in both men and women.

Clinical Features

Most commonly patients complain of a vaginal discharge that may described as foul-smelling and may be yellow-green in color (Table 19.3). Patients also complain of vulvovaginal pruritis or pain and may have dysuria. Up to half of patients complain of dyspareunia. On exam the vaginal wall may be diffusely erythematous and the vulva mildly edematous or excoriated. Vaginal discharge is noted in over half of patients and may be yellow, gray, or yellow-green. The classically described "strawberry cervix" (caused by diffuse punctuate

Table 19.3 Clinical Features: Trichomoniasis

Organism	*Trichomonas vaginalis*
Signs and Symptoms	• Vaginal discharge • Vulvovaginal soreness or fullness • Vulvovaginal pruritis • Dyspareunia • Diffuse erythema of vaginal wall • Strawberry cervix
Laboratory Findings	• Wet mount demonstrating flagellated protozoa • Vaginal fluid pH >4.5 • Many WBCs on wet mount typical

WBC, white blood cell.

tiny hemorrhages) is uncommon and is seen in only 2% of patients.

Laboratory Findings

A vaginal (not endocervical) swab should be sent for wet mount. Because the sensitivity of the wet preparation is 60–70% and decreases rapidly with time after sampling, the wet mount should be examined as soon as possible after obtaining the specimen. Point-of-care tests using immunochromatography or nucleic acid probe testing are available but not widely used. Vaginal culture is considered the most sensitive and specific means of making the diagnosis and can be used in suspected cases not confirmed by other testing.

Diagnosis of trichomoniasis is suggested by the following findings:

- profuse, yellow, homogeneous discharge
- strawberry cervix (colpitis macularis)
- pH greater than 4.5
- motile trichomonads on saline wet mount
- positive whiff test

Treatment

Recommended treatment by the Centers for Disease Control and Prevention is metronidazole or tinidazole (Table 19.4).

Table 19.4 Treatment of Trichomoniasis

Patient Category	Therapy Recommendations
Adults: **Nonpregnant Patient**	**Recommended regimen:** metronidazole 2 g orally as a single dose *or* tinidazole 2 g orally in a single dose **Alternative regimen:** metronidazole 500 mg orally bid × 7 days

Adults:
Pregnant Patient
	Discuss risks and benefits of treatment with
	  patient and her obstetrician
	If treatment used:
	metronidazole 2 g orally as a single dose
	Note: Tinidazole is pregnancy category C and its
	  safety in pregnancy has not been well
	  evaluated

Patients taking metronidazole should be instructed to refrain from consuming alcohol until at least 24 hours after taking the last dose of the medication. Treatment of nonpregnant, asymptomatic women with trichomoniasis is not recommended.

Complications and Admission Criteria

Vaginal trichomoniasis during pregnancy has been associated with adverse pregnancy outcomes, including premature rupture of membranes, preterm delivery, and low birth weight. Unfortunately, treatment with metronidazole does not appear to decrease this risk, although it may relieve symptoms for the woman and may prevent respiratory or genital infection of the newborn during delivery. Treatment of a pregnant woman with trichomoniasis must include discussion of the risks and benefits of treatment and optimally should involve the patient's obstetrician.

Infection Control

Because trichomoniasis is sexually transmitted, sexual partners should be treated. Patients should avoid sex until they and their sexual partners complete a course of therapy and are asymptomatic.

CANDIDIASIS

Epidemiology

Up to 75% of women will have at least one case of vulvovaginal candidiasis (VVC) during their lifetimes. This infection is usually caused by *Candida albicans*, but other *Candida* species and *Torulopsis* species may cause the infection. Normal vaginal flora suppress the growth of the organism; symptomatic infection occurs when an imbalance develops, either by suppression of vaginal flora (often caused by the use of antibiotics) or by overgrowth of the yeast (as seen in patients with diabetes). This infection is not considered a sexually transmitted disease, but it may occur in conjunction with another sexually transmitted disease.

Predisposing factors for candidiasis include antibiotic use, diabetes, pregnancy, oral contraceptive use, and tight, restricted, or poorly ventilated clothing.

Clinical Features

The most common presenting complaint is vulvovaginal itching, which may be severe and can lead to excoriation (Table 19.5). Vaginal pain or burning is common. Vaginal discharge may not be a prominent complaint, and patients may

Table 19.5 Clinical Features: Candidiasis

Organisms	• *Candida albicans* • Other *Candida* species • *Torulopsis* species
Signs and Symptoms	• Vulvovaginal pruritis, soreness, edema, erythema • Vulvovaginal excoriations • Dysuria • Dyspareunia • Discharge, usually white, sometimes curdlike
Laboratory Findings	• Presence of hyphae or pseudohyphae on KOH prep • Vaginal pH <4.5 • Lack of WBCs on wet mount

WBC, white blood cell.

not complain of the "classic" cottage-cheese discharge. Malodor is an uncommon complaint. Dysuria (caused by urine passing over irritated and raw genital tissue) is common, as is dyspareunia. On examination, the vulvae and vaginal walls are erythematous and may be edematous, sometimes significantly. Excoriations may be seen from scratching due to the intense pruritis. Vaginal discharge, when present, is typically white and may have a curdlike, cottage cheese appearance.

Patients with VVC are classified as either uncomplicated or complicated. Uncomplicated VVC is defined as (1) sporadic or infrequent, (2) mild-to-moderate, (3) likely to be due to *Candida albicans*, and (4) occurring in an immunocompetent host. Complicated VVC is defined as (1) recurrent, (2) severe, (3) caused by non-*albicans* species, or (4) occurring in patients who are pregnant, debilitated, or immunocompromised (including those with diabetes or renal disease).

Laboratory Findings

A vaginal swab should be sent to the laboratory for wet preparation, and a Gram stain can also be ordered. Wet mount examination with KOH may show yeast and pseudohyphae, and vaginal pH is typically normal (<4.5). White blood cells (WBCs) are not seen with candidiasis, and their presence suggests another cause or co-infection. Culture should be considered in patients with signs or symptoms highly suggestive of candidiasis with a negative wet mount.

The following findings suggest the diagnosis of VVC:

- scant to moderate white, clumped vaginal discharge adherent to vaginal walls
- pH less than 4.5
- yeast and/or pseudohyphae on wet prep/Gram stain
- negative whiff test
- vaginal and/or vulvar erythema/pruritis

Treatment

Most patients with VVC will respond to a short or long course of topical therapy (Table 19.6). Severe VVC, with extensive erythema, edema, and excoriation should always be treated with a long course. Pregnant patients should be treated only with intravaginal topical azole agents for 7 days.

Complications and Admission Criteria

Admission is rarely indicated for VVC. Vaginal culture is indicated in complicated VVC, as conventional antimycotic therapies are not as effective against the non-*albicans Candida* species and other yeast. These patients often need a longer course of therapy, and referral to a primary care physician or gynecologist is recommended for close follow-up and additional therapy as needed.

Infection Control

Vulvovaginal candidiasis is not usually acquired through sexual contact, so treatment of sexual partners is not recommended. If the patient has recurrent infections, however, treatment of the sexual partners should be considered.

Table 19.6 Treatment of Vulvovaginal Candidiasis

Patient Category	Therapy Recommendations
Adults: Uncomplicated	**Intravaginal agents:** butoconazole 2% cream 5 g intravaginally × 3 days *or* butoconazole 2% cream 5 g (sustained release), single dose *or* clotrimazole 1% cream 5 g intravaginally × 7–14 days *or* clotrimazole 100 mg vaginal tablet × 7 days *or* clotrimazole 100 mg vaginal tablet, 2 tablets × 3 days *or* miconazole 2% cream intravaginally × 7 days *or* miconazole 100 mg vaginal suppository, one × 7 days *or* miconazole 200 mg vaginal suppository, one × 3 days *or* miconazole 1200 mg vaginal suppository, once *or* nystatin 100,000-unit vaginal tablet, one × 14 days *or* tioconazole 0.4% cream 5 g intravaginally × 7 days *or* terconazole 0.4% cream 5 g intravaginally × 7 days *or* terconazole 0.8% cream 5 g intravaginally × 3 days *or* terconazole 80 mg vaginal suppository, one × 3 days **Oral agent:** fluconazole 150 mg orally, single dose
Adults: Complicated	**Recurrent VVC:** intravaginal preparations × 7–14 days *or* fluconazole 100 mg, 150 mg, or 200 mg orally every 3 days for three doses (days 1, 4, 7) Also consider oral maintenance regimen fluconazole (100 mg, 150 mg, or 200 mg) weekly for 6 months **Severe VVC:** topical azole × 7–14 days *or* fluconazole 150 mg orally in two doses 72 hours apart **Non-albicans VVC:** nonfluconazole azole × 7–14 days Referral to a gynecologist or generalist **VVC in pregnancy:** Only use topical intravaginal azole agents × 7 days

Differential Diagnosis of Vulvovaginitis

The differential diagnosis of vulvovaginitis (Table 19.7) includes:

- bacterial vaginosis
- trichomoniasis
- candidiasis (and other yeast infections)

Noninfectious causes include contact vulvovaginitis (from douches, vaginal creams, scented tampons, sexual aids, latex), local inflammatory response to an intravaginal foreign body, atrophic vaginitis, and invasive carcinoma of the cervix.

Table 19.7 Summary of Clinical Features of Vulvovaginitis

	Bacterial Vaginosis	Trichomoniasis	Vulvovaginal Candidiasis
History:			
Vaginal Discharge	20%	50–75%	50%
Vaginal Itching	10%	25–50%	50%
Foul Odor	50%	10–25%	Rare
Dyspareunia	Rare	50%	Common
Lower Abdominal Pain	No	5–10%	No
Dysuria	10–20%	25%	Common
Exam:			
Vulvar Erythema/Edema	Not common	10–30%	Common
Vaginal Erythema	Not common	20–75%	Common
Vaginal Discharge Present	70%	50–75%	Most; not all
Color of Vaginal Discharge	Gray; yellow	Yellow-green	White
Odor	45%	Rare	Rare
Diagnostic Testing:			
pH >4.5	Yes	Yes	No
WBCs	++	+++	No
Clue Cells	Yes	No	No
Trichomonads	No	Yes	No
Yeast Forms	No	No	Yes
Sexually Transmitted?	No	Yes	No
Treat Sexual Partners?	No	Yes	No

PEARLS AND PITFALLS

1. All pregnant women who meet diagnostic criteria for bacterial vaginosis (BV) and are symptomatic or at risk for preterm delivery should be treated.
2. Treatment of asymptomatic pregnant women with bacterial vaginosis and no other risk factors for preterm delivery is somewhat controversial; consider consulting the patient's obstetrician.
3. Treatment regimens for pregnant and nonpregnant patients with trichomoniasis differ; a single dose of 2 g of metronidazole is recommended in pregnant women after a discussion of the risks and benefits of treatment.
4. Intravaginal creams and suppositories are oil-based and may weaken diaphragms and condoms that contain latex. Other forms of birth control should be used during treatment.
5. Vulvovaginal candidiasis may be the first symptom of diabetes; patients should have a rapid blood glucose checked.

REFERENCES

Guise JM, Mohan SM, Aickin M, et al. Screening for bacterial vaginosis in pregnancy. Am J Prev Med 2001;20(3 Suppl):62–72.

Hager WD. Treatment of metronidazole-resistant *Trichomonas vaginalis* with tinidazole. Sex Transm Dis 2004;31:343–5.

Holley RL, Richter HE, Varner RE, et al. A randomized, double-blind clinical trial of vaginal acidification versus placebo for the treatment of symptomatic bacterial vaginosis. Sex Transm Dis 2004;31:236–8.

Kane BG, Degutis LC, Sayward HK, et al. Compliance with the Centers for Disease Control and Prevention recommendations for the diagnosis and treatment of sexually transmitted diseases. Acad Emerg Med 2004;11:371–7.

Schwebke JR. Bacterial vaginosis. Curr Infect Dis Rep 2000;2(1):14–7.

ADDITIONAL READINGS

Centers for Disease Control and Prevention (CDC). Sexually transmitted diseases: treatment guidelines, 2006. MMWR 2006;55(RR-11).

Murtagh J. Vaginal discharge. Aust Fam Physician 1991;20:1050.

20. Male Genitourinary Infections

Esther K. Choo

INTRODUCTION

The male urinary tract is contiguous with the reproductive organs, so infections arising in the urethra, epididymis, testicle and prostate share common symptoms of dysuria, frequency, and urgency. In healthy young or middle-aged men presenting to the acute care setting, these symptoms are unlikely to be caused by simple cystitis and are usually attributable to sexually transmitted disease or prostatitis.

URETHRITIS

Epidemiology

Urethritis affects about 4 million males in the United States each year. The peak incidence is in males age 20–24. It is most often a sexually transmitted disease, caused by *Neisseria gonorrhoeae* (gonococcal urethritis) or *Chlamydia trachomatis* (nongonococcal urethritis, NGU). Other nongonococcal causes include *Ureaplasma urealyticum*, *Mycoplasma hominis*, or *Trichomonas vaginalis* (see Chapter 18, Nonulcerative Sexually Transmitted Diseases). Rare infectious causes of urethritis include lymphogranuloma venereum, herpes genitalis, syphilis, mycobacterium, and adenovirus. Enteric species can cause urethral infection in patients who practice insertive anal intercourse or patients with urethral strictures who develop cystitis.

Clinical Features

Male patients with urethritis may present with dysuria, penile discharge, and a history of unprotected sexual contact (Table 20.1). However, up to half of men are asymptomatic and present only because they were referred by a sexual partner who was diagnosed with a sexually transmitted disease (STD). Gonococcal urethritis is more likely to be symptomatic than nongonococcal urethritis.

Table 20.1 Clinical Features: Urethritis

Organisms	• *Neisseria gonorrhoeae* • *Chlamydia trachomatis* • *Ureaplasma urealyticum* • *Mycoplasma hominis* • *Trichomonas vaginalis*
Incubation period	• Gonococcal: 2–7 days • Nongonococcal: 7–14 days
Signs and Symptoms	• Dysuria • Penile discharge • Asymptomatic
Laboratory Findings	• Gram stain of urethral secretions demonstrating $\geq$5 WBCs per oil immersion field • Positive leukocyte esterase test on first-void urine • $\geq$10 WBCs per high-power field on microscopic urinalysis • Urine or urethral swab testing (culture or DNA) positive for gonorrhea or *Chlamydia*

WBC, white blood cell.

Differential Diagnosis

The differential includes postinstrumentation (traumatic) urethritis, cystitis, pyelonephritis, urethral stricture, and urethral foreign body. Urethritis may occur in conjunction with other local infections, such as epididymitis or prostatitis. Nongonococcal urethritis may present in association with a reactive arthritis (Reiter's syndrome).

Features that raise the possibility of atypical organisms, alternate causes of urethral pain, or urethritis complicated by other conditions include:

• eye and joint complaints
• insertive anal sex practices
• recent instrumentation

- lesions of herpes simplex virus (HSV), syphilis, or lymphogranuloma venereum
- masses or fluctuance along the shaft of the penis
- testicular tenderness
- signs or symptoms of systemic illness (fever, chills, rigors, rash)

Laboratory Findings

The presence of purulent or mucopurulent urethral discharge confirms the diagnosis of urethritis. Laboratory criteria are any of the following:

- Gram stain of urethral secretions demonstrating 5 white blood cells (WBCs) or more per oil immersion field
- positive leukocyte esterase test on first-void urine
- positive first-void urine nucleic acid based test
- microscopic examination of first-void urine sediment demonstrating 10 WBCs or more per high-power field

Gram stain may reveal WBCs with gram-negative intracellular diplococci on urethral smear, consistent with gonorrhea infection. Because gonorrhea and *Chlamydia* often coexist in urethral infection, the clinical or laboratory diagnosis of gonorrhea should prompt treatment of both. Elevated WBCs without gram-negative diplococci suggests a nongonococcal urethritis.

Culture and other tests (direct immunofluorescence, enzyme immunoassay [EIA], nucleic acid hybridization tests, and nucleic acid amplification tests on cervical and urethral swabs and first-void urine) are available for detection of gonorrhea and *Chlamydia*. Nucleic acid amplification tests (NAATs) are FDA approved for use on urine specimens and provide ease of collection and transport. Because of their high sensitivity (90–99%) and specificity (97–99%), amplification tests are preferred when available.

Treatment and Prophylaxis

Antibiotic treatment reduces morbidity and prevents transmission of disease. Selected patients who do not meet criteria for urethritis and who have close follow-up with a primary care provider may await results prior to treatment. However, empiric treatment of symptoms consistent with urethritis is usually appropriate in the acute care setting, particularly in patients at high risk for STDs or those who may be lost to follow-up. Empiric treatment in the absence of laboratory confirmation should cover both gonorrhea and *Chlamydia*.

In many locations, a single dose of a cephalosporin may be used to treat gonococcal urethritis (Table 20.2). *Chlamydia* can be treated with one dose of azithromycin or a 10-day course of doxycycline.

Sexually transmitted infections are often transmitted by asymptomatic males who fail to use barrier protection. All patients evaluated for urethritis should receive education about safe sex practices as an essential part of their management.

Complications and Admission Criteria

Acute complications include urethral abscess, prostatitis, epididymitis, proctitis, disseminated gonococcal infection, and

Table 20.2 Initial Therapy for Urethritis

Patient Category	Therapy Recommendation
Adults	ceftriaxone 125 mg IM *or* cefixime 400 mg PO *plus* azithromycin 1 g PO in a single dose *or* doxycycline 100 mg PO bid × 7 days **Treatment for persistent or recurrent NGU:** metronidazole 2 g PO single dose *or* tinidazole 2 g PO single dose *or* azithromycin 1 g PO single dose (if not used for initial treatment)

Because of a high level of resistance, fluoroquinolones are no longer recommended for treatment of gonorrhea except when antibiotic sensitivities are obtained or when community prevalence of quinolone-resistant *Neisseria gonorrhoeae* (QRNG) is known to be low.

Reiter's syndrome. Patients with urethritis complicated by any of these processes who appear ill should be admitted to the hospital. Patients with uncomplicated urethritis do not require admission. Cases usually resolve spontaneously even without treatment, though treatment is also aimed at reducing transmission rates. Long-term complications include urethral stricture or stenosis or, rarely, infertility.

Infection Control

Antibiotics will be ineffective unless sexual partners are also treated. All partners of patients seen for urethritis should be referred to a health care provider for evaluation and treatment. Patients should be instructed not to engage in sexual activity until all symptoms have resolved and until at least 7 days after initiation of therapy.

Pearls and Pitfalls

1. Urethritis not only indicates unsafe sexual practices that place patients at risk for human immunodeficiency virus (HIV) infection, but also directly facilitates HIV infection. Patients should be referred to an STD clinic or to a primary care provider for testing and counseling for other STDs, including HIV and syphilis.

EPIDIDYMITIS
Epidemiology

Acute epididymitis is the most common cause of scrotal pain presenting to the Emergency Department (ED), occurring in about 1 in 1000 men in the United States each year. It is thought to be caused by the retrograde travel of infected urine from the urethra to the epididymis. It is most common in sexually active young men (<35 years) and often occurs in the setting of urethritis caused by *Neisseria gonorrhoeae* or *Chlamydia trachomatis*. Infection by enteric species may also occur in patients who practice insertive anal intercourse.

Table 20.3 Clinical Features: Epididymitis

Organisms	**<35 years of age:** • *Neisseria gonorrhoeae* • *Chlamydia trachomatis* **>35 years of age or prepubescent boys:** • Enteric species **Immunocompromised:** • Mycobacteria or fungi
Signs and Symptoms	• Unilateral scrotal pain • Dysuria • Penile discharge • Fever
Laboratory and Radiologic Findings	• **Urethral swab:** ≥5 WBCs per oil immersion field or intracellular gram-negative diplococci • **Urinalysis:** leukocyte esterase or ≥10 WBCs per high-power field • **Doppler ultrasound:** generalized inflammation, epididymal enlargement, asymmetrical increase in blood flow and decreased vascular resistance in affected testicle

Mechanical causes of urinary reflux predispose patients to infection with urinary coliforms (*Escherichia coli*). In children, congenital genitourinary anomalies can cause chronic backflow of urine. In older patients, urinary obstruction due to prostatic enlargement, urethral strictures, instrumentation of the urethra, or presence of a chronic indwelling urethral catheter are common causes of epididymitis. Men of any age who Valsalva with a full bladder in the course of performing strenuous activities are also prone to developing epididymitis.

Clinical Features

Epididymitis classically presents with unilateral scrotal pain that is gradual in onset (Table 20.3). Pain may begin in the lower abdomen and then localize to the scrotum. Patients may report concurrent or antecedent dysuria or penile discharge. Urethral symptoms may precede epididymitis by as much as 3–4 weeks. Fever and chills are occasionally present.

On exam, patients have unilateral testicular tenderness and edema. A prominent epididymis and hydrocele may be palpated. Early in the course of the disease, tenderness may localize to the tail of the epididymis, but inflammation may spread to the entire length of the epididymis and to the testicle (epididymo-orchitis). For this reason, epididymitis may be difficult to distinguish from testicular torsion. Prehn's sign, or relief of pain with scrotal elevation, is characteristic of epididymitis.

Differential Diagnosis

The differential diagnosis includes testicular torsion, appendageal torsion, epididymal or testicular abscess, chronic (nonbacterial) epididymitis, primary orchitis, hydrocele, spermatocele, hernia, trauma, or testicular cancer. Epididymitis may be one manifestation of Behçet's disease and can be a dose-dependent side effect of amiodarone.

Persistent symptoms despite a course of empiric therapy may be due to unusual organisms, undertreatment of partners, or a noninfectious cause of testicular pain.

Testicular torsion should be considered as a possibility in all cases of unilateral testicular pain. However, features helpful in distinguishing epididymitis from torsion are:

• gradual onset
• prolonged course
• mild or moderate pain
• normal cremasteric reflex
• urine or urethral testing supportive of epididymitis/urethritis

Isolated orchitis is a sequela of mumps. It occurs in 20% of prepubertal male patients with mumps and should be considered when:

• the diagnosis is supported by a history of mumps or parotitis
• orchitis follows parotitis by 3–7 days
• physical exam shows an enlarged, indurated testicle with a nontender epididymis

Patients infected with brucellosis may develop epididymitis or epididymo-orchitis that can lead to testicular abscess or necrosis. In the United States, where handling of milk and dairy products is tightly regulated, only 100 cases of brucellosis are reported each year, most in California, Texas, Florida, and Virgina; worldwide, however, there are hundreds of thousands of cases. The most common exposures to *Brucella* species are via:

• employment as a slaughterhouse worker, meat inspector, farmer, or shepherd
• recent travel to an endemic country and consumption of unpasteurized dairy products
• laboratory work handling aerosolized bacteria specimens
• veterinary work administering live vaccines to animals

In immunocompromised patients, epididymal infection due to fungal species (blastomycosis, coccidioidomycosis, cytomegalovirus, aspergillosis, and candidiasis) and tuberculosis have been reported.

Laboratory and Radiographic Findings

The work-up for epididymitis is similar to the evaluation for urethritis. Patients should have one of the following:

• Gram stain of urethral secretions demonstrating 5 WBCs or more per oil immersion field
• positive leukocyte esterase test on first-void urine
• microscopic examination of first-void urine sediment demonstrating 10 WBCs or more per high-power field

Culture or DNA testing for gonorrhea and *Chlamydia* should be performed on all patients.

Patients may require imaging for evaluation of testicular torsion. Color Doppler ultrasonography is accurate (sensitivity of 89%, specificity of 94%) in identifying changes consistent with epididymitis: asymmetrically increased blood flow and decreased vascular resistance in the affected testicle.

Table 20.4 Initial Therapy for Epididymitis

Patient Category	Therapy Recommendation
Adults <35 Years	ceftriaxone 250 mg IM once *plus* doxycycline 100 mg PO bid × 10 days
Adults ≥35 Years or Testing for Gonorrhea Negative	levofloxacin 500 mg PO qd × 10 days *or* ofloxacin 300 mg PO qd × 10 days
Adjunctive Therapy	• Reduced activity or bed rest • Scrotal elevation • NSAIDs

NSAID, nonsteroidal anti-inflammatory drug.

Treatment and Prophylaxis

Empiric treatment should be initiated while awaiting test results. The antibiotic regimen is determined by age (Table 20.4). Patients younger than the age of 35 should receive treatment for gonorrhea, with a single intramuscular (IM) dose of ceftriaxone, and for *Chlamydia*, with a 10-day course of doxycycline. Patients 35 years or older require coverage for enteric gram-negative species; a 10-day course of a quinolone is advised.

All patients treated for sexually transmitted infection should receive counseling about safe sex practices as a key part of their acute care management.

Complications and Admission Criteria

Potential complications include epididymo-orchitis, scrotal abscess, testicular infarction, chronic pain, infertility, and sepsis.

Although most genitourinary infections in men can be managed in the outpatient setting, patients may require admission to the hospital if they:

- appear toxic with signs of systemic inflammation
- are unable to take oral medications
- require intravenous pain medications
- are significantly symptomatic despite a course of outpatient therapy
- are elderly or immunocompromised

Infection Control

Patients should be instructed to refer all partners with whom they have had sexual contact within 60 days to be evaluated and treated for STDs. Patients should be referred to an STD clinic or to a primary care provider for testing and counseling for other STDs, including HIV and syphilis.

Pearls and Pitfalls

1. Testicular torsion is a surgical emergency and must be considered in all cases of acute scrotal pain
2. Symptoms of epididymitis should improve between 1 and 3 days after initiating appropriate therapy. Patients should be instructed to seek prompt follow-up for ongoing or escalating symptoms.

ACUTE BACTERIAL PROSTATITIS
Epidemiology

Prostatitis will occur in about 5% of U.S. males during their lifetime. Although only a small percentage of these cases fall under the category of acute bacterial prostatitis, this form presents to the ED in disproportionate numbers because of the rapid and dramatic onset of symptoms. Men 20–45 years of age are at highest risk. Benign prostatic hypertrophy (BPH), urethral catheterization or instrumentation, and urinary tract infection are common risk factors.

Acute bacterial prostatitis is caused by Enterobacteriaceae, usually *E. coli* (75% of cases), and less commonly *Pseudomonas aeruginosa*, *Staphylococcus saprophyticus*, *Staphylococcus aureus*, and *Enterococcus faecalis*. In young sexually active men, *N. gonorrhoeae* and *C. trachomatis* are rare pathogens.

Clinical Features

Patients complain of urinary symptoms (dysuria, frequency, and urgency) and pain in the lower abdomen, perineum, rectum, or genitalia (Table 20.5). Patients may note symptoms of systemic illness, such as fever, chills, arthralgias, and myalgias. Varying degrees of urinary obstruction may also be present.

Patients may appear quite ill, with signs of bacteremia (fever, rigors, tachycardia). Rectal exam reveals an enlarged, warm, indurated, and exquisitely tender prostate.

Table 20.5 Clinical Features: Acute Bacterial Prostatitis

Organisms	• *Escherichia coli* • *Klebsiella* spp. • *Proteus mirabilis* • *Pseudomonas aeruginosa* • *Staphylococcus saprophyticus* • *Staphylococcus aureus* • *Enterococcus faecalis*
Signs and Symptoms	• Dysuria, frequency, urgency • Abdominal, rectal, perineal, or back pain • Fever • Urinary retention
Laboratory	• Pyuria, with large numbers of leukocytes and lipid-laden macrophages • Bacteruria
Treatment	**Outpatient therapy:** ciprofloxacin 500 mg PO bid × 28 days *or* ofloxacin 200 mg bid × 28 days Alternative: TMP-SMX DS PO bid × 28 days **Inpatient therapy:** ceftriaxone 1–2 g IV q12–24h *plus* gentamicin 1.7 mg/kg IV q8h

DS, double strength; SMX, sulfamethoxazole; TMP, trimethoprim.

Differential Diagnosis

The differential diagnosis includes chronic bacterial or chronic nonbacterial prostatitis, proctitis, anal or rectal abscess or fistula, urethritis, cystitis, and prostatic abscess. Acute prostatitis can also be an extrapulmonary manifestation of Wegener's granulomatosis.

Chronic bacterial prostatitis is usually not an acute care diagnosis. It may be suspected in patients with:

- long-standing (months) symptoms of perineal, testicular, lower abdominal, lumbar, or penile pain, ejaculatory pain, dysuria, frequency, urgency, urethral discharge, hematospermia
- history of recurrent urinary tract infections
- few objective abnormal findings on physical examination
- soft, boggy, mild to moderately tender prostate

Because many of the symptoms of chronic bacterial prostatitis overlap with those of urinary tract infection or sexually transmitted genitourinary infections, patients should be evaluated and treated for these as appropriate. They should be referred to their primary care provider or urologist for further evaluation.

Laboratory and Radiographic Findings

Evaluation should include:

- a mid-stream urine sample for urinalysis
- a first-void urine sample for nucleic acid based testing
- urine culture for bacteria and antibiotic sensitivity
- blood cultures for bacteria and antibiotic sensitivity
- complete blood count

Urine will show bacteruria and pyuria, with large numbers of leukocytes and lipid-laden macrophages. Prostatic massage or serial prostate exams should be avoided, as this practice may precipitate bacteremia. If present, pathogens are almost always isolated from the urine in acute bacterial prostatitis, and sterile urine makes this diagnosis unlikely.

If prostate abscess is suspected based on fluctuance on exam, a transrectal ultrasound or a computed tomographic (CT) scan of the pelvis should be obtained. However, there is no need for routine imaging in the work-up of prostatitis.

Treatment and Prophylaxis

Prostatitis is a clinical diagnosis. Treatment should be started empirically and antibiotic therapy can be discontinued or narrowed when culture results become available. Patients who require intravenous (IV) therapy should receive a broad-spectrum cephalosporin plus gentamicin. When oral therapy is suitable, quinolones are effective first-line antibiotics.

Adjunctive therapies include bed rest, antipyretics and anti-inflammatories, stool softeners, hydration, and sitz baths. Acute urinary obstruction must be relieved by a suprapubic catheter to avoid damaging the edematous prostate or precipitating bacteremia.

Complications and Admission Criteria

Complications include prostatic abscess, acute bladder outlet obstruction, chronic bacterial prostatitis, and sepsis.

Criteria for hospitalization and IV antibiotics include:

- toxic appearance
- elderly patient
- immunosuppression
- multiple comorbidities
- failure of outpatient regimen
- inability to take oral medications
- need for IV pain medication

Because of the intense inflammation, intravenous antibiotics penetrate into the prostate well and patients generally respond rapidly. Persistent fever after 48 hours of therapy raises the question of prostatic abscess.

Pearls and Pitfalls

1. Acute bacterial prostatitis can progress to sepsis, septic shock, and death; initiation of treatment in an ill-appearing patient should not await results of urinalysis or urine culture.
2. Failure of antibiotic therapy may be due to unusual organisms (*Pseudomonas*, *Enterococcus*) or the development of a prostatic abscess.
3. Practitioners should obtain a transrectal ultrasound or CT if the patient is poorly responsive to therapy or if fluctuance is felt on the initial prostate exam.
4. Patients with acute bladder obstruction due to prostatitis should receive prompt urology consultation, and will likely require suprapubic catheterization.
5. Bacterial prostatitis can be refractory to treatment. Patients who are discharged from the acute care setting must have close outpatient follow-up.

REFERENCES

Andriole VT. Use of quinolones in treatment of prostatitis and lower urinary tract infections. Eur J Clin Microbiol Infect Dis 1991 Apr;10(4):342–50.

Black CM, Marrazzo JM, Johnson RE, et al. Head-to-head multicenter comparison of DNA probe and nucleic acid amplification tests for *Chlamydia trachomatis* in women performed with an improved reference standard. J Clin Microbiol 2002;40:3757–63.

Brown JM, Hammers LW, Barton JW, et al. Quantitative Doppler assessment of acute scrotal inflammation. Radiology 1995;197:427–31.

Centers for Disease Control and Prevention (CDC). Update to CDC's sexually transmitted diseases treatment guidelines, 2006: fluoroquinolones no longer recommended for treatment of gonococcal infections. MMWR 2007;56(14);332–336.

Chorba T, Tao G, Irwin KL. Sexually transmitted diseases. In: Litwin MS, Saigal CS, eds. Urologic diseases in America.

U.S. Department of Health and Human Services, Public Health Service, National Institutes of Health, National Institute of Diabetes and Digestive and Kidney Diseases. Washington, DC: U.S. Government Printing Office, 2004; NIH Publication No. 04–5512 [pp. 233–82].

Johnson RE, Green TA, Schachter J, et al. Evaluation of nucleic acid amplification tests as reference tests for *Chlamydia trachomatis* infections in asymptomatic men. J Clin Microbiol 2000;38:4382–6.

Nickel JC. Prostatitis: evolving management strategies. Urol Clin North Am 1999;26:737–51.

Van Der Pol B, Ferrero DV, Buck-Barrington L, et al. Multicenter evaluation of the BDProbeTec ET System for detection of *Chlamydia trachomatis* and *Neisseria gonorrhoeae* in urine specimens, female endocervical swabs, and male urethral swabs. J Clin Microbiol 2001;39:1008–16.

ADDITIONAL READINGS

Association for Genitourinary Medicine (AGUM), Medical Society for the Study of Venereal Disease (MSSVD). 2002 national guideline for the management of prostatitis. London: Association for Genitourinary Medicine (AGUM), Medical Society for the Study of Venereal Disease (MSSVD), 2002.

Centers for Disease Control and Prevention (CDC). Sexually transmitted diseases treatment guidelines, 2006. MMWR 2006;55(11):61–2.

Centers for Disease Control and Prevention (CDC). Sexually transmitted disease surveillance 2005 supplement, Gonococcal Isolate Surveillance Project (GISP) annual report 2005. Atlanta, GA: U.S. Department of Health and Human Services, Centers for Disease Control and Prevention, January 2007.

21. Adult Septic Arthritis

James M. Mok and Serena S. Hu

INTRODUCTION

Septic arthritis is a suppurative bacterial infection of a synovial joint. Most commonly, joint infection occurs through hematogenous seeding of the synovium. Less often, joint infection results from joint aspiration or injection, penetrating trauma, or extension into the joint space from adjacent osteomyelitis. Bacterial septic arthritis is considered a medical emergency because permanent destruction of a joint can occur from the resulting inflammatory response to infection. In particular, bacterial invasion of a joint causes activation of a potent host immune inflammatory response. This results in the production of proteolytic enzymes that destroy the extracellular cartilage matrix of the affected joint.

EPIDEMIOLOGY

Populations at increased risk for septic arthritis include individuals older than 60 years of age, those with osteoarthritis or rheumatoid arthritis, and those on corticosteroids or with human immunodeficiency virus (HIV)/acquired immunodeficiency syndrome (AIDS). In particular, individuals with rheumatoid arthritis have a 10-fold greater incidence of septic arthritis than the general population. Individuals with diabetes mellitus or other chronic medical conditions such as renal disease, cirrhosis, granulomatous disease, or malignancy are also at increased risk.

CLINICAL FEATURES

Septic arthritis typically presents with erythema, swelling, tenderness and warmth about the affected joint (Figure 21.1). The patient will display decreased and painful range of motion of the affected joint (Table 21.1). Signs and symptoms of inflammation may be less pronounced in those who are immunosuppressed. The knee joint is the most commonly affected joint, followed by the hip, shoulder, wrist, and ankle. Septic arthritis of the sacroiliac joint and the sternoclavicular joint are seen in intravenous drug users.

DIFFERENTIAL DIAGNOSIS

Key features that may help to distinguish septic arthritis from other arthropathies are:

- Usually single joint involvement.
- Acute onset severe pain, swelling, heat, erythema, inability to bear weight.
- Inability to perform active range of motion.
- Severe pain with passive range of motion.
- Fever and tachycardia.
- Gonococcal arthritis occurs in young healthy adults with a female preponderance and classically presents as a migratory polyarthritis, tenosynovitis, and vesicopapular skin lesions. It usually responds to antibiotics and aspiration alone.

Other conditions to consider are:

- acute exacerbation of chronic arthritis (e.g., rheumatoid), although a high index of suspicion should be maintained
- viral arthritis
- crystal-induced arthritis
- reactive arthritis

Key clinical questions that help to diagnose septic arthritis are:

- age
- history of immunosuppression
- acuity of onset

LABORATORY AND RADIOGRAPHIC FINDINGS

The diagnosis of septic arthritis depends on culturing the causative organism from the synovial fluid of the affected joint (Table 21.2). Antibiotics have been shown to substantially decrease culture yields and should be held until aspiration is performed. The joint fluid should always be sent for aerobic and anaerobic culture and, depending on the clinical situation, for mycobacterial, fungal, and gonococcal culture prior to initiating any antibiotics. All joint fluid samples should also be sent for cell count and examined by polarized light microscopy for negative (gout) and positive (pseudogout) birefringent crystals. Synovial fluid culture will be positive in approximately 90% of nongonococcal septic arthritis cases, and Gram stain will be positive less than 50% of the time. Synovial fluid leukocyte counts are typically greater than 50,000/mm^3 in septic arthritis with polymorphonuclear

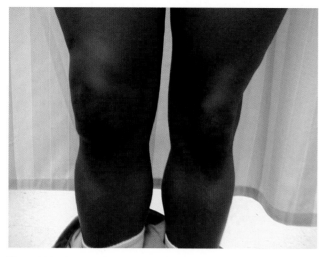

Figure 21.1   Patient with a right knee effusion showing loss of contour of patella and effusion extending into the suprapatellar pouch of joint. From website http://medicine.ucsf.edu. Permission granted to use this image by Dr. Charlie Goldberg and Dr. Jan Thompson.

Table 21.1 Adult Acute Septic Arthritis

Organism	*Staphylococcus aureus* is most common
Clinical Features	• Warmth, erythema, painful range of motion and effusion of affected joint • Fever and malaise
Laboratory and Radiographic Findings	• WBC may be normal, ESR and CRP usually elevated • Blood cultures may be positive in up to 50% • Radiographs usually show soft-tissue swelling and joint effusion • Infected joint fluid will appear purulent, opaque, with variable viscosity; generally has >50,000 WBC/mm^3, >90% PMNs, and a glucose level below blood glucose level
Differential Diagnosis	• Gout • Pseudogout • Viral arthritis (often polyarticular) • Reactive arthritis • Inflammatory arthritis
Treatment	• Hold antibiotics until joint aspiration is performed and cultures are sent • Emergent drainage (surgical incision versus repeat bedside aspiration) • Empiric IV antibiotics after synovial fluid sent for culture and Gram stain* piperacillin-tazobactam 3.375 g IV q6h *or* (for MRSA) vancomycin 10–15 mg/kg IV q12h *plus* ceftriaxone 1 g IV q24h *or* (for gonococcal arthritis) ceftriaxone 1 g IV q24h

*Empiric antibiotics need to cover *Staphylococcus aureus*, so consider administering vancomycin or equivalent antibiotic if MRSA is common in your community.
CRP, C-reactive protein; ESR, erythrocyte sedimentation rate; MRSA, methicillin-resistant *Staphylococcus aureus*; PMNs, polymorphonuclear neutrophil leukocytes; WBC, white blood (cell) count.

Table 21.2 Standard Emergency Department Evaluation for Septic Arthritis

1. Joint fluid for:
    • Gram stain
    • Cell count and differential
    • Culture (aerobic, anaerobic, gonococcal, fungal, mycobacterium)
    • Crystal analysis
2. Blood samples for:
    • ESR
    • CRP
    • WBC
    • Culture
3. Radiographs of affected joint

neutrophil leukocytes (PMNs) of at least 75% and often approaching 90%. However, synovial fluid leukocyte counts less than 50,000/mm^3 can occur in those with septic arthritis who are immunocompromised. Besides obtaining joint fluid, radiographs of the affected joint(s) should be obtained to assess for associated osteomyelitis, preexisting disease, and foreign bodies. The white blood cell count (WBC) and erythrocyte sedimentation rate (ESR) may be elevated but have not been shown to reliably detect septic arthritis. However, the C-reactive protein (CRP) is usually elevated to greater than 100 mg/L. The CRP is also a useful test to track the response to therapy.

TREATMENT AND PROPHYLAXIS

The treatment of septic arthritis involves early drainage of the purulent synovial effusion and treatment with appropriate antibiotics. There is controversy regarding the best method of drainage for purulent joint effusions. Some practitioners prefer daily bedside arthrocentesis because of its convenience and noninvasive nature. Other practitioners consider septic arthritis as a closed-space infection and feel that formal surgical incision and drainage of the affected joint using arthroscopy or open arthrotomy is more appropriate. Unfortunately, there have been no prospective controlled trials comparing serial arthrocentesis with surgical irrigation and debridement. However, surgical incision is the treatment of choice for poorly accessible joints such as the hip and shoulder, joints with thick purulence or loculations, or those not responsive to serial aspiration and antibiotics. If serial joint aspiration is to be attempted, it must be done frequently to prevent stagnation and loculation of pus and must be done utilizing strict sterile technique and a large-bore needle.

COMPLICATIONS AND ADMISSION CRITERIA

Septic arthritis should be considered a surgical emergency requiring urgent surgical or bedside drainage to prevent destruction of the articular cartilage. Serial aspirations may be adequate in some situations. Treatment delay has been shown to correlate with morbidity and mortality.

Intravenous antibiotics should be initiated immediately after aspiration and continued until clinical improvement is observed.

Reports of death from septic arthritis have ranged from 8% to as high as 15%.

PEARLS AND PITFALLS

1. Antibiotics should be held until joint aspiration is performed (this time should be minimized).
2. Aspiration with a large-bore (18 gauge) needle utilizing sterile technique is the most important diagnostic test to perform and should be part of the initial evaluation of a suspected septic joint.
3. High index of suspicion should be maintained in patients with a history of immunocompromise or chronic arthritis.
4. Gram stain of synovial fluid may be negative in up to half of cases and should not be relied on to rule out septic arthritis.

REFERENCES

Goodman SB, Chou LB, Schurman DJ. Management of pyarthrosis. In: Chapman MW, ed, Chapman's orthopedic surgery. Philadelphia: Lippincott Williams & Wilkins, 2001:3561–75.

Manadan AM, Block JA. Daily needle aspiration versus surgical lavage for the treatment of bacterial septic arthritis in adults. Am J Ther 2004;11:412–5.

Shirtliff ME, Mader JT. Acute septic arthritis. Clin Microbiol Rev 2002;15:527–44.

Smith JW, Chalupa P, Hasan MS. Infectious arthritis: clinical features, laboratory findings and treatment. Clin Microbiol Infect 2006;12:309–14.

22. Hand Infections: Fight Bite, Purulent Tenosynovitis, Felon, and Paronychia

Michael Kohn

FIGHT BITE

Introduction – Agents

The most notorious of all nonvenomous bite wounds is the fight bite. As the name implies, this injury occurs when the subject punches an adversary in the teeth, lacerating the dorsum of one or more metacarpal-phalangeal (MCP) joints (Figure 22.1). Other names for this injury, such as "morsus humanus" or "clenched fist injury," have been proposed, though "fight bite" is more descriptive and widely used. The fight bite gave human bites their reputation for being more prone to infection than other animal bites. This has more to do with the location of the bite and the typical delay in treatment than with the mix of organisms in the human mouth. Common fight bite infections include cellulitis, subcutaneous abscesses, septic MCP joint, and purulent tenosynovitis. In the preantibiotic era, fight bite infections commonly necessitated finger and occasionally arm amputations. Fight bite infections are usually polymicrobial and often involve *Streptococcus* species, *Staphylococcus* species, *Eikenella*, and oral anaerobic bacteria.

The first two fight-bite patients reported in the medical literature were described by William H. Peters in 1911. He was primarily concerned with culturing mouth organisms, specifically Fusobacteria, from the infected wounds. Various other studies emphasizing the symbiosis of spirochetes and fusiform organisms in fight bites appeared afterwards. In 1930, Michael L. Mason and Sumner L. Koch published a 34-page study of fight bites emphasizing the importance of the anatomy of the injured area in determining the spread of infection. In 1983 Schmidt identified *Eikenella corrodens*, a microaerophilic gram-negative rod, as an important etiologic agent in fight bite infections.

Clinical Features

Clinicians should be suspicious of a fight bite in any laceration over the dorsal MCP joint, particularly in young male patients, in whom this injury primarily occurs (Table 22.1). An x-ray may reveal air or even a piece of tooth in the MCP joint.

If not, exploration of the skin wound and examination of the extensor hood (with the MCP flexed) are essential to determine whether the joint capsule has been violated. Sometimes adequate visualization of the extensor hood requires extension of the skin wound.

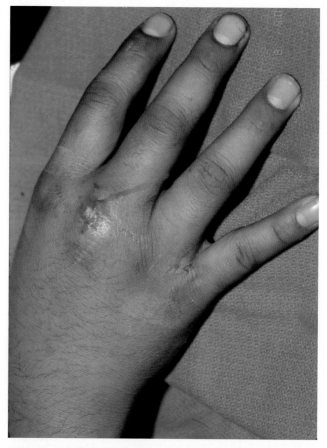

Figure 22.1 Fight bite. Also known as a "clenched fist injury," this serious injury typically is characterized by a laceration on the dorsal metacarpalphalangeal joint. Courtesy of Dr. Alan Bindiger.

Table 22.1 Clinical Features: Fight Bite (Clenched Fist Injury)

Organisms	• *Streptococcus* (predominantly *S. anginosus*) • *Staphylococcus* species • *Eikenella* • Oral anaerobes
Signs and Symptoms	• Laceration over the dorsal MCP joint • Examine with MCP flexed for laceration of the extensor hood
Laboratory and Radiographic Findings	X-ray may reveal air or a retained tooth in the MCP joint
Treatment	**Uninfected, extensor hood intact:** Thorough irrigation, no sutures. Optional short (1- to 3-day course) of: amoxicillin-clavulanate 250–500 PO tid or 875 PO bid *or* gatifloxacin or moxifloxacin 400 PO qd *or* doxycycline 100 mg PO bid **Uninfected, extensor hood violated:** Irrigation of joint, splinting, prophylactic beta lactam/beta lactamase inhibitor, or combination of clindamycin* (300–450 mg PO qid) *plus* penicillin, second- or third-generation cephalosporin, or fluoroquinolone. Admission or next-day follow-up by hand surgeon. **Infected:** Usually requires admission for joint washout and parenteral antibiotics. Ampicillin-sulbactam 1.5–3 g IV q6h; or other beta lactam/beta lactamase inhibitor. If beta lactam allergic, clindamycin* 600 IV q 8h plus gatifloxacin or moxifloxacin 400 mg IV qd.

* E. corrodens is uniformly resistant to clindamycin, so clindamycin must be used in combination with another antibiotic.

Differential Diagnosis

Fight bites should be distinguished from occlusive bites (which are somewhat less prone to infection) and other hand lacerations (which are substantially less prone to infection).

Key features that distinguish fight bite from typical hand lacerations are:

- polymicrobial and more prone to infection
- progression of infection because of delayed diagnosis and treatment
- high suspicion of human bite based on location over the dorsal MCP

Treatment and Prophylaxis

Antibiotic recommendations for prophylaxis and treatment of fight bite infections are based on the susceptibilities of the common infectious agents: *Streptococcus* species (especially *S. anginosus*), *Staphylococcus aureus*, and *Eikenella*. The choice is between a single beta lactam–beta lactamase inhibitor drug such as amoxicillin-clavulanate or a combination of clindamycin with either penicillin, a second- or third-generation cephalosporin, or a fluoroquinolone. Although it is effective

against methicillin-resistant *S. aureus* (MRSA), clindamycin alone is never adequate therapy, as *E. corrodens* is uniformly resistant to clindamycin.

An uninfected fight bite that does not violate the extensor hood should be irrigated thoroughly under pressure and dressed open (no closure by suture, adhesive strips, or glue). There is no evidence regarding prophylactic antibiotics in this situation. Although a short, 1- to 3-day course of antibiotics might be justifiable, thorough irrigation and precautions to return for signs of infection are more important.

Complications and Admission Criteria

An uninfected fight bite that does violate the extensor hood requires thorough irrigation of the joint, splinting, prophylactic antibiotics, and either admission or next-day follow-up. A hand surgeon should usually manage treatment.

An infected fight bite almost always requires hospitalization for intravenous antibiotics and frequently for surgical debridement.

PURULENT TENOSYNOVITIS

Introduction – Agents

An important element of the surgical anatomy of the hand is that the deep and superficial flexors to the digits run through delicate tendon sheaths and utilize a complex system of tissue pulleys. Repairing damage to these sheaths and pulleys requires magnification and the controlled, sterile environment of the operating room. In contrast, the extensor tendons to the digits do not run through sheaths, and damaged extensors may be repaired in the emergency department (ED). That is why the palm and dorsum of the hand are sometimes referred to as the "OR side" and the "ER side," respectively.

Purulent tenosynovitis is a bacterial infection within one of the flexor tendon sheaths (Figure 22.2). The inoculum comes from a puncture wound or laceration to the palmar surface of the hand or finger and spreads rapidly throughout the tendon sheath. As with all skin infections resulting from lacerations or puncture wounds, the primary bacterial pathogens are *Staphylococcus aureus*, *Streptococcus*, and anaerobes.

Clinical Features

Patients with purulent tenosynovitis present with a painful swollen digit anytime from hours to weeks after a palmar wound (Table 22.2). Kanavel's four cardinal signs of purulent tenosynovitis are as follows:

1. slightly flexed finger posture
2. symmetrical swelling
3. pain on passive extension
4. tenderness along flexor tendon sheath

These findings distinguish purulent tenosynovitis from the less serious localized subcutaneous abscess.

Differential Diagnosis

Purulent tenosynovitis can be distinguished from less serious localized subcutaneous abscess by the Kanavel's signs mentioned above.

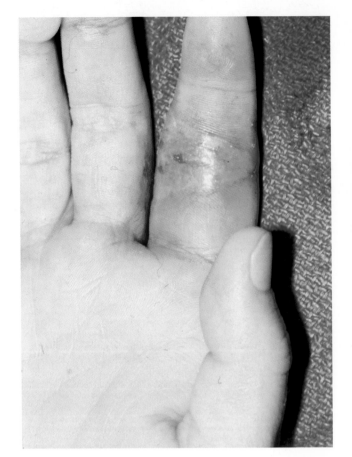

Figure 22.2 Purulent flexor tenosynovitis of the index finger of the right hand. Courtesy of Dr. Alan Bindiger.

Table 22.2 Clinical Features: Purulent Tenosynovitis

Organisms	• *Staphylococcus aureus* (methicillin resistance increasing in the community) • *Streptococcus pyogenes* (group A) • Anaerobes
Signs and Symptoms	**Kanavel's signs:** • Slightly flexed finger posture • Symmetrical swelling • Pain on passive extension • Tenderness along flexor tendon sheath
Laboratory and Radiographic Findings	This is a clinical diagnosis requiring operative irrigation of the tendon sheath, at which time cultures should be obtained.
Treatment	Hospital admission and operative irrigation of the tendon sheath. Antibiotic therapy should be guided by operative cultures. **Empiric IV antibiotics (no MRSA):** cefazolin 0.5–1.5 g IV q6–8h *or* nafcillin 2 g IV q4–6h *plus* penicillin G 2–4 million units q6h *or* ampicillin-sulbactam 1.5–3 g IV q6h **Empiric IV antibiotics (MRSA):** vancomycin 1 g IV q12h *or* clindamycin 600–900 mg IV q8h *or* TMP-SMX 240–480 mg of TMP IV q8h (15 mg/kg/day divided tid) plus rifampin 300 PO bid or tid

MRSA, methicillin-resistant *Staphylococcus aureus*; SMX, sulfamethoxazole; TMP, trimethoprim.

Acute inflammatory reactions to insect bites and stings may present similarly but can usually be identified by history.

Treatment

Prior to the epidemic of community acquired methicillin-resistant *S. aureus* (MRSA), appropriate empiric antibiotic therapy included the following options:

- first-generation cephalosporin (e.g., cefazolin)
- antistaphylococcal penicillin (e.g., nafcillin)
- beta lactam-beta lactamase inhibitor (e.g., ampicillin-sulbactam)

The increasing prevalence of MRSA in skin and soft-tissue infections should lower the threshold for early surgical intervention to obtain cultures to guide antibiotic therapy and to irrigate the tendon sheath. Vancomycin, clindamycin, or trimethoprim-sulfa plus rifampin are reasonable options as empiric therapy in communities with high rates of MRSA.

Complications and Admission Criteria

Patients with purulent tenosynovitis require hospitalization. In early, apparently mild infections, intravenous antibiotics and close observation may suffice. If the infection does not improve within 24 hours of antibiotic treatment, or if the infection is already established or advanced, irrigation of the tendon sheath is required.

ACUTE PARONYCHIA AND FELON

Introduction – Agents

Acute paronychia, a bacterial infection of the skin folds that hold the nail plate in place, is the most common of hand infections (Figure 22.3). A felon is a painful and potentially disabling infection of the fingertip pulp that can progress to tissue necrosis and osteomyelitis of the distal phalanx (Figure 22.4). Except in the very early stages, pus occupies the closed space formed by the fibrous septae of the fingertip. As with purulent tenosynovitis, the infection in both paronychia and felon results from a break in the skin, and the common organisms are *S. aureus* (increasingly methicillin resistant), *Streptococcus* species, and anaerobes.

Clinical Features

The tenderness, erythema, and edema of the felon are all limited to the volar pad of the distal phalanx (Table 22.3). In contrast, the paronychia is limited to the dorsal side of the fingertip. Sometimes there is visible pus under the nail plate. Paronychia and felon are occasionally found together.

Differential Diagnosis

Acute paronychia should be distinguished from chronic paronychia as described below, and from herpetic whitlow, as

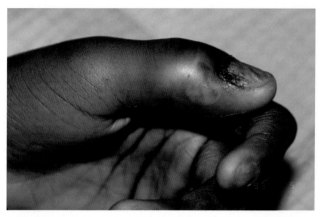

Figure 22.3 Acute paronychia of the left thumb. Courtesy of Dr. Alan Bindiger.

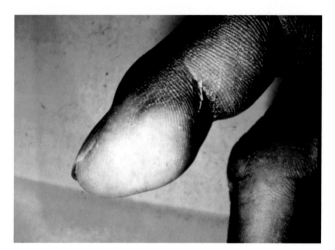

Figure 22.4 Felon. Courtesy of Dr. Alan Bindiger.

Table 22.3 Clinical Features: Felon and (Acute) Paronychia

Organisms	• *Staphylococcus aureus* • *Streptococcus* spp. • Anaerobes
Signs and Symptoms	**Felon (volar pad of distal phalanx):** • Tenderness • Erythema • Tense edema **Paronychia (skin folds around the fingernail):** • Tenderness, erythema, edema • Fluctuance • Look for subungual pus (pus under the nail plate)
Laboratory/ Radiographic Findings	In long-standing felon, x-ray may reveal osteomyelitis of the distal phalanx
Treatment	Primary treatment is incision and drainage **Felon:** • Single lateral longitudinal incision with placement of gauze wick or, occasionally, bilateral longitudinal incisions with placement of a through-and-through wick or drain **Paronychia:** • No subungual pus – elevate the skin fold, drain, and place a small wick • Subungual pus – remove a longitudinal section of the nail plate to drain and maintain drainage **Antibiotics:** Are appropriate but less important than drainage. Must consider MRSA: clindamycin 300–450 mg PO tid *or* TMP-SMX 1–2 DS tabs PO bid If MRSA unlikely: cephalexin 500 mg PO qid *or* dicloxacillin 500 mg PO qid *or* amoxicillin-sulbactam 875 mg PO bid

DS, double strength; SMX, sulfamethoxazole; TMP, trimethoprim.

incision and drainage of herpetic whitlow is contraindicated (see section below).

Chronic paronychia is inflammation of the nail folds of greater than 6 weeks' duration:

- rarely seen in the ED
- results from repeated exposure of hands to water and irritants
- commonly caused by *Candida albicans*
- treat by avoiding exposure to water and irritants
- topical steroids or antifungals also helpful

Treatment

Early incision and drainage is the mainstay of treatment for both felon and paronychia. For a felon, a simple, lateral longitudinal incision is usually adequate. Occasionally, bilateral incisions and passage of a through-and-through wick or drain is necessary. For a paronychia, adequate drainage may be obtained by simply elevating the skin edge. If subungual pus is present, the clinician should resect a longitudinal section of the nail plate on the side of the paronychia. Although drainage is more important, antistaphylococcal antibiotics (with consideration of possible methicillin resistance) are indicated for both paronychia and felon.

Chronic paronychia, rarely seen in the ED, is inflammation of the skin around the nail plate of more than 6 weeks' duration. It is an occupational hazard among bakers, bartenders, dishwashers, and house cleaners whose hands are exposed to water and skin irritants while suffering repeated minor trauma to the nail plates. The etiologic agent is overwhelmingly *Candida albicans* but may also include mycobacteria. Treatment consists of wearing gloves to avoid contact with water and irritants. Topical steroids or antifungals may also be helpful.

Complications and Admission Criteria

Felon is a serious bacterial infection that can progress to osteomyelitis of the distal phalanx and even to sepsis requiring hospitalization.

Table 22.4 Clinical Features: Herpetic Whitlow

Organism	Herpes simplex type 1 or 2
Signs and Symptoms	• Vesicles • Serous, crusting, not purulent discharge • Often associated with perioral cold sores
Laboratory Findings	Though rarely done, Tzanck smear may show multinucleated giant cells
Treatment	Condition is self-limited, but severe cases may be treated with oral acyclovir 400 mg PO tid × 7 days

HERPETIC WHITLOW

Introduction – Agents

Herpetic whitlow is a herpes simplex infection of the finger that can be confused with a paronychia or felon. In children, herpetic infections of the hand are exclusively due to herpes simplex type 1 autoinoculation from the mouth during an episode of gingivostomatitis. In adults, herpetic whitlow is caused by either herpes simplex type 1 or type 2. Herpes simplex type 2 infections occur more frequently in women and are associated with a history of genital herpes. The occurrence of herpetic whitlow in dentists, anesthetists, nurses, and others with occupational exposure to oral secretions has decreased in recent years. As with other herpes infections, herpetic whitlow can recur after the primary infection.

Clinical Features

Herpetic whitlow that involves the fingertip may be distinguished from felon or paronychia by the presence of vesicles, and a serous, crusting, rather than purulent discharge (Table 22.4). The simultaneous presence of cold sores, or a history of previous similar infections, can also make the diagnosis. Though rarely done, a Tzanck smear of the discharge may show multinucleated giant cells. Herpetic whitlow can be associated with lymphangitic streaking up the forearm and swollen epitrochlear or axillary nodes, which may be mistaken as an indication of bacterial infection.

Differential Diagnosis

Distinguish from felon or paronychia by:

- presence of vesicles
- serous, crusting, rather than purulent discharge
- simultaneous presence of cold sores
- history of previous similar infections

Treatment

It is important to distinguish herpetic whitlow from felon or paronychia, because herpetic whitlow should not be incised and drained. Although the infection is usually self-limited, treatment with oral acyclovir is indicated for severe acute cases. In patients with frequent, painful recurrences, maintenance acyclovir therapy may ultimately be necessary.

Complications

Herpetic whitlow can recur after the primary infection.

PEARLS AND PITFALLS

1. Suspect a fight bite in any knuckle laceration. Make sure to inspect the extensor hood, even if it requires extending the wound. Never close a fight bite.
2. *E. corrodens* is uniformly resistant to clindamycin, so clindamycin alone is never adequate treatment for a fight bite.
3. Purulent tenosynovitis is a true hand emergency requiring admission and consultation of a hand surgeon.
4. Distinguish herpetic whitlow from felon and paronychia by the presence of vesicles, a clear and crusting rather than purulent discharge, the simultaneous presence of cold sores, or a history of recurrent infections.

REFERENCES

Boland F. Morsus humanus. JAMA 1941;116:127.

Boles SD, Schmidt CC. Pyogenic flexor tenosynovitis. Hand Clin 1998 Nov;14(4):567–78.

Bowling JC, Saha M, Bunker CB. Herpetic whitlow: a forgotten diagnosis. Clin Exp Dermatol 2005 Sep;30(5):609–10.

Gill MJ, Arlette J, Buchan K. Herpes simplex virus infection of the hand. A profile of 79 cases. Am J Med 1988 Jan;84(1):89–93.

Kanavel AB. Infections of the hand; a guide to the surgical treatment of acute and chronic suppurative processes in the fingers, hand, and forearm, 7th ed. Philadelphia: Lea & Febiger, 1939.

Karanas YL, Bogdan MA, Chang J. Community acquired methicillin-resistant *Staphylococcus aureus* hand infections: case reports and clinical implications. J Hand Surg [Am] 2000 Jul;25(4):760–3.

Mason M, Koch S. Human bite infections of the hand. Surg Gynecol Obstet 1930;51:591–625.

Peters W. Hand infection apparently due to *Bacillus fusiformis*. J Infect Dis 1911;8:455–62.

Rockwell PG. Acute and chronic paronychia. Am Fam Physician 2001 Mar 15;63(6):1113–6.

Schmidt DR, Heckman JD. *Eikenella corrodens* in human bite infections of the hand. J Trauma 1983 Jun;23(6):478–82.

Welch C. Human bite infections of the hand. N Engl J Med 1936;215:901.

ADDITIONAL READINGS

Lamb DW, Hooper G. Hand conditions. New York: Churchill Livingstone, 1994.

Clark DC. Common acute hand infections. Am Fam Physician 2003 Dec 1;68(11):2167–76.

Talan DA, Abrahamian FM, Moran GJ, et al. Clinical presentation and bacteriologic analysis of infected human bites in patients presenting to emergency departments. Clin Infect Dis 2003 Dec 1;37(11):1481–9.

23. Osteomyelitis

Melinda Sharkey and Serena S. Hu

Outline   Introduction
Epidemiology
Clinical Features
Differential Diagnosis
Laboratory and Radiographic Findings
Treatment
Complications and Admission Criteria
Special Considerations: Pressure Ulcers
Pearls and Pitfalls
References

INTRODUCTION

Osteomyelitis is an infectious inflammatory disease of bone, often of bacterial origin. Early diagnosis, antibiotic therapy, and possibly surgical management can control and even eradicate bone infection. Causative organisms vary depending on the portal of entry (direct inoculation versus hematogenous seeding) and the associated health status of the patient.

EPIDEMIOLOGY

Patients with increased susceptibility to osteomyelitis include those with sickle cell anemia, chronic granulomatous disease, diabetes mellitus, and human immunodeficiency virus (HIV)/acquired immunodeficiency syndrome (AIDS). Although *Staphylococcus aureus* is the most common cause of osteomyelitis overall, patients with these chronic medical conditions are especially prone to infection by gram-negative organisms, including *Pseudomonas aeruginosa*, as well as by fungi and atypical mycobacteria.

CLINICAL FEATURES

The most common route of infection is direct inoculation due to injury. Hematogenous osteomyelitis secondary to bacteremia is usually a single organism infection, whereas direct penetration may involve multiple organisms. *S. aureus* is the causative organism in most cases of osteomyelitis.

The inflammatory process causes tissue necrosis and destruction of bony structure. Infection also obliterates vascular channels to the periosteum and intramedullary bone, leading to ischemia and areas of necrotic cortical bone, or sequestra. These sequestra are the hallmark of chronic infection, as the devitalized bone cannot be healed by the body's immune response. Surviving periosteum forms new bone, called an involucrum, which encases the dead bone. Draining sinuses form when purulence tracks to the skin surface through irregularities in the involucrum.

Presentation can vary from an open wound with exposed bone or a draining sinus to swelling and tenderness without any skin changes (Table 23.1). In acute osteomyelitis, defined as less than 6 weeks from onset of infection, patients may present with fevers, chills, and night sweats indicating

intermittent or persistent bacteremia. With progression to a chronic phase, patients complain of chronic pain and drainage with or without low-grade fevers. The white blood cell count (WBC) is usually elevated in acute but not chronic cases. The

Table 23.1 Clinical Features: Osteomyelitis

Organisms	• Hematogenous osteomyelitis: *S. aureus* • Direct penetration: multiple organisms
Signs and Symptoms	**Variable presentation:** • Swelling and tenderness without any skin changes • Draining sinus • Open wound with exposed bone **Acute phase:** • Fever, chills, and night sweats **Chronic phase:** • Drainage, pain, low-grade fevers
Laboratory and Radiologic Findings	• White blood cell count may be normal in chronic cases. ESR and CRP are elevated. • Blood culture may identify organism in hematogenous osteomyelitis. • Plain radiographs lag by 2 weeks and show soft-tissue swelling, periosteal thickening and elevation, and focal osteopenia. • MRI can differentiate between involvement of bone or soft tissue when the region is known. Affected areas appear as low signal on T1 and high signal on T2. • Technetium-99 bone scan shows increased uptake within 48 hours. Indium-labeled white blood cell scan is sensitive for acute and chronic osteomyelitis. • Deep bone biopsy is necessary to identify causative organism in chronic osteomyelitis.
Treatment	IV antibiotics for 4–6 weeks. Initial antibiotic selection should cover *Staphylococcus aureus* and is tailored to culture results: nafcillin 2 g IV q6h *or* cefazolin 2 g IV q8h (high doses are necessary) vancomycin (for MRSA) 10–15 mg/kg IV q12h (serum trough levels should be 15–20) Antibiotics may be sufficient for acute hematogenous osteomyelitis. Operative drainage, debridement, and soft-tissue coverage will likely be necessary for chronic osteomyelitis.

MRI, magnetic resonance imaging; MRSA, methicillin-resistant *Staphylococcus aureus*; ESR, erythrocyte sedimentation rate; CRP, C-reactive protein.

erythrocyte sedimentation rate (ESR) and C-reactive protein (CRP) are elevated in both acute and chronic cases. The CRP is more specific but should not be used alone to rule out osteomyelitis. The white blood cell count, ESR, and CRP should be measured at initial evaluation and followed to track response to treatment.

DIFFERENTIAL DIAGNOSIS

The clinical presentation of chronic osteomyelitis usually consists of nonspecific signs and symptoms such as pain and low-grade fever present for 1 to 3 months.

Key features that may help to distinguish osteomyelitis are:

- swelling and erythema over the involved bone (in acute phase)
- signs of bacteremia such as fever and chills (in acute phase)
- persistent drainage or sinus tracts

Other conditions to consider are:

- tumor
- traumatic or stress fracture
- inflammatory arthritis
- gout
- reactive bone marrow edema
- endocarditis

LABORATORY AND RADIOGRAPHIC FINDINGS

Identification of an organism is the single most important step and depends on a positive culture. In acute osteomyelitis, blood cultures may yield growth, but sampling of affected bone or deep soft tissue will likely be required in more chronic stages. Unless the patient is acutely ill, antibiotics *should not be given until operative or deep-tissue specimens are obtained*. Sinus tract and cutaneous wound cultures do not reliably predict the organisms responsible for the underlying bone infection and should not be sent.

Plain radiographs should be the first imaging performed but radiologic evidence of osteomyelitis often lag 2 weeks behind the infectious process, the earliest changes noted are soft-tissue swelling, periosteal thickening or elevation, and focal osteopenia (Figures 23.1 and 23.2).

Magnetic resonance imaging (MRI), which has a high sensitivity and specificity for detection of osteomyelitis, should be performed for suspicious cases and is useful for evaluating the bone and surrounding soft tissue. Edema appears dark on the T1-weighted sequence and bright on T2. Technetium-99 bone scans are positive within 48 hours of infection (Figure 23.3).

Gallium labels transferrin and is sensitive for inflammation. Indium-labeled white blood cell scan is positive in 80% of cases of acute osteomyelitis. Computed tomographic (CT) scan defines the sequestrum well and can be used for surgical planning.

Standard acute care evaluation for osteomyelitis includes:

- radiographs
- complete blood count (CBC), ESR, CRP
- blood cultures

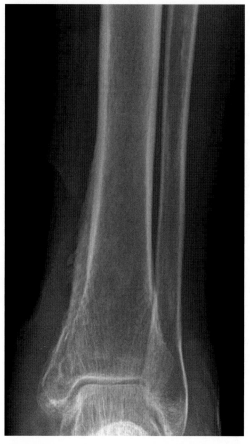

Figure 23.1 AP radiograph of the left ankle in a patient with a chronic ulcer over the medial ankle with underlying chronic osteomyelitis of the medial malleolus and medial distal tibia. Note the periosteal elevation and osteopenia.

- MRI if radiographs unclear
- nuclear medicine studies if MRI not possible or extent of involvement unknown

TREATMENT

Acute osteomyelitis should usually be treated by targeted intravenous antibiotics for 4–6 weeks, although there is evidence that some newer antibiotic regimens have adequate bony penetration with oral administration. Clinical response as well as laboratory markers, such as CRP, should be used to monitor treatment response.

Definitive treatment of chronic or refractory acute osteomyelitis requires drainage of the abscess and debridement of devitalized tissue, obliteration of dead space, tailored antibiotic therapy, and when possible, correction of host comorbidities such as nutrition status, smoking cessation, diabetes control, and reversal of vascular compromise. Management of large defects may require complex reconstructive surgery. Intravenous antibiotics are usually administered for 4–6 weeks based on outcomes of animal studies showing that revascularization of bone takes 4 weeks. A course of oral antibiotics may be given following completion of intravenous antibiotics, especially in patients with poor microvascular circulation (e.g., diabetics). Cure rates better than 90% have been reported. Treatment failure is typically due to

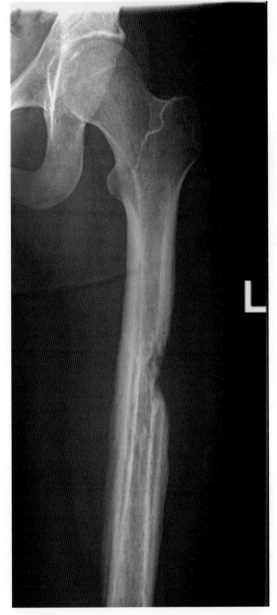

Figure 23.2 AP radiograph of a patient with osteomyelitis of the left femur.

microbial resistance to antibiotics, failure to complete antibiotic regimens, or inadequate debridement.

COMPLICATIONS AND ADMISSION CRITERIA

Complications and admission criteria include:

- bacteremia and sepsis
- persistent infection
- admission is generally necessary for initial diagnostic evaluation, identification of organism, and initiation of antibiotic therapy

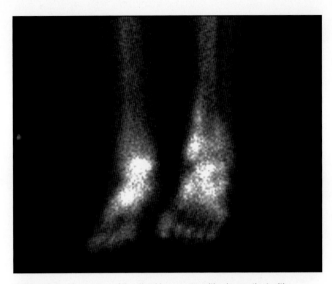

Figure 23.3 Bone scan of the distal lower extremities in a patient with osteomyelitis showing increased uptake in the left medial malleolus and distal tibia compared to the right ankle. This bone scan corresponds to the radiographs in Figure 23.1.

SPECIAL CONSIDERATIONS: PRESSURE ULCERS

Pressure ulcers are a common problem in debilitated and immobilized patients. The incidence of osteomyelitis of pressure ulcers in spinal cord injury and stroke patients has been reported to be 17–32%. Non-healing cutaneous ulcers may indicate an underlying bone infection. Diagnosis requires a positive bone culture and pathological examination demonstrating inflammatory cells in bone marrow tissue. While prevention is the ultimate goal, treatment for osteomyelitis from pressure ulcers consists of a 6- to 8-week course of antibiotics followed by delayed flap coverage.

PEARLS AND PITFALLS

1. Withhold antibiotics until cultures are obtained.
2. Sinus tract cultures and wound swabs are unreliable.
3. Surgical debridement is usually necessary for chronic osteomyelitis.

REFERENCES

Darouiche RO, Landon GC, Klima M, et al. Osteomyelitis associated with pressure sores. Arch Intern Med 1994 Apr 11;154(7):753–8.

Gustilo RB, Gruninger RP, Tsukayama DT. Orthopaedic infection: diagnosis and treatment. Philadelphia: Saunders, 1989.

Lazzarini L, Mader JT, Calhoun JH. Osteomyelitis in long bones. J Bone Joint Surg Am 2004 Oct;86-A(10):2305–18.

Lew DP, Waldvogel FA. Osteomyelitis. Lancet 2004 Jul 24–30;364(9431):369–79.

24. Open Fractures

Melinda Sharkey and Serena S. Hu

INTRODUCTION

Open fractures occur when the involved bone and surrounding soft tissues communicate with the outside environment because of a traumatic break in the overlying skin. Many open fractures are a result of high-energy trauma and are associated with severe soft-tissue injury. Lower energy open fractures occur when the skin break is caused by an "inside-out" injury. This occurs when a fractured end of the bone penetrates the overlying skin.

EPIDEMIOLOGY

Fractures represent a major public health problem. The lifetime risk of fracture up to age 65 years is one in two, and every year, 1 in 118 people younger than 65 years of age sustains a fracture. Approximately 2% of all fractures and dislocations are open.

CLINICAL FEATURES

Open fractures can be classified according to the Gustilo classification system (Figures 24.1, 24.2, and 24.3; Table 24.1).

DIFFERENTIAL DIAGNOSIS

Key clinical questions that may help in the diagnosis of open fractures are:

- Is an open fracture the source of visible bleeding?
- How large is the wound and how severe is the soft-tissue damage?
- Are the joints above and below affected?
- What is the neurovascular status of the affected limb?

TREATMENT AND PROPHYLAXIS

The rate of infection despite antibiotic administration in type I fractures range from 0% to 2%, in type II fractures from 2% to 10%, and in type III fractures from 10% to 50%. Administration of antibiotics for open fractures should not be thought of as a prophylactic measure, but rather as a treatment measure. All open fractures are contaminated with bacteria because of their communication with the outside environment.

Treatment of open fractures includes assessment of the patient and resuscitation as necessary, classification of injury, immediate antibiotic administration and tetanus prophylaxis, wound management, and fracture stabilization. In general, patients with type I and II open fractures should at least receive a first-generation cephalosporin to cover gram-positive bacterial contamination. Often, an aminoglycoside is also administered to cover gram-negative bacteria. For elderly patients or those with renal insufficiency, other antibiotics such as quinolones, aztreonam, or third-generation

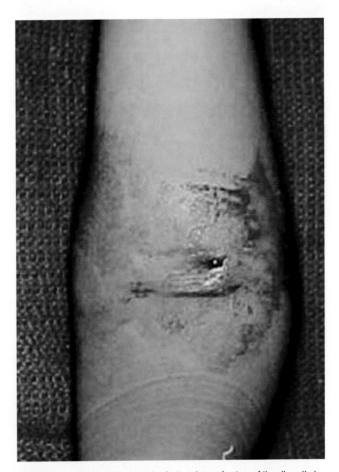

Figure 24.1 Photographic example of a type I open fracture of the elbow that shows a small, less than 1-cm skin opening and minimal soft-tissue damage. Photograph from the Orthopaedic Trauma Association website, http://www.ota.org.

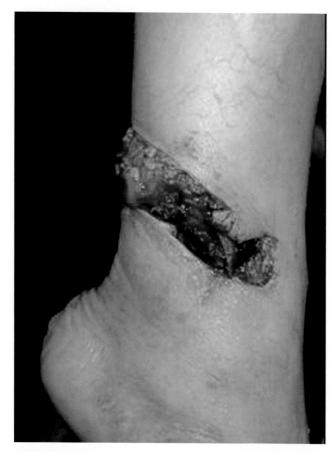

Figure 24.2 Photographic example of a type II open fracture of the distal tibia with a >1-cm skin opening, with moderate to severe soft soft-tissue damage but adequate soft soft-tissue coverage of bone. Photograph from the Orthopaedic Trauma Association website, http://www.ota.org.

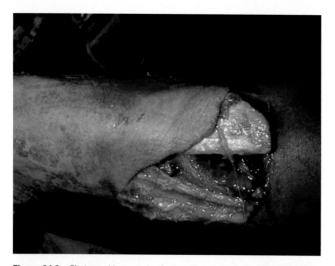

Figure 24.3 Photographic example of a type III open fracture of the tibia. Notice the >10-cm skin break as well as extensive soft-tissue injury including periosteal and muscle stripping from bone. Photograph from the Orthopaedic Trauma Association website, http://www.ota.org.

cephalosporins can also be administered for gram-negative coverage. Antibiotics that are effective against gram-positive and gram-negative organisms such as cefazolin and an aminoglycoside should be administered for type III fractures. Fur-

Table 24.1 Gustilo Classification of Open Fractures

Fracture Type	Soft-Tissue Injury	Bone Injury	Antibiotics*
Type I	<1 cm skin opening, minimal soft-tissue damage	Simple transverse or short oblique fracture	cefazolin 2 g IV q8h
Type II	>1 cm skin opening, moderate to severe soft-tissue damage but adequate bone coverage	Transverse and oblique fractures, minimal comminution	cefazolin 2 g IV q8h

Type III >10 cm skin break with extensive soft-tissue injury, often with a severe crushing component and fracture pattern consistent with a high-energy mechanism.

Fracture Type	Soft-Tissue Injury	Bone Injury	Antibiotics*
Type IIIA	Limited periosteal stripping, bone coverage usually adequate	Segmental fractures, highly comminuted fractures	cefazolin 2 g IV q8h and gentamicin 1.5–1.7 mg/kg/ dose IV q8h Alternative: piperacillin-tazobactam
Type IIIB	Extensive periosteal and muscle stripping from bone, usually severe contamination	Segmental fractures, highly comminuted fractures	cefazolin 2 g IV q8h and gentamicin 1.5–1.7 mg/kg/ dose IV q8h Alternative: piperacillin-tazobactam
Type IIIC	Any open fracture associated with vascular injury requiring surgical repair	Variable	cefazolin 2 g IV q8h and gentamicin 1.5–1.7 mg/kg/ dose IV q8h Alternative: piperacillin-tazobactam

*Penicillin G 2–3 million units IV q4–6h and clindamycin 600–900 mg IV q8h should be added for highly contaminated wounds (i.e., those occurring in a farmyard) to cover *Clostridium perfringens*.

ther, any open fracture that occurs in a highly contaminated environment should additionally be treated with penicillin and clindamycin to cover *Clostridium perfringens*.

In addition to antibiotic administration, initial management should include irrigation of the wound with sterile saline and coverage of the open wound with a sterile dressing. The extremity should then be splinted and radiographs obtained. In addition, a complete neurovascular exam of the injured extremity as well as an exam for compartment syndrome should be performed. After initial acute treatment, the patient will need to be taken to the operating room for formal irrigation and debridement of the wound and fixation of the fracture.

COMPLICATIONS AND ADMISSION CRITERIA

Complications and admission criteria include:

- unrecognized fractures
- compartment syndrome
- vascular injury
- osteomyelitis
- admission for surgical irrigation, debridement, and intravenous antibiotics

PEARLS AND PITFALLS

1. Antibiotics should be initiated immediately on recognition of an open fracture.
2. Following identification and initial irrigation, the wound should be covered with a sterile dressing and repeat examinations avoided.
3. The joint above and below should be examined and imaged to rule out adjacent fractures.
4. Open fractures are usually high-energy injuries with increased risk of neurovascular injury and/or compartment syndrome.
5. Bleeding in the presence of underlying fracture should be considered an open fracture until proven otherwise.

REFERENCES

Gustilo RB, Anderson JT. Prevention of infection in the treatment of one thousand and twenty-five open fractures of long bones. J Bone Joint Surg 1976;58-A:453–8.

Gustilo RB, Mendoza RM, Williams DN. Problems in the management of type III (severe) open fractures: a new classification of type III open fractures. J Trauma 1984;24:742–6.

Patzakis MJ, Harvey JP, Ivler D. The role of antibiotics in the management of open fractures. J Bone Joint Surg 1974;56-A:532–41.

Patzakis MP, Wilkins J. Factors influencing infection rate in open fracture wounds. Clin Orthop 1989;243:36–40.

Zalavras CG, Patzakis MJ. Open fractures: evaluation and management. J Am Acad Orthop Surg 2003;11:212–9.

25. Spinal Infections

James M. Mok and Serena S. Hu

VERTEBRAL OSTEOMYELITIS

Introduction

Pyogenic infections of the spine are most frequently caused by hematogenous spread. Other possible mechanisms are direct inoculation and local extension from a contiguous infection. Involved structures may include the vertebral body, intervertebral disk, spinal canal, or surrounding soft tissues. Because it is an uncommon disease, diagnosis of vertebral body osteomyelitis is often delayed, and late diagnosis may result in collapse of the vertebral body, kyphosis, and spinal instability that can lead to neurologic compromise.

Epidemiology

Vertebral osteomyelitis usually occurs in men older than 50 years of age, though increasing incidence has been noted in younger patients who are injection drug users. The spine is involved in 2% to 4% of all cases of osteomyelitis with the lumbar region most frequently involved. Gram-positive organisms are responsible for the majority of cases, with *Staphylococcus aureus* reported as the causative organism in greater than 50% of cases. Vertebral infection by *Escherichia coli* and *Proteus* has been associated with preceding urinary tract infection, and infection by *Pseudomonas* has been reported in injection drug users. Diabetes mellitus or penetrating trauma may increase susceptibility to anaerobic infection. Patients with sickle cell anemia are at risk for *Salmonella* osteomyelitis. *Staphylococcus epidermidis* and *Streptococcus viridans* cause infections characterized by an indolent course.

Clinical Features

Patients complain of axial back pain, insidious in onset and worsened by motion, which is constant and unrelieved by rest (Table 25.1). Fever is not reliably present. The presentation is usually subacute or chronic in nature. On physical examination, the most common finding is exquisite tenderness to palpation of the affected area due to paraspinal muscle spasm. Although neurologic symptoms are uncommon on initial presentation, the earliest sign of spinal cord involvement is clonus in the ankle. Risk factors include advanced age, intravenous drug use, recent urinary tract infection, trauma, any immunocompromised state due to steroid use, malignancy, chronic illness, or liver disease.

Table 25.1 Clinical Features: Vertebral Osteomyelitis

Organisms	• *Staphylococcus aureus* most common • *Escherichia coli* • *Proteus* • *Pseudomonas* • *Salmonella* • *Staphylococcus epidermidis* • *Streptococcus viridans* • *Bartonella quintana* • *Mycobacterium tuberculosis* • *Histoplasma capsulatum*
Incubation Period	Weeks to months
Signs and Symptoms	• Back pain • Tenderness to palpation • Loss of motion • Pseudoscoliosis • Fever (unreliable)
Laboratory and Diagnostic Findings	• ESR and CRP elevated • Plain radiographs show changes at 2–3 weeks. Initial osteolysis of the vertebral body may progress to disk space narrowing, end plate sclerosis, and vertebral body collapse. • MRI with gadolinium contrast shows hypointense signal on T1-weighted images and hyperintense signal on T2-weighted images within the vertebral body or disk • Core needle biopsy
Treatment	Hold antibiotics until biopsy unless absolutely necessary cefazolin 2 g IV q8h *or* nafcillin 2 g IV q6h *or* vancomycin (for MRSA coverage) 10–15 mg/kg IV q12h (trough should be 15–20)

CRP, C-reactive protein; ESR, erythrocyte sedimentation rate; MRI, magnetic resonance imaging; MRSA, methicillin-resistant *Staphylococcus aureus*.

Differential Diagnosis

Key features that may help to distinguish pyogenic vertebral osteomyelitis from tuberculous osteomyelitis are:

- history of recent travel or residence in tuberculosis-endemic areas
- relative intervertebral disk space sparing in tuberculous osteomyelitis
- thoracic region involvement more frequent in tuberculous osteomyelitis

Other conditions to consider:

- tuberculous vertebral osteomyelitis
- epidural abscess
- neoplasm or metastatic disease
- osteoporotic vertebral compression fracture

Laboratory and Radiographic Findings

Leukocytosis is usually absent, but the erythrocyte sedimentation rate (ESR) and C-reactive protein (CRP) are elevated in most cases. Blood cultures should be obtained but are not reliably positive, although the yield may be better during febrile episodes. A purified protein derivative (PPD) test should be ordered along with an anergy test to rule out tuberculous osteomyelitis.

Plain radiographs should be part of the initial evaluation. Findings such as osteolysis of the vertebral body are nonspecific and first appear 2–3 weeks after infection. Disk space narrowing and adjacent end plate sclerosis characterize more advanced disease that, if left untreated, progresses to eventual collapse of the vertebral body with local kyphosis (Figure 25.1).

Magnetic resonance imaging (MRI) is the imaging study of choice in spinal infections because of its very high sensitivity, specificity, and accuracy. Osteomyelitis appears as areas of hypointense signal on T1-weighted images and hyperintense signal on T2-weighted images within the vertebral body or disk. Gadolinium contrast enables earlier detection as well as improving specificity (Figure 25.2). Technetium-99 bone scan is highly sensitive but because of its poor specificity should be limited to those cases in which MRI is contraindicated.

Core needle biopsy is essential because identification of the organism guides all future treatment. Biopsy should be performed under fluoroscopic or computed tomographic (CT) guidance. Yields as high as 70–100% have been reported, although more commonly it is lower, especially with non-*Staphylococcus* species. Because antibiotics have been shown to significantly decrease the yield rate, whenever possible they should be held until biopsy unless the patient is septic, critically ill, or develops a neurologic deficit. In cases where therapy has already been initiated, antibiotics should be held for 2 weeks prior to biopsy to maximize the likelihood that an organism will be isolated.

Treatment and Prophylaxis

The goals of treatment are to identify the organism and eradicate the infection while maintaining spinal stability and a normal neurologic status. When patients are neurologically

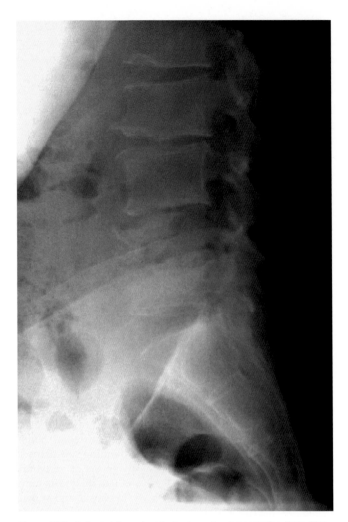

Figure 25.1 Lateral radiograph of the lumbar spine demonstrating destruction of the L4 and L5 vertebral bodies and intervening disk space from bacterial osteomyelitis.

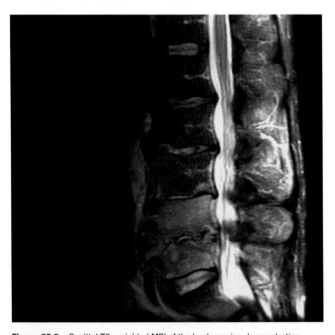

Figure 25.2 Sagittal T2-weighted MRI of the lumbar spine demonstrating destruction of the L4 and L5 vertebral bodies and the intervening disk space from bacterial osteomyelitis. The MRI corresponds to the plain radiograph in Figure 25.1.

intact, nonoperative treatment is successful in the majority of cases. However, patients are often debilitated and have significant comorbidities that contribute to a mortality rate as high as 5–15%. During the course of treatment, neurologic status must be carefully monitored. Intravenous antibiotics are administered for a period of 6–12 weeks. The duration of treatment is ultimately dictated by the patient's clinical progress.

Surgery is indicated when an open biopsy is necessary in order to identify an organism. Indications for surgical debridement also include clinically significant sepsis, failure of nonoperative treatment, cord compression with neurologic deficit, and spinal deformity or instability. Nonoperative treatment is deemed to have failed if symptoms, inflammatory markers, and imaging studies do not improve after 1 month of therapy. Surgical treatment most commonly consists of anterior debridement and fusion.

Special Considerations

TUBERCULOUS OSTEOMYELITIS OF THE SPINE

Pott's disease is characterized by an indolent course with less severe back pain, longer duration of symptoms, and absence of fever. The spine is involved in more than 50% of tuberculous infections of bone. Patients are usually immigrants from countries where the disease is endemic. Plain radiographs may show vertebral body destruction with relative sparing of the disk space, kyphosis, and a large soft-tissue mass with calcifications that is considered pathognomonic. MRI findings include a well-defined abscess spreading anteriorly to adjacent levels (Figure 25.3). The lesion may be confused with a tumor. Treatment is with oral antibiotics consisting of isoniazid, rifampin, ethambutol, and pyrazinamide for the first 2 months followed by a regimen based on sensitivities for an additional 8–10 months. Treatment can last up to 2 years. Surgery is indicated in the presence of a progressive kyphotic deformity or neurologic compromise. (See Chapter 33, Tuberculosis.)

POSTOPERATIVE INFECTION

Postoperative infections are becoming increasingly common as more spinal procedures are performed. Rates are historically higher than other orthopedic procedures. The most common organisms are *Staphylococcus aureus* and *Streptococcus epidermidis*. Instrumented fusion and staged surgery have been identified as independent risk factors. The most common presentation occurs during the second postoperative week with wound discharge and dehiscence. Treatment is surgical irrigation and debridement with primary or delayed closure.

Complications and Admission Criteria

Complications include:

- collapse of vertebral body causing kyphotic deformity
- neurologic compromise
- extension of infection to adjacent structures
- bacteremia and sepsis

Admission is generally necessary to perform a biopsy, identify the organism, and initiate intravenous antibiotic therapy.

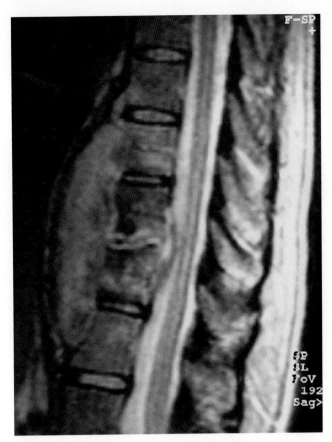

Figure 25.3 Sagittal MRI of the spine of a patient with tuberculosis of the spine. Notice the well-defined large anterior soft-tissue abscess. From: Griffith J, et al. Imaging of musculoskeletal tuberculosis: a new look at an old disease. Clin Orthop 2002 May;398:32–9.

Pearls and Pitfalls

1. Diagnosis of vertebral osteomyelitis is often delayed.
2. Antibiotics should be held until core needle biopsy is performed unless clinically necessary.
3. Neurologic status must be closely monitored over the course of antibiotic therapy.
4. The earliest sign of spinal cord involvement is ankle clonus.
5. Collapse of the vertebral body and local kyphosis seen in advanced disease may be confused for osteoporotic vertebral compression fracture, so a mechanism of injury should be identified.

EPIDURAL ABSCESSES

Introduction

An epidural abscess usually develops in association with vertebral osteomyelitis. It can cause neurologic injury through mechanical compression of the neural elements and ischemic thrombosis of the spinal cord. In the presence of a neurologic deficit, it is considered a surgical emergency requiring urgent decompression. A delay in diagnosis can have devastating consequences including permanent paraplegia.

Epidemiology

Epidural abscesses are estimated to occur in 0.2 to 2 cases per 10,000 hospital admissions and have been increasing over the

Table 25.2 Clinical Features: Epidural Abscess

Organisms	• *Staphylococcus aureus* most common • *Streptococcus* species **After spinal procedure:** *S. aureus*, coagulase-negative staphylococci, gram-negative bacilli (including *Pseudomonas*), *Aspergillus* (after steroid injections) **Immunocompromised host:** *Candida* species, *Aspergillus* species, *Cryptococcus neoformans*, *Nocardia asteroides*, *Mycobacterium tuberculosis*, and other mycobacteria
Signs and Symptoms	• Fever (60–80%) • Focal vertebral pain • Tenderness to percussion • Radicular pain or paresthesias along involved nerve roots • Evidence of spinal cord compression: motor weakness, bowel or bladder dysfunction, sensory changes, paralysis (possible depressed respiratory function if cervical cord involved).
Laboratory and Diagnostic Findings	• Elevated WBC, ESR, and CRP • Plain radiographs may show evidence of osteomyelitis • MRI with gadolinium will demonstrate ring-enhancing lesion in epidural space with or without osteomyelitis
Treatment	Immediate broad-spectrum antibiotics piperacillin-tazobactam 4.5 g IV q6h (*Pseudomonas* dosing) *and* vancomycin 10–15 mg/kg IV q12h Emergent surgical decompression

WBC, white blood (cell) count.

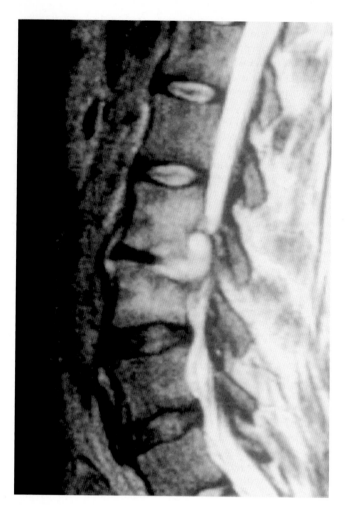

Figure 25.4 Sagittal MRI of the spine of a patient with an epidural abscess.

past decade. Peak incidence is the sixth and seventh decade of life with a 2:1 male predominance. The lumbar spine is usually the affected region. *S. aureus* accounts for approximately 70% of epidural abscesses, followed by *Streptococcus* species with 7% of cases.

Clinical Features

Presentation can be highly variable, and immunocompromised patients should be approached with a high index of suspicion (Table 25.2). Patients usually present with a neurologic deficit and unremitting back pain that is not relieved by rest. Most are febrile. Symptoms progress from localized back pain and radiculopathy to motor weakness, bowel or bladder incontinence, and eventually complete paralysis. Physical examination should include assessment of perineal sensation and anal sphincter tone. A post-void residual urinary volume greater than 100 to 200 mL is indicative of retention. Straight leg raise maneuver may elicit radicular pain. Diminished reflexes are an early neurologic sign, with progression to hyperreflexia, clonus, and positive Babinski response (up-going toes). Risk factors for epidural abscess include any immunocompromised state secondary to diabetes mellitus, renal disease, alcoholism, human immunodeficiency virus (HIV), cancer, chronic steroid use, or sepsis; intravenous drug use; obesity; and trauma. Additional risk factors include recent spinal surgery or epidural injection.

Differential Diagnosis

Other conditions to consider are:

• vertebral osteomyelitis
• intra-abdominal or retroperitoneal abscess
• cauda equina syndrome
• epidural hematoma
• disk herniation
• meningitis
• neoplasm
• cord infarction
• acute viral flaccid paralysis (e.g., West Nile virus, enterovirus)

Laboratory and Radiographic Findings

Elevated white blood cell count, ESR, and CRP are common. Blood cultures may yield the organism in 60% of patients.

Plain radiographs should be assessed for evidence of vertebral osteomyelitis. MRI with gadolinium contrast is the study of choice and should be obtained emergently if epidural abscess is suspected. With addition of contrast, the abscess will appear as a ring-enhancing lesion and can be delineated from the neural elements (Figure 25.4).

Standard laboratory tests to order for epidural abscess are:

- white blood cell count
- ESR and CRP
- MRI with gadolinium

Treatment

Diagnosis of an epidural abscess should be followed immediately by the administration of broad-spectrum antibiotics with activity against *Staphylococcus* and *Streptococcus* and additional coverage for gram-negative organisms if there is a history of immune suppression. If neurologic compromise is present, treatment includes emergent surgical decompression and drainage of the abscess. Surgery is followed by long-term antibiotic therapy with at least 4 weeks of intravenous antibiotics. In patients with no neurologic deficit, percutaneous drainage of the epidural abscess has been reported to have good results.

Complications and Admission Criteria

Complications and admission criteria include:

- cauda equina syndrome: paraplegia, sexual dysfunction, and bowel and bladder incontinence
- bacteremia and sepsis

Pearls and Pitfalls

1. Lumbar puncture is contraindicated in the setting of epidural abscess.
2. Permanent neurologic sequelae are common.
3. The major determinant of outcome is prompt diagnosis.
4. No neurologic recovery is expected if paraplegia has been present for more than 12 hours.

REFERENCES

An HS, Seldomridge JA. Spinal infections: diagnostic tests and imaging studies. Clin Orthop 2006 Mar;444:27–33.

Bluman EM, Palumbo MA, Lucas PR. Spinal epidural abscess in adults. J Am Acad Orthop Surg 2004 May–Jun;12(3):155–63.

Fang A, Hu SS, Endres N, et al. Risk factors for infection after spinal surgery. Spine 2005 Jun 15;30(12):1460–5.

Swanson AN, Pappou IP, Cammisa FP, et al. Chronic infections of the spine: surgical indications and treatments. Clin Orthop 2006 Mar;444:100–6.

Tay BK, Deckey J, Hu SS. Spinal infections. J Am Acad Orthop Surg 2002 May–Jun;10(3):188–97.

Weinstein MA, McCabe JP, Cammisa FP Jr. Postoperative spinal wound infection: a review of 2,391 consecutive index procedures. J Spinal Disord 2000 Oct;13(5):422–6.

26. Prosthetic Joint Infections

James M. Mok and Serena S. Hu

INTRODUCTION

Prosthetic joint infection is a feared complication of total joint replacement surgery and occurs as a result of bacterial contamination of the implant surface. It can occur at any point after the initial operation and is characterized by a slow, indolent course that usually results in a delay in diagnosis. Diagnosis and treatment are difficult, and eradication by nonoperative means is rare if not impossible. The consequences of misdiagnosis are substantial and may lead to unnecessary surgery in the case of a false positive. Delays in diagnosis can make control of the infection more difficult and necessitate removal of the prosthesis, which entails prolonged immobilization and delayed reimplantation.

EPIDEMIOLOGY

Approximately 500,000 primary joint arthroplasties are performed every year in the United States. Infection is relatively rare, occurring in 1–2% of primary surgeries, but represents the second leading cause of failure. Treatment for prosthetic joint infection costs an estimated $250 million annually in the United States. The causative organisms are usually *Staphylococcus aureus* or *Staphylococcus epidermidis*.

CLINICAL FEATURES

Pain is the most common presenting symptom (Table 26.1). Drainage is the second most common and is strongly suggestive of infection if it is present several weeks postoperatively. Fever is rarely present. The presentation is often subacute, and complaints of pain must be approached with a high degree of suspicion for infection. Most prosthetic joint infections occur as late infections.

Prosthetic joint infections are classified by their clinical features as acute, hematogenous, or chronic types. Characteristics of acute infection are acute onset of severe joint pain, effusion, decreased range of motion, warmth, and erythema, accompanied by fevers and chills. Hematogenous infections are usually preceded by an oral, skin, gastrointestinal, or urinary tract infection. Chronic infections are caused by low-virulence organisms and may present as persistent postoperative pain or early loosening of hardware on radiographs. Risk factors for infection include a history of revision surgery, problems with wound healing, rheumatoid arthritis, diabetes mellitus, or malignancy.

DIFFERENTIAL DIAGNOSIS

Key features that distinguish prosthetic joint infection from other conditions are:

- pain localized to joint
- elevated erythrocyte sedimentation rate (ESR) and CRP
- effusion, decreased range of motion (variable)

Other conditions to consider are:

- aseptic loosening
- postoperative hematoma
- implant failure
- periprosthetic fracture

Key clinical questions that help to distinguish postoperative joint infection are:

- Is the ESR or CRP elevated?
- Is there a history of trauma?

Table 26.1 Clinical Features: Prosthetic Joint Infection

Organisms	*Staphylococcus aureus* and *Staphylococcus epidermidis* most common
Signs and Symptoms	• Variable • Severe joint pain with decreased range of motion • Swelling/effusion • Warmth/erythema • Persistent postoperative pain, swelling
Laboratory and Diagnostic Findings	• CRP usually elevated • Plain radiographs usually normal or nonspecific • Synovial fluid white cell count elevated (10,000–50,000/mm^3) • Nuclear medicine studies show increased signal
Treatment	• Hold antibiotics unless absolutely necessary (in order to ensure accurate cultures). • Surgical incision and drainage with retention of implants if <6 weeks of symptoms

CRP, C-reactive protein.

- Has the patient had persistent postoperative pain?
- Is the patient less than 6 weeks postoperative?

LABORATORY AND RADIOGRAPHIC FINDINGS

The ESR and CRP have important roles in the evaluation of the painful joint arthroplasty. An elevated CRP greater than 3 months postoperatively should raise concern for infection. Sensitivity and specificity of ESR greater than 30 mm/hr have been reported as 82% and 85%, and for CRP greater than 10 mg/L as 96% and 92%. A normal ESR and CRP are reassuring for no infection.

Plain radiographs usually appear normal but should be obtained routinely to rule out wear, osteolysis, or fracture. When present, radiographic findings are nonspecific and include periosteal reaction, scattered osteolysis, or bone resorption.

Joint aspiration employing sterile technique is the usual diagnostic technique and should be part of the early evaluation. It can be performed at bedside for superficial joints such as the knee but may require fluoroscopic guidance for deep joints such as the shoulder and hip. Gram stain has poor sensitivity, and sensitivity of bacterial culture ranges from 50% to 93% and is greatly reduced if antibiotics have been administered. Synovial fluid cell counts of 10,000 to 50,000 leukocytes/mm^3 are suggestive of an infection, but no strict threshold exists.

Nuclear studies are frequently used to detect infection or loosening of the implants. Although sensitive, they are not specific. The physician should be aware that the technetium-99m bone scan may remain abnormal for up to 1 year postoperatively. Indium-111 tagged white blood cell scan is an alternative nuclear study but takes 2 days to perform.

Standard tests to order for evaluation of prosthetic joint infections are:

- ESR and CRP
- joint aspiration fluid
- plain radiographs
- nuclear medicine studies

TREATMENT AND PROPHYLAXIS

Treatment of prosthetic joint infection is operative. Unless clinically necessary, antibiotics should be held until an organism is identified. Chronic suppression with antibiotics is reserved for severely debilitated patients who are unable to tolerate additional surgery, as attempts at suppression only lead to more extensive and resistant infection. At surgical incision and debridement, retention of implants may be considered if symptoms have been present for less than 6 weeks. Better outcomes have been reported when incision and drainage are performed early. In the United States, the preferred treatment for prosthetic joint infection is two-stage revision arthroplasty. All implants are removed and replaced with antibiotic-impregnated cement, followed by 6 weeks of intravenous antibiotics. Reimplantation is attempted after eradication of infection is confirmed.

COMPLICATIONS AND ADMISSION CRITERIA

Complications include:

- early implant failure
- persistent infection precluding retention of implants due to delayed diagnosis or intervention

Admission is indicated for bacteremia or sepsis.

PEARLS AND PITFALLS

1. ESR and CRP are useful in evaluation of the painful joint arthroplasty.
2. Antibiotics should be held until joint aspiration is performed unless clinically necessary.
3. Surgical incision and drainage should be performed as early as possible if attempting to retain implants.
4. Painful joint arthroplasty must be approached with a high index of suspicion for infection and should include evaluation by an orthopedic surgeon.

REFERENCES

Bauer TW, Parvizi J, Kobayashi N, Krebs V. Diagnosis of periprosthetic infection. J Bone Joint Surg Am 2006 Apr;88(4):869–82.

Della Valle CJ, Zuckerman JD, Di Cesare PE. Periprosthetic sepsis. Clin Orthop 2004 Mar;(420):26–31.

Hanssen AD, Spangehl MJ. Treatment of the infected hip replacement. Clin Orthop 2004 Mar;(420):63–71.

Larsson S, Thelander U, Friberg S. C-reactive protein (CRP) levels after elective orthopedic surgery. Clin Orthop 1992 Feb;(275):237–42.

Zimmerli W, Trampuz A, Ochsner PE. Prosthetic-joint infections. N Engl J Med 2004 Oct 14;351(16):1645–54.

27. Diabetic Foot Infections

Melinda Sharkey and Serena S. Hu

INTRODUCTION

A diabetic foot infection is defined as any inframalleolar infection in a person with diabetes mellitus, and most arise from diabetic foot ulcers. Diabetic foot ulcers are portals of entry for infection in hosts with impaired immunity as well as physiologic limitations to wound healing. Therefore, all diabetic foot ulcers should be treated as chronic wounds that will not heal on their own – intervention is mandatory. Moreover, it is critical that infected diabetic foot ulcers be recognized and treated promptly because they represent the biggest risk factor for nontraumatic amputations in the diabetic population.

EPIDEMIOLOGY

Diabetic foot infections account for the largest number of diabetes–related hospital bed days. In the United States alone, about 82,000 limb amputations are performed annually in those with diabetes, and an amputation in a diabetic patient is associated with a 5-year mortality rate between 39% and 68%.

CLINICAL FEATURES

Purulent secretions, necrotic tissue, and signs of inflammation including pain, redness, warmth, tenderness and induration indicate infection of a diabetic foot ulcer (Figure 27.1, Table 27.1). All patients seen in the acute care setting with diabetic foot ulcers should undergo a basic peripheral vascular exam including palpation of the peripheral pulses and measurement of the ankle brachial index in each leg. An ankle brachial index is calculated by dividing the blood pressure in the calf of the affected foot by the blood pressure in the upper extremity. An ankle brachial index of 1 is normal. Atherosclerosis can markedly decrease blood flow to the lower extremities and therefore inhibit healing of diabetic foot ulcers. Patients with an ankle-brachial index (ABI) of less than 0.9 require evaluation by a vascular surgeon.

Probing of bone in the depths of an infected diabetic foot ulcer has been shown to strongly correlate with the presence of underlying osteomyelitis. Bone detected on probing has been shown to be 66% sensitive and 85% specific for underlying osteomyelitis. If bone is probed, other tests to diagnose osteomyelitis are unnecessary. Probing of all ulcers should be done on initial assessment using a sterile metal instrument or sterile cotton swab.

DIFFERENTIAL DIAGNOSIS

Key features that may help to distinguish diabetic foot osteomyelitis from acute Charcot arthropathy (noninfectious joint destruction; see Special Considerations) are:

- presence of ulcer with signs of infection
- elevated white blood cell count (WBC) (erythrocyte sedimentation rate [ESR] may be elevated in both conditions)
- systemic inflammatory response is more indicative of infection
- typical radiographic appearance of Charcot arthropathy: dorsal dislocations of toes and midfoot, metatarsophalangeal joint destruction, metatarsal stress fractures, flattened arch, destruction of talus, cuneiform, or cuboid bones

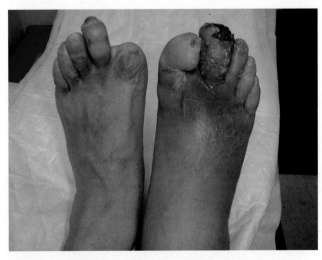

Figure 27.1   Photograph of a diabetic foot infection demonstrates swelling, draining purulence, necrotic tissue and associated cellulitis of the dorsum of the foot. From the website http://medicine.ucsf.edu/cliniclimg/extremities-diabetic-foot-infection.html. Permission granted by Dr. Charlie Goldberg and Dr. Jan Thompson.

Table 27.1 Clinical Features: Diabetic Foot Infections

Organisms	Acute infections are usually monomicrobial, whereas chronic infections are polymicrobial • *Staphylococcus aureus* and beta-hemolytic • *Streptococcus* (especially group B) are most common • Chronic wounds may contain *Enterococcus*, Enterobacteriaceae, anaerobes, *Pseudomonas aeruginosa*, and gram-negative rods • Previous treatment may predispose to resistant organisms such as methicillin-resistant *S. aureus* (MRSA) or vancomycin-resistant *Enterococcus* (VRE).
Signs and Symptoms	• Foot ulcer • Purulent secretion • Redness, warmth, swelling, induration, and/or pain and tenderness • If severe, systemic toxicity possible
Laboratory and Radiographic Findings	• Plain radiographs show osteomyelitis as demineralization, periosteal reaction and bony destruction after 2 weeks • MRI highly sensitive for bone edema • ESR and CRP elevated • Severe hyperglycemia and electrolyte imbalance in severe cases
Treatment	**Empiric therapy for severe infection:** • vancomycin 10–15 mg/kg IV q12h *plus* piperacillin-tazobactam 4.5g IV q8h *or* • ertapenem 1 g IV daily **Empiric therapy for mild infection:** • cephalexin 500 mg PO qid for 10–14 days *or* • dicloxacillin 500 mg PO qid for 10–14 days *or* • clindamycin 300 mg PO tid for 10–14 days • wound care • surgical debridement or amputation

CRP, C-reactive protein; ESR, erythrocyte sedimentation rate; MRI, magnetic resonance imaging; MRSA, methicillin-resistant *Staphylococcus aureus*.

• combined technetium-99 bone scan and indium-labeled leukocyte scan improve specificity
• magnetic resonance imaging (MRI) cannot distinguish bone edema due to neuroarthropathy from osteomyelitis

Key clinical questions that help to distinguish severity of infection are:

• Are there signs of systemic toxicity or metabolic instability?
• What is the stage of the infection: cellulitis, abscess, gangrene?
• What is the depth and tissue involvement of the wound: fascia, muscle, tendon, joint, bone?
• What is the extent of surrounding cellulitis and/or lymphangitic streaking?

LABORATORY AND RADIOGRAPHIC FINDINGS

If there is clinical evidence of infection, a bacterial culture should be obtained prior to empiric antibiotic administration. Generally, superficial wound swabs are not considered reliable and deep-tissue cultures are necessary. Consequently, if

the patient is not systemically infected and will be taken in a timely manner for formal irrigation and debridement, it is better to hold antibiotics until deep tissue cultures can be obtained intraoperatively.

Laboratory tests should include complete blood count with differential, ESR, C-reactive protein (CRP), basic chemistry panel, hemoglobin A1C, prealbumin, and urine microalbumin. Prealbumin is a marker for short-term evaluation of nutrition status and is important because malnutrition is associated with immunodeficiencies that can impair wound healing. Microalbuminuria is used for early detection of diabetic nephropathy but is also a significant risk factor for foot ulcers.

Radiographic imaging of the infected foot is important in diagnosing associated bone infection, as the diagnosis of osteomyelitis will affect surgical planning. Plain radiographs (anteroposterior, lateral, and oblique views) of the involved foot are sufficient in the vast majority of cases to assess for bony involvement and to look for foreign bodies and gas. The radiographic triad of osteomyelitis includes demineralization, periosteal reaction, and bony destruction but may not be evident for up to 2 weeks after infection. If the diagnosis of osteomyelitis is in question, other imaging modalities can be utilized. MRI is very sensitive but not specific in diagnosing osteomyelitis. MRI will clearly show edema and hyperemia of the bone, but this may be caused by surrounding soft soft-tissue infection and not by infection of the bone itself. Bone scans and leukocyte scans can also be utilized.

TREATMENT

The goal of treatment of diabetic foot ulcers in an acute care setting is the identification of infected foot ulcers so the patient can be treated expeditiously and aggressively with necessary debridements and antibiotics. The need for hospitalization should be evaluated based on the severity of the infection. When signs of systemic toxicity are present, the patient should be medically stabilized to restore fluid and electrolyte balances, control hyperglycemia, and treat other comorbidities.

Initial antibiotic therapy is usually empiric, with the choice of antibiotic depending on the severity of the infection. Broad-spectrum intravenous antibiotics are indicated for severe, extensive, or chronic infections and should include activity against gram-positive cocci. Coverage for methicillin-resistant *Staphylococcus aureus* (MRSA) should be considered in areas where community-acquired MRSA is common. Initial empiric treatment for mild and moderate infections is usually adequate using more narrow-spectrum oral antibiotics that cover only aerobic gram-positive cocci. Few clinical trials of antibiotic therapy for diabetic foot infection have been published, and no consensus exists on the most effective single agent or combination therapy.

Indications for surgery include necrotizing fasciitis, gas gangrene, extensive soft-tissue loss, or critical ischemia (ABI <0.5). Urgent amputation is reserved for those cases in which extensive necrosis or life-threatening infection is present. Pus under pressure can rapidly cause irreparable damage and should be drained promptly. Mild infections can be observed to determine the efficacy of medical therapy and demarcate the boundary between necrotic and viable tissue. In the case of dry gangrene, waiting for the necrotic portion to autoamputate is a reasonable option. A dry and adherent heel eschar

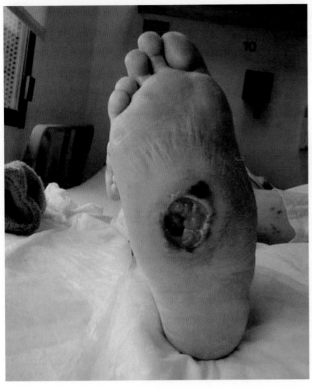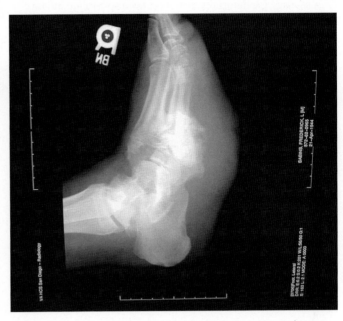

Figure 27.2 Photograph and corresponding radiograph of a patient with neuropathic arthropathy of the foot showing a typical rocker-bottom foot with an associated plantar ulcer. The plain radiograph shows severe bony destruction through the tarsal-metatarsal joint. From the website http://medicine.ucsf.edu/cliniclimg/extremities-neuropathic-ulcer.html. Permission granted by Dr. Charlie Goldberg and Dr. Jan Thompson.

should not be debrided unless it appears to be the source of infection.

SPECIAL CONSIDERATIONS

Osteomyelitis

Diagnosis of osteomyelitis in the diabetic foot can be difficult, and the optimal treatment remains controversial. Osteomyelitis causes impaired wound healing and may act as a focus for recurrent infection. As the size and depth of an ulcer increases, the likelihood of underlying bone infection increases as well. The forefoot is most commonly affected. The presence of osteomyelitis signifies a greater likelihood of surgery, including amputation, and longer duration of antibiotics.

Charcot Arthropathy

Diabetes is the most common cause of neuropathic arthropathy (Charcot arthropathy), a noninfectious condition in which joint destruction occurs secondary to lack of protective sensation. Diagnosis is often clinical, especially in the early stages. In acute Charcot neuroarthropathy, the foot is warm, edematous, and markedly erythematous. Patients will demonstrate a sensory and autonomic neuropathy and may or may not complain of pain. The exact mechanism of progressive joint destruction has yet to be understood. In the foot, neuroarthropathy can affect the forefoot, the midfoot, and the hindfoot. Most commonly, the tarsal-metatarsal joint is affected. Patients with neuroarthropathy need to be followed closely and treated carefully because the associated foot deformities result in a particularly high risk of developing severe diabetic foot ulcers (Figure 27.2).

COMPLICATIONS AND ADMISSION CRITERIA

Admission is indicated for:

- systemic toxicity (e.g., fever and leukocytosis)
- metabolic instability (e.g., severe hypoglycemia or acidosis)
- rapidly progressive or deep-tissue infection with substantial necrosis or gangrene
- presence of critical ischemia (ABI <0.5)
- urgent diagnostic or therapeutic interventions
- inability to care for self or inadequate home support

PEARLS AND PITFALLS

1. Not all diabetic foot ulcers are infected.
2. Infection may be more extensive than the initial appearance because of spread among foot compartments, to the deep plantar space, or along the tendon sheaths.
3. Palpable dorsalis pedis and posterior tibial pulses generally indicate adequate perfusion.
4. Caution must be used when interpreting ABIs in the presence of arterial calcification, which is suggested by ABIs of >1.

5. Suspect underlying osteomyelitis when an ulcer does not heal after 6 weeks of appropriate wound care.
6. Visible or easily palpated bone within an ulcer is likely to be complicated by osteomyelitis.
7. A sausage toe deformity, resulting from soft-tissue inflammation and underlying bony changes, is also highly suggestive of osteomyelitis.
8. Superficial wound cultures have no utility in directing antibiotic therapy and should not be performed. For osteomyelitis, deep tissue and bone cultures are necessary to direct treatment. If patient is clinically stable, antibiotics should be held until such cultures are obtained.

REFERENCES

Brem HB, Sheehan P, Rosenberg HJ, et al. Evidence-based protocol for diabetic foot ulcers. Plast Reconstr Surg 2006;117:193S–209S.

Guyton GP, Saltzman CL. The diabetic foot: basic mechanisms of disease. J Bone Joint Surg 2001;83-A:1083–96.

Lipsky BA, Berendt AR, Deery HG, et al. Diagnosis and treatment of diabetic foot infections. Clin Infect Dis 2004;39:885–910.

Grayson ML, Gibbons GW, Balogh K, et al. Probing to bone in infected pedal ulcers. A clinical sign of underlying osteomyelitis in diabetic patients. JAMA 1995;273:721–3.

28. Plantar Puncture Wounds

Rebeka Barth

Outline   Introduction
                Epidemiology
                Evaluation
                Clinical Features
                Laboratory and Radiographic Findings
                Treatment and Prophylaxis
                Complications and Admission Criteria
                Pearls and Pitfalls
                References

INTRODUCTION

Puncture wounds to the plantar surface of the foot are seemingly innocuous and common injuries but have the potential for serious complications.

EPIDEMIOLOGY

Puncture wounds of the foot are a common problem encountered by the acute care physician. One study showed that plantar puncture wounds constitute 7.4% of lower extremity trauma seen in the emergency department or office setting. In another series, puncture wounds made up 0.8% of all pediatric emergency department visits. These estimates may be deceivingly low as many puncture wounds are self-treated and present once complications have arisen. There is a seasonal variation, with the highest occurrence in incidence seen in the warm months from May through October when children go barefoot and people engage in more outdoor activities. The vast majority of these are caused by nails (98%). Of the remaining cases, a wide variety of other objects have been described including wood, toothpicks, glass, plastic, rock, bones, coral, straw, bullets, wire, and sewing needles. Infection risk is increased in patients with wounds to the forefoot, in patients wearing shoes when the injury occurred, and in patients with diabetes.

EVALUATION

The complication rate of plantar puncture wounds is dependent on multiple factors that must be considered when determining management. See Table 28.1.

CLINICAL FEATURES

Plantar puncture wound infection may present with the five classic signs of inflammation: rubor (erythema), tumor (swelling), dolor (pain), calor (warmth), and functio laesa (loss of function) (Table 28.2). The presence of drainage is also highly suggestive of infection.

The spectrum of infection can span from local wound infection or cellulitis through abscess, septic arthritis, sepsis, or osteomyelitis (see Chapter 43, Bacterial Skin and Soft-Tissue Infections; Chapter 21, Adult Septic Arthritis; Chapter 61, Septic Shock; and Chapter 23, Osteomyelitis). Direct exten-

sion osteomyelitis is a rare but severe complication seen in approximately 1–2% of injuries. Osteomyelitis presents weeks after the injury and may be preceded by a period of clinical improvement. Patients should always be evaluated radiographically for a retained foreign body that may serve as a nidus of infection, especially in cases of relapsing infection despite antibiotics.

LABORATORY AND RADIOGRAPHIC FINDINGS

Complete blood count (CBC) with differential, blood cultures, erythrocyte sedimentation rate (ESR), and/or C-reactive protein (CRP) should be obtained if there is suspicion of systemic infection or osteomyelitis. A normal CRP or ESR, however, does not rule out osteomyelitis or other significant infection. Deep wound swabs after incision and drainage may be sent for Gram stain, culture, and sensitivity, which may be useful for wounds with clinical signs of infection such as purulent drainage, cellulitis, lymphangitis. Superficial swabs are not recommended. Joint aspiration should be obtained for suspected septic arthritis. Bone biopsy is the gold standard for diagnosis of osteomyelitis.

Plain film radiographs are the initial recommended diagnostic modality for puncture wounds and are used to assess fractures, effusions, osteomyelitis, and retained foreign bodies. Their shortcomings include inability to visualize

Table 28.1 History and Examination for Plantar Puncture Wounds

History
- Time elapsed since injury (less than or greater than 24 hours)
- Material and size of the penetrating object as well as depth of penetration
- Environment in which injury occurred (i.e., farmland, industrial area, or aquatic)
- State of the object (e.g., clean or rusty or dirt-covered)
- Type of shoe worn, particularly tennis shoes
- Constitutional symptoms including fever, chills, vomiting
- Presence or absence of diabetes, human immunodeficiency virus (HIV), long-term steroid use, peripheral vascular disease, asplenia, or transplanted organs

Physical Examination
- Depth, extent, and location of wound
- Neurovascular status
- Any signs of local or systemic infection such as fever, tachycardia, erythema, warmth, drainage, fluctuance, lymphangitis, joint effusion

Table 28.2 Clinical Features: Plantar Puncture Wound Infection

Organisms	**Cellulitis:** • *Staphylococcus aureus* (most common) • Beta-hemolytic *Streptococcus* • *Staphylococcus epidermidis* • *Escherichia coli* • *Proteus mirabilis* • *Klebsiella* sp. **Osteomyelitis in nondiabetic patients:** • *Pseudomonas aeruginosa* (>90%) **Osteomyelitis in diabetic patients:** • *Staphylococcus aureus* or polymicrobial
Signs and Symptoms	• Warmth, erythema, tenderness, swelling surrounding puncture site • Antalgic (abnormal) gait • Wound drainage • Fever, chills, vomiting. tachycardia if systemic involvement
Laboratory and Radiographic Findings	• WBC may be elevated • ESR, CRP may be elevated • Superficial wound swabs not recommended • X-rays initially to look for any suspected foreign body • CT if nonradiopaque foreign body or early osteomyelitis suspected • Ultrasound for suspected abscess or nonradiopaque foreign body (operator dependent)

CRP, C-reactive protein; CT, computed tomography; ESR, erythrocyte sedimentation rate; WBC, white blood (cell) count.

nonradiopaque foreign bodies and to detect osteomyelitis in the acute phase. Computed tomography (CT) is useful for nonradiopaque foreign bodies and identification of early osteomyelitis. Ultrasound is most useful for real-time imaging of nonradiopaque foreign bodies and abscesses, facilitating removal and drainage. Magnetic resonance imaging (MRI) is useful for detection of abscess, osteomyelitis, or septic arthritis, but cannot be used for detection of metallic foreign bodies.

Retained foreign body occurs in 3% of all plantar puncture wounds. Broken needles or pins are the most common objects, constituting 30% of all foreign-body retention. Foreign bodies may act as a continued nidus of infection and inflammatory response, preventing proper healing, or may cause persistent discomfort and difficulty with ambulation. Indications for removal of foreign bodies include location near or into bone, joint, or neurovascular structures, infection, or persistent symptoms. Failure to obtain radiographic evaluation is the most frequent cause of missed foreign body, but not all materials appear on plain films. All metal fragments and most glass fragments will appear on x-ray, but wood or plastic may not.

Fluoroscopy is the current method of choice for removal of radiopaque foreign bodies as it is less invasive and does not involve delays with sending patients back to the radiology department. Immediate images can be obtained in a series of exposures while dissecting toward the foreign object.

TREATMENT AND PROPHYLAXIS

Depending on the footwear, the entry of a sharp object into the foot can carry with it particles of dirt, grass, sock, and rubber sole or other shoe material. These wounds should be treated as contaminated and tetanus-prone.

Most puncture wounds heal uneventfully with little or no intervention. Infection risk is increased in patients with wounds to the forefoot, in patients wearing shoes, and in patients with diabetes.

Although there is no current consensus on the appropriate treatment for plantar puncture wounds, initial treatment for all puncture wounds should include (Table 28.3):

- Wound care: Superficial cleansing and debridement of nonviable tissue can be performed for all wounds. Varying recommendations exist regarding more aggressive treatment such as coring, and probing of the wound. These interventions can be painful and difficult to perform but may be worthwhile in deep wounds with gross contamination. Deep pressure irrigation is controversial and may contaminate surrounding tissues.
- Foreign body removal: Whenever possible, foreign bodies should be removed to reduce the risk of complications such as persistent pain or infection. Risks of removal of foreign bodies must be taken into consideration according to location and characteristics of object.
- Tetanus immunization: Plantar puncture wounds are at high risk for tetanus because they are commonly inoculated with *Clostridium tetani* spores and constitute an oxygen-poor environment (see Chapter 63, Tetanus).
- Antibiotics: There is no prospective investigation on the use of prophylactic antibiotics in uncomplicated plantar puncture wounds. Widespread use of prophylactic antibiotics is not recommended. Antibiotics should be considered at initial presentation in the case of gross contamination, wounds deep to bone or joint, or wounds presenting after 24 hours with persistent symptoms.
- The decision to prescribe antibiotics should take into account the nature of the wound as well as any underlying medical issues of the patient. The most common pathogen in cellulitis associated with plantar puncture wounds is *Staphylococcus aureus*. The most common pathogen in osteomyelitis due to puncture wounds is *Pseudomonas aeruginosa*. *P. aeruginosa* should be suspected in patients with a history of a nail puncture wound through a tennis shoe. One series showed that cases of cellulitis or osteochondritis following a nail puncture wound could be treated with intravenous (IV) ciprofloxacin for 24 hours in conjunction with surgical intervention followed by oral ciprofloxacin (750 mg bid) for 7–14 days. There are however, increasing cases of documented fluoroquinolone-resistant *P. aeruginosa*. In addition, fluoroquinolones are not recommended for children. Alternative therapies are ceftazidime or cefepime.
- Follow-up care: All plantar puncture wounds should have follow-up and be instructed to return immediately for persistent pain or any signs of infection. Patients who present with infected wounds should have 48 hour follow-up if they are not admitted.

COMPLICATIONS AND ADMISSION CRITERIA

Complications of plantar puncture wounds include cellulitis, abscess, septic arthritis, sepsis, and osteomyelitis. Infections

Table 28.3 Treatment of Plantar Puncture Wounds

Treatment	• Wound care • Foreign body removal • Tetanus immunization • Antibiotic prophylaxis not recommended for clean wounds in immunocompetent patients • No data on prophylactic antibiotic choice or duration. • Staphylococcus, streptococcus, or pseudomonas coverage for contaminated or deep wounds or immunocompromised patients may prevent complications. **Cellulitis***: • 7 days of therapy with oral staphylococcus and streptococcus coverage with or without additional antipseudomonal coverage • cephalexin 500 mg PO qid for uncomplicated cellulitis. • cephalexin + TMP-SMX DS PO bid or clindamycin 450 mg PO qid for associated abscess or for high-probability MRSA. • ciprofloxacin 500 mg PO bid (poor staph/strep coverage) or moxifloxacin 400 mg + 1 g probenecid PO qd (will cover *S. aureus* [susceptible strains] and *Pseudomonas* [susceptible strains]) **Early bone involvement (osteochondritis)***: • oral ciprofloxacin for 14 days **Osteomyelitis**: • cefepime (2 g IV q12h) or IV ciprofloxacin for anti-pseudomonal coverage or IV-piperacillin-tazobactam dose (should be directed by surgical/bone culture as there is significant pseudomonal resistance in each locality). Treat for 4 to 6 weeks.

*In limited studies, oral therapy of 750 mg bid was preceded by 24 hours of IV ciprofloxacin coupled with surgical intervention.
MRSA, methicillin-resistant *Staphylococcus aureus*; TMP-SMX DS, trimethoprim-sulfamethoxazole double strength.

are commonly associated with retained foreign body. Diabetics are at increased risk for osteomyelitis, as are nondiabetics with puncture wounds through a rubber-soled shoe. Cellulitis or abscess formation is usually seen in presentations greater than 24 hours after injury. These patients present with persistent symptoms of pain and/or drainage and have local or systemic signs of infection on examination.

PEARLS AND PITFALLS

1. Imaging is necessary to look for retained foreign body.
2. Antibiotics should include *P. aeruginosa* coverage for wounds unresponsive to initial therapy and all wounds through rubber-soled shoes.
3. Pressure irrigation of puncture wounds is controversial and may contaminate surrounding tissues

REFERENCES

Baldwin G, Colbourne M. Puncture wounds. Pediatr Rev 1999 Jan;20(1):21–3.

Chachad S, Kamat D. Management of plantar puncture wounds in children. Clin Pediatr 2004;43:213.

Chisholm CD, Schlesser JF. Plantar puncture wounds: controversies and treatment recommendations. Ann Emerg Med 1989 Dec;18(12):1352–7.

Gasink LB, Fishman NO, Weiner MG, et al. Fluoroquinolone-resistant *Pseudomonas aeruginosa*: assessment of risk factors and clinical impact. Am J Med 2006 Jun;119(6):526.e19–25.

Lavery LA, Walker SC, Harkless LB, et al. Infected puncture wounds in diabetic and nondiabetic adults. Diabetes Care 1995 Dec;18(12):1588–91.

Raz R, Miron D. Oral ciprofloxacin for treatment of infection following nail puncture wounds of the foot. Clin Infect Dis 1995 Jul;21(1):194–5.

Schwab RA, Powers RD. Conservative therapy of plantar puncture wounds. J Emerg Med 1995:13:291–5.

29. Periocular Infections

Renee Y. Hsia

INTRODUCTION

The eyelid is the first and foremost defense of the eye, covering the cornea and also distributing and eliminating tears. Understanding of the structures of the eyelid margin area allows easier diagnosis of periocular disorders (Figure 29.1). Anatomically, the eyelid is composed of skin, the orbicularis oculi muscle (innervated by the seventh cranial nerve), and tarsus and conjunctiva. The levator muscle (supplied by the third cranial nerve) and Müller's muscle (sympathetically innervated) open the upper lid. The eyelashes themselves can be affected in an isolated fashion, for example, or the effect may extend to the meibomian glands within the tarsus. Both the nasolacrimal duct and the lacrimal sac can become obstructed, producing dacryocystitis and canaliculitis, respectively. The orbital septum, contiguous with the tarsal plates both superiorly and inferiorly, serves a barrier between the eyelid and posterior orbital structures. An infection that is anterior to this septum is known as preseptal (or periorbital) cellulitis; postseptal infections are known as orbital cellulitis.

BLEPHARITIS AND HORDEOLA

Epidemiology

Blepharitis (Figure 29.2) and hordeola (Figure 29.3), both infections of the eyelids or eyelashes, are often confused with each other. Blepharitis is inflammation of the eyelids and/or eyelash follicles and is a relatively common ocular disorder. It is usually bilateral. The mean age is approximately 40–50 years old, affecting women more than men, and is more common in those with fair skin. It is generally categorized into three categories: seborrheic blepharitis, contact dermatitis blepharitis, and infectious blepharitis.

The first two noninfectious (seborrheic and contact dermatitis blepharitis) causes are due to sloughing skin cells from overfunctioning sebaceous glands and sensitivity to various materials or chemicals (e.g., mascara) and will not be the focus of the discussion here. Infectious blepharitis is most often caused by *Staphylococcus epidermidis*, *Propionibacterium* acnes, and *Corynebacterium* species. It can occur either as a result of

direct infection of the lid or as a reaction to the bacterial antigen and/or exotoxin.

A hordeolum is similar in that it is an infection of the eyelash follicles due to blockage of sebaceous glands (causing an external hordeolum) or secondary infection of the meibomian glands (causing an internal hordeolum). Hordeola are usually unilateral.

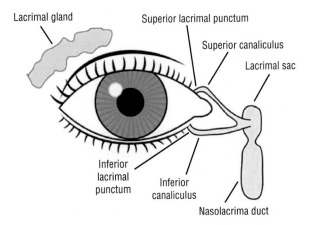

Figure 29.1 Eyelid anatomy. Adapted from drawing by Felipe Micaroni Lalli.

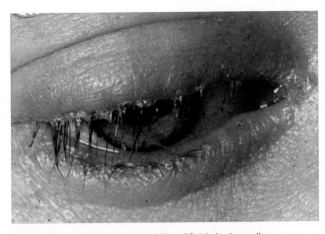

Figure 29.2 Blepharitis. Courtesy of Atlas of Ophthalmology online.

Table 29.1 Clinical Features: Blepharitis and Hordeolum

Organisms	**Blepharitis:** • *Staphylococcus epidermidis* • *Propionibacterium* acnes • *Corynebacterium* species **Hordeolum:** • Most often *Staphylococcus aureus*, but can be infected with organisms similar to those causing blepharitis
Incubation Period	1–7 days (up to 12 days)
Signs and Symptoms	**Blepharitis:** • Usually bilateral and intermittent symptoms • Inflamed eyelid margins • Eyelid itching, burning, or soreness • Mild foreign-body sensation • Crusting and debris of eyelid margins, especially on awakening • With or without misdirection or loss of eyelashes • With or without conjunctival injection • With or without swollen eyelids • With or without light sensitivity **Hordeolum:** • Usually unilateral • Pointing eruption or "pimple-like" lesion on either internal or external side of eyelid • Inflamed eyelid margin • Eyelid itching, burning, or soreness • Crusting and debris of eyelid margins, especially on awakening • With or without conjunctival injection
Laboratory and Radiographic Findings	There are no specific laboratory tests or radiographic findings for these diagnoses. It is possible to do a microbial culture of the eyelid by swabbing the eyelashes but usually not necessary in these diagnoses.

Clinical Features

Table 29.1 summarizes the clinical features that distinguish these two disorders from each other.

Differential Diagnosis

Blepharitis and hordeola are usually fairly straightforward to diagnose. However, a broad initial differential can avoid misdiagnosis:

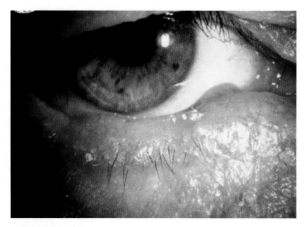

Figure 29.3 Hordeolum. Courtesy of Atlas of Ophthalmology online.

- Orbital cellulitis is distinguished from blepharitis by the presence of more systemic symptoms, tender sinuses, and sometimes limited extraocular movements.
- Squamous cell, basal cell, or sebaceous cell carcinoma of the eyelid are rare but can be missed in those diagnosed with chronic blepharitis; biopsy in these cases can be helpful.
- Viral or bacterial conjunctivitis usually affects the conjunctiva more than the eyelid itself.
- Dry eye syndrome often is associated with blepharitis.
- Chalazia (chronic granulomatous, inflammatory lesions) are painless when palpated.
- Ocular herpes simplex usually presents as a painful red eye and will manifest dendrites on fluorescein staining.
- Herpes zoster ophthalmicus entails inflammation of the conjunctiva and/or cornea and less of the eyelid itself.
- Molluscum contagiosum is characterized by dome-shaped, umbilicated shiny nodules on the eyelid that are usually non-tender.
- Crab lice (infestation with *Phthirus pubis*) may also be in other places on the body.

Treatment and Prophylaxis

Eyelid hygiene is extremely important (e.g., washing eyelids and eyelashes with diluted baby shampoo, eyelid cleanser) (Table 29.2). Clean, warm compresses at the onset of symptoms may limit severity. Those with dry eyes can be given artificial tears (e.g., Hypromellose 0.3%). Many cases of blepharitis and hordeolum will resolve without antibiotic (topical or systemic) treatment.

If inflammation seems to have spread beyond the localized area of the hordeolum or eyelid margin, topical antibiotics can be prescribed (see Table 29.2). For recurrent infection, severe secondary infection, or local cellulitis, systemic antibiotics are indicated. External hordeola are often self-limited but can be drained by lancing the lesion if necessary.

Table 29.2 Treatment of Blepharitis and Hordeolum

Patient Category	Therapy Recommendations
Adults: Preferred Choices	• Eyelid hygiene • Cleanse eyelids bid with cloth soaked in warm water for 5–10 minutes • Wash eyelid margins with diluted baby shampoo, eyelid cleanser, or a teaspoon of sodium bicarbonate in cup of boiled water • Artificial tears (e.g., Hypromellose 0.3%) for those with dry eyes • Topical antibiotics for mild cases of blepharitis and hordeola (e.g., erythromycin ointment 1.25 cm to lid margin qid or eye drops such as chloramphenicol (AK-Clor, Chloroptic, 5 mg/mL) q4h) • Systemic antibiotics (e.g., erythromycin 250 mg PO qid × 7 days, azithromycin 500 mg PO day 1, then 250 mg PO daily on days 2–5) for hordeolum, recurrent staphylococcal blepharitis, severe secondary infection of the meibomian glands, or local cellulitis • External hordeola are often self-limited but can be drained by lancing the lesion if necessary

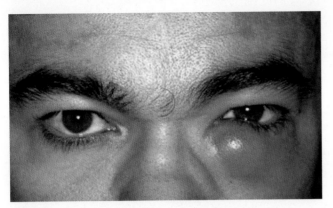

Figure 29.4 Dacryocystitis. Courtesy of Atlas of Ophthalmology online.

Table 29.4 Treatment of Dacryocystitis

Patient Category	Therapy Recommendations
Adults: **Preferred Choices**	Irrigation of the lacrimal sac Warm compresses **Topical antibiotics:** ● Erythromycin ointment 1.25 cm to lid margin qid ● Eye drops such as trimethoprim sulfate and Polymyxin B sulfate ophthalmic solution 1 drop q3h **Oral antibiotics:** ● Pediatric: oral antibiotics: amoxicillin-clavulanate 20–40 mg/kg/day divided tid; cefaclor 20–40 mg/kg/day divided tid ● Adult: cephalexin 500 mg qid or amoxicillin/clavulanate 500 mg bid ● Surgical treatment for dacryoliths, obstruction, or congenital causes

DACRYOCYSTITIS

Epidemiology

Dacryocystitis (Figure 29.4) can be either congenital or acquired; in the acquired form, it can present either acutely or chronically. Congenital dacryocystitis is related to the embryogenesis of the lacrimal excretory system. Dacryocystitis is presumed by some to occur more often on the left rather than the right because of a narrower angle between the nasolacrimal duct and lacrimal fossa on the left. Those at higher risk for acquired dacryocystitis include females, those with flatter noses and narrower faces, and age greater than 40. African Americans seem to have a lower risk of dacryocystitis.

Clinical Features

Table 29.3 summarizes the clinical features of dacryocystitis.

Differential Diagnosis

Dacryocystitis is most often confused with canaliculitis, which is infection of the lacrimal sac as opposed to the nasolacrimal duct. Canaliculitis is primarily due to infection by Actinomyces and can be secondary to solid concretions in the lacrimal sac, known as dacryoliths. These can often be expressed from the sac.

Table 29.3 Clinical Features: Dacryocystitis

Organisms	Usually due to streptococci (including *Streptococcus pneumoniae*) or *Staphylococcus aureus*
Signs and Symptoms	● Pain, swelling, and erythema over inner aspect of lower eyelid (usually nasal aspect) ● Excessive tearing ● With or without fever ● Tenderness in medial canthal region
Laboratory and Radiographic Findings	As in many of these disorders, this is a clinical diagnosis. Other laboratory or imaging modalities may be used to rule out other diseases (e.g., CT scan for mass as a cause of dacryocystitis).

CT, computed tomography.

Other diagnoses to consider are:

● blepharitis
● orbital or preseptal cellulitis
● chalazion
● conjunctivitis
● canalicular laceration

Treatment and Prophylaxis

For mild cases of dacryocystitis without fever, outpatient therapy is the standard of care. This includes irrigation of the lacrimal sac, warm compresses, topical antibiotics (e.g., polymyxin B sulfate–trimethoprim [Polytrim] or ofloxacin [Ocuflox] drops or ointments), and oral antibiotics (Table 29.4). Recommended therapies for pediatric patients are amoxicillin-clavulanate or cefaclor, and for adults are cephalexin or amoxicillin-clavulanate.

Acutely ill patients should be admitted and given broad-spectrum intravenous (IV) antibiotics (e.g., cefazolin) until improved. Imaging should be considered if orbital extension is suspected.

Surgical intervention (dacryocystorhinostomy) in addition to medical therapy may be appropriate for chronic dacryocystitis, or for persistent acute infections after several days of treatment with antibiotics.

Complications and Admission Criteria

Patients who are febrile and appear acutely ill should be hospitalized for IV antibiotics and possible surgical management as mentioned above. Dacryocystitis can progress to orbital cellulitis and has been reported to lead to orbital abscess as well as cavernous sinus thrombosis.

PERIORBITAL AND ORBITAL CELLULITIS

Epidemiology

Periorbital cellulitis is much more common than orbital cellulitis. Both periorbital and orbital cellulitis are more prevalent in children than adults, with the former peaking in much younger children (usually 3–36 months) rather than the

Table 29.5 Clinical Features: Periorbital and Orbital Cellulitis

	Periorbital (Preseptal)	Orbital (Postseptal)
Etiology	Trauma, bacteremia	Sinusitis
Organisms	**Trauma:** • *Staphylococcus aureus* • Group A *Streptococcus* **Bacteremia:** • *Streptococcus pneumoniae*	• *Streptococcus pneumoniae* • *Staphylococcus aureus* • *Moraxella catarrhalis* • Group A *Streptococcus* • Anaerobes (*Haemophilus influenzae* no longer predominant in postvaccination era)
Mean Age	<2 years	12 years
Clinical Findings	• Erythema and induration of periorbital tissues • Tenderness of periorbital tissues • Generally less toxic-appearing (unless bacteremic)	Same symptoms as periorbital cellulitis but may also have: • Proptosis • Conjunctival edema or chemosis • Ophthalmoplegia • Decreased visual acuity • Increased intraocular pressure • Headache

adolescent years. The microbiological causes of each are related to their etiology (Table 29.5).

Clinical Features

Table 29.5 summarizes the clinical features that distinguish these two disorders from each other.

Differential Diagnosis

Distinguishing periorbital cellulitis from orbital cellulitis is difficult. At times, periorbital cellulitis may appear worse than orbital cellulitis, as in Figure 29.5 (periorbital cellulitis caused by a mucormycosis fungal infection in an immunosuppressed patient) and Figure 29.6 (orbital cellulitis caused by *Staphylococcus aureus*). Distinguishing characteristics are discussed in the next section.

Other diagnoses to consider besides orbital and periorbital cellulitis are:

• cavernous sinus thrombosis: usually accompanied by headache and, in later stages, by severe gaze palsies and other eye findings
• neoplasms (e.g., neuroblastoma, rhabdomyosarcoma, retinoblastoma): typically less systemic symptoms
• endocrinopathies (e.g., thyroid ophthalmopathy): usually less erythema, swelling, and tenderness
• hordeolum/blepharitis: generally confined to eyelid margin
• conjunctivitis: normally confined to conjunctiva and less periorbital erythema and swelling

Other presentations of rare disorders include:

• orbital pseudotumor
• periocular dermoid cyst
• Wegener's granulomatosis of the orbit

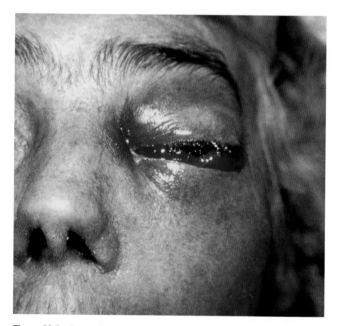

Figure 29.5 Periorbital cellulitis caused by mucormycosis. http://phil.cdc.gov/phil/home.asp, Centers for Disease Control and Prevention / Dr. Thomas F. Sellers / Emory University.

Laboratory and Radiographic Findings

There are no definitive laboratory tests for periorbital and orbital cellulitis. Blood cultures are generally recommended, especially in the pediatric population, where up to one-third of patients may have positive cultures. Cultures of eye secretions may be confusing because there may be many contaminants; in general, cultures should not be used to narrow antibiotic therapy, but rather to identify possible antibiotic-resistant organisms. The most specific cultures are from sinus contents or abscess material if surgically drained.

Because most cases of periorbital and orbital cellulitis occur in children, the recommendation for imaging is generally

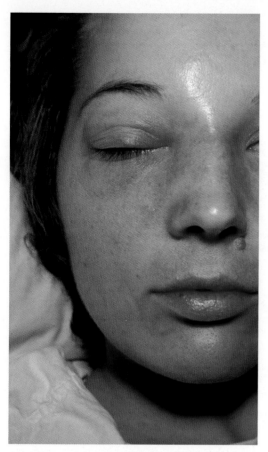

Figure 29.6 Orbital cellulitis caused by *Staphylococcus aureus*. http://phil.cdc.gov/phil/home.asp, Centers for Disease Control and Prevention / Dr. Thomas F. Sellers / Emory University.

based on clinical suspicion. In children where vision cannot be accurately assessed, the threshold for imaging should be lowered. Furthermore, even if one is almost certain of the orbital involvement, imaging may help direct surgical drainage.

High-resolution CT scanning is often considered the most easily available modality to distinguish periorbital from orbital cellulitis, as well as evaluating other competing diagnoses. Importantly, axial and coronal views are necessary: the former to evaluate for brain abscess in the parenchyma, and the latter for any subperiorbital processes.

Magnetic resonance imaging (MRI) can also narrow down the differential but is less available and more difficult to perform in the pediatric population because it requires a longer imaging time.

Orbital ultrasonography is also used in some institutions but is extremely operator dependent. This modality is useful for sequential follow-up of abscesses and in children where the sedation necessary for CT or MRI is contraindicated.

Treatment and Prophylaxis

Although children with periorbital cellulitis were previously hospitalized for observation, the trend is toward outpatient management with close follow-up for patients who do not appear toxic. There are a number of suggested regimens based on the usual organisms found in periorbital cellulitis, with duration of treatment for 7–10 days, with

amoxicillin-clavulanate, cefpodoxime, or cefdinir, as shown in Table 29.6.

Those less than 1 year of age and more ill-appearing patients should be treated as aggressively as those with orbital cellulitis, with IV antibiotics for 1 week (or at least until afebrile and clinically improved). There is limited data regarding the optimal duration of therapy, and the most conservative recommendation is for outpatient antibiotics for 2–3 weeks after clinical improvement from intravenous antibiotics, although many clinicians may choose not to prescribe such a long duration of therapy.

Failure to respond to IV antibiotics warrants repeat imaging and possible surgical drainage.

Complications and Admission Criteria

Any patient with suspected orbital cellulitis should be admitted for IV antibiotics and observation. Untreated orbital cellulitis can be fatal in up to 17% of patients and lead to blindness in the affected eye of approximately 20% of patients. With proper treatment of orbital cellulitis, the rate of visual loss is still 3–10% and mortality 1–2%. Permanent vision loss can occur from orbital cellulitis by two mechanisms: (1) increased intraorbital pressure causing damage to the optic nerve, or (2) direct extension of infection into the optic nerve. Cavernous sinus thrombosis is a potential complication and can be distinguished from orbital cellulitis by cranial MRI.

PEARLS AND PITFALLS

1. Perform a complete examination of the globe, especially the conjunctiva and cornea, for ocular herpes simplex or herpes zoster ophthalmicus.
2. Beware of recurrent blepharitis that does not respond to treatment. An occult malignancy could be the cause.
3. Congenital dacryocystitis should be treated aggressively because of its significant morbidity and mortality. Because the orbital septum is not fully formed in neonates, extension of the infection can lead to brain abscesses and sepsis. This condition can also be associated with amniotocele (when amniotic fluid is retained in the lacrimal sac because of an obstructed nasolacrimal duct) and requires probing of the duct by an ophthalmologist.
4. Severe cases of dacryocystitis can manifest by pupillary dysfunction due to increased intraorbital pressure and its effects on pupillomotor fibers in the orbit.
5. Orbital cellulitis should be strongly considered in the setting of pupillary dysfunction, diplopia, or loss of peripheral vision.
6. Squamous, basal, and sebaceous cell cancers can sometimes be misdiagnosed as chronic dacryocystitis.
7. Consider fungal causes (e.g., *Mucor*, *Aspergillus*) of orbital cellulitis, especially in patients who are immunosuppressed. Fungal orbital cellulitis can be lethal and treatment with amphotericin B must be monitored for both the progression of disease and medication side effects.
8. Patients with altered level of consciousness and ocular infections should be evaluated for meningitis and intracranial abscess formation, which can be extensions of orbital cellulitis.

Table 29.6 Treatment and Prophylaxis for Periorbital and Orbital Cellulitis

Patient Category	Therapy Recommendations

Adults: **Preferred Choices**	**For periorbital cellulitis:**
	• amoxicillin-clavulanate 875 mg PO bid
	• cefpodoxime 200 mg PO bid in adults
	• cefdinir 600 mg PO qd in adults
	For orbital cellulitis:
	• For empiric treatment or polymicrobial infection, vancomycin 1 g IV every 12 hours, if normal renal function, plus one of the following:
	  ○ piperacillin-tazobactam 4.5 g IV every 6 hours
	  ○ ceftriaxone 2 g IV every 12 hours, or
	  ○ cefotaxime 2 g IV every 4 hours
	• For MSSA, nafcillin 2 g IV every 4 hours
	• For MRSA, vancomycin 1 g IV every 12 hours, if normal renal function

Children: **Preferred Choices**	**For periorbital cellulitis:**
	• amoxicillin-clavulanate 90 mg/kg PO (based on amoxicillin component) in two divided doses
	• cefpodoxime 10 mg/kg PO in two divided doses (maximum 400 mg daily)
	• cefdinir 14 mg/kg PO in two divided doses (maximum 600 mg daily)
	For orbital cellulitis:
	• For empiric treatment or polymicrobial infection, vancomycin 15 mg/kg IV q12h, plus one of the following:
	  ○ piperacillin-tazobactam 240 mg/kg IV in three divided doses, maximum 16 g daily
	  ○ ceftriaxone 80 to 100 mg/kg IV in two divided doses, maximum 4 g daily, or
	  ○ cefotaxime 150 to 200 mg/kg IV in three to four equally divided doses, maximum 12 g daily
	• For MSSA, nafcillin 200 mg/kg IV in four or six divided doses, maximum 12 g daily
	• For MRSA, vancomycin 15 mg/kg IV q12h

Pregnant Women	Same as for nonpregnant adults, as all recommended drugs in the table are pregnancy category B. The only exception is for MRSA coverage, where vancomycin is pregnancy category C. In cases where MRSA is highly suspected and/or culture results identify MRSA, the risks of a spreading orbital cellulitis would warrant use of vancomycin, but recommendation is to consult infectious disease service as well.
Immunocompromised	Same as for nonimmunocompromised persons and children, but awareness that other infections (particularly fungal causes) could be present as well. Initial treatment would be the same, but additional fungal cultures should be sent if fungal causes are suspected and then treated with amphotericin B 5 mg/kg IV (single infusion at rate of 2.5 mg/kg/h; contents of infusion should be shaken q2h)

MRSA, methicillin-resistant *Staphylococcus aureus*; MSSA, methicillin-sensitive *Staphylococcus aureus*.

REFERENCES

Blepharitis Preferred Practice Pattern, American Academy of Ophthalmology, 2003.

Frith P, Gray R, MacLennan AH, et al. (eds). The eye in clinical practice, 2nd ed. London: Blackwell Science, 2001.

Gilliland G. Dacryocystitis. Emedicine. February 22, 2005. Retrieved February 21, 2007, from http://www.emedicine.com/oph/topic708.htm.

Givner LB. Periorbital versus orbital cellulitis. Pediatr Infect Dis J 2002 Dec;21:1157–8.

Hurwitz JJ. The lacrimal drainage system. In Yanoff M, Duker JS, Augsburger JJ, et al., eds, Ophthalmology. St. Louis: Mosby, 2004:764.

Nageswaran S, Woods CR, Benjamin DK Jr, et al. Orbital cellulitis in children. Pediatr Infect Dis J 2006;25:695.

Sobol SE, Marchand J, Tewfik TL, et al. Orbital complications of sinusitis in children. J Otolaryngol 2002;31:131.

ADDITIONAL READINGS

Carter SR. Eyelid disorders: diagnosis and management. Am Fam Physician 1998 Jun;57(11):2695–702. Available at: http://www.aafp.org/afp/980600ap/carter.html.

Howe L, Jones NS. Guidelines for the management of periorbital cellulitis/abscess. Clin Otolaryngol Allied Sci 2004;29:725.

30. Conjunctival and Corneal Infections

Renee Y. Hsia

INTRODUCTION

Because infections of the surface of the eye are common, and the consequences of misdiagnosis or delayed referral may be severe, familiarity with the anatomy and variable presentations of these infections is crucial to the acute care physician. The conjunctiva is a well-vascularized, clear membrane that both envelops the globe and wraps underneath the eyelids (Figure 30.1). The former segment is labeled the bulbar conjunctiva, and the latter, the tarsal or palpebral conjunctiva. The conjunctiva, along with the tear film, provides a physical and immunologic barrier against microbes and can produce an antimicrobial environment when its mast cells are activated.

Just below the conjunctiva is the vascularized episclera, and beneath this the sclera, which lies just over the choroid. The choroid and the episclera provide oxygen to the poorly vascularized sclera.

The cornea itself is subject to inflammation, which can be due to noninfectious causes (noninfectious keratitis) or infectious causes (infectious keratitis, including that caused by bacteria, viruses, or fungi).

CONJUNCTIVITIS

Clinical Features

Of all red-eye complaints, conjunctivitis (Figure 30.2) is the most common diagnosis. It can be separated into three categories: bacterial, viral, and allergic (Table 30.1).

Differential Diagnosis

Conjunctivitis is diffuse, not localized. Localized hyperemia may suggest:

- foreign body
- pterygium
- subconjunctival hemorrhage
- episcleritis

Conjunctivitis should inflame both the bulbar and tarsal conjunctiva. Infection of only the bulbar conjunctiva is suggestive of other "red eye" diagnoses, the most serious including:

- keratitis
- iritis
- acute angle closure glaucoma

Laboratory Findings

No cultures are needed for the diagnosis of conjunctivitis, unless *Neisseria gonorrhoeae* (or, less commonly, *Neisseria*

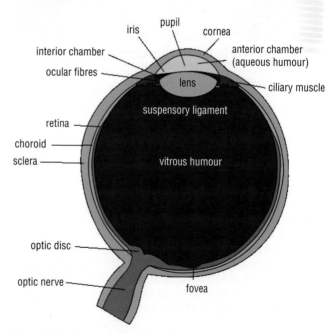

Figure 30.1 Eye anatomy. http://en.wikipedia.org/wiki/Image:Schematic_diagram_of_the_human_eye_with_English_annotations.svg, created by Erin Silversmith, August 30, 2006.

Table 30.1 Clinical Features: Conjunctivitis

	Bacterial	Viral	Allergic
Epidemiology	More common in children than adults (although even in children, most common cause of conjunctivitis is viral)	Most common cause of conjunctivitis in both children and adults	Common in patients with other seasonal allergies or atopy
Organisms	*Staphylococcus aureus* (more common in adults) *Streptococcus pneumoniae* *Haemophilus influenzae* *Moraxella catarrhalis* *Neisseria* (see Pearls and Pitfalls for further discussion)	Most common is adenovirus (many different strains) Herpes simplex virus*	No organisms involved; can be caused by perfume, cosmetics, drugs, other irritants
Signs and Symptoms	Typically unilateral but can be bilateral Thick, purulent discharge throughout the day	Generally bilateral and less purulent; more mucoid and serous Profuse tearing Can be associated with other viral symptoms With or without preauricular node	Distinguished by itchiness Otherwise symptoms similar to those of viral conjunctivitis Patients may have history of other seasonal allergies or atopy

*Usually causes keratitis but can cause conjunctivitis alone.

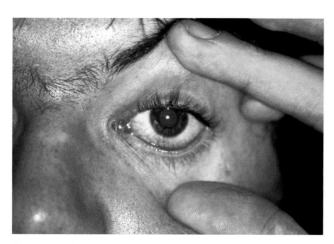

Figure 30.2 Conjunctivitis. http://phil.cdc.gov/phil/home.asp, Centers for Disease Control and Prevention / Joe Miller.

meningitidis) and/or *Chlamydia trachomatis* are suspected. In these cases, Gram stains and culture may be useful.

Treatment and Prophylaxis

As a general rule, all contact lens wearers diagnosed with any ocular complaint should discontinue contact lens use until seen by an ophthalmologist.

Viral and allergic conjunctivitis generally do not require treatment to expedite healing. Symptomatic relief can be obtained with topical antihistamines or decongestants.

Bacterial conjunctivitis is also self-limited in most cases, although antibiotic treatment can reduce the duration of symptoms by 2 to 5 days (Table 30.2). It is important to note that both placebo and treatment groups seem to have good long-term prognoses, with few sight-threatening complications.

Complications and Admission Criteria

Hyperacute bacterial conjunctivitis (e.g., purulent discharge that reaccumulates after being wiped away) should raise

Table 30.2 Initial Therapy for Bacterial Conjunctivitis

Patient Category	Therapy Recommendation

Adults*	• Topical antihistamines or decongestants
	  ○ Visine, Naphcon-A, Ocuhist 1–2 drops qid prn, no longer than 3 weeks
	• Topical antibiotics
	  ○ erythromycin ophthalmic ointment (1.25 cm) or 1–2 drops qid × 5–7 days (then decrease to bid if improved after 3–4 days)
	  or
	  ○ sulfacetamide ophthalmic drops (10%) 1–2 drops qid × 5–7 days

Children	Same as for adults
Pregnant Women	Same as for nonpregnant adults
Immunocompromised	Same as for nonimmunocompromised persons and children

*Contact lens wearers should be additionally covered for *Pseudomonas* infection with fluoroquinolone 1–2 drops qid × 5–7 days. Contact lens wearers (especially those with extended-wear lenses) have a higher risk of developing pseudomonal keratitis. This presents as ulcers and can lead to ocular perforation in as little as 24 hours if not treated appropriately.

concern for *Neisseria* species, especially *N. gonorrhoeae* (Figure 30.3), which can be sight-threatening. Evaluate for coexisting urethritis, although its absence does not exclude *Neisseria* conjunctivitis. *Neisseria* conjunctivitis is characterized by copious purulent discharge and significant chemosis. Suspicion of this diagnosis necessitates immediate consultation with an ophthalmologist, and a confirmed diagnosis requires hospitalization for topical and systemic antibiotics (such as ceftriaxone, or spectinomycin or ciprofloxacin for those who are allergic).

In addition, more than 30% of patients with gonococcal conjunctivitis have coexisting chlamydial infection and all patients should be treated for both infections. Isolated chlamydial infection may present with concomitant asymptomatic

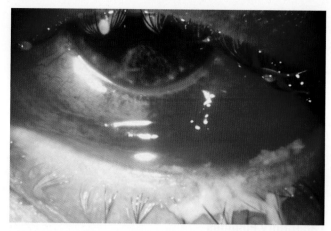

Figure 30.3 Gonorrheal conjunctivitis. http://phil.cdc.gov/phil/home.asp, Centers for Disease Control and Prevention.

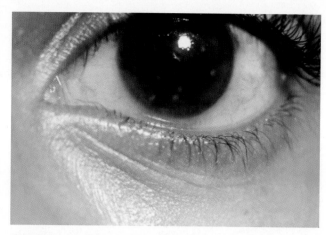

Figure 30.4 Keratitis. http://phil.cdc.gov/phil/home.asp, Centers for Disease Control and Prevention / Susan Lindsley, VD.

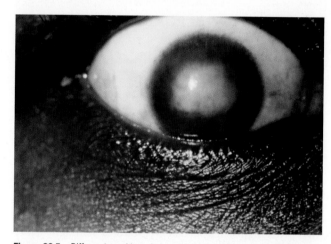

Figure 30.5 Diffuse stromal haze in keratitis. http://phil.cdc.gov/phil/home.asp, Centers for Disease Control and Prevention / Susan Lindsley, VD.

urogenital infection but usually manifests in an indolent fashion and does not respond to traditional topical antibiotics. This diagnosis may also be confirmed with direct fluorescent antibody staining or, if desired, polymerase chain reaction (PCR) of conjunctival smears. Most clinicians, however, treat both empirically and do not routinely send for conjunctival smears for PCR. Coexisting chlamydial infection is treated with systemic antibiotic therapy such as azithromycin or doxycycline.

Pearls and Pitfalls

1. For neonates, conjunctivitis ("ophthalmia neonatorum") from either *N. gonorrhoeae* (usually 3–5 days after birth) or *C. trachomatis* (usually 5–12 days after birth) can be transmitted during passage through the birth canal. Neonatal conjunctivitis can lead to corneal ulceration and perforation, and can be associated with other localized or disseminated infections. Of the two diagnoses, *C. trachomatis* is the more common cause of conjunctivitis in a neonate.

2. In a patient with a red eye who also has decreased visual acuity, ciliary flush (injection that does not spare the limbus), a fixed pupil, corneal opacity, or photophobia, a diagnosis in addition to conjunctivitis should be suspected (e.g., herpes simplex virus [HSV] can cause isolated conjunctivitis, but may also cause keratitis).

3. Aminoglycoside ointment and drops should be generally avoided, as they can damage the corneal epithelium and, after multiple days of use, even cause a reactive keratoconjunctivitis.

KERATITIS

Epidemiology

Infectious keratitis (Figures 30.4 and 30.5) is one of the most common preventable causes of blindness worldwide, and may be bacterial, viral, or fungal. There are an estimated 30,000 cases of bacterial keratitis annually in the United States alone.

Pseudomonas is the most common gram-negative organism found in bacterial keratitis. It is associated with contact lens wearers and is notable for its tendency to cause ulcers, though contact lens wearers as a group are more prone to other gram-negative etiologies, including *Serratia, Escherichia, Klebsiella,* and *Proteus.*

HSV keratitis, with a prevalence of 150 per 100,000 population, deserves attention because it has a high recurrence rate (~60% within 20 years). About 10–20% of patients will have recurrence within 1 year.

Etiologies of noninfectious keratitis can be mechanical (e.g., lid defects), neurologic (e.g., neurotrophic keratitis), immunologic (e.g., collagen vascular disease), dermatologic (e.g., erythema multiforme), and traumatic (e.g., chemical injury).

Clinical Features

The following table summarizes the clinical features of keratitis.

Depending on the type of keratitis, there may be certain distinguishing features (Table 30.3). For example, varicella-zoster virus (VZV) and HSV keratitis are characterized on fluoroscein exam by branching dendritic epithelial lesions that may have "terminal bulbs" at the tips of dendrite branches. VSV lesions typically have a fine and lacy appearance, with linear defects in epithelium; HSV lesions are described as "thick and ropy," with an epithelium that is elevated and appears "painted on."

Table 30.3 Clinical Features: Keratitis

Organisms	**Bacteria:** • *Streptococcus* • *Pseudomonas* • Enterobacteriaceae (including *Klebsiella, Enterobacter, Serratia,* and *Proteus*) • *Staphylococcus* **Viral:** • Herpes simplex (HSV) • Varicella-zoster (VZV) • Epstein-Barr (EBV) • Adenovirus • Cytomegalovirus (CMV) **Fungal:** • *Fusarium* • *Aspergillus* • *Candida*
Signs and Symptoms	Decreased vision, pain, and photophobia Other accompanying signs of infectious keratitis visualized with a slit lamp may include: • Corneal ulcers • Corneal infiltrates • Stromal edema • Lid edema • Conjunctival inflammation • Discharge/purulent exudate • Anterior chamber reaction • Hypopyon • Posterior synechiae
Laboratory Findings	Usually does not require laboratory confirmation

Differential Diagnosis

The differential diagnosis for keratitis is broad, but there are ways to distinguish it from others based on a thorough history and physical:

- blepharitis – a disorder of the eyelids only and should not have corneal involvement
- conjunctivitis – should be limited to conjunctival structures only and not cornea
- scleritis and episcleritis – should not have corneal involvement
- corneal ulcers – should be limited to ulcerated area alone

Most patients with corneal involvement will have a foreign body sensation or have a difficult time keeping the eye open.

Risk factors that should be specifically sought out in the history include:

- previous history of ophthalmologic disorders (e.g., herpetic keratitis)
- congenital/mechanical anomalies (e.g., lacrimal duct malformation)
- use of contact lenses (including lens type, length of wear, disinfection)
- trauma/instrumentation (e.g., previous surgery)
- ocular medications (e.g., topical steroids)

Onchocerciasis ("river blindness") is endemic in many countries in Africa and is an infection from the parasite *Onchocerca volvulus*, transmitted by the black fly. The skin findings of dryness and depigmentation, along with subcuta-neous nodules containing the worms, usually precede the ocular findings. The microfilariae can be identified within the skin and sometimes visualized in the anterior chamber. Blindness is caused by corneal inflammation and scarring. Treatment is one dose of ivermectin (150 micrograms/kg by mouth [PO]) and should be continued yearly.

In developing countries, there should also be a low threshold for suspicion of mycobacterial causes of keratitis (nontuberculous mycobacteria such as *M. fortuitum* and *M. chelonae,* as well as *M. tuberculosis*).

Noninfectious keratitis may be related to chronic epithelial defects, autoimmune disease, and trauma.

Laboratory Findings

The diagnosis of bacterial keratitis is based on history and physical and does not require laboratory confirmation. As the majority (~95%) of cases of bacterial keratitis resolve with initial treatment, Gram stain and culture of initial scrapings are often unnecessary. In most cases, targeting of therapy to culture results is unnecessary.

In cases where bacterial keratitis has not resolved, however, scrapings of the most active parts of the ulcer should be obtained and sent for Gram stains and aerobic and fungal culture. For viral keratitis, the most common viral etiologies – HSV, VZV, Epstein-Barr virus (EBV), and cytomegalovirus (CMV) – can be diagnosed by history and physical, as well as examination of smears with enzyme-linked immunosorbent assay (ELISA) antibodies, viral culture, or PCR. Scrapings should be performed by an ophthalmologist to minimize the risk of perforation.

Treatment and Prophylaxis

Duration of therapy depends on clinical response, as indicated by decreased inflammation in the anterior chamber, decreased stromal infiltrate and edema, and improvement in pain. In general, topical monotherapy with earlier fluoroquinolones (e.g., ciprofloxacin, ofloxacin) has been the mainstay of treatment, as they cover gram-negative bacteria, but patients at higher risk for gram-positive infection should be treated with a newer fluoroquinolone such as gatifloxacin or moxifloxacin. Another recommended regimen is an alternating combination of tobramycin and gentamicin, both of which should be in "fortified" doses (higher than the usual concentrations; see Table 30.4).

In general, systemic antibiotics are rarely used, as they achieve a low concentration within the cornea. Systemic antibiotics are recommended when there is corneal perforation or when an underlying scleritis is suspected.

Furthermore, although steroids can help decrease the amount of inflammation and corneal precipitate, as a general rule, an emergency physician should avoid prescribing steroid eye drops. In some cases (e.g., fungal and herpetic keratitis), steroids can exacerbate the infection, leading to deeper infection and blindness.

Complications and Admission Criteria

A first-time diagnosis of keratitis does not require admission. However, patients who fail to respond to treatment and

Table 30.4 Initial Therapy for Keratitis

Patient Category	Therapy Recommendation
Adults	**Bacterial keratitis:** • Topical antibiotics, such as: ciprofloxacin 0.3% 2 drops q15 minutes × 6 hours, followed by 2 drops q30 minutes × 18 hours, and then tapered based on response *or* gatifloxacin 0.3% 1 drop q30 minutes for 12 doses, then 1 drop qh for the first 24–48 hours; gradually taper off according to clinical response *or* tobramycin (14 mg/mL) 1 drop q1 hour alternating with fortified cefazolin (50 mg/mL) 1 drop q1 hour • Systemic antibiotics – should be used in conjunction with an ophthalmologist • Surgical care • Penetrating keratoplasty • Sclerocorneal patch • Application of cyanoacrylate tissue adhesive **Viral keratitis:** • HSV: acyclovir 400 mg PO five times daily • VZV*: Herpes zoster ophthalmicus (HZO) and disseminated disease: acyclovir 800 mg PO five times a day × 7–10 days, although famciclovir 500 mg PO daily × 7 days and valacyclovir 1000 mg PO tid × 7–10 days have been shown to be even more effective in decreasing the pain of the infection **Fungal keratitis†:** • Amphotericin B 0.15% topical 1 drop q5 min × 5 doses, then q1 hour during day and q2 hours during the night *or* • Fluconazole 0.2% topical 1 drop q5 min × 5 doses, then q1 hour during day and q2 hours during the night
Children	**Bacterial keratitis:** Treatment generally follows that of adults with the caveat that fluoroquinolone eye drops should be avoided when possible **Viral keratitis:** • HSV‡: Systemic acyclovir for first episodes of HSV are dosed as such: <3 months: 60 mg/kg/day IV divided q8h; 3 months–2 years: 15 mg/kg/day IV divided q8h (maximum 60 mg/kg/day); 2–12 years: 1200 mg/day PO divided q8h (maximum 80 mg/kg/day PO); or 15 mg/kg/day IV divided q8h (maximum 60 mg/kg/day IV); >12 years: 1000–1200 mg PO div 3–5×/day (maximum 1200 mg/day PO); or 15 mg/kg/day IV divided q8h (maximum 60 mg/kg/day IV) • VZV*: acyclovir 10–20 mg/kg/dose PO qid **Fungal keratitis†:** Treatment generally follows that of adults
Pregnant Women	**Bacterial keratitis:** Treatment generally follows that of nonpregnant adults with the caveat that fluoroquinolone eye drops should be avoided when possible **Viral keratitis:** Treatment generally follows that of nonpregnant adults with the caveat that all systemic antiviral medications are pregnancy category B; all should be administered with ophthalmologist to weigh risks and benefits **Fungal keratitis†:** Antifungals listed above in nonpregnant adults are pregnancy category C; all should be administered with ophthalmologist to weigh risks and benefits
Immunocompromised	Same as for nonimmunocompromised persons and children, but be aware that they may have a more fulminant and prolonged course of keratitis. IV antivirals are not needed for HIV patients with keratitis, with the exception of those who have acute retinal necrosis, uveitis, or cranial nerve involvement. Even this treatment, however, is evolving, and if these infections are suspected (in HIV and non-HIV patients), ophthalmologic consult should be obtained urgently.

*Systemic corticosteroids also seem to reduce the short-term symptoms of pain, although the long-term post-herpetic neuralgia has not been definitively shown. Because of this, and the risk of further suppressing the immune system, only patients who have low risk of immunocompromise and who are in severe pain should be considered for this therapy.
†Should only be used in conjunction with ophthalmologist; oral antifungals may also be recommended along with topical antifungals depending on response. *DO NOT USE TOPICAL OR ORAL STEROIDS WITH FUNGAL INFECTIONS.*
‡If congenital HSV disease is suspected, these patients should be admitted and given systemic acyclovir therapy (see Complications and Admission Criteria).
HIV, human immunodeficiency virus.

patients with a high risk of visual loss should be referred urgently to an ophthalmologist for further care. Delayed diagnosis can be disastrous in some virulent strains of rapidly progressing keratitis (of any etiology), as destruction of the cornea can occur within 1–2 days.

Neonates who are suspected of having congenital HSV (80% of which is HSV-2 because it is transmitted from maternal genitalia) should be admitted. These patients must be treated with systemic antibiotics (acyclovir).

Major complications of keratitis include:

- formation of scar tissue and neovascularization leading to corneal leukoma
- uneven healing of stroma that results in irregular astigmatism
- corneal perforation causing secondary endophthalmitis and potential loss of the globe
- acute retinal necrosis, particularly in the cases of VZV and HSV keratitis

Pearls and Pitfalls

1. It is generally not recommended to use Gram stains of a corneal scraping to dictate antibiotic treatment of keratitis, as they are sometimes inconsistent with culture results.
2. One in 5 cases of fungal keratitis can be complicated with bacterial co-infection; therefore both should be treated.
3. Have a low threshold to suspect bacterial keratitis, especially in contact lens wearers. Almost half of all patients diagnosed with bacterial keratitis are contact lens wearers.
4. Surgical procedures such as LASIK have made fungal etiologies more common.

REFERENCES

Acyclovir for the prevention of recurrent herpes simplex virus eye disease. Herpetic Eye Disease Study Group. N Engl J Med 1998 Jul 30;339(5):300–6.

Ahmed I, Ai E, Chang E, Luckie, A. Ophthalmic manifestations of HIV. HIV Insite. University of California at San Francisco. August 2005. Available at: http://hivinsite.ucsf.edu/InSite?page = kb-00&doc = kb-04-01-12. Accessed March 12, 2007.

Cheng KH, Leung SL, Hoekman HW, et al. Incidence of contact-lens-associated microbial keratitis and its related morbidity. Lancet 1999;354(9174):181–5.

Galindez OA, Sabates NR, Whitacre MM, et al. Rapidly progressive outer retinal necrosis caused by varicella zoster virus in a patient with human immunodeficiency virus. J Infect Dis 1996;22:149–51.

Goldstein DA, Tessler HH. Episcleritis, scleritis, and other scleral disorders. In Yanoff M, Duker JS, Augsburger JJ, et al., eds, Ophthalmology. St. Louis. MO: Mosby, 2004: 512–8.

Jacobs, DS. Conjunctivitis. UptoDate. Available at: www.uptodate.com. Accessed March 2, 2007.

Morrow GL, Abbot RL. Conjunctivitis. Am Fam Physician 1998 Feb;57(4):735–46. http://www.aafp.org/afp/980600ap/carter.html

Rietveld RP, ter Riet G, Bindels PJ, et al. Predicting bacterial cause in infectious conjunctivitis: cohort study on informativeness of combinations of signs and symptoms. BMJ 2004;329:206.

Rose PW, Harnden A, Brueggemann AB, et al. Chloramphenicol treatment for acute infective conjunctivitis in children in primary care: a randomised double-blind placebo-controlled trial. Lancet 2005;366:37.

Sellitti TP, Huang AJ, Schiffman J, Davis JL. Association of herpes zoster ophthalmicus with acquired immunodeficiency syndrome and acute retinal necrosis. Am J Ophthalmol 1993 Sep;116(3):297–301.

Sheikh A, Hurwitz B. Antibiotics versus placebo for acute bacterial conjunctivitis. Cochrane Database Syst Rev 2006;CD001211.

ADDITIONAL READINGS

McLeod SL. Infectious keratitis. In: Yanoff M, Duker JS, Augsburger JJ, et al., eds, Ophthalmology. St. Louis. MO: Mosby, 2004:466–91.

31. Uvea, Vitreous, and Retina Infections

Renee Y. Hsia

INTRODUCTION

The uvea lies between the corneoscleral layer of the eye and the retina, and is composed of anterior (iris and ciliary body) and posterior (choroid) structures. The term uveitis is generally used to describe *anterior* uveitis, including iritis or anterior chamber infection. Extension of the infection to the ciliary body is termed iridocyclitis. Inflammation of posterior structures can occur without anterior involvement, as in choroiditis, retinitis, and chorioretinitis, all forms of *posterior* uveitis. Endophthalmitis is an infection of the aqueous humor or vitreous (Figure 31.1) within the globe.

UVEITIS AND RETINITIS

Epidemiology

Although uveitis is usually associated with systemic diseases (e.g., vasculitides) this chapter focuses on infectious causes of uveitis. Anterior uveitis accounts for the majority of uveitis (approximately 28–66% of cases), with posterior uveitis causing the rest (representing about 19–51% of cases).

Within anterior uveitis, fewer than 10% of cases are due to infectious causes, most being idiopathic or related to systemic disease. Posterior uveitis is most often attributed to toxoplasmosis (Figure 31.2) and cytomegalovirus (CMV). Although

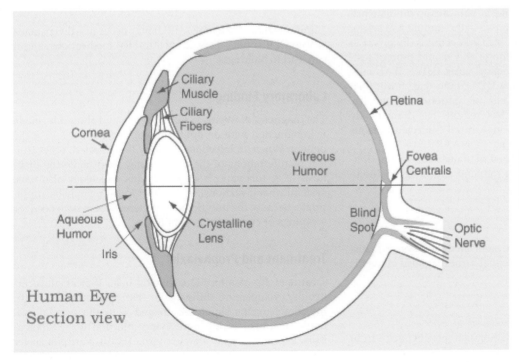

Figure 31.1 Eye anatomy and illustration of eye chambers. http://commons.wikimedia.org/wiki/ Image:Eyesection.gif; Illustration of Human Eye.

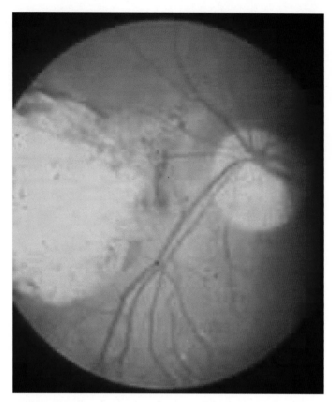

Figure 31.2 Severe chorioretinitis from *Toxoplasmosis gondii*. http://www.dpd.cdc.gov/dpdx/HTML/ImageLibrary/Toxoplasmosis_il.htm.

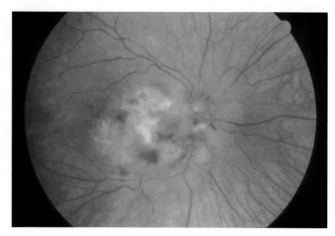

Figure 31.3 CMV retinitis. National Eye Institute, National Institutes of Health, Ref. No. EDA07, http://www.nei.nih.gov/photo/eyedis/index.asp.

- pupillary constriction
- pain (where conjunctivitis, episcleritis, and scleritis may have some irritation, uveitis is typically described as a "deeper pain")

Other conditions to consider that are often known as "masquerade syndromes" are:

- giant retinal tears
- ischemia
- leukemia
- lymphoma (most commonly central nervous system [CNS] B-cell lymphoma)
- ocular melanoma
- pigmentary dispersion syndrome
- retinitis pigmentosa
- retinoblastoma

"Immune recovery uveitis" (IRU) may occur in AIDS patients whose CD4 counts respond well to HIV medications, and it can lead to blindness.

Laboratory Findings

The diagnosis of uveitis is a clinical one and should be made in conjunction with an ophthalmologist who can follow the patient. When an infectious etiology is suspected, other clinical manifestations of the disease may help make the diagnosis (e.g., tuberculosis-related uveitis will likely also have systemic manifestations), and serologic testing may be appropriate. Because the infections are systemic, there is no need for scrapings or cultures as in keratitis.

Treatment and Prophylaxis

Treatment for noninfectious uveitis (e.g., topical glucocorticoids, cycloplegics) differs from that of infectious uveitis. Infectious uveitis should be treated with the general systemic treatment of the underlying infection (e.g., tuberculosis, syphilis, herpes simplex virus [HSV], varicella-zoster virus [VZV], CMV). Uveitis may, in HIV patients in particular, be due to chronic infections such as toxoplasmosis, syphilis, tuberculosis, coccidioidomycosis, and histoplasmosis. Only treatment of the underlying infection can resolve its associated

patients with acquired immunodeficiency syndrome (AIDS) are particularly susceptible to ocular toxoplasmosis due to reactivation, normal hosts with a history of exposure to cats or eating undercooked meats can also develop ocular toxoplasmosis. Ocular toxoplasmosis may occur in infants via vertical transmission from mothers who are infected during pregnancy. In ocular toxoplasmosis, parasites accumulate primarily on the retina and can spread to the choroid and sclera.

Active CMV disease, including CMV retinitis (Figure 31.3) and uveitis, is rare in normal hosts and should prompt testing for human immunodeficiency virus (HIV). It usually occurs in HIV patients with low CD4 counts (e.g., fewer than 50 cells/mL). With the advent of antiretroviral therapy (HAART), the incidence of CMV retinitis has dramatically decreased, though it remains high in HIV-infected persons with low CD4 counts who are not on HAART.

Intermediate uveitis (localized to the vitreous and peripheral retina) and panuveitis are rare and almost never due to infectious causes.

Clinical Features

Since the majority of cases are associated with systemic disease, a complete history is essential to the diagnosis of uveitis (Table 31.1).

Differential Diagnosis

Key features that may help to distinguish anterior uveitis from conjunctivitis, keratitis, episcleritis, and scleritis are:

- "ciliary flush", or perilimbal (the intersection of the sclera and cornea) injection

Table 31.1 Clinical Features: Infectious Uveitis and Retinitis

Organisms	**Bacterial:** ● Atypical mycobacteria ● Brucellosis ● *Bartonella henselae* (cat scratch disease) ● Mycobacterium leprae (leprosy) ● *Borrelia burgdorferi* (Lyme disease) ● *Propionibacterium* ● *Treponema pallidum* (syphilis) ● *Mycobacterium tuberculosis* **Viral:** ● Cytomegalovirus ● Epstein-Barr virus ● Herpes simplex virus ● Varicella-zoster virus ● Human T-cell leukemia virus ● Mumps virus ● Rubeola virus ● Vaccinia virus ● HIV ● West Nile virus **Fungal:** ● *Aspergillus* ● Blastomycosis ● *Candida* sp. ● *Coccidioides* ● *Cryptococcus* ● *Histoplasma* ● Sporotrichosis (*Sporothrix schenckii*) **Parasitic (protozoan/helminthic):** ● *Toxoplasmosis gondii* ● *Acanthamoeba* ● Cysticercosis ● Onchocerciasis ● *Pneumocystis carinii* ● Toxocariasis
Signs and Symptoms	**Anterior uveitis:** ● Pain ● Redness ● With or without visual loss ● With or without keratitic precipitates ● Leukocytes in anterior chamber (e.g., "flare") **Posterior uveitis:** ● Usually painless ● Floaters or debris in visual field ● Typically not red unless accompanied by uveitis ● Macular edema ● Perivascular exudates ● Focal or diffuse retinitis or choroiditis ● Choroidal and retinal neovascularization ● Retinal lesions of CMV often described as having a "pizza pie" appearance ● Gray-white, "fluffy" areas of retinal whitening in ocular toxoplasmosis

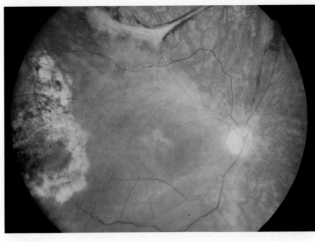

Figure 31.4 Acute retinal necrosis. Courtesy of Dr. Michael Morley.

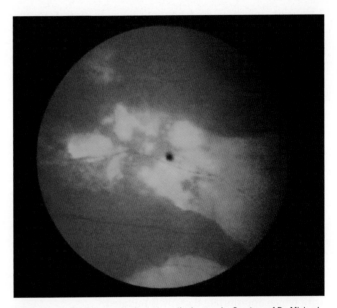

Figure 31.5 Rapidly progressive outer retinal necrosis. Courtesy of Dr. Michael Morley.

uveitis, and no particular ophthalmic treatment is needed. Exceptions are rare cases such as AIDS patients with CMV, where a ganciclovir implant may be recommended. Ophthalmologists should be closely involved in management to monitor the eye infection.

Complications and Admission Criteria

As a general rule, the diagnosis of uveitis/retinitis does not require admission, though exceptions include:

● necrotizing retinitis (also known as acute retinal necrosis)
● rapidly progressive outer retinal necrosis (RPORN)
● associated systemic illness requiring inpatient treatment

Acute retinal necrosis (ARN) (Figure 31.4) can be identified by the triad of retinitis, vitreitis, and vasculitis, which is usually diagnosed by an ophthalmologist or retina specialist. The most common etiology of ARN is viral, either from varicella zoster or, less commonly, HSV-1 and HSV-2.

Treatment should be directed by an ophthalmologist but usually includes intravenous (IV) acyclovir, oral ganciclovir or foscarnet, with or without aspirin, and oral prednisone.

The diagnosis of rapidly progressive outer retinal necrosis (RPORN) (Figure 31.5) should be considered in immunosuppressed patients (e.g., HIV, bone marrow transplant patients) who may have a simple complaint of decreased vision (usually bilateral) and no pain or redness and only minimal anterior chamber/vitreous reaction. The majority of these patients have a history of cutaneous zoster, as varicella is the most common etiology. RPORN can cause retinal disintegration involving the macula and requires immediate high-dose antiviral therapy as well as maintenance therapy from an ophthalmologist.

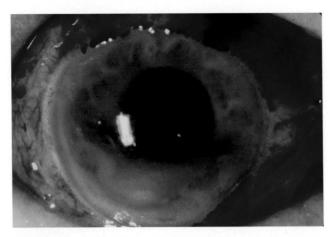

Figure 31.6 Endophthalmitis. Courtesy of Dr. Michael Morley.

Pearls and Pitfalls

1. Uveitis, infectious and non-infectious, is almost always associated with systemic illness.
2. The inflammation of simple conjunctivitis usually spares the limbus; the presence of "ciliary flush" is indicative of uveitis.
3. Patients with a low CD4 count and a complaint of "floaters" in the eye should be evaluated for possible retinal detachment, because it occurs in approximately 30% of patients with CMV retinitis.

ENDOPHTHALMITIS

Epidemiology

Most cases of endophthalmitis (Figure 31.6) are bacterial and present acutely. Rarely, fungus may cause endophthalmitis, but there are no known viral or parasitic causes. Acute bacterial endophthalmitis is a vision-threatening condition and must be managed as an emergency. The clinical outcome depends both on the virulence of the infecting organism and on the speed with which appropriate therapy is initiated.

In the United States, the most common form of endophthalmitis (62%) is acute endophthalmitis after cataract surgery. The surgery requires access to the anterior chamber and can result in an accidental communication with the vitreous. Three-fourths of all cases present within the first week postoperatively. It is a relatively infrequent complication of cataract surgery (less than 0.2% of cases), but the sheer number of cataract operations (more than 2 million per year) mean that the infection is not rare. Risk factors for this infection include diabetes, wound abnormalities, and certain lens implant materials (e.g., polypropylene).

There are other categories of endophthalmitis, including (in decreasing order of frequency):

- post-traumatic (after penetrating globe injury)
- chronic pseudophakic-related endophthalmitis (thought to be a reaction against remaining lens tissue)
- bleb-related (infection of a "filtering bleb," which is an intentional surgical defect created in the sclera to treat severe glaucoma)
- endogenous (extremely rare, from bacteremia) and fungal (also rare but more common in immunocompromised and injection drug users)

Table 31.2 Clinical Features: Endophthalmitis

Organisms	**Bacteria (usually postsurgical):** • Coagulase-negative staphylococci (70%) • *Staphylococcus aureus* (10%) • *Streptococcus* sp. (9%) • Gram-negative organisms (6%) • Other gram-positive organisms (5%) **Fungal:** • *Candida albicans* • Molds (extremely rare) • *Aspergillus* • *Fusarium*
Signs and Symptoms	• Decreased visual acuity • Eye "soreness" with or without pain • With or without conjunctival chemosis • Hypopyon • Inability to see retinal vessels • Cell and flare on slit lamp • Loss of red reflex • Corneal striae or opacity

- risk factors for both endogenous and fungal endophthalmitis include history of bacteremia, endocarditis, recent abdominal surgeries, malignancy, alcoholism, diabetes mellitus, trauma, hemodialysis, use of long-term indwelling catheters

Clinical Features

Table 31.2 summarizes the most important clinical features of endophthalmitis.

Differential Diagnosis

Early endophthalmitis is sometimes misdiagnosed as sterile postoperative inflammation. This benign inflammation often presents on the first postoperative day (as opposed to endophthalmitis, which presents on or after the second day), but this is not a reliable distinguishing feature, and any postoperative inflammation must be approached with a high index of suspicion for infectious etiologies, regardless of time of onset.

Laboratory Findings

As in most ocular disease, the diagnosis of endophthalmitis is made by physical exam. Leukocytosis is not a reliable predictor of serious disease, and the erythrocyte sedimentation rate (ESR) is usually normal. A "B-scan" (ultrasound of the eye) can show increased vitreous echogenicity or debris, and retinochoroidal thickening, but is neither sensitive nor specific. Aqueous or vitreous culture aspiration (or vitrectomy) can be done by an ophthalmologist to obtain cultures that may help direct therapy, though negative cultures do not exclude the diagnosis.

Treatment

Aspiration of the vitreous or vitrectomy, as well as intravitreal antibiotics, are the traditional mainstays of treatment (Table 31.3). Controversial treatments include use of topical

Table 31.3 Initial Therapy for Endophthalmitis

Patient Category	Therapy Recommendation

Adults*	**Bacterial***:
	• Vitrectomy or aspiration of vitreous
	• Vitreous injection of antibiotics
	   ○ vancomycin 1 mg/0.1 mL *plus*
	   ○ either amikacin 200 mcg or 400 mcg/0.1 mL (some sources say 400 mcg)
	• Vitreous injection of steroids is controversial
	Fungal:
	No controlled trials exist, but standard of care includes:
	• Vitrectomy
	• Removal of foreign material (e.g., intraocular lens implant)
	• Intravitreal antifungal agents
	• Amphotericin B 5 mcg or 10 mcg/0.1 mL
	• Intravitreal antifungal agents (too few case reports to provide recommendation)
	• With or without systemic antifungal such as voriconazole 4 mg/kg IV every 12 hours

Children	Treatment generally follows that of nonpregnant adults (always done in conjunction with an ophthalmologist). Not all treatment is well documented or tested in this population because of its rarity of occurrence, but benefits are understood to be greater than risks.
Pregnant Women	Treatment generally follows that of nonpregnant adults (always done in conjunction with an ophthalmologist). Not all treatment is well documented or tested in this population because of its rarity of occurrence, but benefits are understood to be greater than risks.
Immunocompromised	Same as for immunocompetent persons and children, although suspicion for infectious etiologies should be heightened appropriately (e.g., fungal etiologies more common in immunocompromised)

*If *Bacillus* confirmed or after penetrating trauma, clindamycin 0.1 mg/0.1 mL can be used.

or systemic antibiotics and intravitreal steroids. According to the Endophthalmitis Vitrectomy Study, IV antibiotics did not confer any significant benefit to the regimen of "tap (vitreous biopsy) and inject (intravitreal injection of antibiotics)", and thus are not listed in this table. Of note, this study was done before the introduction of fourth-generation antibiotics and certain quinolones (e.g., moxifloxacin, which has good intraocular penetration) some ophthalmologists are beginning to use them, but it is not considered standard of care at this time.

Complications and Admission Criteria

All patients with suspected endophthalmitis require emergent ophthalmology consult and admission if the diagnosis is confirmed.

Endophthalmitis is an emergency, as undiagnosed and untreated cases often result in loss of vision; overall 10% of patients, even some who have been treated promptly, will be left with compromised vision.

Pearls and Pitfalls

1. Endophthalmitis should be high in the differential for any eye complaint in a patient who has had cataract surgery within a week.
2. Almost 10% of penetrating globe trauma may be complicated by endophthalmitis; post-traumatic endopthalmitis is most commonly caused by *Bacillus cereus* and can have a fulminant course. Systemic intravenous antibiotics should be considered in addition to vitrectomy and intravitreal antibiotics.

REFERENCES

Dugel PU. Syphilitic uveitis. In Yanoff M, Duker JS, Augsburger JJ, et al., eds, Ophthalmology. St. Louis. MO: Mosby, 2004:1135–8.

Durand ML. Bacterial endophthalmitis. UptoDate. March 23, 2006. Available at: www.uptodate.com. Accessed March 12, 2007.

Forster, DJ. General approach to the uveitis patient and treatment strategies. In Yanoff M, Duker JS, Augsburger JJ, et al., eds, Ophthalmology. St. Louis. MO: Mosby, 2004:1108–12.

Kauffman CA, Durand ML. Fungal endophthalmitis. UptoDate. July 21, 2006. Available at: www.uptodate.com. Accessed March 12, 2007.

Results of the Endophthalmitis Vitrectomy Study. A randomized trial of immediate vitrectomy and of intravenous antibiotics for the treatment of postoperative bacterial endophthalmitis. Endophthalmitis Vitrectomy Study Group. Arch Ophthalmol 1995;113:1479.

ADDITIONAL READINGS

Ahmed I, Ai E, Chang E, et al. Ophthalmic manifestations of HIV. HIV Insite. University of California at San Francisco. August 2005. Available at: http://hivinsite.ucsf.edu/InSite?page=kb-00&doc=kb-04-01-12. Accessed March 12, 2007.

32. Community-Acquired Pneumonia

Bradley W. Frazee and Rachel L. Chin

Outline   Introduction
               Epidemiology
               Clinical Features
               Differential Diagnosis
               Laboratory and Radiographic Findings
               Treatment and Prophylaxis
               Complications and Admission Criteria
               Special Considerations – Pneumonia in Nursing Home Residents
               Pearls and Pitfalls
               References

INTRODUCTION

Community-acquired pneumonia (CAP) is defined as an infection of the pulmonary parenchyma, acquired in the community. The definition of CAP excludes patients who are hospitalized, have been hospitalized in the 14 days prior to the onset of symptoms, or who reside in long-term care facilities, including nursing homes. This chapter focuses on CAP in immunocompetent adults. See Chapter 35, HIV-Associated Respiratory Infections, for a discussion of pulmonary infections in immunocompromised patients and Chapter 49, Pediatric Respiratory Infections, for a discussion on pediatric pulmonary infections.

Streptococcus pneumoniae is the most important CAP pathogen, accounting for 35–55% of cases of CAP, and two-thirds of deaths from CAP. Current *S. pneumoniae* resistance to both to penicillins and macrolides, as well as the possibility of future widespread resistance to fluoroquinolones, drives current recommendations for empiric therapy. The risk factors for infection with drug-resistant *S. pneumoniae*, include significant medical comorbidities and use of antimicrobials within the prior 3 months.

The so-called atypical bacterial causes of CAP, which cannot be seen on Gram stain or cultured on typical media, include *Mycoplasma pneumoniae*, *Chlamydophila* (formerly *Chlamydia*) *pneumoniae*, and *Legionella pneumophila*. *M. pneumoniae* and *C. pneumoniae* are common causes of CAP in ambulatory patients younger than 50. No rapid diagnostic tests exist for *M. pneumoniae* and *C. pneumoniae*, and although they are associated in general with a less severe disease, pneumonia caused by these organisms cannot be distinguished on clinical grounds. *Legionella*, by contrast, often causes severe pneumonia and is associated with outbreaks linked to contaminated water. A urinary antigen test for *Legionella* serogroup 1 (responsible for ~70–80% of cases) is available. Treatment guidelines recommend antibiotics with activity against atypical bacteria (macrolide/azalide, doxycycline, and fluoroquinolones) be included in all empiric CAP therapy.

Haemophilus influenzae and *Moraxella catarrhalis* are relatively common causes of CAP in elderly patients, smokers, and patients with chronic obstructive pulmonary disease (COPD). CAP caused by enteric gram-negative organisms is generally limited to patients with multiple comorbidities (e.g., congestive heart failure [CHF], other chronic lung disease, or cancer), residents of long-term care facilities, or patients with recent broad-spectrum antibiotic exposure. *Pseudomonas* rarely causes pneumonia in immunocompetent patients outside of a hospital setting. *Staphylococcus aureus* pneumonia is more common in injection drug users, elderly patients, and children with recent influenza. Cases of community-associated methicillin-resistant *S. aureus* (CA-MRSA) pneumonia have recently been reported in previously healthy adults, concomitant with the rise in CA-MRSA skin and soft-tissue infections. Oral anaerobes are associated with aspiration pneumonia and lung abscess. Respiratory viruses, such as influenza and respiratory syncytial virus (RSV), are a common cause of CAP and may be clinically indistinguishable from bacterial pneumonia. Finally, tuberculosis and fungal pneumonia (e.g., coccidioidomycosis and histoplasmosis), although typically indolent in onset, may be mistaken for bacterial pneumonia and should remain on the differential diagnosis when faced with clinical CAP that does not respond to antibiotic therapy.

EPIDEMIOLOGY

CAP is the leading cause of death from infectious disease in the United States and the sixth leading cause of death overall. It accounts for approximately 1 million hospitalizations. Mortality rates are less than 1–5% in the outpatient setting, but as high as 12% in hospitalized patients. The incidence of CAP is highest in the winter months and in elderly patients.

CAP is not generally thought of as a contagious or transmissible infection. Rather, in most cases, it involves inoculation of the normally sterile pulmonary parenchyma by the patient's own oropharyngeal flora. However, drug-resistant *S. pneumoniae* strains are known to pass among close contacts, such as within families, day care centers and nursing homes, and outbreaks of pneumococcal pneumonia occasionally occur in these settings. Furthermore, infection with mycobacteria tuberculosis, which is highly transmissible, often presents clinically as CAP.

CLINICAL FEATURES

Common clinical features of CAP include productive cough, fever, pleuritic chest pain, and dyspnea (Table 32.1).

Table 32.1 Clinical Features: Community-Acquired Pneumonia

Organisms	**Common and covered in all empiric treatment regimens**: • *Streptococcus pneumoniae* • *Mycoplasma pneumoniae* • *Chlamydophilae (formerly Chlamydia) pneumoniae* • *Legionella pneumophila* • *Haemophilus influenzae* • *Moraxella catarrhalis* • Respiratory viruses **Less common, predominantly occur in special at-risk populations**: • Enteric gram-negative bacteria • *Pseudomonas aeruginosa* • *Staphylococcus aureus*
Signs and Symptoms	Cough, sputum production, dyspnea, pleurisy, GI symptoms, altered mental status, fever, tachypnea, low oxygen saturation, rales or evidence of consolidation
Laboratory and Radiographic Findings	• Chest x-ray demonstrates an infiltrate • Blood count: leukocytosis; left shift (bands); leukopenia is associated with severe disease • Blood cultures (2 sets, prior to antibiotics; obtain in patients requiring hospitalization): positive in 5–14% • Sputum culture and Gram stain (in most patients requiring hospitalization; all intubated patients) • Legionella urinary antigen test (obtain in severe disease) • Pneumococcal urinary antigen test • Rapid antigen tests for influenza virus (during outbreaks)

GI, gastrointestinal.

Table 32.2 Non-CAP Causes of Cough and Infiltrates on Chest X-Ray

Uncommon infectious causes of pneumonia:
• Tuberculosis
• Coccidioidomycosis
• Histoplasmosis
• *Pneumocystis*
• Hantavirus pulmonary syndrome
• Anthrax (bioterrorism)
• Plague (bioterrorism)
• Tularemia (bioterrorism)

Noninfectious causes:
• Malignancy
• Pulmonary hemorrhage
• Pulmonary edema
• Interstitial lung disease

Gastrointestinal symptoms, including nausea, vomiting, and diarrhea, may be prominent. Mental status changes can be seen, particularly in the elderly, and indicate a worse prognosis. Chest pain occurs in 30% of cases, chills in 40–50%, and rigors in 15%. Because of the rapid onset of symptoms, most individuals seek medical care within a week of infection.

On physical examination, approximately 80% of patients are febrile, although fever may be absent, especially in the elderly. A respiratory rate above 24 breaths/minute is noted in 45–70% of patients and may be the most sensitive sign in the elderly. Tachycardia is common. Careful chest examination usually reveals rales or evidence of consolidation, but this can easily be missed. Oxygen saturation is often decreased, though patients with good cardiopulmonary reserve can maintain normal saturation with significant disease, and normal pulse oximetry by no means excludes pneumonia. At the same time, oxygen saturation as low as 90–92% is well tolerated by otherwise healthy patients, and this finding alone does not mandate hospital admission. (See Admission Criteria, below.)

No constellation of signs and symptoms has been found to predict with certainty whether or not a patient has pneumonia. Nonetheless, in non-elderly patients with normal vital signs and no abnormal findings on chest auscultation radiographic pneumonia is very unlikely. In such patients, a chest x-ray may not be necessary to exclude CAP.

Finally, it is critical to recognize the clinical features, such as respiratory rate above 30, which are correlated with severe

CAP and worse prognosis. These features are enumerated under Complications and Admission Criteria.

DIFFERENTIAL DIAGNOSIS

Among ambulatory patients with acute cough and signs and symptoms of infection, often the main differential diagnosis is between acute bronchitis (almost always viral) and CAP (defined by an infiltrate on chest x-ray). However, less common but serious diagnoses can easily be mistaken for CAP (Table 32.2).

LABORATORY AND RADIOGRAPHIC FINDINGS

The diagnosis of pneumonia generally relies on a constellation of clinical findings, as well as radiographic evidence. The presence of an infiltrate on plain chest radiograph is considered the "gold standard" for the diagnosis of CAP, when clinical features are supportive. Acute care practitioners should maintain a low threshold for obtaining a chest x-ray to assess for possible CAP. The radiographic appearances of CAP include lobar consolidation, interstitial infiltrates, cavitation, and pleural effusion. False negative results are possible and may be due to dehydration or presentation within the first 24 hours of infection. Correlation between a particular chest x-ray finding and certain pathogens is not reliable. Multilobar involvement and parapneumonic effusion are associated with a worse prognosis and generally require hospitalization. Chest computed tomographic (CT) scan is more sensitive than chest x-ray for small infiltrates, occult multilobar involvement, adenopathy, and effusion, but there is no evidence that routine CT scanning improves management or outcome. In many cases, chest x-ray is the only diagnostic test required in the evaluation of CAP.

Leukocytosis with a left shift is the major blood test abnormality found in CAP. Leukopenia (white blood cell [WBC] count less than 4000 cells/mm^3) also can occur and connotes a worse prognosis. In addition to complete blood count, thorough assessment of severity requires serum chemistries and an assessment of oxygenation.

Diagnostic tests to determine the etiologic organism in CAP may include sputum Gram stain and culture, blood cultures, urinary antigen tests, and serologic tests. However, in outpatients, initial empiric treatment is almost always successful. In one study of more than 700 ambulatory patients with CAP treated with empiric antibiotics, only 1% required hospitalization due to failure of the outpatient regimen.

Performing etiological testing in all hospitalized patients, although controversial, is widely recommended. Although these studies almost never change initial acute care management, they can be crucial to later hospital management and are important for public health surveillance. In general, the more severe the pneumonia, the more likely that sputum and blood cultures will lead to a change in management. Blood cultures prior to antibiotics are recommended in all hospitalized patients. Sputum studies are reserved for patients with cavitary lesions, those able to produce a good expectorated specimen, and those with severe pneumonia requiring intensive care unit (ICU) admission.

Urine antigen assays are available for the diagnosis of *Legionella* serogroup 1 and *S. pneumoniae* infection. These tests are recommended in cases of severe CAP. With their high specificity and a turnaround time of less than 1 hour, these tests offer the possibility of rapid etiologic diagnosis. Urine antigen tests often remain positive even when specimens are collected after antibiotic therapy is started.

Rapid antigen testing for influenza is recommended during flu season, particularly in patients requiring hospitalization. A positive test for influenza has a number of implications: establishing the diagnosis is important for epidemiologic purposes; there may be hospital infection control implications; it might reduce unnecessary antibiotic use; and it may prompt antiviral therapy (if symptoms have been present less than 48 hours). See Chapter 75, Microbiology Laboratory Testing for Infectious Diseases, and Chapter 34, Influenza.

TREATMENT AND PROPHYLAXIS

Numerous resources are available to assist in the selection of initial antibiotic therapy for CAP. Frequently-updated treatment guidelines based on hospital-specific bacterial susceptibility data are preferred. Treatment guidelines are based on the principles listed in Table 32.3. Outpatient and inpatient therapies are summarized in Tables 32.4 and 32.5.

Beta-lactam and macrolide/azalide resistant *S. pneumoniae* is a significant problem in the United States, with resistance rates around 25% for both antibiotic classes. Recent antibiotic therapy with any drug from a class is a major risk factor for resistance to that class. Comorbidities, advanced age, and having a child in day care also increase the risk of a drug-resistant strain. Penicillin resistance has leveled off since the

Table 32.3 General Principles of CAP Treatment

Initial antibiotic selection in the acute care setting is always empiric (versus pathogen-directed).
Antibiotic selection begins with categorizing the patient with regard to severity and site of care (outpatient, hospital ward, intensive care unit)
For outpatient therapy (Table 32.4), antibiotics with activity against drug-resistant *S. pneumoniae* are necessary only in patients at risk, based on comorbidities and recent (within 3 months) antibiotic use.
For inpatient therapy (Table 32.5), activity against drug-resistant *S. pneumoniae* is always provided.
All antibiotic regimens should ensure activity against atypical pathogens.
Activity against enteric gram-negative pathogens, *Pseudomonas*, *S. aureus*, and anaerobes is reserved for patients at increased risk.
Consider drug allergy history and pregnancy status.

Table 32.4 Initial Therapy for Outpatient: Community-Acquired Pneumonia

Patient Category	Therapy Recommendation
Adults: Previously healthy and no use of antimicrobials within the previous 3 months.	**A macrolide or doxycycline:** azithromycin 500 mg PO day 1, then 250 mg qd days 2–5 or 2 g (sustained release) PO × 1 dose *or* clarithromycin XR 1 g PO qd or 500 mg bid PO × 7 days *or* doxycycline 100 mg bid PO × 7–10 days
Presence of comorbidities such as chronic heart, lung, liver or renal disease; diabetes; alcoholism; malignancies; asplenia; immunosuppressive drugs; or use of antimicrobials within the previous 3 months (an alternative from a different class should be selected)	**A respiratory fluoroquinolone or a beta-lactam plus a macrolide:** levofloxacin 750 mg PO qd × 5 days *or* moxifloxacin 400 mg PO qd × 7 days *or* amoxicillin 1 g PO tid *plus* azithromycin 500 mg PO qd × 3 days or 2 g PO × 1 dose or clarithromycin XR 1 g PO qd or 500 mg bid PO × 7 days
Pregnant women	Same as for nonpregnant adults except avoid doxycycline and fluoroquinolones

introduction of the conjugated pneumococcal vaccine for children in the year 2000, whereas macrolide resistance continues to rise, and clinical treatment failure due to macrolide resistance appears to be more significant than with penicillins. Fluoroquinolone resistance remains less than 5% in most regions of the United States, and limiting use of fluoroquinolones is recommended in an effort to prevent a future rise in resistance to this class.

An important treatment issue in the emergency department (ED) is how soon antibiotics are administered to patients requiring hospitalization for CAP. A time to first dose of antibiotics of 4 hours or less is considered a benchmark for quality care and is monitored by federal agencies. How rapidly the chest x-ray is obtained and interpreted and blood cultures drawn is an important determinant of time to first antibiotic dose. Interestingly, there is only limited retrospective data supporting the notion that giving antibiotics within 4 hours improves outcome.

An important means of reducing morbidity and mortality from CAP is appropriate use of pneumococcal vaccines in target populations (Table 32.6) and widespread use of the annual influenza vaccine.

COMPLICATIONS AND ADMISSION CRITERIA

A critical task of the emergency physician in evaluating CAP is to correctly assess need for hospitalization. Hospital admission is costly and can lead to further iatrogenic complications, so inappropriate admission must be minimized. Furthermore, practitioners must recognize signs of occult disease requiring ICU level care. The pneumonia severity index (PSI) (Figure 32.1; Tables 32.7 and 32.8) and CURB-65 score (Table 32.9) provide an objective means to assess prognosis and aid in disposition and treatment decisions.

The PSI is based on age, comorbidities, vital sign abnormalities and laboratory and chest x-ray findings. Non-elderly patients without major comorbidities or major vital sign

Table 32.5 Initial Therapy for Inpatient: Community-Acquired Pneumonia

Patient Category	Therapy Recommendation
Adults: Non-ICU	**A respiratory fluoroquinolone or a beta-lactam plus a macrolide:** levofloxacin 750 mg IV qd *or* moxifloxacin 400 mg IV qd *or* ceftriaxone 1–2 g IV qd *plus* azithromycin 500 mg IV qd
ICU Patients	**A beta-lactam plus either a respiratory fluoroquinolone or azithromycin (same doses as for non-ICU patients):** respiratory fluoroquinolone *plus* aztreonam 2 g IV q6h or vancomycin 1 g IV q12h
Special Considerations: **Aspiration Pneumonia**	clindamycin 600 mg IV q8h *plus* a respiratory fluoroquinolone
***Pseudomonas* Infection**	antipseudomonal beta-lactam: piperacillin-tazobactam 4.5 g IV q6h or cefepime 2 g IV q12h, or imipenem 500 mg q6h *plus* either a respiratory fluoroquinolone *or* gentamicin or tobramycin 5 mg/kg q24h *plus* azithromycin 500 mg IV qd
CA-MRSA Infection*	Add vancomycin 1 g IV q12h or linezolid 400–600 mg IV bid*
Suspected Influenza (and Symptoms Present <48 hours)	Add oseltamivir 75 mg PO bid × 5 days

*Community-acquired methicillin-resistant *Staphylococcus aureus*.
Adapted from the IDSA/ATS Guidelines for CAP in Adults, CID, Mandell et al. (2007).

Table 32.6 Recommendation for Vaccine Prevention of Community-Acquired Pneumonia

Factor	Pneumococcal Polysaccharide Vaccine
Route of Administration	IM injection
Recommended Groups	All persons ≥65 years of age High-risk persons 2–64 years of age
Specific High-Risk Indications for Vaccination	Chronic cardiovascular, pulmonary, renal, or liver disease; diabetes mellitus; CSF leaks; alcoholism; asplenia; immunocompromising conditions/medications; Native Americans and Alaska natives; long-term care facility residents
Revaccination Schedule	One-time revaccination after 5 years for (1) adult >65 years of age, if the first dose is received before age 65 years; (2) persons with asplenia; and (3) immunocompromised persons

Adapted from the IDSA/ATS Guidelines for CAP in Adults, CID, Mandell et al. (2007).
CSF, cerebrospinal fluid.

The CURB-65 severity assessment tool, published by the British Thoracic Society, is attractive because it is simple to remember and can be calculated using a bedside assessment plus a blood urea nitrogen level (Table 32.9). However, it is not as well studied or validated as the PSI. The CURB-65 tool may be particularly useful in identifying patients who require ICU admission, such as those with a score of 3, 4 or 5, in whom the combined hospital mortality is 22% (Table 32.10).

Additional signs of severe pneumonia that do not appear in the PSI or CURB-65 indexes are multilobar disease evident on chest x-ray, severe hypoxemia, leukocytosis in excess of 20 cells/mm^3 or leukopenia (<4 cells/mm^3), and elevated serum lactate. A reasonable practice is to send a serum lactate in any CAP patient in whom blood cultures are drawn. A lactate level greater than 4 mmol/L in this setting indicates likely tissue hypoperfusion from sepsis, need for aggressive resuscitation, and consideration of ICU-level care.

The major complications of CAP that may require ED intervention are ventilatory failure, sepsis syndrome, and pleural complications. Parapneumonic effusion is present in 20–40% of CAP requiring hospitalization, and empyema complicates 5–7% of cases. Diagnostic paracentesis is recommended for an effusion measuring greater than 10 mm on lateral decubitus chest x-ray, and pleural fluid should be obtained prior to administering antibiotics, if possible. Indications for definitive drainage are complex, but pleural fluid with a pH less than 7.2 is the best single indicator. The extent to which practitioners are involved in managing pleural complications of CAP will depend greatly on the practice setting, but diagnostic thoracentesis can be rapidly and safely performed with ultrasound guidance.

SPECIAL CONSIDERATIONS – PNEUMONIA IN NURSING HOME RESIDENTS

Pneumonia occurring in residents of long-term care facilities (LTCFs) and those undergoing dialysis is categorized as

abnormalities are assigned to class 1 without the need for blood tests. (See Figure 32.1.) For patients not satisfying PSI class 1 criteria, a scoring system based on 22 clinical and laboratory elements is used to assign patients to class 2–5 (Table 32.8). Classes 1 and 2 have a 30-day mortality of 0.1% and 0.6%, respectively, and are usually candidates for outpatient management. Class 3 is associated with a 0.9–2.8% mortality, suggesting that hospitalization is appropriate, and classes 4 and 5 are associated with 8.2–9.3% and 27–31.1% mortality and thus almost always require admission. Performance of the PSI in determining prognosis has been validated in more than 50,000 patients and, when used consistently by practitioners, leads to a decreased CAP hospitalization rate without adversely affecting outcome. It is important to recognize that the PSI has limitations and should contribute to, but not supersede, physician judgment. Reasons to hospitalize patients assigned to class 1–3 include the following: poor oxygenation (SpO$_2$ <90), pleural complications, psychosocial issues (psychiatric illness, alcoholism, poor home situation); inability to take antibiotics by mouth; and patient preference.

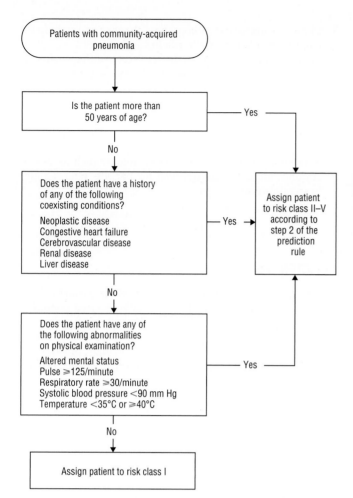

Figure 32.1 Pneumonia Severity Index. Identifying patients in risk class I in the derivation of the prediction rule. In step 1 of the prediction rule, the following were independently associated with mortality: an age of more than 50 years, five coexisting illnesses (neoplastic disease, congestive heart failure, cerebrovascular disease, renal disease, and liver disease), and five physical-examination findings (altered mental status; pulse, ≥125 per minute; respiratory rate, ≥30 per minute; systolic blood pressure, <90 mm Hg; and temperature, <35°C or >40°C). In the derivation cohort, 1372 patients (9.7%) with none of these 11 risk factors were assigned to risk class I. All 12,827 remaining patients were assigned to risk class II, III, IV, or V according to the sum of the points assigned in step 2 of the prediction rule. Reprinted from Fine MJ, Auble TE, Yealy DM, et al. A prediction rule to identify low-risk patients with community-acquired pneumonia. N Engl J Med 1997;336(4):243–50. Copyright 1997 Massachusetts Medical Society. All rights reserved.

Table 32.7 Pneumoria Severity Index. Point Scoring System for Step 2 of the Prediction Rule for Assignment to Risk Classes II, III, IV, and V

Characteristic	Points Assigned*
Demographic factor	
Age	
Men	Age (yr)
Women	Age (yr) − 10
Nursing home resident	+10
Coexisting illnesses†	
Neoplastic disease	+30
Liver disease	+20
Congestive heart failure	+10
Cerebrovascular disease	+10
Renal disease	+10
Physical-examination findings	
Altered mental status‡	+20
Respiratory rate ≥30/min	+20
Systolic blood pressure <90 mm Hg	+20
Temperature <35°C or ≥40°C	+15
Pulse ≥125/min	+10
Laboratory and radiographic findings	
Arterial pH <7.35	+30
Blood urea nitrogen ≥30 mg/dl (11 mmol/liter)	+20
Sodium <30 mmol/liter	+20
Glucose ≥250 mg/dl (14 mmol/liter)	+10
Hematocrit <30%	+10
Partial pressure of arterial oxygen 60 mm Hg§	+10
Pleural effusion	+10

*A total point score for a given patient is obtained by summing the patient's age in years (age minus 10 for women) and the points for each applicable characteristic.

†Neoplastic disease is defined as any cancer except basal- or squamous-cell cancer of the skin that was active at the time of presentation or diagnosed within one year of presentation. Liver disease is defined as a clinical or histologic diagnosis of cirrhosis or another form of chronic liver disease, such as chronic active hepatitis. Congestive heart failure is defined as systolic or diastolic ventricular dysfunction documented by history, physical examination, and chest radiograph, echocardiogram, multiple gated acquisition scan, or left ventriculogram. Cerebrovascular disease is defined as a clinical diagnosis of stroke or transient ischemic attack or stroke documented by magnetic resonance imaging or computed tomography. Renal disease is defined as a history of chronic renal disease or abnormal blood urea nitrogen and creatinine concentrations documented in the medical record.

‡Altered mental status is defined as disorientation with respect to person, place, or time that is not known to be chronic, stupor, or coma.

§In the Pneumonia PORT cohort study, an oxygen saturation of less than 90 percent on pulse oximetry or intubation before admission was also considered abnormal.

Reprinted from Fine MJ, Auble TE, Yealy DM, et al. A prediction rule to identify low-risk patients with community-acquired pneumonia. N Engl J Med 1997;336(4):243–50. Copyright 1997 Massachusetts Medical Society. All rights reserved.

health care associated (versus community acquired), as such patients are at increased risk for drug-resistant pathogens and require expanded empiric antibiotic coverage. Pneumonia is up to 10 times more common in LTCF residents, compared to elderly patients in the community. Factors associated with an increased risk of pneumonia include older age, immobility, difficulty swallowing, inability to take oral medications, and presence of a feeding tube. Diagnosis can be very difficult in this population because localizing signs such as cough are often absent and chest x-ray interpretation may be hampered by chronic changes, dehydration, and patient positioning. Elevated respiratory rate may be the best early sign. Pathogens responsible for pneumonia in LCTF residents include *S. aureus* (including methicillin-resistant *S. aureus*), multidrug resistant gram-negative species, and *Legionella*. Recommended empiric regimens generally combine an antipseudomonal beta-lactam plus an antipseudomonal fluoroquinolone. Vancomycin or linezolid is added if there is a high local incidence of methicillin-resistant *S. aureus*. Acute hospitalization, which is costly and associated with declines in quality of life and functional status, is usually, but not invariably, necessary in LTCF residents diagnosed with pneumonia. Return to the nursing home for further treatment, after blood cultures and a dose of parenteral antibiotic, may be considered in those who can eat and drink, have relatively normal vital signs (e.g., respiratory rate <30), and adequate oxygenation.

Table 32.8 Pneumonia Severity Index–Based Mortality Prediction for Community-Acquired Pneumonia

Class	Points	Mortality	Disposition
1	<51	0.1%	Outpatient
2	51–70	0.6%	Outpatient
3	71–90	0.9%	Inpatient briefly vs. outpatient
4	91–130	9.5%	Inpatient
5	>130	26.7%	Inpatient, possible ICU

Table 32.9 The CURB-65 Severity Assessment Tool

C	onfusion
U	rea (BUN ≥7 mmol/L or approximately ≥20 mg/dL)
R	espiratory rate ≥30 breaths/min
B	lood pressure (SBP <90 mm Hg or DBP ≤60 mm Hg)
65	years old or greater

One point is assigned for each CURB-65 criteria that is present.
BUN, blood urea nitrogen; DBP, diastolic blood pressure; SBP, systolic blood pressure.

Table 32.10 CURB-65 Score and Mortality Prediction

Score	30-Day Mortality Rate	Patient Disposition
0–1	1.5%	Outpatient
2	9.2%	Outpatient vs. brief inpatient
3–5	22%	Inpatient; consider ICU if 4 or 5 points

PEARLS AND PITFALLS

1. Chest x-ray is required for the diagnosis of CAP in the acute care setting.
2. A normal chest x-ray in a well-appearing young patient with respiratory symptoms usually signifies bronchitis that does not require antibiotics.
3. A normal chest x-ray in an ill-appearing or elderly patient could signify a false negative test for CAP, but should prompt a search for other sources of fever or respiratory symptoms.
4. Chest x-ray opacities may be caused by serious noninfectious problems (such as heart failure) and uncommon infectious diseases (such as tuberculosis or fungi) that may masquerade as CAP.
5. Clinical features and radiographic changes do not help to identify the etiologic pathogen in CAP.
6. Initial antibiotic therapy in the acute care setting is almost always empirical, dictated by disease severity, recent antibiotic use, and comorbidities.
7. Careful and structured severity assessment (using the pneumonia severity index or CURB-65 score) is recommended in order to reduce unnecessary hospitalization and to identify occult severe CAP.
8. Microbiologic tests to determine etiology, such as blood cultures, are generally reserved for patients who require hospitalization.

REFERENCES

Fine MJ, Auble TE, Yealy DM, et al. A prediction rule to identify low-risk patients with community-acquired pneumonia. N Engl J Med 1997;336(4):243–50.

Kennedy M, Bates DW, Wright SB, et al. Do emergency department blood cultures change practice in patients with pneumonia? Ann Emerg Med 2005;46(5):393–400.

Lim WS, van der Eerden MM, Laing R, et al. Defining community acquired pneumonia severity on presentation to hospital: an international derivation and validation study. Thorax 2003;58(5):377–82.

Loeb M, Carusone SC, Goeree T, et al. Effect of a clinical pathway to reduce hospitalizations in nursing home residents with pneumonia: a randomized controlled trial. JAMA 2006;295(21):2503–10.

Mandell LA, Wunderink RG, Anzueto A, et al. Infectious Diseases Society of America/American Thoracic Society consensus guidelines on the management of community-acquired pneumonia in adults. Clin Infect Dis 2007;44(Suppl 2):S27–72.

Marie TJ, Lau CY, Wheeler SL, et al. A controlled trial of a critical pathway for treatment of community-acquired pneumonia. CAPITAL Study Investigators. Community-Acquired Pneumonia Intervention Trial Assessing Levofloxacin. JAMA 2000;283:749.

Metlay JP, Kapoor WN, Fine MJ. Does this patient have community-acquired pneumonia? Diagnosing pneumonia by history and physical examination. JAMA 1997;278:1440.

Shapiro NI, Howell MD, Talmor D, et al. Serum lactate as a predictor of mortality in emergency department patients with infection. Ann Emerg Med 2005;45(5):524–8.

33. Tuberculosis

Adithya Cattamanchi and Payam Nahid

INTRODUCTION – AGENT

Mycobacterium tuberculosis is a large, nonmotile, curved rod that causes the vast majority of human tuberculosis cases. *M. tuberculosis* and three very closely related mycobacterial species (*M. bovis*, *M. africanum*, and *M. microti*) all cause tuberculous disease, and they comprise what is known as the *M. tuberculosis* complex. *M. tuberculosis* is an obligate aerobe, accounting for its predilection to cause disease in the well-aerated upper lobes of the lung. However, *M. tuberculosis* can persist in a dormant state for many years even with a limited oxygen supply. The organisms also persist in the environment and are resistant to disinfecting agents.

Mycobacterium species are classified as acid-fast organisms because of their ability to retain certain dyes when heated and treated with acidified compounds. Humans are the only known reservoir of infection.

EPIDEMIOLOGY

Tuberculosis is the second leading cause of death related to an infectious disease. Nearly one-third of the world's population is infected with *Mycobacterium tuberculosis*. In 2005, the World Health Organization (WHO) estimated there were 8.8 million new cases of tuberculosis and 1.6 million deaths due to the disease. Tuberculosis is the leading cause of death among human immunodeficiency virus (HIV)-infected persons, accounting for 12% of worldwide deaths. Whereas the average person infected with *Mycobacterium tuberculosis* has a 10% lifetime chance of developing active disease, immunocompromised patients can have their risk jump to that same percentage *annually*.

Drug resistance is of increasing concern, particularly among high-risk populations such as persons born in countries with high rates of drug resistance and those with a prior history of tuberculosis treatment. Multidrug-resistant tuberculosis (MDR-TB), defined as *Mycobacterium* tuberculosis resistant to at least isoniazid and rifampin (the two most powerful anti-tuberculosis drugs), accounted for approximately 5% of new tuberculosis cases worldwide. Extensively drug-resistant tuberculosis (XDR-TB), defined as MDR-TB with additional resistance to a fluoroquinolone and at least one injectable second-line anti-tuberculosis drug, has been documented in every country surveyed.

In the United States, following a resurgence in the 1980s, the incidence of tuberculosis has been declining since 1993 and is currently at an all-time low. However, the rate of decline has slowed since 2000. In addition, wide disparities persist. The rate of tuberculosis in 2006 among foreign-born person was 9.5 times higher relative to the rate among U.S.-born persons. Although urban areas tend to show greater rates of tuberculosis than rural areas, these rates vary significantly with socioeconomic status, with the poor and recent immigrants being disproportionately affected. In 2006, MDR-TB accounted for 1.2% of all tuberculosis cases, with 81.5% of MDR-TB cases arising in foreign-born populations.

Tuberculosis cases develop either through exogenous infection with rapid progression to clinical illness or through endogenous reactivation of latent infection. In the developing world, where the burden of disease is high, the majority of new cases arise from transmission through contact with active cases of tuberculosis. In low-incidence countries, the majority of new cases arise from reactivation of latent infection. Molecular epidemiologic data from low-incidence countries has shown that up to 90% of all tuberculosis cases are due to reactivation of latent infection. Thus, identification and treatment of persons with latent infection is a major priority.

Pathogenesis and Risk Factors

The development of tuberculosis can be thought of as a two-phase process: the acquisition of *M. tuberculosis* infection and the subsequent development of active tuberculosis. Infection occurs when a susceptible individual is exposed to a person with active tuberculosis. The most common route of transmission is inhalation of aerosolized particles of approximately 1–5 μm generated when a person with active disease coughs. In heavily exposed individuals, there is a 30% chance of infection; it is estimated that as few as five viable bacilli delivered to a terminal alveolus can cause infection.

In the majority of cases, infected patients with an intact immune system will experience few or no symptom after the initial exposure. Both innate and adaptive host defense mechanisms prevent active disease in the majority of persons but are unable to eliminate the tubercle bacilli, leading to a "latent" infected state. Though little is known about this pathologic state, histopathological animal model studies have demonstrated that granulomas are formed through the sensitized immune response at approximately 4 weeks: lymphocytes surround the initial macrophage and neutrophil responders to the mycobacterial infection, and sequester the bacilli. Some bacilli may escape this initial immune response and disseminate to organs outside of the lungs producing other latent foci of infection. Mycobacteria have also been shown to adapt to the immune response through decreased metabolism and develop resistance to hostile environmental elements, which may help explain how latent bacteria can remain viable for decades.

Approximately 3–5% of immunocompetent individuals will bypass a latent infection and develop active tuberculosis within 1 year of becoming infected, with an additional 3–5% progressing to active tuberculosis within their lifetime after a prolonged latent infection. Thus, 90% of infected, healthy persons will never develop clinical manifestations of tuberculosis.

The likelihood of developing active tuberculosis is related to both host and environmental factors. HIV infection is clearly the strongest risk factor for the development of active tuberculosis. The annual risk of developing active tuberculosis is 5–8% and the lifetime risk is 20% or greater in HIV-infected persons with a positive tuberculin skin test. The likelihood of disseminated disease is also increased in this population. In the United States, 20% of extrapulmonary tuberculosis cases are in HIV-infected patients, and 50% of tuberculosis infections in HIV patients have extrapulmonary foci. In addition, active tuberculosis has also been shown to accelerate the course of HIV infection.

Other conditions associated with impaired cell-mediated immunity also increase the risk of tuberculosis. Examples include nutritional deficiencies, hematologic malignancies, chemotherapy, and treatment with tumor necrosis factor alpha (TNF-alpha) inhibitors. Conditions such as diabetes mellitus and uremia are also associated with increased risk. Pulmonary silicosis increases the risk of tuberculosis, presumably because of the effects of silica on alveolar macrophage function. In addition to associated medical conditions, age has a marked effect on the development of tuberculosis. The elderly and young children are at increased risk for developing tuberculosis and disseminated disease. The majority of child cases occur between the ages of 1 and 4, with 1 of 4 infections manifesting as extrapulmonary. Children under 4 years of age are more likely to experience hematogenous dissemination of mycobacteria and are at an increased risk of tubercular meningitis.

CLINICAL FEATURES

Current guidelines recommend targeted screening of persons at high risk for the development of active tuberculosis. The guidelines emphasize that a decision to screen implies a decision to treat if the screening test is positive. Persons who should be considered for screening include those who may have recently acquired infection: contacts of active tuberculosis cases, recent immigrants from high-prevalence countries, infants and young children, immunocompromised persons (HIV infection, diabetes, etc.), health care personnel, and institutionalized persons (see Table 33.1).

Table 33.1 Clinical Features: Tuberculosis

Incubation Period	Variable
Organism	*Mycobacterium tuberculosis*
Signs and Symptoms	• Cough is the most common symptom • Night sweats, fever, malaise, and weight loss • Hemoptysis and pleuritic chest pain
Laboratory and Radiographic Findings	• Laboratory studies are often normal • There may be anemia, leukocytosis, leukopenia, or hyponatremia • **Acute primary TB CXR** – middle or lower lung infiltration with ipsilateral hilar lymphadenopathy • **Reactivation TB CXR** – upper lobe infiltration or cavitation are present unilaterally or bilaterally or in a miliary pattern • **Advanced HIV CXR** – cavitation rare; lower lung or diffuse infiltration with intrathoracic lymphadenopathy • **Pediatric population** – cavitation rare; intrathoracic lymphadenopathy with occasional lower lung infiltration

CXR, chest x-ray; TB, tuberculosis.

General Manifestations of Tuberculosis

The clinical presentation of tuberculosis varies tremendously depending on the affected site or sites of disease, the effectiveness of host defense mechanisms in containing the infection, and the presence of associated diseases. The systemic symptoms associated with active tuberculosis include fever, night sweats, malaise, anorexia, and weight loss. Fever is the most common systemic complaint, occurring in approximately 35–80% of cases. All of the systemic symptoms are thought to be mediated by the production of cytokines, particularly TNF-alpha, in response to the presence of *M. tuberculosis* antigens.

The systemic manifestations of tuberculosis may be obscured or modified by the presence of associated conditions including alcohol and drug abuse, HIV infection, diabetes, and chronic kidney disease. For unclear reasons, neuropsychological changes such as depression and hypomania have also been reported in association with active tuberculosis. As these factors may obscure typical presenting symptoms, a high index of suspicion is often necessary to make the diagnosis of tuberculosis.

Pulmonary Tuberculosis

Pulmonary involvement is the most common manifestation of tuberculosis, occurring in approximately 80% of cases.

Cough is the most common symptom and may initially be nonproductive. As the disease progresses and tissue necrosis occurs, the cough typically becomes productive. Hemoptysis is common with more extensive involvement. Pleuritic chest pain may result from inflammation of lung parenchyma adjacent to a pleural surface, pleural effusion, or an empyema. Physical findings are nonspecific and generally not helpful in distinguishing tuberculosis from other pulmonary infections. Crackles can be heard in areas of pulmonary involvement, and bronchial breath sounds may indicate areas of consolidation.

Extrapulmonary Tuberculosis

Extrapulmonary involvement is more common in infants and HIV-infected persons. Following initial infection with *M. tuberculosis* in the lung, failure to contain the infection can result in hematogenous dissemination of bacilli and the establishment of latent foci of infection in almost any organ of the body. Extrapulmonary disease occurs in approximately 15% of active tuberculosis cases and can involve virtually any organ system. Common sites of extrapulmonary infections include lymph nodes (granulomatous lymphadenitis, which is often painless and can be with or without fever), pleura (pleural effusion causing shortness of breath and pleuritic chest pain), genitourinary tract, joints, and bones (most classically spinal osteomyelitis, or Pott's disease). Life threatening disease can occur involve the meninges, brain parenchyma, and pericardium.

Depending on the site of involvement, patients with extrapulmonary tuberculosis may present with painless lymphadenopathy, abdominal pain, dysuria, monoarticular joint swelling, back pain, headache, cranial nerve impairments, altered mental status, focal neurological symptoms, or seizures, in addition to or instead of cough. Very rarely, tuberculosis can present acutely as bacteremia or sepsis.

Latent Tuberculosis Infection

Latent tuberculosis infection is a clinical condition characterized by evidence of prior *M. tuberculosis* infection and lack of clinical or radiological signs of active tuberculosis. Consequently, persons with latent tuberculosis infection are asymptomatic and have normal chest radiographs. The only evidence of tuberculosis infection is an immune response to tuberculosis antigens demonstrated through a tuberculin skin test or through newer whole-blood interferon gamma release assays.

DIFFERENTIAL DIAGNOSIS

The differential diagnosis of tuberculosis is broad and depends on the suspected site of infection.

There are no key features that can reliably distinguish tuberculosis from other pulmonary infections. The following can be suggestive of tuberculosis, but their absence does not rule out the diagnosis:

- chest x-ray (CXR) is typically abnormal (except in HIV-infected persons) and classically shows upper-lobe thick-walled cavitation with surrounding consolidation
- symptoms are subacute to chronic and usually are constitutional in nature
- patient typically has demographic characteristics that place them at risk for tuberculosis

Other conditions to consider:

- other bacterial pneumonia may cause cavitary pulmonary lesions (e.g., gram-negative rods, *Staphylococcus aureus*, and anaerobes)
- other mycobacterial pneumonias (e.g., *M. kansasii*)
- carcinoma (e.g. squamous cell, melanoma, and sarcoma)
- autoimmune disease (Wegener's granulomatosis, sarcoidosis)
- septic emboli

LABORATORY AND RADIOGRAPHIC FINDINGS

Though laboratory studies are often normal, there are a few nonspecific abnormalities that may be associated with active tuberculosis. The most common hematologic abnormalities in tuberculosis are an elevation in the peripheral blood leukocyte count and anemia, which occurs in 10% of patients without bone marrow involvement. Anemia is more common in advanced or disseminated infection. Other reported hematologic abnormalities include leukopenia and elevations in the peripheral blood monocyte and eosinophil counts. Hyponatremia is a fairly common metabolic effect of tuberculosis, occurring in up to 11% of patients in one report.

Radiographic Features

The chest radiograph is abnormal in nearly all cases of pulmonary tuberculosis. One exception is with HIV-related pulmonary tuberculosis in which up to 11% of chest radiographs have been reported to be normal.

In acute primary tuberculosis, chest radiography commonly shows middle or lower lung zone infiltrates with ipsilateral hilar lymphadenopathy. Atelectasis may be seen because of airway compression. Cavitation may occur if the primary process persists (progressive primary tuberculosis).

In reactivation tuberculosis, abnormalities are typically present in the upper lobe of one or both lungs. The most common sites of involvement are the apical and posterior segments of the right lung and the apical-posterior segment of the left lung. Involvement of the anterior segment alone is rare. Cavitation secondary to destruction of lung tissue is often present. The development of a fibrotic scar with loss of lung parenchymal volume and calcification is seen with healing of tuberculous lesions. A miliary pattern of involvement may be seen when a tuberculous focus erodes into lymph or blood vessels allowing for dissemination of tuberculous bacilli.

In HIV-infected persons, particularly those with advanced disease, cavitation is less common, and lower lung zone or diffuse infiltrates along with intrathoracic lymphadenopathy are more often seen.

Although recognition of the classic findings in primary and reactivation tuberculosis remains important, the time from acquisition of infection to development of clinical disease may not reliably predict the radiographic appearance of tuberculosis.

Latent Tuberculosis Infection

The tuberculin skin test remains the gold standard for diagnosis of latent tuberculosis infection. The test demonstrates a delayed type hypersensitivity reaction to purified protein derivative (PPD), a crude mixture of mycobacterial antigens. The test is performed by the Mantoux method – intradermal injection of 0.1 mL (5 TU) of PPD typically on the volar surface of the forearm. Reading of the test is conventionally done after 48–72 hours, but may be delayed up to 1 week.

Reaction size is determined by measuring the diameter of induration and is recorded in millimeters. Recommended cut-offs for a positive test vary with the population being tested (see Table 33.2).

Table 33.2 Criteria for Positive Tuberculin Skin Test

Reaction ≥5 mm of Induration	Reaction ≥10 mm of Induration	Reaction ≥15 mm of Induration
1. HIV-positive persons 2. Recent contacts of TB case patients 3. Fibrotic changes on chest radiograph consistent with prior TB 4. Patients with organ transplants and other immunosuppressed patients (receiving the equivalent of 15 mg/day of prednisone for 1 month or more)	1. Recent immigrants (i.e., within the last 5 years) from high-prevalence countries 2. Injection drug users 3. Residents and employees of high-risk congregate settings including health care facilities, prisons and jails, long-term care facilities, and homeless shelters 4. Mycobacteriology laboratory personnel 5. Persons with silicosis, diabetes mellitus, chronic renal failure, hematologic disorders (e.g., leukemias and lymphomas), other specific malignancies (e.g., carcinoma of the head or neck and lung), weight loss of >10% of ideal body weight, gastrectomy, and jejunoileal bypass 6. Children younger than 4 years of age or infants, children, and adolescents exposed to adults at high risk	1. Persons with no TB risk factors

Adapted from Centers for Disease Control and Prevention. Screening for tuberculosis and tuberculosis infection in high risk populations: recommendations of the Advisory Council for the Elimination of Tuberculosis. MMWR 1995;44(No. RR-11):19–34.
TB, tuberculosis.

- **Highest risk persons** (immunodeficient states, infants, contacts of tuberculosis cases) have the lowest cutoff of 5 mm.
- **Intermediate-risk persons** (health care workers, residents of correctional facilities or nursing homes, homeless persons) have a cutoff of 10 mm.
- **Low-risk persons** (routine job screening) have the highest cutoff of 15 mm and in general should not be tested.

Although widely used, the tuberculin skin test has problems with both specificity and sensitivity. False positive results are seen in populations with high background rates of nontuberculous mycobacterial infections and bacille Calmette-Guérin (BCG) vaccination. False negative tests are seen in HIV infection and in other conditions of decreased cell-mediated immunity.

The QuantiFERON-TB Gold is a newer blood test to detect latent tuberculosis infection that may be available through some local tuberculosis control programs and hospital laboratories. The test incorporates antigens that are more specific than PPD for *Mycobacterium tuberculosis*. Unlike the tuberculin skin test, interpretation of test results is the same regardless of the population being tested. Test results are typically available within 24 hours. The test is currently recommended for use in the same population as the tuberculin skin test, although data are insufficient to recommend use in children and HIV-infected persons.

Pulmonary Tuberculosis

The definitive diagnosis of pulmonary tuberculosis is most often made through the isolation of *M. tuberculosis* in sputum culture or by the amplification of specific nucleic acid sequences from sputum samples. A minimum of three sputum samples should be collected at least 8 hours apart during the initial evaluation of suspected cases of pulmonary tuberculosis. Single, early-morning specimens have the highest yield.

In patients who are not producing sputum, several options exist. The most effective is induction of sputum by the inhalation of a concentrated (3–5%) saline mist produced by an ultrasonic nebulizer. Sputum induction is generally well tolerated and inexpensive and has a similar sensitivity to bronchoalveolar lavage. Pulmonary secretions containing tuberculous bacilli are frequently swallowed and can be recovered from the gastric contents. In young children who cannot voluntarily expectorate sputum, sampling of gastric contents via a nasogastric tube is ofen performed, though sputum induction has been shown to be safe and to have a higher yield than nasogastric lavage even in very young children. Fiberoptic bronchoscopy is the next diagnostic modality if sputum inductions are negative or cannot be performed.

The diagnosis of pulmonary tuberculosis can also be made clinically in the absence of positive cultures, although this approach does not allow for the determination of drug susceptibility and is not standard of care. In a high-risk patient with a positive tuberculin skin test or interferon gamma release assay, resolution or improvement of radiographic changes following antituberculosis chemotherapy is sufficient to make the diagnosis of pulmonary tuberculosis and to necessitate a complete course of therapy. In general, a clinical response should be seen within 2 months of initiating treatment.

Extrapulmonary Tuberculosis

The diagnosis of extrapulmonary tuberculosis is challenging. Sites of infection may be difficult to access and often contain

Table 33.3 Recommended Dosages for First-Line Antituberculosis Drugs Used for Initial Treatment in Children and Adults

Drug	Type of Administration	Dosage Frequency*		
		Daily	2 Days/Week†	3 Days/ Week†
Isoniazid	Oral, intra-muscular, or intravenous			
Children		10 mg/kg	20–30 mg/kg	–
Adults		5 mg/kg	15 mg/kg	15 mg/kg
Maximum		300 mg	900 mg	900 mg
Rifampin	Oral or intravenous			
Children		10–20 mg/kg	10–20 mg/kg	–
Adults		10 mg/kg	10 mg/kg	10 mg/kg
Maximum		600 mg	600 mg	600 mg
Rifabutin	Oral			
Adults		5 mg/kg	5 mg/kg	5 mg/kg
Maximum		300 mg	300 mg	300 mg
Pyrazinamide	Oral			
Children		15–30 mg/kg	50 mg/kg (2 g max)	–
Adults		25 mg/kg	50 mg/kg	35–40 mg/kg
Maximum		2 g	4 g	3 g
Ethambutol	Oral			
Children		15–20 mg/kg (1 g max)	50 mg/kg (2.5 g max)	–
Adults		15–25 mg/kg	50 mg/kg	25–30 mg/kg
Maximum		1600 mg	2400 mg	4000 mg

*Doses per weight are based on ideal body weight. Children weighing >40 kg should receive adult doses.
†Must be administered by directly observed therapy only.
Adapted with permission from the American Medical Association. Blumberg HM, Leonard MK Jr, Jasmer RM. Update on the treatment of tuberculosis and latent tuberculosis infection. JAMA 2005;293:2776–84.

Table 33.4 Treatment of Latent Tuberculosis Infection

Drug Regimen	Duration	Oral Dose (mg/kg) (max dose)			
		Daily		Twice Weekly*	
		Adults	Children	Adults	Children
Isoniazid	9 months 6 months†	5 (300)	10–20 (300)	15 (900)	20–40 (900)
Rifampin	4 months	10 (600)	10–20 (600)	10 (600)	–

*Therapy must be directly observed when given twice weekly.
†Therapy for 6 months not recommended in HIV-infected persons.

relatively few bacilli. The cornerstone of diagnosis remains isolation of tuberculous bacilli from suspected sites of infection. Multiple samples from all affected sites should be sent for culture to maximize the diagnostic yield for both smear and culture analysis. If possible, fluid from the suspected site of infection should be aspirated – it takes 5000 to 10,000 mycobacteria bacilli per mL for detection with a smear; some more sensitive culture methods can detect as few as 10 bacilli per mL. Surgical procedures are often needed to obtain adequate tissue samples. CSF analysis will often show a neutrophilic predominance, mononuclear cells and a low glucose level in mycobacterial meningitis.

TREATMENT

The treatment of active tuberculosis and latent infections are reviewed in Tables 33.3 and 33.4. National, evidence-based guidelines for the treatment of tuberculosis and latent infections have been published in joint statements by the American

Thoracic Society, Infectious Diseases Society of America, and the Centers for Disease Control and Prevention (CDC).

General Principles

Tuberculosis treatment differs from that of many other infectious diseases in that the responsibility for treatment completion is shifted to the treating clinician. For each individual patient, special consideration should be given to the specific clinical and social context in which tuberculosis treatment is being administered. The goals of antituberculosis therapy include achieving cure without relapse of disease, stopping transmission of *M. tuberculosis*, and preventing the emergence of drug-resistant strains.

Directly observed therapy (providing medications and watching the patient swallow them) is recommended for all patients and has been shown to increase compliance and completion of therapy. Tuberculosis is generally treated through public health agencies because of the significant infrastructure and cost of administering directly observed therapy. Tuberculosis should never be treated with a single drug, and a single drug should never be added to a failing regimen because of the risk of acquiring drug resistance. Thus, multidrug therapy is always required.

The efficacy of treatment should be monitored by obtaining sputum for acid-fast bacillus (AFB) smear and culture at least monthly until two consecutive cultures are negative. Cultures should always be obtained after 2 months of treatment because positive cultures at this stage predict a high risk of relapse and mandate prolongation of therapy. Drug susceptibility testing should be performed on the initial culture and again if cultures remain positive after 3 months of treatment.

Tuberculosis treatment with combination chemotherapy can be complicated by both mild and serious adverse reactions (see Table 33.5). Mild adverse reactions can generally be managed with conservative therapy aimed at controlling symptoms, whereas with more severe reactions the offending drug or drugs must be discontinued. Managing serious adverse reactions frequently necessitates expert consultation. Although it is important to recognize the potential for adverse effects, first-line drugs should not be discontinued without adequate justification.

Treatment of Drug-Susceptible Disease

Tuberculosis treatment is generally divided into two phases: the initiation (bactericidal) phase, which lasts 2 months, and

Table 33.5 Monitoring Recommendations and Adverse Reactions for First-Line Antituberculosis Drugs

Medication	Monitoring	Adverse Reactions
Isoniazid	• No routine monitoring • Hepatic enzymes if preexisting liver disease, HIV infection, or pregnancy	• Hepatic enzyme elevation, hepatitis, and fatal hepatitis • Peripheral neuropathy and CNS effects • Increased phenytoin levels • Lupus-like syndrome
Rifampin	• No routine monitoring • Check for drug interactions	• Pruritis with or without rash (typically self limited) • Nausea, anorexia, abdominal pain • Flulike syndrome • Hepatotoxicity • Orange discoloration of bodily fluids (sputum, urine, sweat, tears) • Drug interactions due to induction of hepatic microsomal enzymes
Rifabutin	• Similar to rifampin	• Hematologic toxicity such as neutropenia • Uveitis • Orange discoloration of bodily fluids • Polyarthralgias • Pseudo-jaundice (skin discoloration with normal bilirubin) • Hepatotoxicity
Pyrazinamide	• Hepatic enzymes if preexisting liver disease or when used with rifampin for latent tuberculosis treatment • Serum uric acid measurements serve as a surrogate marker for compliance	• Hepatotoxicity • Hyperuricemia, gouty arthritis • Polyarthralgia (usually responds to nonsteroidal anti-inflammatory agents) • Nausea, vomiting, abdominal discomfort • Transient morbilliform rash (usually not an indication for discontinuation)
Ethambutol	• Monthly color and acuity vision check	• Decreased visual acuity or decreased red-green color discrimination (dose related) should prompt immediate and permanent discontinuation • Rash

the continuation phase, which lasts 4 to 7 months for patients with drug-susceptible disease (see Figure 33.1). Antituberculosis treatment should be administered following bacteriologic confirmation of tuberculosis or empirically when there is a high clinical suspicion for disease prior to culture confirmation and, in certain cases, prior to the availability of AFB smear microscopy results. Treatment is generally initiated with an empiric four-drug regimen consisting of isoniazid, rifampin, ethambutol, and pyrazinamide. Recommended dosages and dosing schedules for first line anti-tuberculosis medications are shown in Table 33.3.

A special warning is needed about the use of fluoroquinolones in empirically treating infections in the acute care setting. Fluoroquinolones have recently been under study

as potential first-line agents for tuberculosis. Moxifloxacin and gatifloxacin are believed to have the greatest activity in vitro against *M. tuberculosis*, followed by levofloxacin and ofloxacin. To minimize the potential development of fluoroquinolone-resistant tuberculosis, this class of medication should be avoided in patients in whom tuberculosis is part of the differential diagnosis and in whom a trial of empiric antibiotics is planned.

Treatment of Latent Tuberculosis Infection

Prior to initiating treatment for latent infection, it is important to exclude the presence of active tuberculosis. Isoniazid (INH) given for 9 months is the preferred treatment for latent infection (see Table 33.4). The reported efficacy of INH treatment in preventing active tuberculosis has varied considerably from 25% to 92%. However, the efficacy is closer to 90% when the analysis is restricted to patients compliant with therapy. INH can be given as a single daily dose (300 mg for adults, 5 to 10 mg/kg for children) or twice weekly (15 mg/kg) when therapy is directly observed.

Hepatotoxicity and peripheral neuropathy are the major adverse events associated with INH therapy. Asymptomatic elevations in liver enzymes are relatively common, but the rate of symptomatic hepatitis is low (1 to 3 per 1000 persons treated). Alcohol consumption has been shown to significantly increase the risk of INH-induced hepatitis. Routine monitoring of liver enzymes is not currently recommended except for patients who are HIV-infected, pregnant, or taking other hepatotoxic medications and those with chronic liver disease and alcohol abuse. Patients predisposed to the development of peripheral neuropathy (such as patients with diabetes mellitus, malnutrition, renal failure, and HIV infection) should be given pyridoxine 25–50 mg/day concurrently with INH.

The only recommended alternative regimen for the treatment of latent infection is rifampin 10 mg/kg (maximum dose 600 mg) alone for 4 months (see Table 33.4). Rifampin was well tolerated with very low rates of hepatotoxicity. Given the limited clinical trial data, rifampin is best reserved for the treatment of persons with suspected INH-resistant tuberculosis infection.

HIV Infection and Tuberculosis Treatment

The treatment of patients co-infected with HIV and *M. tuberculosis* is complicated by overlapping toxicity profiles of some medications and complex drug interactions. The optimal timing of initiating antiretroviral medication in patients being treated for tuberculosis has not been clearly established. Drug interactions resulting in altered serum drug levels are common between antiretroviral and antituberculosis medications. Updated guidelines, specific interactions, and dosage recommendations for most antiretroviral medications are published by the CDC at http://www.cdc.gov/tb/TB_HIV_Drugs/default.htm.

Tuberculosis treatment regimens are similar in HIV-infected patients with the following exceptions. There is an unacceptably high risk of relapse and acquired rifamycin resistance when a once-weekly isoniazid and rifapentine regimen is used. Thus, it is recommended that HIV-infected patients with a low CD4+ T-lymphocyte count receive antituberculosis medications daily or at least three times weekly.

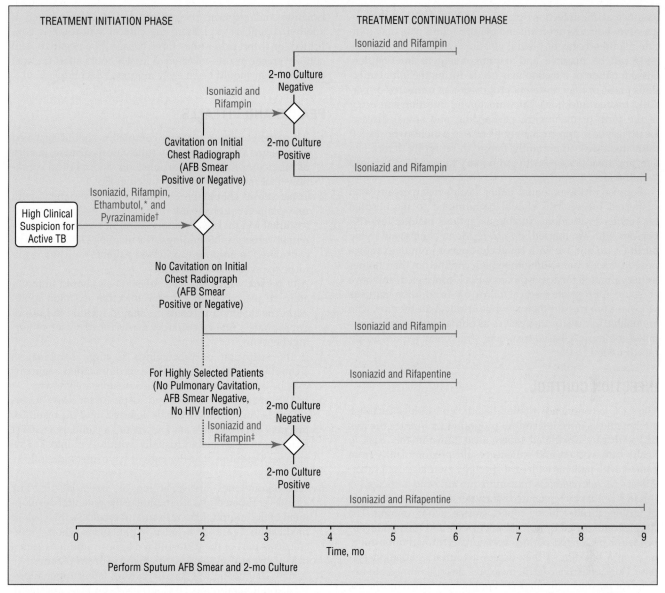

Figure 33.1 Treatment algorithm for drug-susceptible pulmonary tuberculosis. In patients with suspected drug susceptible tuberculosis, treatment is initiated with isoniazid (INH), rifampin (RIF), pyrazinamide (PZA), and ethambutol (ETH) for the initial 2 months of therapy. Further treatment decisions are based on the presence of cavitation on the initial chest radiograph and the results of repeat acid-fast bacilli (AFB) smear and culture performed after the initial 2 months of drug treatment. Treatment is continued with INH and RIF for a total of 6 months when cavitation was not present on the initial chest radiograph and when cavitation was present but the repeat tuberculosis culture is negative after the initial 2 months of therapy. The continuation phase should be extended 3 months (total treatment duration 9 months) if cavitation was present on the initial chest radiograph and the repeat tuberculosis culture is positive. In highly selected patients (HIV-negative, no cavitation on chest radiograph, negative sputum AFB smears performed after the initial 2 months of therapy), treatment with once-weekly INH and rifapentine can be considered as an alternative to INH and RIF. Asterisk indicates ETH may be discontinued when results of drug susceptibility testing indicate no drug resistance. Dagger indicates PZA may be discontinued after it has been taken for 2 months. Double dagger indicates rifapentine should not be used in patients who have HIV and tuberculosis or in patients with extrapulmonary tuberculosis. Section symbol indicates therapy should be extended to 9 months if the 2-month culture was positive. Reproduced with permission from the American Medical Association. Blumberg HM, Leonard MK Jr, Jasmer RM. Update on the treatment of tuberculosis and latent tuberculosis infection. JAMA 2005;293:2776–84.

Treatment of Extrapulmonary Tuberculosis

Extrapulmonary tuberculosis is treated with the same drug regimens as pulmonary tuberculosis. Treatment duration is 6 months for every site except the meninges. Meningeal tuberculosis should be treated for a minimum of 9 to 12 months. The addition of corticosteroids is recommended for the treatment of pericardial and meningeal tuberculosis only. However, data showing a significant decrease in morbidity or mortality are limited, particularly in HIV-infected patients.

Drug-Resistant Tuberculosis

Treatment of drug-resistant tuberculosis is complex and should only be done in consultation with an expert.

COMPLICATIONS AND ADMISSION CRITERIA

One of the most serious complications of untreated tuberculosis is the risk of transmission in the community. Clinical complications of tuberculosis include progressive hypoxia and dyspnea as the infection spreads in the lungs. Rapidly progressive shortness of breath and pleuritic chest pain may indicate pneumothorax or pleural effusion. Occasionally hemoptysis can be massive and require emergent intervention. Dissemination of infection may occur during the initial infectious phase or may represent progression of untreated or partially treated infections. Life-threatening infection can occur in the form of meningitis, pericarditis, and spinal disease. Death results in approximately 40–60% of patients who are left untreated. Most importantly, failure to promptly detect, isolate, and treat persons with pulmonary tuberculosis can lead to outbreaks.

Because of the potential public health risk, persons with suspected tuberculosis should be admitted to the hospital for further evaluation. Notable exceptions include low-risk persons who are housed, do not reside in congregate living facilities, do not live with small children or immunocompromised persons, are willing to remain confined in their homes until evaluation for active tuberculosis is completed, and have access to appropriate medical follow-up. In addition, patients who have progressive disease while on adequate therapy, who are unable to care for themselves as outpatients, or who have failed community-based treatment efforts may require hospital admission.

INFECTION CONTROL

The CDC recommends that all health care settings establish a tuberculosis infection control program to minimize the risk of health care associated tuberculosis transmission. Risk to health care workers and patients results predominantly from contact with patients with unsuspected or undiagnosed tuberculosis. *M. tuberculosis* is transmitted in airborne particles 1–5 μm in size that are generated when persons with pulmonary or laryngeal tuberculosis cough, sneeze, shout, or sing. The droplets are carried by normal air currents and can remain airborne for prolonged periods and spread throughout a room or even a building if they access a central ventilation system. Thus, effective control measures include immediate isolation of persons with suspected pulmonary tuberculosis, use of respiratory isolation rooms (negative pressure ventilation room with a minimum of 6–12 air exchanges per hour with an approved exhaust filtration mechanism), appropriate use of airborne infection precautions during contact with suspected cases, decontamination of patient care areas following triage of suspected cases, and both routine monitoring and postexposure evaluation of health care staff.

The risk of tuberculosis transmission in health care settings varies according to the specific setting, tuberculosis prevalence in the community, effectiveness of tuberculosis control measures, and the characteristics of the specific exposure. Patients with cough, cavitary disease, or positive AFB smears and those undergoing aerosol-generating procedures (sputum induction, bronchoscopy) are more likely to be infectious. Tuberculosis transmission is also increased when the exposure occurs in a small, enclosed setting and when inadequate ventilation fails to dilute or remove infectious droplet nuclei. Any person with suspected tuberculosis should immediately be placed in an airborne infection isolation room, when available. Airborne infection precautions should immediately be instituted including the use of appropriately fitted respiratory masks for all persons entering the room. Both respiratory

isolation and airborne precautions can be discontinued if another diagnosis explaining the clinical syndrome is confirmed, or if the patient has three consecutive negative AFB sputum smear results collected at least 8 hours apart (at least one specimen should be an early morning specimen).

PEARLS AND PITFALLS

1. All patients with respiratory complaints should be asked about signs and symptoms of tuberculosis disease, history of tuberculosis exposure or infection, and medical conditions that increase the risk of tuberculosis.

2. Tuberculosis should be considered in any patient with unexplained cough greater than 2 weeks in duration, unintentional weight loss, hemoptysis, night sweats, or characteristic radiographic findings. The diagnosis should also be considered in immunosuppressed patients with any respiratory or systemic complaints.

3. Any person with suspected tuberculosis should immediately be placed in an airborne infection isolation room. Airborne infection precautions should include the use of appropriately fitted respiratory masks for all persons entering the room.

4. If the suspicion of tuberculosis is high, combination chemotherapy using one of the recommended regimens may be initiated before AFB smear results are known.

5. If AFB smears are negative and suspicion for active tuberculosis is low, treatment can be deferred until the results of mycobacterial cultures are known and a comparison chest radiograph is available (usually within 2 months). This approach requires that the patient have adequate follow-up.

6. Fluoroquinolones are emerging as potential first-line agents for tuberculosis. To minimize the potential development of fluoroquinolone-resistant tuberculosis, this class of medication should be avoided in patients in whom tuberculosis is part of the differential diagnosis and in whom a trial of empiric antibiotics for other reasons is planned.

7. A new diagnostic test for diagnosing latent tuberculosis infection (Quantiferon TB Gold) has been FDA approved. As with the tuberculin skin test, a negative Quantiferon TB Gold does not rule out active tuberculosis.

REFERENCES

American Thoracic Society and the Centers for Disease Control and Prevention (CDC). Targeted tuberculin testing and treatment of latent tuberculosis infection. Am J Respir Crit Care Med 2000 Apr;161:S221–47.

American Thoracic Society, Centers for Disease Control and Prevention and Infectious Disease Society of America. Treatment of tuberculosis. MMWR 2003;52(RR-11).

Blumberg HM, Burman WJ, Chaisson RE, et al. American Thoracic Society/Centers for Disease Control and Prevention/Infectious Diseases Society of America: treatment of tuberculosis. Am J Respir Crit Care Med 2003;167: 603–62.

Blumberg HM, Leonard MK Jr, Jasmer RM. Update on the treatment of tuberculosis and latent tuberculosis infection. JAMA 2005;293:2776–84.

Cattamanchi A, Hopewell PC, Gonzalez LC, et al. A 13-year molecular epidemiological analysis of tuberculosis in San Francisco. Int J Tuberc Lung Dis 2006;10:297–304.

Hass DW, Des Prez RM. Tuberculosis and acquired immunodeficiency syndrome: a historical perspective on recent developments. Am J Med 1994;96:439–50.

Havlir DV, Barnes PF. Tuberculosis in patients with human immunodeficiency virus infection. N Engl J Med 1999;340:367–73.

Hopewell PC. Tuberculosis and other mycobacterial diseases. In: Mason RJ, Broaddus C, Murray JF, Nadel JA, eds, Murray and Nadel's textbook of respiratory medicine, 4th ed. Philadelphia: Elsevier Saunders, 2005:979–1043.

Horsburgh CR, Jr. Priorities for the treatment of latent tuberculosis infection in the United States. N Engl J Med 2004;350:2060–7.

Jasmer RM, Nahid P, Hopewell PC. Clinical practice. Latent tuberculosis infection. N Engl J Med 2002;347:1860–6.

Jensen PA, Lambert LA, Iademarco MF, et al. Guidelines for preventing the transmission of Mycobacterium tuberculosis in health-care settings, 2005. MMWR Recomm Rep 2005;54(17):1–141.

Marais BJ, Gie RP, Schaaf HS, et al. Childhood pulmonary tuberculosis: old wisdom and new challenges. Am J Respir Crit Care Med 2006;173:1078–90.

Mayosi BM, Ntsekhe M, Volmink JA, et al. Interventions for treating tuberculous pericarditis. Cochrane Database Syst Rev 2002(4):CD000526.

Mazurek GH, Jereb J, Lobue P, et al. Guidelines for using the QuantiFERON-TB Gold test for detecting Mycobacterium tuberculosis infection, United States. MMWR Recomm Rep 2005;54(RR-15):49–55.

Nahid P, Daley CL. Prevention of tuberculosis in HIV-infected patients. Curr Opin Infect Dis 2006;19:189–93.

Nahid P, Pai M, Hopewell PC. Advances in the diagnosis and treatment of tuberculosis. Proc Am Thorac Soc 2006;3:103–10.

Piessens WF, Nardell EA. The pathogenesis of tuberculosis. In: Reichman LB, Hershfield ES, eds, Tuberculosis: a comprehensive international approach, 2nd ed. rev. New York: Marcel Dekker, 2000:241–60.

Prasad K, Volmink J, Menon GR. Steroids for treating tuberculous meningitis. Cochrane Database Syst Rev 2000(3):CD002244.

Pratt R, Robison V, Navin T, et al. Trends in tuberculosis incidence – United States 2006. MMWR 2007;56(11):245–50.

Trenton AJ, Currier GW. Treatment of comorbid tuberculosis and depression. Primary care companion. J Clin Psychiatry 2001;3:236–43.

Small P, Fujiwara P. Management of tuberculosis in the United States. N Engl J Med 2001 Jul 19;345(3):189–200.

ADDITIONAL READINGS

Iseman MD. A clinician's guide to tuberculosis. Philadelphia: Lippincott Williams & Wilkins, 2000.

Raviglione MC, ed. Reishman and Hershfield's tuberculosis: a comprehensive international approach, 3rd ed. New York: Informa Healthcare, 2006.

34. Influenza

Asim A. Jani and Timothy M. Uyeki

INTRODUCTION

Influenza is an acute respiratory disease caused by influenza viruses transmitted primarily by droplets expelled during coughing and sneezing. Influenza type A and B virus infections can cause substantial human disease and mortality worldwide. Patients present with variable signs and symptoms depending on age and the presence of underlying chronic disease. Seasonal winter influenza epidemics in temperate countries can have a substantial impact on the emergency department (ED), but travelers may present with influenza illness acquired in other countries year-round. Rarely, the emergence of a novel influenza A subtype virus can lead to a global influenza pandemic.

Influenza viruses are single-stranded negative sense RNA viruses of the family Orthomyxoviridae. Three types (A, B, and C) of influenza viruses infect humans. Type A and B viruses are known to cause significant human disease. The genome contains eight gene segments that code for 11 proteins, including the two main surface glycoproteins, hemagglutinin (HA) and neuraminidase (NA). Type A viruses are further classified into subtypes based on their HA and NA proteins. Currently circulating human influenza A subtypes include A (H1N1) and A (H3N2) viruses. Human influenza viruses bind to and replicate primarily in epithelial cells of the upper respiratory tract.

Influenza viruses are evolving continuously through a process called "antigenic drift" in which random point mutations in the HA gene result in changes to the HA surface protein. Minor changes in the genetic composition of influenza viruses can create new virus strains that are not prevented by existing vaccines. Humoral immunity is based largely on strain-specific HA antibodies and is reduced in young children and in immunosuppressed, immunocompromised, and elderly persons. Antigenic drift is the reason that influenza virus strain surveillance must be conducted worldwide year-round; vaccine strains must be updated each year, and thus, annual influenza vaccination is needed.

"Antigenic shift," as opposed to "drift," is the emergence of a novel influenza A subtype virus in humans. If the novel influenza A virus acquires the ability for sustained human-to-human transmission, a pandemic can result. This can occur through direct mutation from an avian influenza A virus (such as the H1N1 pandemic virus that caused the 1918–19 "Spanish flu" resulting in an estimated 20–100 million deaths) or genetic reassortment between human and avian influenza A viruses. The natural reservoir for all influenza A virus subtypes is in wild aquatic ducks and geese. The 1957–58 "Asian influenza" H2N2 and 1968–69 "Hong Kong influenza" H3N2 pandemic viruses originated through genetic reassortment between human influenza A and low pathogenic avian influenza A viruses. See Chapter 71, Avian Influenza A (H5N1).

EPIDEMIOLOGY

Seasonal influenza epidemics of unpredictable and variable severity occur during winter months in temperate climates of the Northern (October to April) and Southern (May to September) Hemispheres. In temperate climates, communities may experience high influenza activity for 6–8 weeks, although influenza virus infections may occur for several weeks longer. Attack rates are usually highest in schoolchildren, generating high rates of visits to outpatient clinics and EDs. In the United States, an estimated average of more than 200,000 hospitalizations and 36,000 deaths attributable to complications from influenza occur each year. Those at highest risk for complications from influenza are the very young, persons with chronic underlying conditions (e.g., cardiopulmonary diseases), and the elderly.

In tropical and subtropical countries, influenza activity can occur year-round and may increase during cooler months or rainy seasons. Worldwide, influenza outbreaks with high attack rates can occur at any time, especially among nursing home residents, children at boarding schools and camps, and travelers in large organized tour groups such as cruise ship passengers. Thus, a returned traveler from any part of the world with influenzalike illness should be evaluated for possible influenza.

CLINICAL FEATURES

Following infection of the upper respiratory tract, the incubation period is generally 2 days (ranging from 1 to 4 days).

Table 34.1 Signs and Symptoms of Uncomplicated Influenza in Patients Without Underlying Conditions

	Infants and Young Children	School-Age Children	Adults	Elderly
Fever (subjective and objective)	Often high fever; or fever alone	+	+	Absent or low grade
Chills		+	+	+
Headache		+	+	+
Rhinorrhea	+	+	+	+
Nasal congestion	+	+	+	+
Sore throat		+	+	+
Myalgia		+	+	+
Cough, nonproductive		+	+	+
Chest discomfort or pain		+	+	+
Abdominal pain		+		
Vomiting			+	
Diarrhea	+	+		
Malaise		+	+	+
Fatigue		+	+	+

+, may be present.

Table 34.2 Clinical Features: Uncomplicated Influenza

Incubation Period	Generally 2 days, range 1–4 days Viral shedding occurs the day prior to onset of clinical symptoms and continues for 4–5 days
Signs and Symptoms*	Initially, systemic symptoms predominate: • Fever (duration 3 days, range 2–8 days) and nonproductive cough • Chills, malaise, headache, myalgias, sore throat, rhinorrhea, nasal congestion, anorexia Convalescent period can last 1–3 weeks depending on baseline health status: • Cough, fatigue, and malaise
Laboratory and Radiographic Findings	• WBC often normal (unless secondary bacterial process) • Sputum Gram stain unremarkable • CXR usually normal in uncomplicated influenza

*Differs by age and underlying conditions. Young infants may have fever without respiratory symptoms; young children may have abdominal pain and diarrhea; adults may complain of chest pain and vomiting; elderly patients may not always have fever.
WBC, white blood (cell) count.

Most infected children and adults shed influenza viruses from the day prior to illness onset for approximately 4–5 days. Young infants can shed influenza viruses for 1–3 weeks and immunosuppressed or immunocompromised persons can shed viruses for longer periods.

Signs and symptoms of influenza vary by age, underlying conditions, and whether complications are present (Table 34.1). Uncomplicated influenza in adults is characterized by abrupt onset of high fever and other systemic symptoms – chills, myalgias, fatigue, malaise, and headache – and respiratory symptoms such as nonproductive cough, nonexudative pharyngitis, rhinorrhea, and nasal congestion (Table 34.2). Adults may also complain of chest pain. Elderly patients with influenza may not always manifest fever. Young infants can present with high fever and a "sepsis-like" syndrome without respiratory findings. Gastrointestinal symptoms (diarrhea) can occur in young children and are more common with influenza B, whereas schoolchildren may occasionally complain of abdominal pain. Mild illness and asymptomatic infection can occur, and a wide range of clinical complications are associated with influenza (Table 34.3).

The clinical diagnosis of influenza is challenging because influenzalike illness can be caused by many co-circulating pathogens (respiratory viruses, atypical bacteria, or fungi). In general, high fever and cough are frequently associated with influenza. A clinical diagnosis is most accurate during peak community influenza activity. Influenza vaccination is not 100% effective, and some vaccinated persons can develop influenza.

DIFFERENTIAL DIAGNOSIS

The differential diagnosis of uncomplicated acute influenzalike illness in a patient without underlying conditions includes infection with:

- respiratory viruses (influenza viruses, parainfluenza viruses, respiratory syncytial virus, rhinoviruses, adenoviruses, human metapneumovirus, non-SARS [severe acute respiratory syndrome] coronaviruses, bocavirus)
- atypical bacteria (*Legionella pneumophila*, *Mycoplasma pneumoniae*, *Chlamydophila pneumoniae*)
- community-acquired bacteria (e.g., *Streptococcus pneumoniae*, *Haemophilus influenzae*, *Bordetella pertussis*)

Fungal (*Histoplasma*, *Cryptococcus*, *Coccidioides*) and parasitic causes of influenzalike illness are less common. Rare human infection with other infectious agents such as *Bacillus anthracis*, SARS-associated coronavirus, and avian influenza A (H5N1) virus can present initially with influenzalike illness, but a good exposure history, radiographic and laboratory testing results can help to distinguish the features of these rare diseases from human influenza. Immunocompromised and immunocompetent patients can present with influenzalike illness caused by opportunistic pathogens such as *Mycobacterium tuberculosis* and fungi. The patient's medical history, exposure history, and a travel history may be very helpful in formulating the differential diagnosis.

LABORATORY DIAGNOSIS

Influenza can be confirmed by a variety of testing methods (Table 34.4). It is important to obtain the appropriate upper respiratory specimens during the time of viral shedding. The best clinical specimens are nasopharyngeal or nasal swabs or aspirates collected from acutely ill patients as close to illness

Table 34.3 Clinical Complications Associated with Influenza

Infants and Young Children
Fever without respiratory complications, "sepsis-like syndrome"
Otitis media
Bronchiolitis
Croup
Reactive airway disease
Pneumonia
Myocarditis, pericarditis
Rhabdomyolysis
Febrile seizures
Encephalopathy and encephalitis
Invasive bacterial infection (sepsis, pneumonia: MRSA, MSSA, *Streptococcus pneumoniae*, Group A *Streptococcus*, *Haemophilus influenzae*)
Reye syndrome (with aspirin use)
Sudden death (may be related to cytokine dysregulation)
Exacerbation of chronic disease

School-Age Children
Bronchitis
Sinusitis
Reactive airway disease
Pneumonia
Myocarditis, pericarditis
Myositis (bilateral gastrocnemius, soleus)
Rhabdomyolysis
Encephalopathy and encephalitis
Invasive bacterial infection (sepsis, pneumonia: MRSA, MSSA, *Streptococcus pneumoniae*, Group A *Streptococcus*, *Haemophilus influenzae*)
Reye syndrome (with aspirin use)
Toxic shock syndrome
Sudden death (may be related to cytokine dysregulation)
Exacerbation of chronic disease

Adults
Bronchitis
Sinusitis
Reactive airway disease
Pneumonia
Myocarditis, pericarditis
Myositis
Rhabdomyolysis
Invasive bacterial infection (sepsis, pneumonia: MRSA, MSSA, *Streptococcus pneumoniae*, Group A *Streptococcus*, *Haemophilus influenzae*)
Toxic shock syndrome
Exacerbation of chronic disease

Elderly Patients
Pneumonia
Invasive bacterial infection (sepsis, pneumonia: MRSA, MSSA, *Streptococcus pneumoniae*, Group A *Streptococcus*, *Haemophilus influenzae*)
Myositis
Exacerbation of chronic disease

Special Groups: Pregnant Women
Dehydration
Pneumonia
Cardiopulmonary disease

Special Groups: Immunocompromised, Immunosuppressed
Infectious and noninfectious complications associated with influenza observed in immunocompetent persons are possible

MRSA, methicillin-resistant *Staphylococcus aureus*; MSSA, methicillin-sensitive *Staphylococcus aureus*.

Table 34.4 Laboratory Tests Available for Diagnosis of Influenza

Rapid Diagnostic Test	**Enzyme immunoassay** (utilizes monoclonal antibodies against influenza viruses) or **neuraminidase detection assay** • Can yield results in 10–30 minutes • Sensitivity 50–75%, specificity 90–99% compared to RT-PCR or viral culture • Influenced by prevalence of circulating influenza viruses in the population tested (how much influenza activity is occurring) • False negative results can occur during peak influenza activity • False positive results can occur during low influenza activity
Immunofluorescence	**DFA or IFA staining** (use monoclonal antibodies against influenza viruses) • Can yield results in 2–4 hours • Requires fluorescent microscope • Moderately high sensitivity, high specificity compared to RT-PCR or viral culture • Collect nasopharyngeal and nasal specimens as close to illness onset as possible (within 4 days) • Influenced by prevalence of circulating influenza viruses in the population tested (how much influenza activity is occurring)
RT-PCR	• Can yield results in 6–8 hours or longer • Very high sensitivity and specificity
Viral Culture	**Usually considered "gold standard" influenza test** • Tissue cell culture requires 2–10 days • Shell vial cell culture requires 1–3 days

Collect nasopharyngeal and nasal swab or aspirate specimens as close to illness onset as possible (within 4 days) for all tests. Serological testing for human influenza is not recommended.
Source: Centers for Disease Control and Prevention http://www.cdc.gov/flu/professionals/labdiagnosis.htm#role.
DFA, direct fluorescent antibody; IFA, indirect fluorescent antibody.

scriptase polymerase chain reaction (RT-PCR) and viral culture may be available at some hospitals, but results will likely not be available for timely clinical management.

Rapid influenza diagnostic tests are screening tests that can yield results in less than 30 minutes and include tests that only detect influenza A, tests that detect (but do not distinguish between) influenza A and B, and tests that detect and distinguish between influenza A and B. The most important factor influencing the accuracy of rapid tests is how prevalent influenza activity is among the patient population being tested. The sensitivities of rapid influenza tests are moderate compared to viral culture. Positive test results are most likely accurate and negative results are frequently inaccurate during peak community influenza activity.

Persons who received intranasally administered live attenuated influenza virus (LAIV) vaccine can shed virus in the nasal passages for 7 days after vaccination and may test positive by rapid tests and other influenza tests if tested within 7 days of LAIV vaccination.

The peripheral white blood cell count (WBC) may reveal leukopenia and lymphopenia but may also be normal or slightly elevated. Transaminases may be mildly elevated.

onset as possible, and ideally within 4 days after fever onset. Throat and sputum specimens are more likely to yield false negative results.

Tests that are most useful for the ED setting include rapid influenza diagnostic tests and immunofluorescence (direct and indirect fluorescent antibody staining) tests. Reverse tran-

Table 34.5 Recommended Antiviral Medications for Treatment and Chemoprophylaxis of Influenza

	Adamantanes		Neuraminidase Inhibitors	
	Amantadine* (Symmetrel and generic)	**Rimantadine* (Flumadine and generic)**	**Oseltamivir* (Tamiflu)**	**Zanamivir (Relenza)**
Route	Oral	Oral	Oral	Inhalation
Activity	Influenza A	Influenza A	Influenza A and B	Influenza A and B
Treatment† (5 Days Duration)	≥1 year old 1–9 years: 5 mg/kg/day divided bid 10–64 years: 100 mg PO bid ≥65 years: ≤100 mg PO/day	≥1 year old 1–9 years: 5 mg/kg/day divided bid 10–64 years: 100 mg PO bid ≥65 years: ≤100 mg PO/day	≥1 year old ≤15 kg: 30 mg/day PO bid >15 kg–23 kg: 45 mg PO bid >23–40 kg: 60 mg PO bid >40 kg: 75 mg PO bid Adults: 75 mg PO bid	≥7 years old 10 mg (2 inhalations of 5 mg each) bid
Chemoprophylaxis†	Same as treatment dose	Same as treatment dose	Same as treatment dose, but only once daily	≥5 years; same as treatment dose, but only once daily
Primary Adverse Effects	GI and CNS effects	GI and CNS (less than amantadine)	Nausea, vomiting	Bronchospasm
Contraindications	Documented hypersensitivity; seizure disorders, psychiatric disorders, renal failure	Documented hypersensitivity; seizure disorders, psychiatric disorders, renal failure	Documented hypersensitivity	Documented hypersensitivity; underlying airway disease (asthma, COPD)

*Antiviral treatment of influenza A with amantadine or rimantadine is not recommended in the United States because of the high frequency of resistance to these drugs. Increased resistance to oseltamivir among influenza A (H1N1) viruses was reported in many countries in 2008; these viruses were susceptible to zanamivir. Reduced susceptibility or resistance to oseltamivir has been reported in previous seasons for a small number of influenza A (H1N1), (H3N2), and B viruses in Japan.
†Physicians should consult the package insert for each antiviral medication for drug interactions, contraindications, adverse events, and dosage – especially for pediatric and renal insufficiency patients.
Antiviral treatment should be initiated within 48 hours of illness onset; recommended duration of treatment is 5 days. Duration of antiviral chemoprophylaxis depends on duration of exposure to persons with influenza.
Oseltamivir dosage should be reduced for persons with creatinine clearance of 10–30 mL/min. Prescribing physicians should consult the oseltamivir package insert for guidance. Health care professional should also be contacted immediately if a patient taking oseltamivir shows any signs of unusual behavior. Neuropsychiatric reports of self-injury and delirium have been reported.
CNS, central nervous system; GI, gastrointestinal.

TREATMENT

Outpatient antiviral treatment of influenza A or influenza B with neuraminidase inhibitor drugs (oseltamivir or zanamivir) is recommended for patients with uncomplicated influenza who present within 48 hours of illness onset (Table 34.5). This treatment can decrease the signs and symptoms of influenza by approximately 1 day compared to placebo. The main adverse events are the following: Oseltamivir is associated with nausea and vomiting; zanamivir is associated with bronchospasm and is not recommended for persons with underlying airway disease. No antiviral medications are approved for treatment of influenza in children younger than 1 year old. Antiviral treatment of uncomplicated influenza can decrease the occurrence of some mild to moderate complications associated with influenza such as otitis media in children and sinusitis in adults. Otherwise, treatment of uncomplicated influenza is supportive. Antiviral treatment of influenza A with amantadine or rimantadine is not recommended in the United States because of the high frequency of resistance among A (H3N2) viruses to these drugs. In 2008, increased resistance to oseltamivir was reported for influenza A (H1N1) viruses in many countries.

Patients and their families should be cautioned about possible complications. Aspirin (salicylic acid) and salicylate-containing products are contraindicated in patients younger than 18 years because of the risk of Reye syndrome.

Treatment of mild to moderate complications can be done on an outpatient basis with good follow-up. Treatment of patients with exacerbation of underlying conditions should focus on stabilization of chronic disease because it is unknown whether antiviral treatment may be beneficial.

COMPLICATIONS AND ADMISSION CRITERIA

Minor to moderate complications of influenza may not require hospital admission, but severe complications can be potentially life-threatening and require hospitalization. Minor to moderate complications include otitis media in young children and sinusitis and bronchitis in children and adults. School-age children can experience painful bilateral myositis of the soleus and gastrocnemius muscles; associated bronchiolitis and croup in young children may require hospitalization. Severe complications include myocarditis, pneumonia (viral or secondary bacterial pneumonia), respiratory failure, encephalopathy, encephalitis, seizures, myositis with compartment syndrome, rhabdomyolysis, sepsis, toxic shock syndrome, and Reye syndrome. Fulminant illness and sudden death can occur in children and adults with influenza without co-infection and with secondary invasive bacterial infections after antecedent influenza virus infection.

Viral pneumonia is more likely to occur in elderly persons, pregnant women, and patients with chronic cardiovascular disease. Chest x-rays can reveal rapid progression from bilateral interstitial infiltrates to acute respiratory distress syndrome (ARDS). Secondary bacterial pneumonia can develop shortly after the onset of influenza illness or after uncomplicated influenza symptoms are resolving. The most common invasive bacterial pathogens associated with influenza include *Streptococcus pneumoniae*, *Staphylococcus aureus*, Group A *Streptococcus* (*S. pyogenes*), and *Haemophilus influenzae*. Fulminant progression and high fatality occurs with *Staphylococcus aureus*, especially with methicillin-resistant (MRSA) invasive infections. A less well-recognized severe complication associated with influenza is meningitis from *Neisseria meningitidis* infection.

Neurological complications of influenza are more common in children than in adults. Febrile and complex seizures may occur. Fulminant and severe influenza-associated acute encephalopathy and encephalitis (with unremarkable cerebrospinal fluid [CSF] findings) occur shortly after illness onset and can result in severe disability and death. Postinfectious encephalopathy and demyelinating syndrome can occur approximately 1–2 weeks after onset of influenza. Reye syndrome, characterized by hypoglycemia, hyperammonemia, and encephalopathy, is associated with aspirin use and may follow influenza onset by 1–2 weeks.

Other severe extrapulmonary complications of influenza include toxic shock syndrome, myocarditis, rhabdomyolysis, and pericarditis. Hypotension and hypothermia have also been reported in pediatric influenza patients with fatal outcomes. A sepsislike syndrome without respiratory findings may occur in young infants with influenza.

Exacerbation of chronic underlying diseases is common with influenza. Influenza can precipitate worsening of cardiopulmonary disease such as congestive cardiac failure and coronary artery disease, chronic obstructive pulmonary disease, and asthma. Persons with neurological diseases that limit breathing or clearance of respiratory secretions are at high risk of respiratory complications, including pneumonia.

Unstable patients should be hospitalized, including those with severe dehydration, hypotension, respiratory distress (hypoxia, hypoxemia, pneumonia), prolonged seizures, encephalopathy or encephalitis, severe myositis, rhabdomyolysis, myocarditis or pericarditis, invasive bacterial infections, sepsis, and exacerbation of underlying chronic conditions.

Special Groups

Pregnant women may experience severe dehydration and cardiopulmonary complications with influenza. Elderly persons may present with malaise and altered mental status without predominant respiratory symptoms but have high frequencies for influenza complications such as pneumonia. Elderly nursing home residents are at particularly high risk for pneumonia and death from influenza. Immunocompromised persons

Table 34.6 Infection Control Measures for Seasonal Influenza

There are several other infection control measures that are appropriate to the ED and hospital setting in order to prevent transmission of influenza infection and control outbreaks:
Surveillance (active): looking for cases of respiratory illness among patients and staff
Education: educating hospital staff about the clinical presentation of influenza, prevention / control strategies and indications for specific laboratory testing
Influenza testing: establishing a systematic plan to collect and process appropriate specimens and conduct tests
Promoting respiratory hygiene and cough etiquette: through the use of flyers, posters, accessible hand-washing sinks, abundant and strategically placed hand-sanitizer stations, maintaining 3 feet distance between people who are coughing
Encouraging adherence to **Standard and Contact Precautions:** gloves and gowns
Encouraging adherence to **Droplet Precautions:** wearing surgical mask on entering a suspect patient's room; encouraging the patient to wear a surgical mask in patient transport
Antiviral chemoprophylaxis: following recommendations to provide antivirals according to standard of care
Restrictions for ill visitors and ill health care personnel – placing patients in private rooms or cohorting similar patients suspected of influenza infection; restricting visitors and monitoring

Derived from
http://www.cdc.gov/flu/professionals/infectioncontrol/healthcarefacilities.htm;
http://www.pandemicflu.gov/plan/maskguidancehc.html

may experience a variety of infectious and noninfectious complications from influenza requiring hospitalization.

It is also important to consult with your hospital's infectious disease specialist to obtain input on management and chemoprophylaxis for influenza outbreaks.

INFECTION CONTROL

Infection control in the ED focuses on prevention of influenza among health care workers and prevention of nosocomial transmission (Table 34.6). All health care workers in the ED should receive annual influenza vaccination. Triage in the ED should rapidly separate persons with influenzalike illness from others. Patients with suspected influenza should be isolated or cohorted if possible. Strict adherence to hand washing and standard respiratory hygiene and cough protocols should be emphasized. Standard, contact, and droplet precautions should be followed for patients with suspected and confirmed influenza.

PUBLIC HEALTH AND INFLUENZA VACCINE

Annual trivalent influenza vaccination is recommended for persons at high risk for complications from influenza, for their household contacts, and for all health care providers (Table 34.7). Each year, the three influenza virus vaccine strains (influenza A [H1N1], A [H3N2], and influenza B) may be updated based on global strain surveillance data. Live attenuated influenza virus vaccine for intranasal administration is available in the United States for healthy individuals aged 2–49 years. When significant antigenic drift in circulating strains distinct from vaccine strains occurs, influenza vaccine

Table 34.7 Recommended Groups for Annual Influenza Vaccination, United States

- All children aged 6–59 months*
- Children aged 6 months to 18 years who are receiving long-term aspirin therapy
- Persons 5–49 years old with certain chronic underlying medical conditions†
- Women who will be pregnant during influenza season
- All persons aged 50 years and older
- Household contacts and caregivers of children <5 years old and persons at high risk for severe complications of influenza‡
- All health care workers

*Beginning in 2008, all children aged 6 months through 18 years are recommended to receive annual influenza vaccination in the United States.
†Chronic pulmonary (including asthma) or cardiovascular disease (excluding hypertension), persons who have required regular medical follow-up or hospitalization during the preceding year because of chronic metabolic disease (including diabetes mellitus), renal dysfunction, hemoglobinopathies, or immunodeficiency (including immunodeficiency caused by medications or HIV); persons who have any condition (e.g., cognitive dysfunction, spinal cord injuries, seizure disorders, or other neurological disorders) that can compromise respiratory function or the handling of respiratory secretions or that can increase the risk for aspiration.
‡Persons at high risk for severe complications of influenza include children aged 6–23 months, children aged 6 months to 18 years who are receiving long-term aspirin therapy; women who will be pregnant during influenza season; persons 5–49 years old with certain chronic underlying medical conditions, residents of nursing homes and other chronic-care facilities that house persons of any age who have chronic medical conditions, persons aged 65 years and older.
Source: Centers for Disease Control and Prevention (CDC). Prevention and control of influenza. Recommendations of the Advisory Committee on Immunization Practices (ACIP). MMWR 2007;56:RR-5:1–54.

effectiveness is reduced. Acute care physicians should not discount the possibility of influenza in persons who have received influenza vaccine.

PEARLS AND PITFALLS

1. Close follow-up of influenza patients who are discharged from the ED is critical. Patients and family members must be educated that complications of influenza can develop and that further medical care may be needed for worsening symptoms, especially in patients with chronic medical conditions. Although most deaths from influenza complications occur in the elderly and persons with chronic medical problems, previously well children and adults have died from fulminant influenza-associated complications.

2. Elderly patients with influenza may not have fever and can present with confusion or altered mental status without typical respiratory symptoms. Such patients can progress rapidly to viral pneumonia.

3. The best way to prevent influenza is to receive annual influenza vaccination. However, influenza vaccination is not 100% effective for multiple reasons (decreased immunogenicity in young infants and elderly persons; "antigenic drifted" strains different than vaccine strains). Do not assume that a person who received influenza vaccination cannot have influenza virus infection.

4. Health care workers can be a source of transmission of influenza viruses to coworkers and to patients. Annual influenza vaccination and adherence to infection control precautions should be emphasized regularly prior to and during seasonal epidemics.

5. To prevent Reye syndrome, avoid aspirin and salicylate-containing products in persons younger than 18 years old.

6. If invasive bacterial co-infection is suspected, empiric treatment should cover MRSA with vancomycin or linezolid until antimicrobial susceptibility data are available, especially in areas where MRSA is prevalent. Fulminant disease and rapid death after a brief influenza illness can occur with invasive MRSA infections.

7. Exacerbation of underlying chronic conditions, including cardiopulmonary diseases is common with influenza.

8. Influenza is unpredictable, and the timing, severity, distribution, and evolution of circulating virus strains are uncertain.

9. Oseltamivir treatment of hospitalized elderly patients with influenza may reduce the duration of hospitalization or mortality.

10. Physicians should check the latest information about influenza vaccination, antiviral treatment, and antiviral resistance issued by medical and public health organizations (e.g., websites of the Centers for Disease Control and Prevention, World Health Organization, and European Centre for Disease Prevention and Control).

REFERENCES

Babcock HM, Merz LR, Fraser VJ. Is influenza an influenza-like illness? Clinical presentation of influenza in hospitalized patients. Infect Control Hosp Epidemiol 2006;27:266–70.

Brankston G, Gitterman L, Hirji Z, et al. Transmission of influenza A in human beings. Lancet Infect Dis 2007;7:257–65.

Bridges CB, Kuehnert MJ, Hall CB. Transmission of influenza: implications for control in health care settings. Clin Infect Dis 2003;37:1094–101.

Call SA, Vollenweider MA, Hornung CA, et al. Does this patient have influenza? JAMA 2005;293:987–97.

Centers for Disease Control (CDC). Prevention and control of influenza: recommendations of the Advisory Committee on Immunization Practices (ACIP). MMWR 2007;56(RR-5):1–54.

De Clercq E. Antiviral agents active against influenza A viruses. Nat Rev Drug Discov 2006 Dec;5(12):1015–25.

Monto AS, Gravenstein S, Elliott M, et al. Clinical signs and symptoms predicting influenza infection. Arch Int Med 2000;160:3243–7.

Nicholson K, Wood J, Zambon M. Influenza. Lancet 2003;362:1733–45.

Poehling KA, Edwards KM, Weinberg GA, et al. The under-recognized burden of influenza in young children. N Engl J Med 2006 Jul 6;355(1):31–40.

Thompson WW, Shay DK, Weintraub E, et al. Influenza-associated hospitalizations in the United States. JAMA 2004;292:1333–40.

ADDITIONAL READINGS

American College of Emergency Medicine (ACEM). Emergency department utilization during outbreaks of influenza. Ann Emerg Med 2005;45:686.

Bonner BB, Monroe KW, Talley LI, et al. Impact of the rapid diagnosis of influenza on physician decision-making and patient management in the pediatric emergency department: results of a randomized, prospective, controlled trial. Pediatrics 2003;112;363–7.

Bourgeois FT, Valim C, Wei JC, et al. Influenza and other respiratory virus–related emergency department visits among young children. Pediatrics 2006;118;1–8.

Monmany J, Rabella N, Margall N, et al. Unmasking influenza virus infection in patients attended to in the emergency department. Infection 2004;32: 89–97.

Ploin D, Gillet Y, Morfin F, et al. Influenza burden in febrile infants and young children in a pediatric emergency department. Pediatr Infect Dis J 2007;26:142–7.

35. HIV-Associated Respiratory Infections

Matthew Fei and Laurence Huang

INTRODUCTION

Shortness of breath is a common presenting complaint in human immunodeficiency virus (HIV)–infected patients, and the relevant differential diagnosis is broad. Etiologies include both infectious and noninfectious causes related and unrelated to underlying HIV infection and range from the minor (e.g., viral upper respiratory infection) to the life-threatening (e.g., *Pneumocystis* pneumonia [PCP]). Although the list of potential diseases may seem overwhelming, an understanding of the most commonly encountered pulmonary complications and their characteristic presentations will help narrow the differential diagnosis.

EPIDEMIOLOGY

The rate of bacterial pneumonia is between 5- and 25-fold higher in HIV-infected patients than in the non-HIV infected population. Although its prevalence has declined after the introduction of highly active anti-retroviral therapy (HAART), PCP is still a common acquired immunodeficiency syndrome (AIDS)-defining illness and is seen almost exclusively in immunocompromised persons. Globally, *Mycobacterium tuberculosis* (TB) pneumonia is the major pulmonary infection complicating the HIV epidemic. HIV-infected patients who have latent TB infection face a 10% *annual* risk of progressing from latent to active tuberculous disease compared to an approximately 10% *lifetime* risk in non-HIV-infected individuals. (See Chapter 33, Tuberculosis.)

CLINICAL FEATURES

The clinical presentations of common HIV-associated pulmonary infections often overlap. The goal of a thorough history and physical is to narrow the differential diagnosis, recognize constellations of particular symptoms and signs, and guide diagnostic testing and therapy.

All of the HIV-associated pulmonary diseases can present with cough, shortness of breath, and decreased exercise tolerance, though there are some characteristic presentations that

may point to a particular diagnosis (Table 35.1). Purulent sputum is typically associated with bacterial pneumonia, whereas a dry, nonproductive cough is typically associated with PCP. The duration of symptoms can also be useful in differentiating between infections. Bacterial pneumonia characteristically presents with an acute onset over 3 to 5 days, whereas PCP and TB present with a more indolent course over weeks to occasionally months. Although patients with any pulmonary infection may complain of pleuritic chest pain, persistent and severe pleuritic pain should raise the suspicion for a pneumothorax, particularly in patients with cysts and pneumatoceles secondary to PCP.

The presence of extrapulmonary symptoms must also be noted, because these may be related to a primary pulmonary infection and suggest a unifying diagnosis. A chronic history of constitutional symptoms such as night sweats and weight loss is common with TB infection. Lymphadenopathy, abdominal complaints, and organomegaly suggest infiltrative, granulomatous infection such as TB, nontuberculous mycobacteria, or endemic fungal disease. New-onset confusion, headache, or focal neurologic findings may indicate both neurologic and pulmonary involvement by *Cryptococcus neoformans* or *Toxoplasma gondii*. Visual complaints and odynophagia may herald concurrent cytomegalovirus (CMV) retinitis, esophagitis, and pneumonitis. In these settings, biopsy of a peripheral lymph node, lumbar puncture, or dilated funduscopic examination may yield the correct diagnosis.

Finally, it must be emphasized that more than one infectious agent may present concurrently in HIV-infected patients. Some patients will have characteristics of dual respiratory infection with symptoms suggestive of both a bacterial process and PCP or TB. For example, a patient who develops a cough productive of purulent sputum over several days may also complain of several weeks of fevers and dyspnea. Such a patient may have bacterial pneumonia superimposed on PCP. In these cases of suspected dual infection, empiric treatment for both processes is appropriate pending etiologic testing.

A thorough physical examination with emphasis on cardiopulmonary findings will help narrow the differential diagnosis for an HIV-infected patient with respiratory symptoms.

Table 35.1 Clinical Features: HIV-Associated Pulmonary Infections

Clinical Features	Bacterial Pneumonia	*Pneumocystis* Pneumonia	Tuberculosis
Organisms	• *Streptococcus pneumoniae* • *Haemophilus* species • Gram negatives and anaerobes (predisposing factors: alcohol use, aspiration)	• *Pneumocystis jirovecii*	• *Mycobacterium tuberculosis*
Signs and Symptoms	• Cough with purulent sputum • Fever, chills, rigors • Acute onset, symptoms <1 week	• Nonproductive cough • Dyspnea • Fever • Gradual onset, symptoms >1 week	• Cough • Fever, night sweats • Weight loss • Gradual onset, symptoms >2 weeks • Lymphadenopathy
Laboratory and Radiographic Tests	• Any CD4+ cell count • Elevated WBC • Chest radiograph: focal alveolar consolidation, with or without associated pleural effusion	• CD4+ cell count: <200 cells/μL • Elevated serum LDH • Chest radiograph: interstitial or granular pattern • HRCT: ground glass opacities	• Any CD4+ cell count • Chest radiograph: alveolar pattern (often with cavitation), miliary pattern, nodules, intrathoracic adenopathy, pleural effusion

HRCT, high-resolution computed tomography; LDH, lactate dehydrogenase; WBC, white blood (cell) count.

Patients with HIV-associated pulmonary infections are typically febrile, tachycardic, and tachypneic. A decreased oxygen saturation is often noted and is a common and appropriate indication for admission. If outpatient follow-up is being considered, postambulation pulse oximetry should be checked, because some patients will manifest hypoxia only after exertion.

Patients with bacterial pneumonia will often have a focal lung examination suggestive of lobar consolidation with or without an accompanying pleural effusion. In contrast, patients with PCP may have diffuse and nonspecific findings, such as bilateral rales. Of note, it is common for patients with PCP to have a normal lung examination. The presence of diffuse wheezes can suggest an exacerbation of asthma, whereas decreased breath sounds may indicate chronic obstructive pulmonary disease (COPD). The unilateral absence of breath sounds may suggest a pneumothorax in a patient complaining of pleuritic chest pain.

The remainder of the physical examination can be helpful in assessing a patient's underlying immune status as well as the etiology of his or her respiratory symptoms. PCP, bacterial pneumonia, and TB are often the HIV-identifying illnesses in patients who are unaware of their HIV infection, and a history of potential HIV risk factors (men who have sex with men, injection drug use [IDU], or heterosexual sex for drugs or with sex workers) may help guide diagnosis. Lymphadenopathy may suggest disseminated mycobacterial or fungal disease, whereas skin and oropharyngeal examinations may reveal lesions consistent with Kaposi's sarcoma (KS) or fungal disease.

LABORATORY AND RADIOGRAPHIC FINDINGS

The CD4+ cell count is essential in formulating a differential diagnosis in HIV-infected patients with respiratory symptoms. In cases where the patient is unaware of a recent CD4+ cell count, the total lymphocyte count can be obtained rapidly and serve as a surrogate marker, helping to estimate the degree of immune suppression. It is important to note that acute illness can suppress the CD4+ cell count below the true

Table 35.2 Standard Acute Care Evaluation for HIV-infected Patients with Suspected Pulmonary Infection

All Patients:
• CD4+ cell count (if unknown or last value >6 months ago)
• Complete blood count with differential and metabolic panel
• Chest radiograph (PA and lateral)
• Electrocardiogram

Selected Patients:
• Room-air arterial blood gas (if patient has mild to moderate respiratory compromise or if PCP is suspected)
• Serum LDH (if PCP is suspected)
• Sputum Gram stain and culture (if bacterial pneumonia is suspected)
• Blood cultures (two sets prior to antibiotic administration if bacterial pneumonia is suspected)
• Serum cryptococcal antigen (if CD4+ cell count <200 cells/μL)

PA, posteroanterior.

baseline value, and a repeat CD4+ cell count after resolution of the acute illness may be indicated.

A room-air arterial blood gas (ABG) should be drawn in any patient with mild to moderate respiratory compromise or suspected PCP. A PaO_2 less than 70 mm Hg or an alveolar-arterial oxygen gradient greater than 35 mm Hg is an indication for adjunctive corticosteroid treatment in PCP. Serum lactate dehydrogenase (LDH) is another laboratory test that has prognostic import in PCP. LDH is frequently, but not invariably, elevated in patients infected with PCP, and the degree of elevation correlates with prognosis. Serial LDH values can help assess severity and progression of illness. In addition to these and other more common laboratory tests (e.g., complete blood count and metabolic panels), an electrocardiogram should be obtained to evaluate for cardiac disease as a potential etiology of respiratory symptoms (Table 35.2).

All HIV-infected patients who present with suspected pulmonary infections should have two sets of blood cultures drawn prior to the initiation of antibiotic therapy. As in non-HIV infected patients, *Streptococcus pneumoniae* is the most common cause of bacterial pneumonia in HIV-infected patients, and bacteremia is more frequent in patients

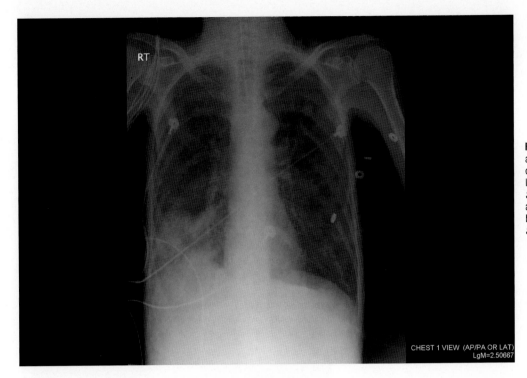

Figure 35.1 Chest radiograph of an HIV-infected patient, CD4+ cell count less than 200 cells/μL, with lobar consolidation from *S. pneumoniae*. This patient was also found to have *S. pneumoniae* bacteremia, meningitis, and *Staphylococcus aureus* bacteremia.

with lower CD4+ cell counts. Positive blood cultures with subsequent antibiotic susceptibility testing will help guide appropriate antimicrobial therapy. In addition, HIV-infected patients may have more than one concomitant bacterial process, given their immunosuppression and high rates of other infection risk factors (e.g., IDU).

If a bacterial respiratory infection is suspected, a sputum sample should be sent from the emergency department (ED) for Gram stain and culture. Prior antibiotic administration can decrease the sensitivity of sputum culture, but the Gram stain may still yield useful information. Although the sensitivity of a sputum culture for bacterial pneumonia is low (~40%), isolating a pathogen from sputum can help guide therapy.

In addition to bacterial Gram stain and culture, the sputum should be sent for PCP and acid-fast bacilli (AFB) in the proper clinical scenarios. Most patients with PCP alone (without a superimposed bacterial pneumonia) will have a nonproductive cough and are unable to produce a spontaneously expectorated sputum sample. In these cases, sputum induction using nebulized hypertonic saline should be performed. Sputum induction has a sensitivity of 60–92% for PCP. In patients suspected of having TB, spontaneously expectorated or induced sputum should be collected daily for 3 consecutive days while the patient is in respiratory isolation. The sensitivity of sputum AFB smears for *M. tuberculosis* ranges from 50% to 60% and can approach 90% in those with disseminated disease. Three negative AFB smears do not rule out active TB, but the likelihood of airborne transmission to other patients and health care providers is significantly decreased. Therefore, after three negative sputums (sampled 8 hours apart and including at least one early morning specimen), these patients can be removed from respiratory isolation while awaiting the results of AFB culture.

There are limitations to the diagnosis of pulmonary infection by sputum studies. Patients who have been recently diagnosed with PCP and have undergone a complete course of

treatment may continue to have positive sputum stains for PCP despite resolution of infection. This can make the diagnosis of recurrent respiratory complaints problematic, as sputum studies may not help distinguish between inadequately treated PCP and a new infectious process. A positive sputum AFB smear is not synonymous with *M. tuberculosis* and can be due to colonization or infection by nontuberculous mycobacteria such as *Mycobacterium avium* complex (MAC). Nevertheless, any positive AFB smear must be treated as if it represents *M. tuberculosis* until a definitive diagnosis is made.

Chest Radiograph

Although there are characteristic chest radiograph findings for the common HIV-associated pulmonary infections, overlap does occur between different disease processes. A basic interpretation of the chest radiograph can be accomplished in the acute care setting by assessing the following:

- pattern of disease (e.g., alveolar, interstitial, nodular)
- distribution of disease (e.g., unilateral or bilateral, focal or diffuse)
- associated findings (e.g., pleural effusion, mediastinal or hilar adenopathy, pneumatocele, or cavitation)

Because HIV-infected patients may present with multiple respiratory infections over time and may have residual radiographic findings, it is critical to compare the current radiograph against prior radiographs, especially the most recent ones.

Bacterial pneumonia is the most common pulmonary infection in HIV-infected patients in the United States. Characteristic findings are similar to those in the HIV-uninfected population, with focal, lobar, or segmental alveolar infiltrates predominating (Figure 35.1). In contrast, *Haemophilus influenzae* pneumonia seems to have a higher likelihood of presenting with an interstitial pattern that mimics PCP.

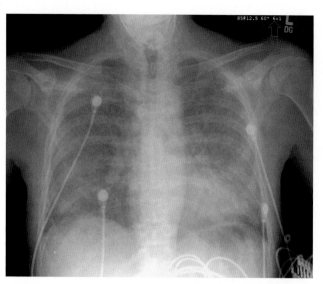

Figure 35.2 Chest radiograph of an HIV-infected patient, CD4+ cell count less than 200 cells/μL, demonstrating the bilateral, reticular pattern characteristic of PCP.

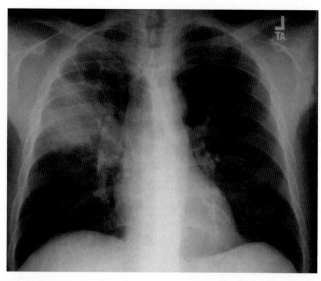

Figure 35.3 Chest radiograph of an HIV-infected patient, CD4+ cell count greater than 200 cells/μL, revealing right upper lobe infiltrate with areas of cavitation. Sputum AFB stain was positive and multiple sputum AFB cultures grew *Mycobacterium tuberculosis*. Courtesy of Dr. L. Huang.

The characteristic radiograph in PCP typically shows bilateral, diffuse interstitial, reticular, or granular opacities (Figure 35.2). The findings can be unilateral or asymmetric. Patients with PCP present with pneumatoceles in 10–20% of cases or can develop them as treatment progresses. Pneumatoceles will vary in number and size and place the patient at increased risk for pneumothorax. A normal chest radiograph or one with focal lobar consolidation does not rule out PCP. In fact, PCP should be high on the differential diagnosis in an HIV-infected patient with a CD4+ cell count less than 200 cells/μL and hypoxemia with a normal chest radiograph. In addition, an apical pattern mimicking TB can be seen in PCP, classically in patients on aerosolized pentamidine prophylaxis. However, intrathoracic adenopathy and pleural effusions are rare in PCP, and these findings should prompt a search and treatment for an alternate (or coexisting) process.

Like PCP, *M. tuberculosis* can present with a variety of radiographic findings including a normal chest radiograph. The specific pattern seen often correlates with the patient's degree of immune suppression, so knowledge of the most recent CD4+ cell count is helpful. TB developing early in the course of HIV infection (i.e., with high CD4+ count) typically presents with a pattern of classic reactivation disease, with cavitary infiltrates in the upper lung zones (Figure 35.3). TB developing in the later stages of HIV infection (i.e., with low CD4+ count) often presents with middle and lower lung zone infiltrates mimicking a bacterial pneumonia and less frequently presents with cavitation (Figure 35.4).

Chest computed tomography (CT) can be very useful in the diagnosis of suspected PCP when the plain radiograph is normal or unchanged. In this setting, high-resolution CT is a sensitive diagnostic study for PCP. Patients with PCP and a normal chest radiograph will usually have patchy areas of ground-glass opacity on high-resolution CT (Figure 35.5). Although the presence of ground-glass opacity is nonspecific, its absence strongly argues against a diagnosis of PCP.

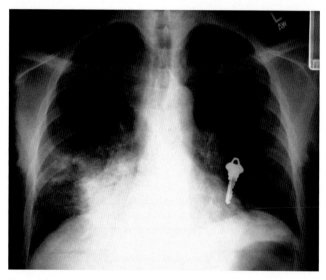

Figure 35.4 Chest radiograph of an HIV-infected patient, CD4+ cell count less than 200 cells/μL, revealing right lower lung consolidation with air bronchograms. Sputum AFB cultures grew *Mycobacterium tuberculosis* that was mono-rifampin resistant. In this case, the key to the diagnosis of TB was knowledge of the patient's CD4+ cell count and an understanding that TB can present in this manner in such an individual. Courtesy of Dr. L. Huang.

DIFFERENTIAL DIAGNOSIS

When evaluating HIV-infected patients with respiratory symptoms, one must consider both infectious and noninfectious causes of cough, dyspnea, and hypoxia. Exacerbations of underlying asthma or COPD are common. HIV can be a cause of cardiac dysfunction, and HIV-associated cardiomyopathy or pulmonary arterial hypertension are important diagnoses to consider in a patient with suggestive findings on examination (e.g., elevated jugular venous pressure and rales) and chest radiography (e.g., cardiomegaly and pulmonary edema).

The distinction between infectious and noninfectious causes of pulmonary disease in HIV-infected patients usually

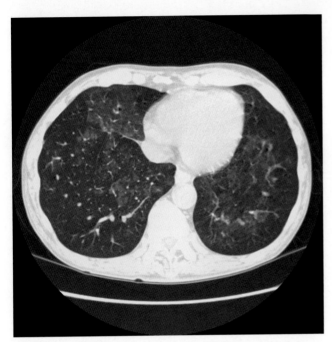

Table 35.3 Differential Diagnosis of Respiratory Infections in HIV and AIDS

Any CD4+ Cell Count	• Bacterial pneumonia (most commonly *S. pneumoniae* or *H. influenzae*) • *M. tuberculosis* pneumonia (TB)
CD4+ <200 Cells/μL	• *Pneumocystis* pneumonia (PCP) • *Cryptococcus neoformans* pneumonia • Bacterial pneumonia complicated by bacteremia • Extrapulmonary or disseminated TB
CD4+ <100 Cells/μL	• *Pseudomonas aeruginosa* pneumonia • *Toxoplasma gondii* pneumonia • Pulmonary Kaposi's sarcoma
CD4+ <50 Cells/μL	• *Histoplasma capsulatum* or *Coccidioides immitis* pneumonia, usually associated with disseminated disease • Cytomegalovirus pneumonia, usually associated with disseminated disease • *Mycobacterium avium* complex pneumonia, usually associated with disseminated disease • *Aspergillus* species pneumonia

Figure 35.5 Chest CT scan of an HIV-infected patient, CD4+ cell count less than 200 cells/μL with ground glass opacities characteristic of PCP.

becomes evident after a thorough history, physical examination, and basic diagnostic tests. Distinguishing among infectious causes can present a greater challenge, as patients with common and uncommon pulmonary infections may complain of fever, cough (with or without purulent sputum), dyspnea, night sweats, fatigue, decreased exercise tolerance, and weight loss of varying duration. The most common causes of pulmonary infection necessitating an ED visit and admission in HIV-infected patients are bacterial pneumonia followed by PCP, both of which are significantly more common than the next most common diagnoses: TB, pulmonary KS (associated with human herpes virus-8 [HHV-8]), and various fungal infections.

A patient's social and travel history also affect the likelihood of a particular etiology. The probability of presenting with certain fungal pneumonias is increased by living in or traveling to endemic areas. Other respiratory diseases can be associated with mode of HIV transmission. KS is almost exclusively seen in men who have sex with men. Primary or reactivation *M. tuberculosis* infection is associated with homelessness, incarceration, recent immigration from an endemic country, and recent conversion to a positive tuberculin skin test, defined as induration of 5 mm or greater in HIV-infected persons. Injection drug users have a higher rate of bacterial pneumonia and TB than do persons with no history of injection drug use.

CD4+ Cell Count

An essential component in formulating a differential diagnosis is the patient's most recent CD4+ cell count (Table 35.3) and their history of prior opportunistic infections (OIs). Equally important to narrowing the differential diagnosis is the patient's medication history, including HAART and OI prophylaxis.

Some pulmonary infections, such as bacterial pneumonia and TB, can occur at any CD4+ count, but both are more frequent and have an increasing complication rate as the CD4+ cell count declines. At lower CD4+ cell counts, bacterial pneumonia is increasingly complicated by bacteremia, and TB is often disseminated. At a CD4+ cell count less than 200 cells/μL, PCP and cryptococcal pneumonia enter the differential diagnosis, whereas neither is commonly seen at higher counts. At a CD4+ cell count less than 100 cells/μL, pulmonary KS, *Toxoplasma gondii*, and *Pseudomonas aeruginosa* pneumonias can be seen. As the CD4+ cell count drops below 50 cells/μL, the endemic fungi (*Histoplasma capsulatum*, *Coccidioides immitis*), *Aspergillus* species, CMV, and nontuberculous mycobacteria become considerations. All CD4+ cell count cutoffs should serve as a general guideline, because exceptions can occur.

Unfortunately, patients presenting to the acute care setting may not have had a recent CD4+ cell count. Besides using the total lymphocyte count as a rough indicator of T-cell levels, the acute care physician should look for surrogate clinical markers of suppressed immune function. For example, oropharyngeal thrush (candidiasis) may be an indication of underlying immunocompromise, and a history of thrush increases the risk of subsequent PCP.

Prior Respiratory Illness and Use of Opportunistic Infection Prophylaxis

Many of the HIV-associated OIs recur. Recurrent bacterial pneumonia (i.e., two or more episodes in a 12-month period) was added to the list of AIDS-defining illnesses in the 1993 U.S. Centers for Disease Control and Prevention Expanded Surveillance Case Definition for AIDS. Patients with a history of PCP and fungal infections (cryptococcosis, coccidioidomycosis, and histoplasmosis) are also at high risk for recurrent illness, especially if they fail to take secondary prophylaxis or maintenance therapy. The high likelihood of relapse makes a careful infection history crucial to the evaluation of pulmonary complaints in the HIV-infected patient.

HIV-infected patients, especially those with the lowest CD4+ cell counts, may develop an OI despite the use of antimicrobial prophylaxis. CD4+ cell counts and adherence to OI prophylaxis should serve only as a general guide as to which pulmonary infections are most likely to occur in a patient.

Key features that may help distinguish PCP from bacterial pneumonia are:

- chest radiograph with diffuse interstitial or granular pattern
- nonproductive cough
- gradual onset and slow evolution of symptoms
- pronounced dyspnea and hypoxemia
- CD4+ cell count less than 200 cells/μL and no PCP prophylaxis

Key features that may help distinguish *M. tuberculosis* are:

- gradual onset of fevers, night sweats, weight loss
- systemic lymphadenopathy
- chest radiograph with upper lung zone infiltrate, cavitary or miliary pattern
- history of positive tuberculin skin test (PPD)

TREATMENT

The symptoms, physical findings, and radiographic imaging of the most common HIV-associated pulmonary infections are nonspecific and can often overlap. Therefore, it is very common for medical providers to begin empiric therapy for a suspected pulmonary infection before a definitive diagnosis has been made. Empiric therapy is entirely appropriate, provided that studies for definitive diagnosis have been initiated.

Determining appropriate initial treatment depends on the pretest probabilities of various diseases, based on the patient's history, physical examination, CD4+ cell count, and imaging studies. Because the most common causes of HIV-associated pulmonary infection are bacterial pneumonia and PCP, empiric therapy for one or both is often implemented. A typical patient with bacterial pneumonia may present with CD4+ cell count greater than 200 cells/μL, a chest radiograph with a noncavitating focal, segmental or lobar infiltrate, and a history of 3 to 5 days of fevers, rigors, and cough productive of purulent sputum. Other suggestive factors include focal findings on lung examination, leukocytosis, and a history of cigarette smoking, IDU, or prior bacterial pneumonia. Given this constellation of findings, the pretest probability of bacterial pneumonia is significantly higher than that of PCP or TB, and empiric therapy for bacterial pneumonia alone would be appropriate pending further diagnostic testing (Tables 35.4 and 35.5).

The ATS and IDSA consensus guidelines for management of community-acquired pneumonia make antimicrobial therapy recommendations for patients with bacterial pneumonia and can be used as a guide for HIV-infected patients as well. In general, a hospitalized patient with mild to moderate respiratory compromise should be treated with an extended-spectrum cephalosporin (ceftriaxone or cefotaxime) and a macrolide or doxycyline, or an antipneumococcal fluoroquinolone. For patients with severe respiratory

Table 35.4 Management of Respiratory Infection in Patients with HIV/AIDS and CD4+ Cell Count (Known or Suspected) Less Than 200 cells/μL

Acute Symptoms (<1 Week)	
Normal CXR	• Symptomatic treatment for URI • Arrange follow-up with primary provider • If symptoms persist or progress, consider repeat chest radiograph or high resolution CT to evaluate for PCP
Abnormal CXR	• Bacterial pneumonia > PCP, TB • Consider admission for bacterial pneumonia treatment and further evaluation for PCP or TB if risk factors present (e.g., prior PCP, homeless) or mixed clinical picture (e.g., nonproductive cough, severe dyspnea that are more suggestive of PCP)
Chronic Symptoms (>1 Week)	
Normal CXR or Interstitial Infiltrate	**Nonproductive cough:** • PCP > bacterial pneumonia, TB • Evaluate for PCP (and possibly TB) with induced sputum, bronchoscopy • Empiric treatment for PCP while awaiting diagnostic testing **Productive cough:** • Mixed clinical picture: consider empiric treatment for both bacterial pneumonia and PCP while awaiting further diagnostic testing
Alveolar Infiltrate	**Nonproductive cough:** • Mixed clinical picture: consider empiric treatment for both bacterial pneumonia and PCP while awaiting further diagnostic testing **Productive cough:** • Bacterial pneumonia > PCP or TB • Consider treatment with antibiotics for bacterial pneumonia and further evaluation for PCP and TB

CXR, chest x-ray; URI, upper respiratory infection.

compromise or patients requiring intensive care unit (ICU) admission, combination therapy with an extended-spectrum cephalosporin and either a macrolide (e.g., azithromycin) or fluoroquinolone should be instituted, with a goal of providing optimal therapy for the two most commonly identified causes of lethal pneumonia (*S. pneumoniae* and *Legionella* species). These recommendations should be tailored to local resistance patterns, when this information is available.

In cases where the clinical scenario suggests a bacterial pneumonia but TB is still on the differential, multiple guidelines recommend avoiding the use of fluoroquinolones until TB has been ruled either in or out. In published studies of multidrug-resistant TB, defined as infection with an organism resistant to isoniazid and rifampin, concomitant HIV infection is seen in disproportionate numbers. In patients with multidrug-resistant TB, fluoroquinolones are a mainstay of therapy, and all efforts must be made to prevent the development of fluoroquinolone resistance.

As the CD4+ cell count declines, the number of possible diagnoses increases, though bacterial pneumonia and PCP still remain the two most common etiologies. Even in a

Table 35.5 Treatment of Common HIV-Related Pulmonary Infections

Infection	Preferred Therapy	Alternative Therapies and Other Issues
Pneumocystis jirovecii pneumonia (PCP)	1. TMP/SMX: 15–20 mg TMP/kg body weight daily IV divided q6–8h *or* 2. same daily dose of TMP/SMX (based on TMP) PO divided q8h *or* 3. TMP/SMX DS 2 tablets PO q8h Total duration 21 days *and* prednisone 40 mg bid days 1–5, 40 mg daily days 6–10, then 20 mg daily days 11–21, if PaO$_2$ <70 mm Hg at room air or alveolar-arterial O$_2$ gradient >35 mm Hg	1. primaquine 15–30 mg (base) PO daily and clindamycin 600–900 mg IV q6–8h or clindamycin 300–450 mg PO q6–8h *or* 2. dapsone 100 mg PO daily and TMP 5 mg/kg PO q8h *or* 3. atovaquone 750 mg PO bid *or* 4. pentamidine 3–4 mg/kg IV daily
Mycobacterium tuberculosis pneumonia	INH 5 mg/kg (max: 300 mg) PO daily and rifampin 10 mg/kg (max: 600 mg) PO daily and PZA and EMB; PZA and EMB dose based on weight*	Urgent initiation of TB therapy in the ED is rarely necessary Consultation with infectious disease specialist or pharmacist recommended because of multiple drug interactions between TB therapy and HAART
Bacterial pneumonia	Empiric therapy targeting *Streptococcus pneumoniae* and *Haemophilus influenzae* Mild to moderate disease: 1. second- or third-generation cephalosporin plus macrolide or doxycycline *or* 2. antipneumococcal respiratory fluoroquinolone alone Severe disease: 1. second- or third-generation cephalosporin plus macrolide or antipneumococcal respiratory fluoro-quinolone	Minimize use of fluoroquinolones unless there is no suspicion of TB; quinolones should be reserved for treatment of drug-resistant TB and in TB patients with liver disease

*Pyrazinamide dose: <55 kg, 1000 mg; 56–75 kg, 1500 mg; >75 kg, 2000 mg; ethambutol dose: <55 kg, 800 mg; 56–75 kg, 1200 mg; >75 kg, 1600 mg.
DS, double strength; EMB, ethambutol; HAART, highly active antiretroviral therapy; INH, isoniazid; PZA, pyrazinamide; SMX, sulfamethoxazole; TMP, trimethoprim.

Table 35.6 Indications for Admission for HIV-Infected Patients with Suspected Pulmonary Infection

High Risk for Clinical Deterioration	• Tachypnea with respiratory rate >25 breaths per minute • Hypotension with systolic blood pressure persistently <90 mm Hg after initial fluid resuscitation • Hypoxia with decreased PaO$_2$, elevated alveolar-arterial oxygen gradient, or requiring supplemental oxygen • Decreased exercise tolerance with limited ability to perform independent daily activities • General ill appearance • Coexisting medical or psychiatric disease that potentially increases severity of pulmonary infection or decreases likelihood of outpatient treatment adherence • Marginal social situation (e.g., homeless, substance abuser)
Potential for Infection Transmission	• Any patient with suspected active tuberculosis and with risk of transmission to other individuals at place of residence
Other	• Inability to provide appropriate follow-up (e.g., no primary care provider) • Inability to schedule necessary diagnostic testing (e.g., sputum induction, bronchoscopy)

cough, PCP is the most likely diagnosis. Empiric therapy with trimethoprim-sulfamethoxazole and corticosteroids (for PaO$_2$ less than 70 mm Hg on room air or alveolar-arterial oxygen gradient greater than 35 mm Hg) should be initiated while arranging for sputum induction or bronchoscopy to diagnose PCP. In reality, it is quite common for patients to present with features of both a bacterial pneumonia and PCP (e.g., subacute onset of fevers, but cough productive of purulent sputum). Therefore, it is reasonable to begin empiric therapy for both bacterial pneumonia and PCP while awaiting further testing to arrive at a definitive diagnosis.

ADMISSION CRITERIA

A patient who has an established primary care physician, a CD4+ cell count significantly greater than 200 cells/μL, and normal pulse oximetry after ambulation and who is suspected to have bacterial pneumonia by history and radiographic imaging could potentially be discharged home on appropriate empiric antibiotic therapy with close follow-up.

However, all patients with CD4+ cell count less than 200 cells/μL and a history or imaging studies suspicious for PCP or TB should be admitted for diagnostic work-up, unless outpatient diagnostic testing (sputum induction and potentially bronchoalveolar lavage) can be arranged in an expedited manner. Discharging a patient on empiric therapy for a presumed diagnosis of PCP without any plans to establish a definitive microbiologic diagnosis is seldom justified (Table 35.6).

ISOLATION AND INFECTION CONTROL

The transmission of infectious respiratory disease such as *M. tuberculosis* between HIV-infected patients and to health care workers (HCWs) in the hospital is a significant concern. An active cough, as well as certain medical

patient with a CD4+ cell count less than 200 cells/μL, if the chest radiograph shows a focal alveolar infiltrate and other findings are consistent with bacterial pneumonia, empiric treatment for common bacterial pathogens alone is reasonable. If the chest radiograph reveals bilateral interstitial, reticular, or granular opacities, the LDH is elevated, and the patient describes a subacute onset of fevers, dyspnea, and dry procedures (e.g., endotracheal intubation, sputum induction, and bronchoscopy) increases the burden of airborne bacilli and thus infectious risk. As we have described, the clinical and radiographic presentations of pulmonary TB in the setting of HIV infection are myriad. The acute care clinician must assess all HIV-infected patients with respiratory symptoms for the possibility of active pulmonary TB. All suspected cases of TB must be placed in respiratory isolation (preferably negative pressure respiratory isolation). Appropriate precautions, such as use of N-95 face masks, should be implemented by hospital staff in contact with suspected cases of TB until three separate sputum specimens have been examined and are negative for AFB. Given the myriad radiographic and clinical presentations of tuberculosis in HIV-infected patients, the acute care physician must have a low threshold for placing suspected patients in respiratory isolation.

PEARLS AND PITFALLS

1. When evaluating a patient with HIV and respiratory symptoms, the differential diagnosis is broad and includes both infectious and noninfectious causes that can be related or unrelated to underlying HIV infection.
2. A patient's CD4+ cell count, history of prior OI, and adherence to HAART and OI prophylaxis are essential in helping to narrow the differential diagnosis for HIV-associated pulmonary infections.
3. *M. tuberculosis* and bacterial pneumonia can occur with any CD4+ cell count.
4. The two most common HIV-associated pulmonary infections are bacterial pneumonia and PCP.
5. The classic chest radiograph for PCP is a diffuse, bilateral interstitial infiltrate. However, *Pneumocystis* can also manifest as a focal airspace opacity or a normal chest radiograph.
6. When considering criteria for admission, the acute care physician must remember that establishing a definitive diagnosis is preferable to empiric outpatient therapy for most HIV-associated pulmonary infections, given the likelihood for rapid respiratory decompensation in this patient population.
7. Fever, hypoxemia, dry cough, and a normal chest x-ray in a patient with CD4+ cell count below 200 cells/μL is highly suggestive of PCP. Further evaluation is recommended with HRCT, sputum induction, or bronchoscopy.
8. Indolent fevers, night sweats, and weight loss in a patient with either diffuse lymphadenopathy or a cavitary or miliary pattern on chest x-ray is highly suggestive of infection with TB or endemic fungal disease.

REFERENCES

American Thoracic Society and the Centers for Disease Control and Prevention. Targeted tuberculin testing and treatment of latent tuberculosis infection. Am J Respir Crit Care Med 2000;161(4 Pt 2):S221–47.

Blumberg HM, Burman WJ, Chaisson RE, et al. American Thoracic Society/Centers for Disease Control and Prevention/Infectious Diseases Society of America: Treatment of tuberculosis. Am J Respir Crit Care Med 2003;167:603–62.

Centers for Disease Control and Prevention (CDC). 1993 revised classification system for HIV infection and expanded surveillance case definition for AIDS among adolescents and adults. JAMA 1993;269(6):729–30.

Centers for Disease Control and Prevention (CDC). Treating opportunistic infections among HIV-infected adults and adolescents: recommendations from CDC, the National Institutes of Health, and the HIV Medicine Association/Infectious Diseases Society of America. MMWR 2004;53(No. RR-15).

Feikin D, Feldman C, Schuchat A, Janoff E. Global strategies to prevent bacterial pneumonia in adults with HIV disease. Lancet Infect Dis 2004;4:445–55.

Greenberg SD, Frager D, Suster B, et al. Active pulmonary tuberculosis in patients with AIDS: spectrum of radiographic findings (including a normal appearance). Radiology 1994;193(1):115–9.

Gruden JF, Huang L, Turner J, et al. High-resolution CT in the evaluation of clinically suspected *Pneumocystis carinii* pneumonia in AIDS patients with normal, equivocal, or nonspecific radiographic findings. AJR Am J Roentgenol 1997;169(4):967–75.

Hirschtick RE, Glassroth J, Jordan MC, et al. Bacterial pneumonia in persons infected with the human immunodeficiency virus. Pulmonary Complications of HIV Infection Study Group. N Engl J Med 1995;333(13):845–51.

Huang L, Schnapp LM, Gruden JF, et al. Presentation of AIDS-related pulmonary Kaposi's sarcoma diagnosed by bronchoscopy. Am J Respir Crit Care Med 1996;153(4 Pt 1):1385–90.

Huang L, Stansell JD. AIDS and the lung. Med Clin North Am 1996;80(4):775–801.

Huang L, Stansell JD. Pulmonary complications of human immunodeficiency virus infection. In: Mason RJ, Broaddus VC, Murray JF, Nadel JA, Murray and Nadel's textbook of respiratory medicine, 4th e-dition, http://intl. elsevier-health.com/catalogue/title.cfm?ISBN=1416024735. Elsevier Saunders, 2005:2111–62.

Kaplan JE, Masur H, Holmes KK. Guidelines for preventing opportunistic infections among HIV-infected persons – 2002. Recommendations of the U.S. Public Health Service and the Infectious Diseases Society of America. MMWR Recomm Rep 2002;51(RR-8):1–52.

Kennedy CA, Goetz, MB. Atypical roentgenographic manifestations of *Pneumocystis carinii* pneumonia. Arch Intern Med 1992;152(7):1390–8.

Mandell LA, Wunderink RG, Anzueto A, et al. Infectious Diseases Society of America/American Thoracic Society consensus guidelines on the management of community-acquired pneumonia in adults. Clin Infect Dis 2007;44:S27–72

Moreno S, Martinez R, Barros C, et al. Latent *Haemophilus influenzae* pneumonia in patients infected with HIV. AIDS 1991;5(8):967–70.

Niederman MS, Mandell LA, Anzueto A, et al. Guidelines for the management of adults with community-acquired pneumonia. Diagnosis, assessment of severity, antimicrobial therapy, and prevention. Am J Respir Crit Care Med 2001;163(7):1730–54.

O'Donnell WJ, Pieciak W, Chertow GM, et al. Clearance of *Pneumocystis carinii* cysts in acute *P. carinii* pneumonia: assessment by serial sputum induction. Chest 1998;114(5):1264–8.

Smith RL, Yew K, Berkowitz KA, Aranda CP. Factors affecting the yield of acid-fast sputum smears in patients with HIV and tuberculosis. Chest 1994;106(3):684–6.

Stansell JD, Osmond DH, Charlebois E, et al. Predictors of *Pneumocystis carinii* pneumonia in HIV-infected persons. Pulmonary Complications of HIV Infection Study Group. Am J Respir Crit Care Med 1997;155(1): 60–6.

36. Arthritis in the Acute Care Setting

Jeffery Critchfield

INTRODUCTION

Musculoskeletal complaints are common in the acute care setting. A systematic approach is critical to determine whether the patient is afflicted with a potentially joint-damaging infection or can be safely referred back to their primary provider or a specialist for further work-up and management. The first step in evaluating a patient who complains of joint pain is to establish that the patient does in fact have true arthritis, consisting of pain (arthralgia) and swelling at the affected joint. Periarticular pain also can arise from bursitis, tendonitis, ligamentous damage, and skin pathology such as a cellulitis. Once a diagnosis of true arthritis has been established, the clinician can organize an approach by addressing a few key questions.

- Is the arthritis acute or nonacute?
- What is the pattern of the joint involvement?
  - How many joints are affected?
  - What is the distribution of the joint involvement?
- Are there hints of systemic disease?

Acute arthritis is defined by the onset of symptoms over hours to several days. Development and persistence of symptoms and signs over many days to weeks indicates a subacute process. The full musculoskeletal exam will reveal a monoarticular (involving one joint), oligoarticular (involving two to four joints), or polyarticular (involving five or more joints) arthritis. When addressing an oligo- or polyarticular process, determine whether the arthritis is unilateral or symmetric (e.g., affecting both wrists or the small joints of the fingers of both hands). The history and examination must also include an evaluation for systemic illness. Arthritis in the setting of fever, weight loss, skin lesions, and a new cardiac murmur, for example, may trigger a more aggressive work-up and greatly influence the admission decision.

MONOARTHRITIS

Epidemiology

In the acute care setting, monoarticular, acute arthritis is a bacterial infection until proven otherwise. Among the general population, the reported incidence of septic arthritis ranges from 2 to 5 per 100,000 individuals. Certain chronic, immunosuppressive conditions greatly increase the incidence of arthritis, including connective tissue diseases, particularly rheumatoid arthritis, diabetes mellitus, human immunodeficiency virus (HIV)/acquired immunodeficiency syndrome (AIDS), and the use of immunosuppressive therapy. Septic arthritis occurs most often secondary to hematogenous spread of bacteria. Physical conditions that predispose to hematogenous seeding include penetrating trauma into the joint or periarticular tissues, injection drug use, therapeutic intra-articular injections, recurrent skin infections, and breaks in the skin on the limb of the affected joint.

Clinical Features

Acute arthritis is characterized by a history of joint pain from hours to several days with accompanying warmth and swelling of the periarticular tissue. The appearance of the joint may be normal or demonstrate erythema and edema that can be difficult to distinguish from cellulitis. The presence of pain that greatly curtails range of motion is not specific enough to distinguish bacterial infection from crystal arthropathy, or trauma. In both children and adults, the joints most commonly involved in suppurative arthritis are, in descending order, the knee, hip, shoulder, wrist, and ankle. Clinicians must maintain a high index of suspicion for septic hips and shoulders because the exam so rarely reveals overlying cutaneous evidence of infection, the condition is rapidly progressive, and morbidity is high. Fever is neither sensitive nor specific, as it is seen in fewer than half of patients with septic arthritis and has been well described in patients with gout. Table 36.1 distinguishes between acute and nonacute monoarthritis.

Differential Diagnosis

For acute, monoarticular arthritis the three leading diagnoses include:

- infection
- crystalline arthropathy
- trauma

Table 36.1 Clinical Features: Monoarthritis

	Acute	**Nonacute**
Etiology	**Bacterial infection:** • *Staphylococcus aureus* • *Streptococcus* group A • *Streptococcus pneumoniae* • Gram-negative bacillus • *Neisseria gonorrhoeae* **Crystalline arthropathy:** • Monosodium urate (gout) • Calcium pyrophosphate dehydrate (pseudogout) **Trauma hemarthrosis**	**Infection:** • *Neisseria gonorrhoeae* • *Mycobacteria* species • Lyme disease • Fungi **Crystalline arthropathy:** • Monosodium urate (gout) • Calcium pyrophosphate dehydrate (pseudogout) **Trauma:** • Degenerative joint disease • Meniscal damage • Charcot joint **Uncommon:** • Osteonecrosis • An atypical form of systemic rheumatic condition, e.g., reactive arthritis
Signs and Symptoms	• Decreased range of motion limited by pain • Warmth, erythema, swelling (only for superficial joints) • Signs on exam indicating skin breakdown suggest infection	• Arthralgia • Possibly warmth, erythema, swelling (only for superficial joints)

Table 36.2 Laboratory Diagnosis of Monoarthritis

	Nongonococcal Arthritis	**Gonococcal Arthritis**	**Uric Acid Arthritis**
Synovial WBC (PMN Predominance)	Typically >50,000/mm³ (can be less)	Typically 20–35,000/mm³	Typically >25,000/mm³ (can be >100,000/mm³)
Gram Stain	Positive for organism in 50–75% of cases	Positive for organism in 20–35% of cases	Negative
Crystals	Negative	Negative	Needle like, negatively birefringent (increased specificity if within a PMN)
Peripheral Blood Leukocytosis	May be present	May be present	May be present

PMN, polymorphonuclear neutrophil leukocyte.

Acute monoarticular arthritis is a bacterial infection until proven otherwise. Crystalline arthropathies, particularly gout, can mimic the appearance of a septic joint. Arthritis from calcium pyrophosphate dihydrate crystals, also known as pseudogout, more frequently presents as a subacute oligoarticular process and rarely as a single erythematous, warm septic joint. Clinical history will usually reveal any traumatic etiology, though in the setting of substance use or psychiatric illness, history may be limited.

Rarely, nonacute monoarticular arthritis, persisting for days to weeks, can still be infectious. For example, gonococcal infections can progress over 3–5 days to a septic arthritis, most commonly involving the knee. Slow-growing organisms such as *Mycobacteria* species and fungi must be considered in certain immunocompromised patients. In the appropriate geographic region, Lyme disease can present as a nonacute knee arthritis. Post-traumatic changes such as degenerative joint disease from distant injuries can present similarly. A broad differential also includes less common entities such as hemarthrosis in the setting of anticoagulation or hemophilia; osteonecrosis of the hip or knee; or an atypical monoarticular presentation of what is usually an oligoarticular or polyarticular systemic rheumatic condition, such as rheumatoid arthritis, lupus, or a spondyloarthropathy.

Laboratory and Radiographic Findings

Sampling of synovial fluid of affected joints is the foundation of any evaluation of an unexplained arthritis. The basic studies must include cell counts with differential, Gram stain, and cultures for bacterial, mycobacterial, and fungal pathogens,

as well as analysis for crystals (Table 36.2). In the acute care setting, cultures will be too delayed to guide initial management. Gram stains are positive in roughly 50–75% of nongonococcal suppurative arthritides, and in only 20–35% of gonococcal arthiritis (Figure 36.1). Clearly, these studies are useful if positive, though negative studies do not exclude the possibility of infection. A synovial fluid white blood cell count (WBC) in excess of 50,000/mm³ strongly suggests a suppurative process, particularly with nongonococcal pathogens, unless urate crystals are observed. The synovial WBC must be interpreted in clinical context because gonococcal septic

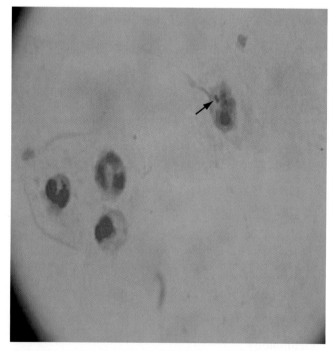

Figure 36.1 Fluid from a knee arthrocentesis demonstrating intracellular gram-negative diplococci, consistent with a *Neisseria* septic joint. Courtesy of Margaret Margaretten and Jon Graf.

Table 36.3 Treatment of Acute Monoarticular Arthritis

Empiric Antibiotics for Nongonococcal Infectious Arthritis	If the Gram stain is negative in the immunocompetent host, initiate vancomycin 10–15 mg/kg IV q12h (correct for renal insufficiency, check trough levels) given the high rates of methicillin-resistant *S. aureus*. In the immunocompromised host, add to the above ceftriaxone 2 g IV, q24h. If gram-negative bacilli are present on Gram stain, initiate ceftriaxone 2 g q24h.
Empiric Antibiotics for Presumed Gonococcal Infectious Arthritis	Ceftriaxone 1 g IV q24h is the cornerstone of therapy. Test and treat for *Chlamydia* and syphilis as well.
Uric Acid Arthropathy (Gout)	Use any available NSAID starting at its highest recommended dose and continued until symptoms resolve. Additionally may offer intra-articular injection with 10–40 mg of triamcinolone or prednisone. If NSAIDs are contraindicated, offer prednisone, 20–40 mg orally for 3 days then tapered off over 7–10 days. Note: There is no role for allopurinol in the acute care setting.

joints typically present with cell counts in the 20–35,000/mm^3 range, whereas nongonococcal or partially treated infections can occasionally present with less inflammatory fluid. Peripheral cell counts may be normal or elevated with septic or crystalline arthropathy. The erythrocyte sedimentation rate has no diagnostic value in the acute setting because any of the processes on the differential diagnosis can generate an abnormal value. If gonococcal infection is suspected, perform pharyngeal and urethral/cervical swabs for culture or nucleic acid testing.

In the acute care setting when trauma is suspected, radiographs are essential for diagnosing fractures or displacements. An infectious process will present only as an effusion on x-ray because the bony changes associated with arthritis are not detectable on plain radiography for at least 2–3 weeks. A nonacute arthritis, particularly one of greater than 3 weeks' duration, might yield characteristic bone changes to suggest an infection, gout, or degenerative pathology.

Treatment and Prophylaxis

If a septic joint is suspected, following arthrocentesis and blood cultures, empiric antibiotics should be initiated to prevent significant morbidity due to joint damage (Table 36.3) (see Chapter 21, Adult Septic Arthritis). Because ongoing therapy will include frequent drainage of the affected joint either by serial arthrocentesis or surgical drainage, an orthopedic surgery consult is indicated. If gout is diagnosed, an intra-articular steroid injection, or a systemic anti-inflammatory agent such as prednisone or a nonsteroidal anti-inflammatory (NSAID) is indicated.

Complications and Admission Criteria

Septic arthritis must be approached as a medical urgency with a low threshold for initiation of antibiotics and admis-

sion because the diagnosis carries a mortality rate of 5–15%. Determination of a septic joint by Gram stain and high white count in the synovial fluid warrants consultation with orthopedic surgery to ensure appropriate ongoing drainage of the joint. An unexplained synovial white count greater than 50,000/mm^3 is sufficient grounds for admission even absent a positive Gram stain. Synovial cell counts less than 50,000/mm^3 can also reflect suppurative processes and, with evidence of systemic illness, are sufficient grounds for admission.

Pearls and Pitfalls

1. Acute monoarticular arthritis is a septic joint until an alternative diagnosis can be established.
2. Perform a complete musculoskeletal exam on all patients complaining of arthritis because a limited exam of the most painful joint may miss a more widespread process.
3. Inquire about signs or symptoms of systemic disease – for example, fevers, weight loss, sweats, skin lesions.
4. A negative Gram stain does not rule out the possibility of a septic joint.

OLIGOARTHRITIS

Epidemiology

Patients presenting with acute arthritis affecting two to four joints must still be considered at risk for an infectious process. Although less than 20% of nongonococcal infectious arthritis presents as an oligoarticular process, gonococcal arthritis commonly involves multiple and asymmetric joints. In addition the seronegative spondyloarthropathies, comprising ankylosing spondylitis, inflammatory bowel associated arthritis, psoriatic arthritis, and reactive arthritis, become more likely. The spondyloarthropathies can be either acute or nonacute in presentation because they frequently do not cause enough morbidity to precipitate an early visit to the emergency department (ED). Oligoarticular gout occurs, but rarely, and almost exclusively in patients with a longstanding diagnosis of gout.

Clinical Features

Disseminated gonococcal infection (DGI) presents in an acute or subacute manner (Table 36.4). Patients typically complain of 3–5 days of arthralgias that localize on exam to an arthritis affecting several joints, most often the knees, wrists, and fingers in an asymmetric manner. Symptoms may be caused by either a frank arthritis or a migratory tenosynovitis of the fingers, wrists, or ankles. Scattered pustules or purpura (often fewer than 10 or 20 lesions) are common.

The spondyloarthropathies classically cause an asymmetric oligoarthritis, often nonacute, with tenosynovitis of the ankles, fingers, and wrists. These patients often present with Achilles tendonitis, plantar fasciitis, and low back pain suggesting sacroiliac involvement. Evidence of psoriatic skin lesions markedly increases the possibility of psoriatic arthritis or reactive arthritis with keratoderma blennorrhagicum, which mimics psoriasis. The presence of dactylitis, swelling of an entire digit, is very suggestive of these entities (Figure 36.2). In their most acute phase these rheumatic diseases can cause fevers, sweats, and weight loss.

Table 36.4 Clinical Features: Oligoarthritis

	Acute	Nonacute
Etiology	**Bacterial infection:** • *Neisseria gonorrhoeae* in its disseminated form • Nongonococcal suppurative arthritis (<20% of time) **Spondyloarthropathies:** • Reactive arthritis (intestinal or venereal) • Psoriatic arthritis • Ankylosing spondylitis • Inflammatory bowel disease associated **Atypical presentation of a systemic connective tissue disease, e.g., RA crystalline arthropathy:** • Monosodium urate (in patients with known gout) • Calcium pyrophosphate dehydrate (pseudogout)	**Infection:** • *Neisseria gonorrhoeae* in its disseminated form • Subacute bacterial endocarditis **Spondyloarthropathies:** • Reactive arthritis (intestinal or venereal) • Psoriatic arthritis • Ankylosing spondylitis • Inflammatory bowel disease associated **Atypical presentation of a systemic connective tissue disease, e.g., RA crystalline arthropathy:** • Monosodium urate (in patients with known gout) • Calcium pyrophosphate dehydrate (pseudogout) **Osteoarthritis**
Signs and Symptoms	• Decreased range of motion limited by pain • Warmth, erythema, swelling (only for superficial joints) • Tenosynovitis at ankles, fingers, wrists • Characteristic skin lesions accompanying DGI, reactive arthritis, psoriatic arthritis	• Arthralgia • Possibly warmth, erythema, swelling (only for superficial joints) • Tenosynovitis at ankles, fingers, wrists • Characteristic skin lesions accompanying DGI, reactive arthritis, psoriatic arthritis

RA, rheumatoid arthritis.

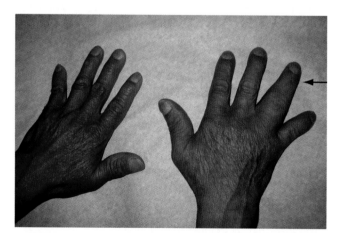

Figure 36.2 The arrow indicates dactylitis of the right fourth finger. This can be seen with psoriatic arthritis and in other seronegative spondyloarthropathies. Courtesy of Margaret Margaretten and Jon Graf.

Differential Diagnosis

Diagnosis of infection remains the priority. Nongonococcal septic joints present only rarely as oligoarthritis, yet remain devastating if overlooked. Nonacute, oligoarticular arthropathies can be caused by infections, such as DGI or Lyme disease, or seen with subacute bacterial endocarditis, which can cause an immune complex mediated oligo- or polyarthritis. The seronegative spondyloarthropathies commonly present as nonacute processes of greater than several weeks' duration, but it can be difficult to distinguish between DGI and the spondyloarthropathies, particularly reactive arthritis. Reactive arthritis, caused by venereal exposure to *Chlamydia* or invasive enteric bacteria such as *Salmonella*, *Shigella*, or *Campylobacter* in the past several weeks, often affects a patient demographic similar to that at risk for DGI. The synovial fluid findings in reactive arthritis can be similar to those in DGI, with moderate WBC counts and negative Gram stains.

For nonacute oligoarthritis, the spondyloarthropathies ultimately are the most common diagnosis (see Table 36.4). Persistent back discomfort without a clear mechanism could point to a spondyloarthritis-associated sacroiliitis that is detectable on plain radiography. Persistent constitutional signs and symptoms are seen with the spondyloarthropathies but should also prompt a full physical exam with consideration of a systemic infection such as subacute endocarditis.

Gout presenting in an oligoarticular manner is well described in patients with previous gouty attacks. Pseudogout affecting multiple joints, particularly wrists, fingers, and knees, is well described.

Also on the differential are early presentations of systemic connective tissue disease that have not yet matured into their full polyarticular form. Rheumatoid arthritis in its early stages can appear very similar to DGI. Noninflammatory, nonacute processes, including osteoarthritis and degenerative joint disease, may also present in an oligoarticular manner.

Laboratory and Radiographic Findings

For acute oligoarthritis, please see the section on monoarticular arthritis. The same considerations apply.

For arthritis of greater than several weeks' duration, plain radiography of the affected joint or the sacroiliac joints in symptomatic patients can yield changes characteristic of the spondyloarthropathies. Proliferative periosteal bone changes along the heel spur or affected joints occur in patients with spondyloarthritis. Ankylosing spondylitis patients may have delicate bone spurs that bridge the vertebral bodies (syndesmophytes). The erosive changes of psoriatic arthritis may be seen in the distal fingers and toes. Gout, if longstanding, causes sclerotic erosions along the margins of the joint line that leave overhanging edges. Laboratory diagnoses of oligoarthritis are listed in Table 36.5.

Treatment and Prophylaxis

If a septic joint is suspected, empiric antibiotics must be initiated (Table 36.6) following arthrocentesis and blood cultures. Ongoing therapy will include frequent drainage of the affected joint either by serial arthrocentesis if possible or by surgical drainage. (See Table 36.3.)

The diagnosis of a spondyloarthropathy should trigger initiation of analgesia and an appropriate anti-inflammatory agent such as an NSAID if there are no contraindications. Avoid administering systemic steroids in the acute care setting because there is a risk of exacerbating an infectious cause. Follow-up with a rheumatologist is critical.

Table 36.5 Laboratory Diagnosis of Oligoarthritis

	Nongonococcal Arthritis	DGI Arthritis	Spondyloarthritis
Synovial WBC (PMN Predominance)	Typically >50,000/mm³ (can be less)	Typically 20–35,000/mm³	13–30,000/mm³
Gram Stain	Positive for organism 50–75%	Positive for organism 20–35%	Negative
Peripheral Blood Leukocytosis	May be present	May be present	Less likely

PMN, polymorphonuclear neutrophil leukocyte.

Table 36.6 Treatment of Oligoarthritis

Empiric Antibiotics for Nongonococcal Infectious Arthritis	If the Gram stain is negative in the immunocompetent host, initiate vancomycin 10–15 mg/kg IV q12h (correct for renal insufficiency, check trough levels) given the high rates of methicillin-resistant *S. aureus*. In the immunocompromised host, add to the above ceftriaxone 2 g IV, q24h. If gram-negative bacilli are present on Gram stain, initiate ceftriaxone 2 g q24h.
Empiric Antibiotics for Presumed Gonococcal Infectious Arthritis	Ceftriaxone 1 g IV q24h is the cornerstone of therapy. Test and treat for *Chlamydia* and syphilis as well.
Spondyloarthropathy	Use any available NSAID starting at its highest recommended dose and continued until symptoms resolve. Send ANA, rheumatoid factor, and anti-CCP antibodies and arrange close follow-up with a rheumatologist.

ANA, antinuclear antibody; CCP, cyclic citrullinated peptide.

Complications and Admission Criteria

Septic arthritis must be approached as a medical urgency with a low threshold for initiation of antibiotics and admission. All the considerations noted with monoarthritis apply in this situation as well. Patients with spondyloarthropathies may require admission to treat debilitating pain and inflammation.

Pearls and Pitfalls

1. Disseminated gonococcal infection and reactive arthritis have similar presentations.
2. Nongonococcal infections present with oligoarthritis less than 20% of the time.
3. When evaluating a person with oligo- or polyarthritis, always closely examine the skin for pustules or papules.
4. Complaints of "arthritis" may be due to tenosynovitis or fasciitis.
5. Subacute bacterial endocarditis can present as a nonacute oligo- or polyarticular arthritis.

6. Calcium pyrophosphate dihydrate (CPPD) commonly presents as oligoarticular, inflammatory arthritis affecting both wrists or knees.
7. Gout presents as an oligo- or polyarthritis only if well established, rarely as the initial presentation.

POLYARTHRITIS

Epidemiology

Systemic viral infections and systemic connective tissue diseases are the most common diagnoses among patients presenting with arthritis in five or more joints. The prevalence of rheumatoid arthritis in women older than 65 years is as high as 5%, though clinicians must maintain a high level of suspicion for infectious causes.

Clinical Features

Acute polyarthritis most commonly represents a viral infection such as parvovirus B19, which is most prevalent in the winter and late spring (Table 36.7) in patients exposed to children and may present with severe pain. The characteristic "slapped cheeks" skin lesion is rare in adults. Acute rubella may cause polyarthritis of the fingers in addition to the characteristic skin lesions. Acute hepatitis B often presents with a polyarthritis accompanied by urticaria and may be preceded by a disease resembling serum sickness. Symmetric arthritis affecting wrists, fingers, and knees can be seen. Abnormal liver enzymes and serologies (see the Laboratory and Radiographic Findings section) will inform this diagnosis.

While rheumatoid arthritis can present acutely with polyarthritis of the fingers, wrists, and shoulders, only about

Table 36.7 Clinical Features: Polyarthritis

	Acute	Nonacute
Etiology	**Viral infection:** • Parvovirus B19 • Hepatitis B • Rubella • Acute HIV **Connective tissue disease:** • Rheumatoid arthritis • Systemic lupus erythematosus • Spondyloarthropathies • Other systemic connective tissue diseases, e.g., Still's disease **Crystalline arthropathy:** • Polyarticular, destructive gout	**Viral infection:** • Parvovirus B19 • Hepatitis B • Hepatitis C • HIV **Subacute bacterial endocarditis** **Connective tissue disease:** • Rheumatoid arthritis • Systemic lupus erythematosus • Spondyloarthropathies • Other systemic connective tissue diseases **Crystalline arthropathy:** • Polyarticular, destructive gout • CPPD (pseudogout) **Osteoarthritis**
Signs and Symptoms	• Decreased range of motion limited by pain • Warmth, erythema, swelling (only for superficial joints) • Tenosynovitis at ankles, fingers, wrists	• Arthralgia • Possibly warmth, erythema, swelling (only for superficial joints) • Tenosynovitis at ankles, fingers, wrists

10% of patients with rheumatoid arthritis present with sudden onset of symptoms, and the presence of high fevers should suggest an alternative diagnosis.

Nonacute polyarthritis is most commonly rheumatoid arthritis or a systemic connective tissue disease such as lupus. Rheumatoid arthritis may be accompanied by rheumatoid nodules on the extensor surfaces of the upper extremities or evidence of dry, red eyes (keratoconjunctivitis). Patients with lupus may describe photosensitivity rashes or malar rash or have pigmented raised discoid lupus lesions on exam. Evidence of systemic disease might include sharp pleuritic chest pain or a cardiac rub suggesting serositis. The seronegative arthritides, while more commonly oligoarticular, may present with five or more affected joints. These entities tend to have an asymmetrical presentation, for example involving several toes, one knee, several fingers, and a wrist or elbow.

Differential Diagnosis

In the acute care setting, it is difficult to differentiate between a viral process and acute rheumatoid arthritis. As symptoms persist longer than 6 weeks, the likelihood of viral infection falls and the most common etiologies are connective tissue diseases or osteoarthritis. For this reason, a duration of arthritic symptoms greater than 6 weeks is included in the diagnostic criteria for rheumatoid arthritis. Acute viral syndromes typically present with polyarthralgias out of proportion to true polyarthritis. Myalgias and high fevers are also common in the acute phase.

Both parvovirus B19 and hepatitis B polyarthritis or arthralgia syndromes can last from 2 to 8 months, with well-described cases lasting for years with parvovirus B19. However, the great majority of the time, nonacute polyarthritis points to a systemic connective-tissue disease. The pattern of the joint involvement, the presence of characteristic symptoms and signs, and the pattern of autoantibodies are critical in identifying the specific disease entity. This is best done in the context of a referral to a rheumatologist or with the primary provider. In the acute clinical setting it is most important to initiate the work-up and make a referral.

Osteoarthritis most commonly presents as a nonacute, non-inflammatory polyarthritis that, although present in many elderly patients in the ED, is rarely the chief complaint. Septic polyarthritis is rare and usually occurs in the setting of an ill, bacteremic patient. The reactive arthritis caused by subacute bacterial endocarditis can mimic the presentation of rheumatoid arthritis, and polyarticular gout can be a terrific mimicker of rheumatoid arthritis.

Laboratory and Radiographic Findings

When hepatitis B associated polyarthritis is suspected, check hepatitis B surface (HBS) antigen levels, which should be high, and anti-hepatitis B core antigen IgM titers, which if present, indicate acute disease. The viral DNA levels can be evaluated in follow-up. Parvovirus B19 acute infection is diagnosed by a positive anti-B19 IgM antibody. The sole presence of the anti-B19 IgG antibody is not sufficient to make this diagnosis, as many individuals exposed during childhood will have these antibodies. Diagnosis of acute HIV syndrome requires viral load testing because the serology will be negative during acute infection.

Table 36.8 Laboratory Diagnosis of Polyarthritis

Laboratory Tests	Viral	Rheumatoid Arthritis	Lupus
ESR, CRP	High	High	High
Rheumatoid Factor	+/−	Present in 50% of patients	+/−
ANA	Negative	+/−	100% (very sensitive, not specific for lupus)
Parvovirus B19 Serology	Anti-B19 IgM antibodies positive	Negative	Negative
Hepatitis B Serology	• HBS antigen high level • HBV DNA positive	Negative	Negative
Other Tests	• Elevated AST/ALT		Look for abnormalities in CBC, urinalysis, anti-phospholipid tests

ALT, alanine aminotransferase; AST, aspartate aminotransferase; HBV, hepatitis B virus.

After infectious causes, the systemic connective tissue disorders and the seronegative spondyloarthropathies must be considered. Although not useful to guide therapy in the acute setting, key serological tests will make the follow-up clinical evaluations of greater yield. Rheumatoid factor is eventually present in 80% of patients with rheumatoid arthritis while the anti-cyclic citrullinated peptide (anti-CCP) is insensitive but carries a specificity of greater than 95% for rheumatoid arthritis. Antinuclear antibodies (ANAs) are present in essentially 100% of patients with lupus. The autoantibody pattern may suggest additional diagnoses such as scleroderma, or mixed connective tissue disease. The erythrocyte sedimentation rate (ESR) and C-reactive protein (CRP), though nonspecific, will provide a quantitative baseline for degree of inflammation. If the clinical scenario strongly suggests lupus, given the systemic nature of this illness, it is important to test for evidence of organ pathology by checking urinalysis, serum creatinine, a complete blood count (CBC), and coagulation studies. For chest or pulmonary complaints in the setting of a clinical picture that suggests lupus, a chest x-ray and electrocardiogram (ECG) should be done to evaluate for serositis.

For the nonacute processes, radiography can be extremely valuable. Rheumatoid arthritis has characteristic erosive changes that distinguish it from gout, whereas lupus, scleroderma and mixed connective tissue disease should have no erosions accompanying the arthritis. It is essential to order bilateral x-rays of hands and feet to allow for comparison. Table 36.8 helps to distinguish the different types of polyarthritis based on laboratory findings.

Treatment and Prophylaxis

Acute viral polyarthritis requires symptomatic treatment most often with NSAIDs or acetaminophen (Table 36.9). For

Table 36.9 Treatment of Polyarthritis

Acute or Nonacute Viral Syndrome	Use any available NSAID starting at its highest recommended dose and continued until symptoms resolve.
Spondyloarthropathy, RA, Lupus	Use any available NSAID starting at its highest recommended dose and continued until symptoms resolve. Arrange close follow-up with a rheumatologist.
RA, rheumatoid arthritis.	

both acute and nonacute connective tissue disorders, symptomatic treatment with NSAIDs and other analgesics with close rheumatology follow-up is sufficient.

Complications and Admission Criteria

Patients with acute polyarthritis from viral infections can usually be discharged with symptomatic treatment. The presence of polyarthritis does not impact the decision to admit patients with acute hepatitis B or HIV unless admission is required for symptom management.

The arthritis of rheumatoid arthritis, lupus, or the spondyloarthropathies will rarely require admission for management of pain or morbidity due to debilitating inflammation. Any of these conditions, particularly lupus, can trigger an admission when there is evidence of significant systemic illness or organ pathology, such as lupus nephritis. The degree of arthritis rarely influences this decision.

Pearls and Pitfalls

1. Acute viral polyarthritis may be indistinguishable from rheumatoid arthritis.

2. The history will aid in determining the viral etiology – for example, if there has been exposure to ill children, consider parvovirus B19.
3. Parvovirus B19 does not present with a "slapped cheeks" rash in adults.
4. Polyarticular, erosive gout can be a mimicker of rheumatoid arthritis.
5. X-rays are particularly valuable with nonacute polyarthritis and should always be bilateral.

REFERENCES

Hootman JM, Helmick CH, Schappert SM. Magnitude and characteristics of arthritis and other rheumatic conditions on ambulatory medical care visits, United States 1997. Arthritis Rheum 2002;47(6):571–81.

Li SF, Cassidy C, Change C, et al. Diagnostic utility of laboratory tests in septic arthritis. Emerg Med J 2007;24:75–7.

Smith JW, Chalupa P, Shabaz M. Infectious arthritis: clinical features, laboratory findings and treatment. Clin Microb Infect 2006;12(4):309–14.

ADDITIONAL READINGS

Mies Richie A, Francis ML. Diagnostic approach to polyarticular joint pain. Am Fam Physician 2003;68(6):1151–60.

Rice PA. Gonococcal arthritis (disseminated gonococcal infection). Infect Dis Clin North Am 2005;19(4):853–61.

Siva C, Velazquez C, Mody A, Brasington R. Diagnosing acute monoarthritis in adults: a practical approach for the family physician. Am Fam Physician 2003;68(1):83–90.

37. Lower Urinary Tract Infection in Adults

Jessica A. Casey and Fredrick M. Abrahamian

INTRODUCTION

Symptomatic acute lower urinary tract infection (LUTI), also known as acute bacterial cystitis, can be described as complicated or uncomplicated. In uncomplicated LUTI, there are no signs and symptoms of upper urinary tract infection (UTI) such as fever, chills, or flank pain. Uncomplicated LUTI is a common diagnosis in healthy, young, nonpregnant females with normal renal function, no underlying structural defect in urinary anatomy, and no condition causing immunocompromise, such as diabetes or human immunodeficiency virus (HIV) infection.

LUTI is considered complicated in the setting of a functional or anatomic abnormality of the urinary tract, nephrolithiasis, neurogenic bladder, diabetes mellitus, other immunosuppression, pregnancy, indwelling urinary catheter use, or recent urinary tract instrumentation. UTI in a patient with a history of pyelonephritis or symptoms lasting more than 14 days also qualifies as complicated. All UTIs in men are considered complicated, as these are almost associated with other conditions requiring specific therapy.

The majority of uncomplicated infections do not require extensive diagnostic tests and are effectively treated with short-term antimicrobial regimens. Complicated infections often require additional diagnostic tests, are treated with longer duration antimicrobial therapy, and may have a higher risk of treatment failure and complications.

EPIDEMIOLOGY

UTI affects half of all women at least once during their lifetime, and during any given year, 11% of women report having had a UTI. The incidence increases with age and sexual activity. The prevalence of UTI in otherwise healthy adult males younger than 50 is less than 1%. In this population, the symptoms of dysuria or urinary frequency are usually due to sexually transmitted diseases (STDs). In men older than 50, the incidence of LUTI increases dramatically because of enlargement of the prostate and associated urinary retention or instrumentation of the urinary tract. All UTIs in men are considered complicated because most of them occur in association with other conditions such as STDs, nephrolithiasis, urologic anatomic abnormalities, prostatitis, or urinary tract instrumentation. The occurrence of UTI in men of any age is best referred to a urologist for further evaluation.

The incidence of LUTI in women has been shown to increase as a result of the following risk factors: increased frequency of intercourse in the past month; spermicide or diaphragm use; a new sexual partner within the past 12 months; and occurrence of first UTI at 15 years of age or younger. Among elderly women living in long-term care facilities, the risk of LUTI increases with age and debility, especially in those with conditions associated with impaired voiding or poor perineal hygiene.

The infecting organism in LUTI generally arises from enteric flora that colonize the perineum and urethra. In uncomplicated UTIs, *Escherichia coli* is responsible for the majority of infections. Other organisms include *Staphylococcus saprophyticus*, *Klebsiella* species, enterococci, and *Proteus mirabilis*. Complicated infections may be due to the same or more resistant strains of the organisms causing uncomplicated UTIs, or unusual pathogens such as *Pseudomonas aeruginosa* or *Serratia marcescens*.

CLINICAL FEATURES

Symptoms of UTI can include dysuria, urinary frequency, hematuria, urgency, and suprapubic discomfort (Table 37.1). Symptoms of dysuria and frequency in women without vaginal discharge or irritation increase the pretest probability of LUTI. The presence of symptoms similar to those of a prior LUTI also increases the probability of infection.

LUTI can also be associated with mild back pain or costovertebral angle tenderness due to referred pain from the bladder. However, moderate-to-severe back pain or costovertebral angle tenderness, especially if associated with fever, chills, or nausea, is indicative of an upper UTI.

DIFFERENTIAL DIAGNOSIS

Other conditions to consider include:

- pyelonephritis
- vaginal infections (e.g., bacterial vaginosis, *Trichomonas vaginitis*, candidiasis)
- pelvic inflammatory disease
- genital herpes infection

Table 37.1 Clinical Features: Lower Urinary Tract Infection in Adults

Organisms	**Uncomplicated infections:** *Escherichia coli* is responsible for the majority of infections. Other organisms may include: • *Staphylococcus saprophyticus* • *Klebsiella* • *Enterococcus* species • *Proteus mirabilis* **Complicated infections:** May be due to the same or more resistant strains of the organisms causing uncomplicated UTIs, or unusual pathogens such as: • *Pseudomonas* • *Serratia* • *Citrobacter* • *Enterobacter*
Signs and Symptoms	Dysuria, urinary frequency, hematuria, urgency, and suprapubic discomfort
Laboratory Findings	**Urine dipstick:** Positive leukocyte esterase and nitrite test **Urine microscopy:** Presence of pyuria and bacteriuria **Urine culture:** Isolation of $\geq 10^3$ CFU/mL of a single uropathogen
Antimicrobial Treatment (always review local susceptibility)	**Acute uncomplicated LUTI:** **If local *E. coli* resistance to TMP-SMX <20%:** TMP-SMX DS (160/800 mg) 1 tab PO bid × 3 days *or* nitrofurantoin (Macrodantin) 50–100 mg PO qid × 7 days *or* nitrofurantoin (Macrobid) 100 mg PO bid × 7 days **If local *E. coli* resistance to TMP-SMX $\geq$ 20%:** ciprofloxacin 250–500 mg PO bid × 3 days *or* ciprofloxacin ER 500 mg PO daily × 3 days *or* levofloxacin 250–500 mg PO daily × 3 days *or* nitrofurantoin (Macrodantin) 50–100 mg PO qid × 7 days *or* nitrofurantoin (Macrobid) 100 mg PO bid × 7 days *or* cephalexin 500 mg PO qid × 7 days **LUTI in pregnancy:** nitrofurantoin (Macrodantin) 50–100 mg PO qid × 7 days *or* nitrofurantoin (Macrobid) 100 mg PO bid × 7 days *or* cephalexin 500 mg PO qid × 7 days *or* amoxicillin-clavulanate 875/125 mg PO bid × 7 days **Complicated LUTI:** ciprofloxacin 500 mg PO bid × 7 days *or* levofloxacin 500 mg PO daily × 7 days **Complicated LUTI and fluoroquinolone allergy:** amoxicillin/clavulanate 875/125 mg PO bid × 14 days *or* cephalexin 500 mg PO qid × 14 days *or* TMP-SMX DS (160/800 mg) 1 tab PO bid × 14 days

DS, double strength; TMP-SMX, trimethoprim-sulfamethoxazole.

• noninfectious causes (e.g., trauma, irritant, allergy)
• prostatitis, orchitis, epididymitis, urethritis, benign prostatic hypertrophy
• urolithiasis
• pregnancy
• ovarian cyst or torsion
• appendicitis
• bladder carcinoma
• diverticular disease
• abdominal aortic aneurysm
• inflammatory bowel disease

Key features that may help to distinguish LUTIs are:

• symptoms of dysuria and frequency in women without vaginal discharge or irritation increase the pretest probability of LUTI
• moderate-to-severe back pain or costovertebral angle tenderness, especially if associated with fever, chills, and nausea, is indicative of an upper UTI

LABORATORY FINDINGS

Urine Collection Methods

The initial step in the diagnosis of a UTI is careful collection of urine for urinalysis and potentially a urine culture. In most adults, the midstream voiding specimen is adequate. Catheterization is indicated if the patient cannot void spontaneously, is too ill or immobilized to provide an adequate specimen, is unable to follow instructions, is extremely obese, or has vaginal discharge or bleeding. Regardless of the collection method, any study of urine must be performed immediately after collection. Urine specimens that are allowed to sit become alkaline, with subsequent dissolution of the cellular elements and multiplication of bacteria.

Urine Dipstick

Pyuria, as indicated by a positive leukocyte esterase dipstick test, is found in the vast majority of patients with UTI. Urine dipstick testing for leukocyte esterase has shown a sensitivity of 75–96% and a specificity of 80–90%. However, low-level pyuria (6–20 white blood cells [WBCs] per high-power field [hpf] microscopy on a centrifuged specimen) can be associated with false-negative leukocyte esterase dipstick test results.

A positive result on the nitrite test is highly specific for UTI (>90%) because of urease-splitting organisms, such as *Proteus* species and, occasionally, *E. coli*. However, it is an insensitive screening test, as only 25% of patients with UTI have a positive nitrite test result. In symptomatic patients, a negative leukocyte esterase or nitrite test on dipstick test cannot reliably rule out an infection and should be followed by urine microscopy.

Urine Microscopy

The diagnosis of a UTI is confirmed if pyuria and bacteriuria are detected on a microscopic examination of the urine. The definition of pyuria varies based on the laboratory counting technique. Pyuria defined as more than 10 WBCs/mm^3 by hemocytometer or more than 5 WBCs/hpf by centrifuge, and microscopy has generally been found to be over

80% sensitive and specific for UTI. The sensitivity of the finding of pyuria appears to be decreased with low bacterial count infections, and specificity appears to be less among women who also have vaginal symptoms. The presence of visible bacteria on microscopic examination increases the specificity to 85–95%.

Urine Culture

The traditional reference standard for diagnosing UTI is defined as the isolation of at least 10^5 colony-forming units (CFU)/mL of a single uropathogen. However, one third to one half of the cases of acute cystitis are characterized by low bacterial concentration (10^2 to 10^4 CFU/mL), which has been termed the *urethral syndrome*. It has been postulated that women with a traditionally negative urine culture ($<10^5$ CFU/mL) have infection localized to the urethra. Recent studies have shown that using a definition of at least 10^3 CFU/mL has the best combination of sensitivity (95%) and specificity (85%) for diagnosing acute UTI.

Uncomplicated infections can be treated empirically without the need to perform a urine culture. A urine culture should be performed in all males being examined for UTI, as well as for individuals with suspected complicated LUTIs. Cultures are also warranted in women whose symptoms either do not resolve with therapy, or recur within 2 to 4 weeks after the completion of treatment.

Asymptomatic Bacteriuria

The prevalence of asymptomatic bacteriuria varies with age, sex, and the presence of genitourinary abnormalities (e.g., healthy, premenopausal women: <5%; postmenopausal women aged 50–70 years: 2.8–8.6%; pregnant women: 2–10%; diabetic women: 9–27%). Rates of asymptomatic bacteriuria in elderly women and men living in long-term care facilities are 25–50% and 15–40%, respectively. Asymptomatic bacteriuria is very common in patients with long-term indwelling catheter use.

The diagnosis of asymptomatic bacteriuria is based on the results of a urine culture, and not the presence of pyuria. For women, bacteriuria is defined as two consecutive voided urine specimens with isolation of the same bacterial strain in quantitative counts of at least 10^5 CFU/mL. For men, a single, clean-catch voided urine specimen with one bacterial species isolated in a quantitative count of at least 10^5 CFU/mL identifies bacteriuria. A single catheterized urine specimen with one bacterial species isolated in a quantitative count of at least 10^2 CFU/mL identifies bacteriuria in women or men.

TREATMENT

Uncomplicated LUTI

The long-standing treatment of choice for uncomplicated LUTIs has been trimethoprim-sulfamethoxazole (TMP-SMX), whereas the fluoroquinolones (e.g., ciprofloxacin, levofloxacin) have been reserved as alternate second-line agents. However, current recommendations are to avoid TMP-SMX as the first-line empiric agent of choice when local resistance of *E. coli* to TMP-SMX is 20% or greater. Among the fluoroquinolones, moxifloxacin should not be used for the treatment of UTIs, because of inadequate urine concentrations.

Most uncomplicated LUTIs can be managed with a short course of antibiotic therapy. Three days of therapy has been shown to be equivalent in efficacy to longer durations of treatment (i.e., 7 or 10 days) in studies of TMP-SMX and ciprofloxacin for uncomplicated LUTIs. Other options for therapy can include nitrofurantoin for 7 days or fosfomycin as a single dose. In comparison to longer durations of treatment with TMP-SMX or fluoroquinolones, single-dose therapy is less effective against eradicating bacteriuria. Oral beta-lactams (e.g., cephalexin) are appropriate agents in areas with increased TMP-SMX and fluoroquinolone-resistant *E. coli*. Beta-lactams should always be prescribed for at least 7 days.

Patients with moderate-to-severe dysuria may also benefit symptomatically from the use of phenazopyridine (Pyridium or Uristat). A potential but rare side effect of phenazopyridine can include hemolytic reaction in patients with glucose-6-phosphate dehydrogenase deficiency.

Complicated LUTI

Short-course antimicrobial regimens are not suitable for the treatment of complicated LUTIs (including those in elderly and pregnant patients). Uncomplicated or complicated infections due to *S. saprophyticus* should also be treated with at least 7 days of antimicrobial therapy. In general for complicated infections, fluoroquinolones (e.g., ciprofloxacin, levofloxacin) prescribed for a duration of seven days are considered first line agents. Other alternatives may be oral cephalosporins (e.g., cephalexin), amoxicillin-clavulanate, or TMP-SMX for 14 days.

LUTI in Pregnancy

(See also Chapter 53, Fever in Pregnancy.)

In pregnant women, options for antimicrobial therapy are more restricted because of the potential adverse effects of the drugs to the fetus. Nitrofurantoin (Pregnancy Category B) and oral cephalosporins (e.g., cephalexin: Pregnancy Category B) are considered safe in pregnancy and are commonly used for the treatment of LUTI in pregnant women. Short-course antimicrobial regimens are not appropriate, and therapy should continue for at least 7 days. TMP-SMX should be avoided in early pregnancy and within 2 weeks of expected delivery date (because of a theoretical increased risk of neonatal hyperbilirubinemia). The quinolones are contraindicated in pregnancy because of adverse effects on fetal bone and cartilage development.

Asymptomatic Bacteriuria

Antimicrobial treatment of asymptomatic bacteriuria during pregnancy decreases the significant 20–30% risk of pyelonephritis and the frequency of low-birth-weight infants and preterm delivery. The recommended duration of antimicrobial therapy is 3–7 days. Patients should be instructed to follow up for periodic screening for bacteriuria after completion of therapy.

Treatment of asymptomatic bacteriuria is not recommended in premenopausal, nonpregnant women, diabetic women, elderly institutionalized residents of long-term care facilities, and patients with an indwelling urethral catheter.

COMPLICATIONS AND ADMISSION CRITERIA

The majority of women with uncomplicated LUTIs have improvement of their symptoms within 72 hours after the initiation of antimicrobial therapy. Complications (e.g., progression to pyelonephritis, papillary necrosis) and long-term adverse effects of LUTI are rare, even in women with frequent recurrences. Recurrence of infection within a few months can be observed in 10–20% of women, which may be due to the original strain or a new strain. Failure of resolution of symptoms should raise the possibility of the improper antimicrobial choice, presence of resistant or unusual organism, or incorrect working diagnosis. Urine cultures should always be sent in cases of recurrent UTI.

Symptomatic infections in elderly, diabetic, or immunocompromised patients and in those with indwelling catheters carry a higher risk of complications, which can include progression to upper UTI, perinephric abscess formation, and urinary tract obstruction.

Patients with isolated LUTIs are stable by definition, with no evidence of systemic toxicity, and can be managed on an outpatient basis. The presence of nausea, vomiting, and fever are clues to an upper UTI (see Chapter 38, Pyelonephritis in Adults, for admission criteria).

PEARLS AND PITFALLS

1. All LUTIs in men are considered complicated.
2. A urine culture should be performed in all complicated or recurrent LUTIs.
3. The diagnosis of asymptomatic bacteriuria is based on results of culture, not the presence of pyuria.
4. Short-course (i.e., 3 days) antimicrobial regimens are not suitable for the treatment of complicated LUTIs (including elderly and pregnant patients).
5. Asymptomatic bacteriuria during pregnancy should be treated with a 3- to 7-day course of antimicrobial therapy, because it has been associated with preterm labor, and the risk of progression to pyelonephritis is significant.

REFERENCES

Gupta K, Hooton TM, Stamm WE. Increasing antimicrobial resistance and the management of uncomplicated community-acquired urinary tract infections. Ann Intern Med 2001;135:41–50.

Hooton TM. Recurrent urinary tract infection in women. Int J Antimicrob Agents 2001;17:259–68.

Hooton TM, Scholes D, Hughes JP, et al. A prospective study of risk factors for symptomatic urinary tract infection in young women. N Eng J Med 1996;335:468–74.

Hooton TM, Stamm WE. Diagnosis and treatment of uncomplicated urinary tract infection. Infect Dis Clin North Am 1997;11:551–81.

Nicolle LE. Urinary tract infection in long-term care facility residents. Clin Infect Dis 2000;31:757–61.

Reid G. Potential preventive strategies and therapies in urinary tract infection. World J Urol 1999;17:359–63.

Ronald AR, Harding GK. Complicated urinary tract infections. Infect Dis Clin North Am 1997;11:583–92.

Scholes D, Hooton TM, Roberts PL, et al. Risk factors for recurrent urinary tract infection in young women. J Infect Dis 2000;182:1177–82.

ADDITIONAL READINGS

Bent S, Nallamothu BK, Simel DL, et al. Does this woman have an acute uncomplicated urinary tract infection? JAMA 2002;287:2701–10.

Fihn SD. Acute uncomplicated urinary tract infection in women. N Eng J Med 2003;349:259–66.

Nicolle LE, Bradley S, Colgan R, et al. Infectious Diseases Society of America guidelines for the diagnosis and treatment of asymptomatic bacteriuria in adults. Clin Infect Dis 2005;40:643–54.

Talan DA, Stamm WE, Hooton TM, et al. Comparison of ciprofloxacin (7 days) and trimethoprim-sulfamethoxazole (14 days) for acute uncomplicated pyelonephritis in women: a randomized trial. JAMA 2000;283:1583–90.

Warren JW, Abrutyn E, Hebel JR, et al. Guidelines for antimicrobial treatment of uncomplicated acute bacterial cystitis and acute pyelonephritis in women. Clin Infect Dis 1999;29:745–58.

38. Pyelonephritis in Adults

Parveen K. Parmar and Fredrick M. Abrahamian

INTRODUCTION

Acute pyelonephritis, an upper urinary tract infection, describes a clinical syndrome of bacteriuria associated with fever, chills, flank pain or tenderness, and lower urinary tract symptoms (e.g., frequency, urgency, dysuria). Uncomplicated infections are those in healthy, nonpregnant females aged 18–40 years, without underlying comorbidities, structural defects in urinary anatomy, or renal dysfunction. Criteria for complicated infection include extremes of age, male gender, immunosuppression (e.g., diabetes, malignancy), pregnancy, presence of a urinary catheter, an anatomic or functional abnormality, obstruction, or history of instrumentation, or the presence of an unusual or resistant organism.

EPIDEMIOLOGY

There are approximately 250,000 cases of acute pyelonephritis annually in the United States, and it is estimated that 30% of these patients are hospitalized. The prevalence of disease is greater in women than men. Men are at higher risk for pyelonephritis if they are uncircumcised, have an enlarged prostate causing urinary stasis, participate in rectal intercourse, or have undergone recent urologic instrumentation or surgery.

Other populations at risk for acute pyelonephritis include those with urinary catheters, spinal cord injury, neurogenic bladder, or fistulae involving the bladder or ureters, or who have undergone renal transplantation. Pregnant women, especially during the second trimester, are also at higher risk for pyelonephritis because of hormonally induced changes in the urinary system. Potential complications of acute pyelonephritis during pregnancy include septicemia, premature labor and low-birth-weight infants.

CLINICAL FEATURES

The organism that is responsible for the vast majority of all acute pyelonephritis is *Escherichia coli* (Table 38.1). Uncomplicated infections may also be due to *Proteus mirabilis*, *Klebsiella* species, *Enterococcus* species, and rarely *Staphylococcus saprophyticus*. Complicated infections may also be caused by *Proteus mirabilis*, *Klebsiella* species, enterococci, *Pseudomonas*

aeruginosa, *Enterobacter* and *Citrobacter* species, and rarely *Staphylococcus aureus*. Mixed infections are common in inpatients and in those with indwelling catheters, recent instrumentation, or urinary tract structural abnormalities. A history of recent antibiotic exposure, recurrent infections, recent instrumentation of the urinary tract, or repeated hospitalizations places a patient at higher risk of harboring a resistant organism as a cause of urinary tract infection.

Clinically, pyelonephritis presents as a combination of fever, chills, flank pain, or costovertebral angle tenderness in association with urinary frequency, dysuria, or hematuria. The spectrum of disease can range from mild illness to fulminant sepsis. The pain associated with pyelonephritis can occasionally present at atypical locations such as the epigastric region or right or left upper abdominal quadrants.

Table 38.1 Clinical Features: Acute Pyelonephritis in Adults

Organisms	The organism that is responsible for the vast majority of uncomplicated and complicated cases of acute pyelonephritis is *Escherichia coli*. Uncomplicated infections may also be due to: • *Proteus mirabilis* • *Klebsiella* species • *Enterococcus* species • *Staphylococcus saprophyticus* (rare) The microbiologic etiology of complicated infections, in addition to *E. coli*, may also be: • *Proteus mirabilis* • *Klebsiella* species • *Enterococcus* species • *Pseudomonas aeruginosa* • *Enterobacter* species • *Citrobacter* species • *Staphylococcus aureus* (rare)
Signs and Symptoms	Fever, chills, flank pain, or costovertebral angle tenderness in association with urinary frequency, dysuria, or hematuria
Laboratory Findings	**Urine dipstick:** Positive leukocyte esterase and nitrite test (Note: Cephalexin can cause false-negative urine dipstick test for leukocytes) **Urine microscopy:** Presence of pyuria and bacteriuria **Urine culture:** Isolation of $\geq 10^3$ CFU/mL of a single uropathogen

The presentation of pyelonephritis is particularly challenging in the elderly, where it can often present with any number of symptoms including abdominal pain, altered mental status, or sepsis. Fever in this population may be low-grade or absent.

Urinary tract infection in men should raise suspicion for acute prostatitis. Gram-negative enteric organisms (e.g., *E. coli*) are the most frequent cause; however, *Neisseria gonorrhoeae* and *Chlamydia trachomatis* may also be culprits (especially in younger patients). In patients with acquired immunodeficiency syndrome, the prostate may be the focus of *Cryptococcus neoformans* infection. The clinical presentation of acute prostatitis is similar to pyelonephritis and includes symptoms of urinary tract infection (e.g., frequency, urgency, dysuria), fever, chills, and perineal and low back pain. Bladder outlet obstruction may result in urinary retention. On physical examination, the prostate gland is swollen and tender. The acutely infected prostate gland should not be massaged because there is potential for precipitating bacteremia. Similarly, urethral instrumentation should be avoided.

DIFFERENTIAL DIAGNOSIS

Other conditions to consider include:

- nephrolithiasis with or without infection
- pelvic inflammatory disease
- ectopic pregnancy
- ovarian cyst or torsion
- acute prostatitis
- renal abscess, carcinoma
- abdominal pathology (e.g., pancreatitis, abdominal aortic aneurysm)
- renal artery stenosis or vein thrombosis
- pulmonary pathology (e.g., pneumonia)

Key features that may help distinguish pyelonephritis are:

- bacteriuria associated with fever, chills, flank pain or tenderness, and lower urinary tract symptoms (e.g., frequency, urgency, and dysuria)
- sudden-onset colicky back and flank pain associated with nausea and vomiting should raise suspicion for nephrolithiasis

LABORATORY FINDINGS

The laboratory diagnosis of pyelonephritis is made through urinalysis and urine culture and specimens should be obtained prior to the initiation of antibiotic therapy. Urinary tract infection is confirmed if pyuria (defined as >10 white blood cells [WBC]/mm^3 of midstream urine by hemocytometer) and bacteriuria are detected on microscopy. Pyuria and positive urine cultures are present in the large majority of symptomatic patients

In uncomplicated infections, blood cultures, when positive, seldom vary from urine cultures and rarely change therapy. Discrepancies between blood and urine cultures are often due to contamination by skin flora. Similar findings have also been demonstrated in pregnant patients with pyelonephritis. Blood cultures are best reserved for patients with complicated infections.

Common imaging modalities used to evaluate renal pathologies include ultrasound and computed tomography (CT) scan. Uncomplicated infections do not require routine radiographic evaluation. However, in complicated cases, in patients who have failed initial empiric therapy, or in patients with an uncertain diagnosis, imaging studies can provide crucial information.

Renal ultrasound, which can be done at the bedside, can demonstrate complications such as hydronephrosis with high sensitivity. Additionally, renal or extrarenal abscesses and distal hydroureter (e.g., ureterovesical or uteropelvic junction) can be visualized by ultrasound. Upper and midureter dilatations are difficult to visualize by ultrasound, ultrasound has a lower sensitivity than CT for the detection of urinary stones.

CT scan is considered the imaging modality of choice in most renal pathologies. Unenhanced helical CT scan of the abdomen and pelvis is the best imaging study for the evaluation of urinary stones. In addition, CT scan can demonstrate hydronephrosis and hydroureter at all levels, and precisely localize gas and abscess. Contrast enhanced CT scan delineates abscess from other structures and provides insight into renal perfusion (e.g., identifying renal infarction from renal artery occlusion or renal vein thrombosis).

TREATMENT

The choice of initial empiric antimicrobial therapy is best directed toward the most likely microbiologic etiology and knowledge of local susceptibility patterns (Table 38.2). Most uncomplicated infections can be managed on an outpatient basis with a 7-day course of a fluoroquinolone (e.g., ciprofloxacin, levofloxacin, ofloxacin). Moxifloxacin or gemifloxacin should not be used for the treatment of urinary tract infections because they do not achieve adequate urine concentrations.

Other options for therapy include oral cephalosporins (e.g., cephalexin), amoxicillin-clavulanate, or trimethoprim-sulfamethoxazole double strength (TMP-SMX DS) for 14 days. In the United States, approximately 30% of *E. coli* is currently resistant to ampicillin and amoxicillin, and increasing *E. coli* resistance to fluoroquinolones and trimethoprim-sulfamethoxazole is a concern.

Intravenous antimicrobial therapy for patients requiring hospitalization may include a fluoroquinolone (e.g., ciprofloxacin, levofloxacin), a third- or fourth-generation cephalosporin (e.g., ceftriaxone or cefepime), antipseudomonal penicillin (e.g., piperacillin-tazobactam, ticarcillin-clavulanate), ampicillin-sulbactam, and ertapenem. A combination therapy may include ampicillin and an aminoglycoside (e.g., gentamicin). Because of the inconsistent in vitro activity of any one class of antimicrobials, in severely ill patients (e.g., those with severe sepsis or septic shock) it is best to use a combination of antimicrobials to ensure adequate coverage for potential resistant pathogens. In such patients, combination therapy may include piperacillin-tazobactam and gentamicin. The recommended duration of therapy for hospitalized patients is 14 days.

The quinolones are contraindicated in pregnancy because of adverse effects on fetal bone and cartilage development (Pregnancy Category C). Inpatient therapy for pyelonephritis during pregnancy may include a third-generation cephalosporin (e.g., ceftriaxone, cefotaxime) or antipseudomonal penicillin (e.g., piperacillin-tazobactam,

Table 38.2 Initial Empiric Therapy for Acute Pyelonephritis in Adults*

Patient Category	Therapy Recommendation
Acute Uncomplicated Pyelonephritis	**Outpatient therapy**: ciprofloxacin 500 mg PO bid × 7 days *or* ciprofloxacin ER 1000 mg PO daily × 7 days *or* levofloxacin 250–500 mg PO daily × 7 days *or* ofloxacin 400 mg PO bid for × 7 days *or* cephalexin 500 mg PO qid × 14 days *or* amoxicillin-clavulanate 875/125 mg PO bid × 14 days *or* amoxicillin-clavulanate 500/125 mg PO tid × 14 days *or* TMP-SMX DS (160/800 mg) 1 tab PO bid × 14 days (**Note**: Do not use TMP-SMX if local *E. coli* resistance to TMP-SMX ≥10%) **Inpatient therapy** (treat for **14 days**): ciprofloxacin 400 mg IV q12h *or* levofloxacin 500 mg IV daily *or* ceftriaxone 1–2 g IV daily *or* piperacillin-tazobactam 3.375 g IV q6h *or* ticarcillin-clavulanate 3.1 g IV q6h *or* ampicillin-sulbactam 3 g IV q6h *or* ertapenem 1 g IV daily
Severely Ill Patients (e.g., Severe Sepsis or Septic Shock)	piperacillin-tazobactam 3.375 g IV q6h *plus* gentamicin 5 mg/kg IV daily
Complicated Pyelonephritis (e.g., Catheter Related, Obstruction, Renal Transplant) (Total Duration of Therapy 2–3 Weeks)	levofloxacin 500 mg IV daily *or* ciprofloxacin 400 mg IV q12h *or* piperacillin-tazobactam 3.375 g IV q6h *or* ticarcillin-clavulanate 3.1 g IV q6h *or* imipenem 0.5 g IV q6h *or* meropenem 1 g IV q8h
Acute Prostatitis (Total Duration of Therapy 2–4 Weeks)	ciprofloxacin ER 500 mg PO daily *or* levofloxacin 750 mg PO daily *or* TMP-SMX DS (160/800 mg) 1 tab PO bid (**Note**: Do not use TMP-SMX if local *E. coli* resistance to TMP-SMX ≥10%) *or* ciprofloxacin 400 mg IV q12h *or* levofloxacin 750 mg IV daily *or* ampicillin-sulbactam 3 g IV q6h *or* ceftriaxone 1–2 g IV daily *or* cefotaxime 2 g IV q8h *or*

Table 38.2 (*cont.*)

Patient Category	Therapy Recommendation
	ticarcillin-clavulanate 3.1 g IV q4–6h *or* piperacillin-tazobactam 3.375 g IV q6h **Note**: If *N. gonorrhoeae* and *C. trachomatis* are suspected as the cause of prostatitis (e.g., young patients), treat with ceftriaxone 250 mg IM × 1 and then doxycycline 100 mg PO bid × 10 days. Fluoroquinolones are no longer recommended for the treatment of gonococcal infections in the United States.
Pyelonephritis in Pregnancy (× 14 Days)	ceftriaxone 1 g IV daily *or* piperacillin-tazobactam 3.375 g IV q6h *or* ticarcillin-clavulanate 3.1 g IV q6h *or* cephalexin 500 mg PO qid *or* amoxicillin-clavulanate 875/125 mg PO bid

*The choice of initial empiric antimicrobial therapy is best directed toward the most likely microbiologic etiology and local susceptibility patterns.

ticarcillin-clavulanate). Oral therapy can include cephalexin or amoxicillin-clavulanate.

Acute prostatitis responds well to oral antimicrobial therapy. Fluoroquinolones, TMP-SMX, and cephalosporins have good penetration into prostatic tissue. The duration of therapy is 2–4 weeks. Urethral instrumentation should be avoided, and suprapubic catheterization is indicated for acute urinary retention. Complications of acute prostatitis can include prostatic abscess formation and should be suspected in patients failing antimicrobial therapy. The diagnosis can be made by CT scan or transrectal ultrasonography, and requires surgical drainage because antimicrobial therapy alone is not sufficient for cure.

If sexually transmitted diseases (e.g., *N. gonorrhoeae* and *C. trachomatis*) are suspected as the cause of prostatitis, treatment should include ceftriaxone and doxycycline. Fluoroquinolones should be avoided and are no longer recommended for the treatment of gonococcal infections in the United States.

Treatment of urinary tract infection in the presence of an indwelling catheter includes intravenous antimicrobial therapy and replacement or removal of the catheter if possible. Antimicrobial therapy should be directed against Enterobacteriaceae, *Pseudomonas aeruginosa*, and enterococci. Suggested monotherapies include ciprofloxacin, levofloxacin, piperacillin-tazobactam, ticarcillin-clavulanate, imipenem, or meropenem. Combination therapy may include ampicillin and gentamicin. The recommended duration of antimicrobial therapy for urinary tract infection associated with an indwelling catheter is 2–3 weeks.

COMPLICATIONS AND ADMISSION CRITERIA

The majority of patients with pyelonephritis will have improvement of their symptoms within 72 hours after the initiation of antimicrobial therapy. Failure of resolution of symptoms should raise the possibility of a resistant or unusual organism, or an incorrect working diagnosis (e.g., nephrolithiasis is commonly misdiagnosed as pyelonephritis). Treatment failure may also be due to the presence of complications such as urinary obstruction, papillary necrosis, intrarenal or perinephric abscess formation, or emphysematous pyelonephritis.

The clinical presentation of intrarenal or perinephric abscess can be similar to pyelonephritis. Predisposing factors to abscess formation include diabetes mellitus and urinary tract obstruction due to calculi, and *E. coli* and other gram-negative enteric bacilli are the usual causative agents. *Staphylococcus aureus* may be a culprit, often from hematogenous seeding (i.e., in the setting of staphylococcal bacteremia and/or endocarditis). In about 30% of patients with perinephric abscess the urinalysis is normal, and 40% have sterile urine cultures. The diagnosis is often suspected in patients who do not respond to initial antimicrobial therapy. Ultrasound and CT scan are both capable of demonstrating perinephric and renal abscess. Emergency department management involves initiation of intravenous broad-spectrum antibiotics and urologic consultation for definitive surgical drainage (e.g., percutaneous or open surgical drainage).

Emphysematous pyelonephritis is a severe necrotizing form of infection that results in the formation of gas in the renal parenchyma and collecting tissues. It is a rare condition that is generally seen in the setting of diabetes with poor glycemic control. It is most often associated with *E. coli* and *Klebsiella* and *Proteus* species. The presentation can be nonspecific and similar to pyelonephritis, although these patients are often very sick on presentation. CT scan of the abdomen and pelvis is the best imaging modality for the evaluation of emphysematous pyelonephritis. The precise localization of gas is important in the differentiation of emphysematous pyelonephritis from other potential sources such as emphysematous pyelitis, perinephric emphysema, or abscess. Early surgical intervention (e.g., drainage or nephrectomy) in combination with broad-spectrum antibiotics has shown to decrease mortality from emphysematous pyelonephritis. Emergency department management involves the initiation of intravenous broad-spectrum antibiotics and urologic consultation for definitive surgical management.

Xanthogranulomatous pyelonephritis is a rare, severe suppurative reaction to chronic renal infection in which dead renal tissue is replaced by granulomas. Predisposing factors include urinary obstruction by tumor or calculi, renal ischemia, dyslipidemia, diabetes, and immunocompromise. The prevalence is higher in women, with the peak incidence between the fifth and seventh decades. Common microbiologic culprits include *Proteus* species and *E. coli*. The presentation can be nonspecific and similar to pyelonephritis. CT scan may show low-attenuation masses with destruction of the renal parenchyma and possibly the presence of a staghorn calculus. Definitive diagnosis requires biopsy, and treatment includes partial or complete nephrectomy.

Indications for hospitalization in patients with acute pyelonephritis include hemodynamic instability, the presence of severe sepsis or septic shock, persistent vomiting or inability to tolerate fluids, failure of outpatient therapy, the presence of complications (e.g., obstruction, emphysematous pyelonephritis), poor social support (e.g., inability to purchase medications, follow-up), immunocompromised states (e.g., diabetes mellitus, cancer), and the presence of indwelling catheters. In addition, patients older than 60 and pregnant patients are also best managed as inpatients because of the high risk of complications. If deemed appropriate for outpatient therapy, these patients require extremely close follow-up. Studies investigating outpatient therapy of pyelonephritis in pregnant patients often included a short hospitalization period with initiation of an intravenous antibiotic regimen for 48 hours. No outpatient trials have been conducted in which oral therapy was used alone. In all cases, regardless of the decision to admit or discharge, it is best to initiate antimicrobial therapy with an intravenous first dose in the emergency department.

PEARLS AND PITFALLS

1. The pain associated with pyelonephritis may present in atypical locations such as the epigastric region or right or left upper abdominal quadrants.
2. Urinary tract infection in men should raise suspicion for acute prostatitis.
3. Urine culture should be performed on all patients with pyelonephritis.
4. In uncomplicated infections, blood cultures seldom vary from urine cultures and do not result in a change in antimicrobial therapy.
5. In severely ill patients, it is best to use a combination of antimicrobials to ensure adequate coverage for potential resistant pathogens.
6. Treatment failure may be due to the presence of complications such as urinary obstruction, abscess formation, or emphysematous pyelonephritis.
7. Consider the diagnosis of emphysematous pyelonephritis in severely ill diabetic patients presenting with a clinical syndrome compatible with pyelonephritis.

REFERENCES

Brown P, Ki M, Foxman B. Acute pyelonephritis among adults: cost of illness and considerations for the economic evaluation of therapy. Pharmacoeconomics 2005;23:1123–42.

Hill JB, Sheffield JS, McIntire DD, et al. Acute pyelonephritis in pregnancy. Obstet Gynecol 2005;105:18–23.

Liu H, Mulholland SG. Appropriate antibiotic treatment of genitourinary infections in hospitalized patients. Am J Med 2005;118(Suppl 7A):14S–20S.

Scholes D, Hooton TM, Roberts PL, et al. Risk factors associated with acute pyelonephritis in healthy women. Ann Intern Med 2005;142:20–7.

Sheffield JS, Cunningham FG. Urinary tract infection in women. Obstet Gynecol 2005;106(5 Pt 1):1085–92.

Song EK, Zwanger M. Xanthogranulomatous pyelonephritis. J Emerg Med 2001;21:63–4.

Talan DA, Klimberg IW, Nicolle LE, et al. Once daily, extended release ciprofloxacin for complicated urinary tract infections and acute uncomplicated pyelonephritis. J Urol 2004;171(2 Pt 1):734–9.

Wing DA, Park AS, Debuque L, et al. Limited clinical utility of blood and urine cultures in the treatment of acute pyelonephritis during pregnancy. Am J Obstet Gynecol 2000;182:1437–40.

ADDITIONAL READINGS

Talan DA, Stamm WE, Hooton TM, et al. Comparison of ciprofloxacin (7 days) and trimethoprim-sulfamethoxazole (14 days) for acute uncomplicated pyelonephritis in women: a randomized trial. JAMA 2000;283:1583–90.

Velasco M, Martinez JA, Moreno-Martinez A, et al. Blood cultures for women with uncomplicated acute pyelonephritis: are they necessary? Clin Infect Dis 2003;37:1127–30.

Warren JW, Abrutyn E, Hebel JR, et al. Guidelines for antimicrobial treatment of uncomplicated acute bacterial cystitis and acute pyelonephritis in women. Clin Infect Dis 1999;29:745–58.

Wing DA, Hendershott CM, Debuque L, et al. Outpatient treatment of acute pyelonephritis in pregnancy after 24 weeks. Obstet Gynecol 1999;94(5 Pt 1):683–8.

39. Fever and Headache: Meningitis and Encephalitis

Anita Koshy

INTRODUCTION

Although there is a broad differential in a patient presenting with fever and headache, a few infectious diagnoses must be ruled in or out immediately. Acute bacterial meningitis is a critical diagnosis because delay of appropriate antimicrobial therapy increases morbidity and mortality. Distinguishing among bacterial, viral, and more chronic meningitides requires the integration of multiple clinical and laboratory findings.

EPIDEMIOLOGY

The Centers for Disease Control and Prevention (CDC) estimates that from 1988 to 1999, more than 800,000 people were hospitalized for meningitis. The majority of these hospitalizations were for viral (50%) and bacterial meningitis (23%). Fungal meningitis accounted for 9% of the hospitalizations and unspecified for 18%. The highest incidence of nonfungal meningitis was in infants younger than 1 year old, whereas fungal meningitis was more common in young adults. Because these numbers describe only hospitalized patients, they underrepresent the actual incidence, especially of viral meningitis.

CLINICAL FEATURES

Meningitis is classically characterized as a triad of fever, neck stiffness, and altered mental status, though it may be more appropriate to consider the triad of fever, headache, and meningismus (Table 39.1). Fewer than half of the patients with bacterial meningitis will present with the complete "classic" triad, though most present with headache. In retrospective studies, fever is the most common symptom, though many of these did not evaluate headache as a clinical feature of meningitis. In the only prospective study of adults with bacterial meningitis, headache was the most common complaint (87%), then neck stiffness (83%), fever (77%), and altered status (69%). Of the patients studied, 95% had at least two of these four symptoms, and 99% had at least one. A petechial rash can be seen in more than 50% of cases of meningitis caused by *Neisseria meningitidis* but can also be seen in *Streptococcus pneumoniae*, *Staphylococcus aureus*, group B *Streptococcus*, and *Rickettsia rickettsii* meningitis.

In infants and children, the presentation of bacterial meningitis is often less specific than in adults, though fever does tend to be a cardinal symptom. Neonates can appear septic and may present with hypotension and apnea, and young children may present with fever and irritability or lethargy. About one-third of children with *S. pneumoniae* or *Haemophilus influenza* B (HIB) meningitis will present with seizures. Clinicians should have a high index of suspicion for meningitis in febrile children, even in the absence of localizing complaints. See also Chapter 45, Work-Up of Newborn Fever, and Chapter 46, The Febrile Child.

Viral meningitis and infectious causes of chronic meningitis also often present with fever and headache. Viral meningitis is usually relatively abrupt in onset, but the patients are less symptomatic than those with bacterial meningitis and should not have an alteration in mentation. Chronic meningitis is characterized by more gradual onset of symptoms and an indolent course. Any meningitis can present with cranial neuropathies, though these neuropathies are more commonly described with basilar meningitides, such as tuberculous, Lyme, fungal, or sarcoid meningitis.

Table 39.1 Clinical Features: Meningitis

Children: Signs and Symptoms	• Fever • Neonates can appear septic • Irritability or lethargy • Seizures (1/3 of children with *S. pneumoniae* or *Haemophilus influenza* B (HIB) meningitis) • Petechial rash (favors *N. meningitidis* but can be present with any organism that causes meningitis)
Adults: Signs and Symptoms	• Fever, headache, neck stiffness, altered mental status • Seizures are very rare • Petechial rash (favors *N. meningitidis* but can be present with any organism that causes meningitis)

DIFFERENTIAL DIAGNOSIS

Table 39.2 summarizes the differential diagnosis of bacterial meningitis.

Table 39.2 Differential Diagnosis of Bacterial Meningitis

Etiology	Key Features
Meningitis	• Fever, headache, meningismus • May have history of otitis media or sinusitis • See the rest of chapter to distinguish acute bacterial, viral, and chronic
Sinusitis	• Sinus headache, facial pain, nasal congestion, • Purulent nasal drainage • Subacute symptoms
Bacterial Brain Abscess	• Progressive headache • History of pulmonary hereditary hemorrhagic telangiectasia • History of recent dental abscess or procedure • Subacute symptoms • May have focal neurologic findings and fever • Poor dentition when oropharynx is examined
Encephalitis	• Headache • Altered mental status • Seizures • Fever
Subarachnoid Hemorrhage	• Acute onset headache, often severe • No fever or meningismus early on (later can develop central fever and will develop meningismus) • Can have focal neurologic findings, including cranial neuropathies

Bacterial Meningitis

Causes of bacterial meningitis vary by age. Neonates acquire organisms such as group B *Streptococcus*, *Escherichia coli*, or less commonly, *Listeria monocytogenes*, from passage through the mother's birth canal. Beyond the first month of life, the most common organisms are *N. meningitidis* (meningococcus) and *S. pneumoniae*, with age-dependent differences in incidence (see Table 39.3).

STREPTOCOCCUS PNEUMONIAE

Since the advent of the HIB vaccine, *S. pneumoniae* has emerged as the most common cause of bacterial meningitis in patients older than 1 month. *S. pneumoniae* is a gram-positive bacterium that forms diplococci or very short chains (Figure 39.1). It is ubiquitous and can cause severe disease in any patient. The morbidity and mortality of pneumococcal meningitis is approximately 30%. The incidence of invasive pneumococcal disease is declining in the setting of widespread vaccination in many countries.

NEISSERIA MENINGITIDIS

N. meningitidis is a gram-negative diplococcus that can be observed intracellularly or extracellularly (see Figure 39.2). It is the second most common cause of bacterial meningitis and usually causes disease in a bimodal age distribution: in infants younger than 12 months of age, and then again in young adults. Meningococcal disease frequently (50%) presents with a petechial rash. The mortality rate of meningococcal meningitis without associated sepsis is approximately

Table 39.3 Bacterial Meningitis

Organism	Gram Stain	Associated Risks
Streptococcus pneumoniae	• Gram-positive coccus that forms diplococci or very short chains	• Most common cause of bacterial meningitis in patients older than 1 month • Declining overall incidence since advent of vaccine, with an increase in cases caused by strains not targeted by the vaccine
Neisseria meningitidis	• Gram-negative coffee-bean diplococcus • Can be intracellular or extracellular	• Second most common cause of bacterial meningitis • Bimodal age distribution: <1 year of age and young adults in close proximity (college, military) • Most common cause of petechial rash associated with meningitis
***Haemophilus influenzae* B (HIB)**	• Gram-negative coccobacillus	• Generally affects children <6 years old • Declining incidence since advent of vaccine
Listeria	• Gram-positive rod	• Age >50, on steroids or other immunosuppressant drugs, history of alcohol abuse, pregnancy, or cancer • Outbreaks have been associated with contaminated coleslaw, raw vegetables, unpasteurized milk or cheese
Rickettsia rickettsii	• Intracellular pathogen that requires special staining • Small gram-negative rod (when cultured)	• Acquired by a tick bite • High mortality rate if not treated • Most commonly found in the South Atlantic United States but has been reported in majority of United States • Presents late spring to early fall • Generally affects children <16 years old • Rash beginning on wrist, ankles around 3–5 days, often involves palms and soles

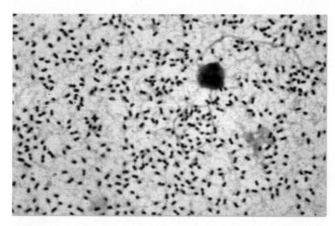

Figure 39.1 *S. pneumoniae* in the CSF. Courtesy of Dr. Ellen Jo Baron, Stanford University.

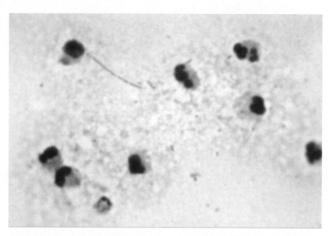

Figure 39.3 *H. influenzae* B in CSF. Courtesy of Dr. Ellen Jo Baron, Stanford University.

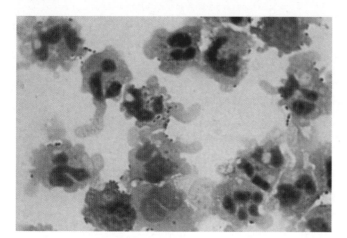

Figure 39.2 Intracellular gram-negative diplococcus from a cytospin. Courtesy of Dr. Ellen Jo Baron, Stanford University.

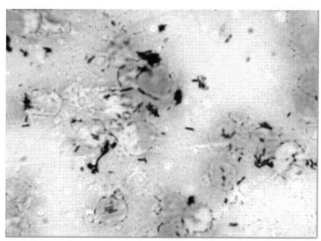

Figure 39.4 *L. monocytogenes* in blood. Courtesy of Dr. Ellen Jo Baron, Stanford University.

7%, and close contacts should receive chemoprophylaxis (see later discussion of infection control).

HAEMOPHILUS INFLUENZAE B (HIB)

Haemophilus influenzae B is a gram-negative coccobacillus that accounted for 45–58% of bacterial meningitis cases in the United States (see Figure 39.3) prior to the widespread introduction of the HIB vaccine in the late 1980s, since which time its prevalence has declined to 7%. Chemoprophylaxis for contacts of a patient with HIB meningitis is described in the Infection Control section.

LISTERIA MONOCYTOGENES

L. monocytogenes is a gram-positive rod commonly found in soil, dust, water, and sewage (see Figure 39.4). It is responsible for approximately 8% of bacterial meningitis cases. It occurs more commonly in neonates, older adults, and patients with a history of immunosuppressive therapy, alcohol abuse, or cancer. Outbreaks of listeriosis have been traced to contaminated coleslaw, raw vegetables, and unpasteurized milk products. In patients with any of these risk factors, ampicillin should be included in the empiric antibiotic regimen.

RICKETTSIA RICKETTSII

R. rickettsii is a tick-borne intracellular pathogen, and more than 50% of infected patients will recall a tick bite. Although a relatively rare cause of meningitis, the mortality rate is greater than 20% if not treated. In the United States, it is found most commonly in the South Atlantic region but has been reported in most states. It usually presents in late spring to early fall and most often affects those under 16 years of age. In most cases, it presents with fever, nausea, vomiting, and headache. A petechial rash that begins on the extremities (often including the palms and soles) and moves centrally may develop several days after the onset of fever. Doxycycline is the treatment of choice.

Key features that distinguish acute bacterial from viral or chronic meningitis include:

- sepsis
- altered mental status
- petechial rash

Aseptic Meningitis

Aseptic meningitis refers to patients who have signs and symptoms of meningitis without evidence of purulent bacterial infection. Thus, aseptic meningitis encompasses viral meningitis, atypical bacterial meningitis, chemical meningitis, carcinomatosis meningitides, granulomatous disease (such as sarcoid), and fungal meningitis. The majority of these entities will present with an indolent course.

Table 39.4 Viral Meningitis

Organism	Signs and Symptoms	Associated Risks
Nonpolio Enteroviruses	• Prodrome of flulike illness and sore throat • Nausea, vomiting, fever, meningismus, and possible viral exanthem	• Causes up to 70% of viral meningitis • Found worldwide • Presents in summer and autumn in temperate climates and year-round in tropical and subtropical climates • Children infected most often **Treatment:** Supportive
Polio	• Symptoms same as above • Can affect motor and ANS neurons leading to permanent paralysis	• Rare cause of meningitis in vaccinated countries • Important cause of aseptic meningitis in endemic areas of Central Africa and West Asia • Anticipated eradication if immunization universal **Treatment:** Supportive
Flavivirus – includes Japanese encephalitis complex, St. Louis encephalitis (SLE) virus, tick-borne encephalitis virus, and West Nile Virus	• CNS involvement depends on the virus • Most infections asymptomatic or mild febrile illnesses without CNS involvement	• Each complex has a general geographic distribution and seasonality • SLE is seen in the south and southeastern states • WNV follows bird migrations and is now found throughout the United States • Older (age >50) and immunocompromised patients generally have the most severe disease • Vector-borne (mosquito or tick) **Treatment:** Supportive
HIV	• Acute HIV infection is often associated with fever, pharyngitis, lymphadenopathy, and rarely a rash	• Risk factors would be unprotected sex and sharing of contaminated needles **Treatment:** supportive, but close follow-up necessary to determine appropriate time to start HAART
Herpes Viruses – includes HSV-1 and -2, VZV, CMV, EBV, and HHV-6	• Fever, headache, neck stiffness • Altered mental status, seizures, focal neurologic findings define meningoencephalitis	• In immunocompetent patients, HSV-2 is the most common cause • Usually associated with a primary genital outbreak • In immunocompromised patients, any of these viruses can be seen **Treatment:** • Immunocompetent patients – no treatment guidelines for meningitis • Immunocompromised patients or any patient with meningoencephalitis: HSV and VZV, acyclovir 10 mg/kg q8h, and for CMV, ganciclovir 5 mg/kg q12h; ganciclovir appropriate for EBV or HHV-6
Lympthocytic Choriomeningitis (LCMV)	• Rarely fever, headache, myalgias	• Can cause congenital hydrocephalus, micro- or macrocephaly, chorioretinitis, intracranial calcifications, and nonimmune hydrops • Risk factors: exposure to rodents such as lab workers, pet owners, and those living in nonhygienic conditions, and transplant recipients on immunosuppressive drugs **Treatment:** Supportive
Mumps	• Fever, headache, neck stiffness • Can be associated with parotitis, precede parotitis, or be the only manifestation of an infection	• Present in winter and spring and usually infects unimmunized and partially immunized children • Affects males more often than females **Treatment:** Supportive

ANS, autonomic nervous system; CMV, cytomegalovirus; EBV, Epstein-Barr virus; HAART, highly active antiretroviral therapy; HHV, human herpesvirus; HSV, herpes simplex virus; VZV, varicella-zoster virus.

Viral Meningitis

The etiology of viral meningitis is identified in 55–70% of cases. The herpes viruses, enteroviruses, flaviviruses, and retroviruses have all been implicated (Table 39.4). The treatment of viral meningitis is generally supportive. Viral *encephalitis*, however, may present with focal features, such as seizures, hallucinations, aphasia, and hemiparesis, and requires emergent antiviral therapy to limit morbidity and mortality. See Chapter 40, Fever and Focal Cerebral Dysfunction.

ENTEROVIRUSES

The most common causes of viral meningitis are the nonpolio enteroviruses. These viruses are found worldwide and cause disease in summer and autumn in temperate climates, and year-round in tropical and subtropical climates. They most often affect children, but epidemics in adults and adolescents have been reported. A prodrome of a flulike illness and sore throat is not unusual and is often followed by nausea, vomiting, fever, headache, meningismus, and occasionally a viral exanthem. In immunocompetent patients, the morbidity and mortality of enteroviral meningitis is very low, though recently enterovirus 71 has been associated with a poliomyelitis-like syndrome as well as encephalitis. In patients with agammaglobulinemia, enteroviruses can cause a severe, chronic meningoencephalitis. In neonates, especially those less than 2 weeks old, enteroviral meningitis or encephalitis can present with severe sepsis.

POLIO VIRUS

Polio is an enterovirus but is a very rare cause of viral meningitis in the developed world where vaccinations are routinely given. The oral live attenuated form of the polio vaccine can rarely cause an aseptic meningitis, but currently in the United States, only the injected form is used. In the unimmunized who live in or have recently traveled to endemic areas of Central Africa and West Asia, polio is still an important, although infrequent, cause of aseptic meningitis.

FLAVIVIRUSES

This family includes Japanese encephalitis complex, St. Louis encephalitis (SLE) virus, tick-borne encephalitis virus, and West Nile virus (WNV). Most often, infection with these viruses is asymptomatic or causes a mild febrile illness without central nervous system (CNS) involvement. In the United States, SLE is seen in the southern and southeastern states. West Nile virus is present in all continental United States, although the majority of cases in the past few years have been in the Rocky Mountain states and on the West Coast. The likelihood of CNS involvement depends on the viral strain and the immune status of the host. Older adults (age >50) or those who are immunocompromised are at increased risk for severe infection.

HUMAN IMMUNODEFICIENCY VIRUS

In the acute phase of infection, human immunodeficiency virus (HIV) can invade the CNS and cause an aseptic meningitis. Usually, this meningitis is accompanied by an acute retroviral (ARS) syndrome which includes fever, pharyngitis, lymphadenopathy, and sometimes a rash. In a patient with risk factors, serum HIV screening should be considered.

HERPES VIRUSES

Herpes simplex virus (HSV) 1 and 2, varicella-zoster virus (VZV), cytomegalovirus (CMV), and Epstein-Barr virus (EBV) have all been associated with aseptic meningitis. In an immunocompetent host, the most likely to cause aseptic meningitis is HSV-2, usually in association with a primary genital outbreak. Herpes zoster (VZV) has been associated with aseptic meningitis, and *zoster sine herpete* is VZV reactivation causing viral meningitis without the cutaneous lesions. CMV, EBV, and now human herpesvirus (HHV)-6 have been associated with meningitis, though all are much better known for causing encephalitis in the immunocompromised.

Although it is clear that in HSV encephalitis, treatment with acyclovir decreases the morbidity and mortality, there are no trials examining the role of antivirals in immunocompetent patients with herpesvirus meningitis. In the immunocompromised or in those with evidence of encephalitis, generally, it is recommended to treat HSV and VZV with acyclovir, and CMV with ganciclovir. Acyclovir or ganciclovir would treat EBV, and ganciclovir or foscarnet would be appropriate for HHV-6. Treatment is also recommended in patients diagnosed with Mollaret's meningitis, a recurrent aseptic meningitis associated with HSV-2 outbreaks, as prophylactic acyclovir may prevent recurrence.

LYMPHOCYTIC CHORIOMENINGITIS VIRUS (LCMV)

This arenavirus is a rare cause of aseptic meningitis in individuals with exposure to rodents: lab workers, pet owners, and those living in unhygienic conditions. It is most common in the fall. Although the affected patient rarely suffers sequelae, a devastating congenital infection can occur. Lethal infections have been recently described in organ transplant recipients that are treated with potent immunosuppressive drugs.

MUMPS

Prior to the introduction of widespread vaccination, mumps was a relatively common cause of aseptic meningitis. It occurs most often in winter and spring and usually infects children, although there have been recent U.S. outbreaks even among vaccinated and partially vaccinated adolescents and young adults. The meningitis can be associated with parotitis, precede parotitis, or be the only manifestation of an infection. The disease is generally benign in terms of neurologic outcomes. The vaccine has rarely (1–10/10,000 vaccinations) been associated with aseptic meningitis.

Key features that may help to distinguish viral from bacterial or chronic meningitis are:

- patients are generally not obtunded or truly altered
- not septic
- acute onset

Chronic Meningitis

Chronic meningitis can present with fever, headache, and mild meningismus, but as the name implies, it is chronic or subacute in nature. In general, chronic meningitis will present with a monocytic pleocytosis, a normal or mildly elevated protein, and a normal or low glucose.

FUNGAL MENINGITIS

Though fungal meningitis occurs most commonly in the immunocompromised or in patients with a prolonged hospital stay, there are several fungi which can also infect immunocompetent hosts (Table 39.5). In general, fungal meningitis presents with a mild cerebrospinal fluid (CSF) pleocytosis and an abnormally low CSF glucose level. The clinical presentation is often a basilar meningitis, which can affect cranial nerves or cause hydrocephalus.

Cryptococcus neoformans is distributed worldwide and can infect immunocompetent patients, but more commonly infects patients with acquired immunodeficiency syndrome (AIDS) or a history of prolonged, high-dose steroid use. In the immunosuppressed patient, the inflammatory response can be blunted, although fever is usually part of the presentation. Immunocompromised patients may lack a pleocytosis, which is a negative prognostic indicator. As increased intracranial pressure is a common feature, when suspicion for *C. neoformans* meningitis is high, and the opening pressure on lumbar puncture (LP) is between 250 mm H_2O and 400 mm H_2O,

Table 39.5 Fungal Meningitis

Fungus*	Associated Risks
Cryptococcus neoformans	• Found worldwide and can infect immunocompetent patients • Most commonly found in patients with AIDS or prolonged high-dose steroid use • Subacute symptoms common in all immunocompromised hosts: headache with or without fever and no nuchal rigidity • CSF can lack a pleocytosis, which is a bad prognostic sign • If the opening pressure is >250 mm H$_2$O, CSF should be drained to <200 mm H$_2$O or half of opening pressure • Diagnosis is made with the CSF cryptococcal antigen test, which is highly sensitive
Coccidioides immitis (Coccidioidomycosis)	• Most often seen in immunocompetent patients of certain ethnic groups (Filipinos, African Americans, and Latinos) • CSF eosinophilia is a hallmark • Diagnosis requires serum and CSF serology, which, if positive, should be confirmed with complement fixation titers
Candida spp.	• Seen in neonates, premature infants, neutropenic patients, those exposed to long courses of broad-spectrum antibiotics, and those with ventricular shunts • Neonates with candidemia have a higher risk of meningeal involvement compared to adults • Patients with CNS prosthetics such as shunts are predisposed to candidal meningitis without candidemia
Rare Fungal Infections in Severely Immunocompromised Hosts	• *Aspergillus* spp., *Histoplasmosis capsulatum*, *Pseudallescheria boydii* • Zygomycetes (*Rhizopus* spp.) in diabetics after a bout of DKA

*Fungal infections of the CNS often present with basilar meningitis, which can affect cranial nerves or cause hydrocephalus, leading to decreased levels of consciousness.

enough CSF should be drained to decrease the opening pressure to below 200 mm H$_2$O. If the opening pressure is higher than 400 mm H$_2$O, the closing pressure should be no lower than half the original opening pressure. Lowering the intracranial pressure will reduce complications such as cranial neuropathies, herniation, and death. CSF cryptococcal antigen testing is highly sensitive and specific for this disease and can be analyzed within 24 hours at most institutions.

Coccidioides immitis, a dimorphic fungus endemic to the southwestern United States, Mexico, and Central and South America, usually causes an asymptomatic or mildly symptomatic pulmonary infection, but can disseminate and cause meningitis in immunocompetent patients. Certain ethnic groups- Filipinos, African Americans, and Latinos are much more likely to have disseminated coccidioidomycosis than Caucasians. Testing for coccidioidomycosis requires serum and CSF serology, which, if positive, should be confirmed with complement fixation titers. The complement fixation titers help determine the likelihood of disseminated disease and can be followed for treatment effectiveness. CSF eosinophilia is common.

Meningitis caused by *Candida* species is seen most often in those who are at risk for invasive candidiasis: neonates, prematurely born infants, neutropenic patients, and those exposed to long courses of broad-spectrum antibiotics. Neonates with candidemia appear to have a much higher risk of meningeal involvement than adults with candidemia. Patients with ventricular shunts are predisposed to candidal meningitis without concomitant candidemia.

In the severely immunocompromised host, such as the immunosuppressed transplant patient or AIDS patient, meningitis can be caused by relatively unusual fungi, including *Aspergillus* species, *Histoplasma capsulatum*, and *Pseudallescheria boydii*. Zygomycete meningitis, such as *Rhizopus* species, can be seen secondary to invasion from the sinuses in poorly controlled diabetics, classically after an episode of diabetic ketoacidosis (DKA).

Chronic Bacterial Meningitis

TUBERCULOUS MENINGITIS

Tuberculosis (TB) is the most common cause of chronic bacterial meningitis worldwide. Risk factors include immigration from a country with a high rate of TB, homelessness, history of TB exposure, and history of incarceration. The CSF in tuberculous meningitis is characterized by a monocytic pleocytosis, occasionally a mild eosinophilia, low glucose, and moderately elevated protein. Definitive diagnosis is made by CSF PCR for TB DNA or culture for acid-fast bacilli, which requires 10 mL of CSF. If clinical suspicion is high enough and the CSF compatible with a diagnosis of tuberculous meningitis, initiating empiric four-drug therapy with or without adjunct steroids in consultation with an infectious disease specialist is appropriate.

Other rare causes of chronic meningitis include *Borrelia burgdorferi*, *Leptospirosis* spp., *Brucella* spp., *Francisella tularensis*, *Treponema pallidum*, and rickettsial diseases (other than Rocky Mountain spotted fever, which presents acutely).

Parasitic Meningitis

Taenia solium is the etiologic agent of cysticercosis, and thus neurocysticercosis, which is the most common cause of seizures worldwide. Although neurocysticercosis usually presents as a new seizure secondary to active or degenerating cysts in the parenchyma, cysts can develop in the ventricular system and produce subacute meningitis. If the cyst ruptures in the ventricle, a more acute decline can ensue. Neurocysticercosis meningitis is often accompanied by typical parenchymal lesions (Table 39.6). Treatment recommendations are beyond the scope of this chapter and should be made in consultation with a neurologist or infectious disease specialist.

Angiostrongylus cantonensis is found in Southeast Asia and the Pacific basin, which including Hawaii. It generally presents as an acute meningitis, often accompanied by cranial neuropathies and paresthesias in the limbs, trunk, or face. Treatment is supportive.

Both of these entities tend to produce CSF eosinophilia.

Noninfectious Chronic Meningitis

There are a variety of noninfectious causes of chronic meningitis (Table 39.7). These causes often present with the same

Table 39.6 Parasitic Meningitis

Etiology	Associated Risks
Taenia solium	• Found in various areas of the world, but not common in the United States • Etiologic agent of cysticercosis and neurocysticercosis • Cysts can develop in the ventricular system and produce subacute meningitis
Angiostrongylus cantonensis	• Found in Southeast Asia and the Pacific basin, including Hawaii • Generally presents as an acute meningitis • Often causes cranial neuropathies and paresthesias in the limbs, trunk, or face

Table 39.7 Noninfectious Chronic Meningitis

Noninfectious* Causes of Meningitis	Etiology
Chemical	• NSAIDs • Antibiotics (trimethoprim, amoxicillin, cephalosporins) • Immunosuppressants (azathioprine, cytarabine, OKT3 antibody)
Rheumatologic	• SLE • Sarcoid (often as basilar meningitis) • Wegener's granulomatosis • Behçet's
Tumor	• Carcinomatous meningitides – often the glucose is very low and cytology shows atypical cells • Send large volume (some recommend approximately 20 mL) for cytology, which should be done on same day as LP
Intrathecal	• Contrast • Chemotherapy

*Except for vasculitis and lymphoma, these noninfectious etiologies will generally not present with fever.
NSAID, nonsteroidal anti-inflammatory drug; SLE, systemic lupus erythematosus.

Table 39.8 IDSA Guidelines for Imaging Prior to Lumbar Puncture for Adults with Suspected Bacterial Meningitis

Head Imaging Prior to Lumbar Puncture	Age ≥60 History of CNS disease (mass lesion, stroke, focal infection) Immunocompromised History of seizure ≤1 week before presentation Abnormal neurologic exam*
Immunocompetent Immunocompromised	Noncontrast image sufficient Image with and without contrast to evaluate for parenchymal enhancing lesions

*Abnormal level of consciousness, inability to answer two consecutive questions or follow two consecutive commands, gaze palsy, abnormal visual fields, facial palsy, arm and/or leg drift, abnormal language.
IDSA, Infectious Diseases Society of America.

Table 39.9 Suggested CSF Studies

Routine Studies on All CSF	Cell count, glucose, protein, routine bacterial culture
Acute Aseptic Meningitis Immunocompromised	Consider enterovirus PCR, WNV IgM, WNV RT-PCR Same list as above, and VZV, CMV, EBV, HHV-6
Chronic Aseptic Meningitis: Immunocompetent Immunocompromised	VDRL, coccidioidomycosis serology and complement fixation, cryptococcal antigen, MTB (minimum 10 mL), cytology (minimum 10–20 mL) Same list as above and consider infectious disease or neurology consult
Eosinophilic Meningitis*	Consider cysticercosis serology, coccidioidomycosis serology and CF titer, MTB in appropriate patient

*Defined as >10 eosinophils and/or >10% eosinophils on cell count.
CF, complement fixation; MTB, *Mycobacterium tuberculosis*; RT-PCR, reverse transcriptase polymerase chain reaction; VDRL, venereal disease research laboratory.

subacute complaints as infectious chronic meningitis, except most lack fever as one of the presenting signs.

Key features that may help to distinguish chronic meningitis from viral or bacterial meningitis are:

• time course (subacute in chronic meningitis, acute in bacterial or viral meningitis.)
• mild meningismus
• immunocompromised patients may be afebrile

LABORATORY AND RADIOGRAPHIC FINDINGS

A lumbar puncture should be done in all patients with suspected meningitis. Imaging prior to LP is recommended in patients who are immunocompromised, who present with focal neurologic deficits or recent seizures, who present with moderate-to-severe impairment of consciousness, and, according to some sources, patients age 60 years or older and patients who have a history of CNS lesion(s) (Table 39.8).

CSF Studies

Ideally, the LP should be performed with the patient in a lateral decubitus position, so that an accurate opening pressure can be measured. After measuring and recording the opening pressure, we recommend collection of 2 mL of fluid in tubes 1 and 2, 6 mL in tube 3, and 10 mL in tube 4. Tube 1 is typically sent for cell count, tube 2 for protein and glucose, and tube 3 for microbiologic studies (Table 39.9). Tube 4 can be used for a second cell count to assess whether the tap was traumatic, for cytology, or for extra cultures, serologies, or PCR studies.

Interpreting the CSF

Generally, in acute bacterial meningitis, the white blood cell (WBC) count is elevated, often above 1000, with a neutrophilic predominance (Tables 39.10 and 39.11). Mildly elevated WBC counts (>5) can be seen in healthy premature infants and neonates, and chronic HIV infection can cause a mild, clinically asymptomatic CSF pleocytosis. Lymphocytic predominance can be seen in *Listeria* meningitis, neonatal gram-negative rod meningitis, and in both partially and fully treated

Table 39.10 General Guidelines for CSF Parameters in Different Diagnoses

Etiology	OP (mm)	Cell Count	Differential	Protein (mg/dL)	Glucose (mg/dL)	Other
Normal: Term* Child* Adult	80–110 <200	0–22 0–7 0–5	61% PMN 5% PMN 0%–rare	20–170 5–40 <45	34–119 40–80 >55	
Acute Bacterial Meningitis	Elevated	>1000†	PMNs predominate	Elevated	Low (CSF: serum ratio often <0.31)	Gram stain +
Viral Meningitis	Normal to mildly elevated	<1000	Monocytic‡	Normal to mild elevation	Normal to mildly low	Patient not septic or obtunded
Fungal or MTB	Often elevated	<500	Monocytic	Mild to highly elevated	Low	High volume for culture

*Adapted from Robertson J. Blood chemistry and body fluids. In: Robertson J, Shilkofski N, eds, Harriet Lane Handbook: a manual for pediatric housestaff, 17th ed. Philadelphia: Elsevier Mosby; 2005:table 25–3.
†Can be low to absent in the immunocompromised.
‡Refers to all cells that are not polymorphonuclear.
MTB, *Mycobacterium tuberculosis*; OP, opening pressure; PMN, polymorphonuclear neutrophil leukocyte.

Table 39.11 Differential Diagnoses of CSF Findings

Cell	Differential	Protein	Glucose	Differential Diagnosis
>1000	PMNs mostly	Elevated	Low	Bacterial meningitis, very early viral (generally <1000 cells)
<1000	Monocytic	Normal or mildly elevated	Normal or mildly low	Viral, partially treated bacterial, parameningeal focus (usually <100 cells), TB meningitis (though usually protein very elevated, glucose low), carcinomatous meningitides (atypical cells in cell count or cytology)
<1000	>10 absolute, and/or >10% eosinophils	Normal to elevated	Low	*A. cantonensis, C. immitis,* neurocysticercosis, sarcoidosis, MTB

MTB, *Mycobacterium tuberculosis*; PMN, polymorphonuclear neutrophil leukocyte.

bacterial meningitis. In acute bacterial meningitis, the protein is usually greater than 100 mg/dL, and the glucose is usually less than 40 mg/dL. When the patient has a very elevated serum blood glucose, estimating the CSF:serum glucose ratio can be helpful. Generally, ratios below 0.31 are more likely to indicate bacterial meningitis.

In viral meningitis, a milder lymphocytic pleocytosis (often 10–1000), with no or only mildly elevated opening pressure, is the rule. The protein is also mildly elevated, usually ranging between 50 and 80, whereas glucose is generally normal, above 40, and the CSF:serum ratio generally is greater than 0.31.

TREATMENT

The rapid administration of appropriate antibiotics is the most important step in the treatment of bacterial meningitis (Table 39.12), and although antibiotics should be given after blood cultures are drawn, they should not be significantly delayed for any reason. If brain imaging is required prior to LP, empiric antibiotics should be given immediately after blood cultures are drawn but prior to imaging and LP. The CSF pleocytosis will persist, though the likelihood of recovering a bacterial organism from the CSF culture decreases with the time from antibiotic administration.

Steroids

In 2002 a prospective, double-blinded, randomized study of adults with bacterial meningitis showed an overall benefit from treatment with 4 days of dexamethasone initiated with or before the first dose of antibiotics.

Several criticisms have been made of this study, including that all of the *S. pneumoniae* organisms tested were penicillin sensitive, and that the benefit was seen only in the *S. pneumoniae* group. Despite these and other concerns, as this study showed no detrimental effects from giving the dexamethasone to any group of patients, the IDSA guidelines recommend, in adults, giving dexamethasone 0.15 mg/kg intravenous (IV) with or before the first dose of antibiotics and every 6 hours thereafter to patients with suspected or proven bacterial meningitis, except for those who are in septic shock. There is no clear consensus on whether or not to continue the steroids in patients who are found not to have pneumococcal meningitis. Dexamethasone may decrease the CSF penetration of vancomycin, and some experts advocate adding

Table 39.12 Treatment of Bacterial Meningitis

Patient Category	Organism	Empiric Treatment
Neonates (<1 month)	• Group B Streptococcus • Escherichia coli, Klebsiella pneumoniae • Listeria monocytogenes	ampicillin: 0–7 days old: 150 mg/kg/day IV (divided q8h) 8–28 days: 200 mg/kg/day IV (divided q6–8h) plus 0–7 days: cefotaxime 100–150 mg/kg/day IV (divided q8–12h) 8–28 days: 150–200 mg/kg/day IV (divided q6–8h) or aminoglycoside amikacin: 0–7 days: 15–20 mg/kg/day IV (divided q12h) 8–28 days: 30 mg/kg/day IV (divided q8h) gentamicin or tobramycin 0–7 days: 5 mg/kg/day IV (divided q12h) 8–28 days: 7.5 mg/kg/day IV (divided q8h)
1 month–5 years	• Neisseria meningitidis • Streptococcus pneumoniae • Haemophilus influenza B	vancomycin 60 mg/kg IV (divided q6h) plus ceftriaxone 80–100 mg/kg IV (divided q12–24h) or cefotaxime 225–300 mg/kg IV (divided q6–8h)
6–50 years	• Neisseria meningitidis • Streptococcus pneumoniae	vancomycin Pediatric: see previous box Adult: 500–1000 mg IV q8–12h plus ceftriaxone Pediatric: see previous box Adult: 2g IV q12h or cefotaxime Pediatric: see previous box Adult: 2 g IV q4–6h
>50 years	• Streptococcus pneumoniae • Neisseria meningitidis • Listeria monocytogenes	vancomycin (dose as above) plus ceftriaxone or cefotaxime (dose as above) plus ampicillin 2 g IV q4h Consider rifampin 300 PO/IV q8–12h instead of vancomycin if steroids are administered

rifampin to the regimen if dexamethasone is to be used with vancomycin.

In the pediatric population, dexamethasone given before or with the first dose of antibiotics decreased the incidence of hearing loss or neurologic complications, especially in children with HIB meningitis. Thus in children with HIB, the recommendation is to give 0.15 mg/kg every 6 hours for 2–4 days. The evidence is less clear for pneumococcal meningitis, and the current recommendation is to consider dexamethasone in children with pneumococcal disease. For infants less than 6 weeks old, there are not enough data to make a recommendation for or against adjuvant dexamethasone.

If steroids are given, they should be given prior to or simultaneously with antibiotics.

SPECIAL CONSIDERATIONS

Shunt Infections

Generally the diagnosis of CSF infections secondary to internalized shunts, such as ventriculoperitoneal or ventriculoatrial shunts, will require tapping of the shunt. The patients often present with shunt malfunction and signs of increased intracranial pressure such as headache, nausea, and decreased level of consciousness or lethargy. They may or may not have fever. Infecting organisms are often coagulase-negative Staphylococcus, Staphylococcus aureus, P. acnes, E. coli, Klebsiella, Proteus, or Pseudomonas aeruginosa. Given this range of organisms, the recommendation is to start vancomycin, and a cephalosporin (e.g., ceftazidime or cefepime) or carbapenem (e.g., meropenem) with anti-pseudomonal activity. In general, these patients should be managed in consultation with neurosurgery and infectious disease specialists. In general, infected shunts must be removed.

Skull Fractures, Penetrating Trauma, or History of Neurosurgical Procedure

There are no data to support prophylactic antibiotics to prevent meningitis in patients with basilar skull fractures. If a patient with a known history of skull fracture or CSF leak presents with symptoms consistent with meningitis, then empiric antibiotics should again include vancomycin and a cephalosporin or carbapenem with anti-pseudomonal activity.

Immunocompromised Patients

Immunocompromised patients include those with HIV and CD4 count below 500 or AIDS, those with a history of transplant who are on immunosuppressive therapy, and those taking chronic steroids above 20 mg daily. Immunocompromised patients have a blunted inflammatory response and may lack meningismus or fever in the setting of meningitis. All immunocompromised patients should have neuroimaging with contrast prior to LP. Additionally, because immunocompromised patients may have meningitis without an associated pleocytosis, the general guidelines for evaluating CSF may not apply. Finally, viral meningitis in the immunocompromised can be life-threatening.

COMPLICATIONS AND ADMISSION CRITERIA

Any patient with proven or highly suspected bacterial meningitis should be admitted. Patients with viral meningitis may require admission if they are unable to keep down food and liquids or require IV medications for pain control. A patient with suspected viral meningitis may be discharged when there is a friend or family member available to monitor the patient for signs or symptoms requiring return to the

Table 39.13 Chemoprophylaxis

Organism	Contact	Antibiotic Regimen
Neisseria meningitidis	• All household contacts • Child care or school contacts • Contacts with exposure to secretions of index case (including health care workers) • Contact in above categories occurring ≤7 days prior to onset of illness in index case	rifampin*: Neonate: 5 mg/kg PO qd × 2 days ≥1 mo: 10 mg/kg PO qd × 2 days ceftriaxone: <16 years 125 mg IM once <16 years 250 mg IM once ciprofloxacin: <18 years: 500 mg PO once
Haemophilus influenzae B	• All household contacts, if household includes any susceptible child† • Nursery or child care contacts if contain susceptible children *and* if there have been ≥2 cases at the nursery or child care facility within 60 days • Index case if ≤2 years old or has a susceptible household member *and* index case treated with antibiotics other than ceftriaxone or cefotaxime	rifampin*: Neonates: 10 mg/kg PO qd × 4 days ≥1 month old: 20 mg/kg PO qd × 4 days

*Maximum rifampin daily dose: 600 mg.
†Unimmunized or partially immunized children <4 years old or immunocompromised children regardless of age and immunization status. Adapted from American Academy of Pediatrics. *Haemophilus influenzae* infections. In: Pickering LK, Baker CJ, Long SS, McMillan JA, eds. Red book: 2006 report of the Committee on Infectious Disease, 27th ed. Elk Grove Village, IL; American Academy of Pediatrics, 2006:310–8.

emergency department (not improving in 24–48 hours, unable to keep down food or liquids, increasing lethargy or altered mental status). Patients with chronic meningitis who do not appear to have hydrocephalus or other concerns for increased intracranial pressure can also be discharged from the ED if they have reliable follow-up.

Increased intracranial pressure (ICP) can be a complication of any form of meningitis, though it is generally not seen in viral meningitis. Uncontrolled increased ICP can lead to permanent neurologic sequelae or death. Several mechanisms can lead to elevated ICP, including diffuse inflammation associated with bacterial meningitis, or hydrocephalus associated with arachnoiditis in subacute meningitis. Symptoms of elevated ICP include headache, lethargy, nausea, and vomiting, all of which are progressive. Measures used to control ICP include hyperventilation, IV mannitol, hypertonic saline, or removal of CSF by repeat lumbar punctures or external ventricular drainage.

INFECTION CONTROL

In general, most etiologies of meningitis do not require contact isolation. The only exceptions are *N. meningitidis* and tuberculous meningitis. Patients with meningococcal disease will need to be in contact isolation, and close contacts will need chemoprophylaxis as described in Table 39.13. Patients with HIB meningitis do not need isolation precautions, but chemoprophylaxis may be necessary.

Patients with proven or suspected tuberculous meningitis should be placed in respiratory isolation until an active respiratory infection can be ruled out. Depending on state-specific guidelines, these cases may require reporting to the department of public health, who may initiate contact screening.

In general, patients with viral meningitis do not need to be isolated, though contact precautions should be considered in cases associated with severe enterovirus diarrhea.

PEARLS AND PITFALLS

1. Never delay appropriate antibiotic therapy for neuroimaging.
2. In neonates and infants, meningitis can present with fever and nonspecific signs.
3. Viral meningitis does not cause obtundation or sepsis (except rarely in neonates and the immunocompromised).
4. Immunocompromised patients with meningitis can present with relatively mild symptoms, and they may have a very mild or no CSF pleocytosis.
5. If a lumbar puncture is considered, it should probably be done.
6. Give steroids prior to or with antibiotics.

REFERENCES

Centers for Disease Control and Prevention (CDC). Rocky Mountain spotted fever. Available at: http://www.cdc.gov/ncidod/dvrd/rmsf/index.htm. Accessed May 18, 2006.

Chadwick DR. Viral meningitis. Brit Med Bull 2005;75–76:1–14.

Chang L-Y, Huang L-M, Gau SS-F, et al. Neurodevelopment and cognition in children after enterovirus 71 infection. N Engl J Med 2007;356:1226–34.

Chavez-Bueno S, McCracken GH. Bacterial meningitis in children. Pediatr Clin North Am 2005;52:795–810.

Davis LE. Subacute and chronic meningitis. Continuum 2006;12: 27–57.

Fishman RA. Cerebrospinal fluid in diseases of the nervous system, 2nd ed. Philadelphia: WB Saunders, 1992.

Gottfredsson M, Perfect JR. Fungal meningitis. Semin Neurol 2000;20:307–22.

Khetsuriani N, Quiroz ES, Holman RC, Anderson LJ. Viral meningitis-associated hospitalizations in the United States, 1988–1999. Neuroepidemiology 2003;22:345–52.

Lo Re III V, Gluckman SJ. Eosinophilic meningitis due to *Angiostrongylus cantonensis* in a returned traveler: case report and review of the literature. Clin Infect Dis 2001;33:e112–5.

Rotbart HA. Viral meningitis. Semin Neurol 2000;20:277–92.

Trunkel AR, Hartman BJ, Kaplan SL, et al. Practice guidelines for the management of bacterial meningitis. Clin Infect Dis 2004;39:1267–84.

Tunkel AR, Scheld WM. Acute meningitis. In: Mandell GL, Bennett JE, Dolin R, eds, Principles and practice of infectious disease, 6th ed. Philadelphia: Churchill Livingstone, 2005:1084–126.

van de Beek D, de Gans J, Spanjaard L, et al. Clinical features and prognostic factors in adults with bacterial meningitis. N Engl J Med 2004;351:1849–59.

ADDITIONAL READINGS

DeBiasi RL, Tyler KL. Viral meningitis and encephalitis. Continuum 2006;12:58–94.

de Gans J, van De Beek. Dexamethasone in adults with bacterial meningitis. N Engl J Med 2002;347:1549–56.

Garcia HH, del Butto OH. Neurocysticercosis: updated concepts about an old disease. Lancet Neurol 2005;4:653–61.

Ginsburg L. Difficult and recurrent meningitis. J Neurol Neurosurg Psychiatry 2004;75(Suppl 1):i16–i21.

Saag MS, Graybill RJ, Larsen RA, et al. Practice guidelines for the management of cryptococcal disease. Clin Infect Dis 2000; 30:710–8.

40. Fever and Focal Cerebral Dysfunction

Serena S. Spudich

INTRODUCTION

A focal cerebral neurological finding in the presence of fever suggests infection or inflammation of the brain or surrounding tissues, or a cerebral complication of systemic infection. Asymmetrical motor or sensory findings, such as one-sided weakness or numbness, or language dysfunction, are more obvious findings. Perceptual deficits such as deficits in reading comprehension, visual field cuts, apraxias, ataxia, and confusion may be more subtle presentations of focal cerebral disease. Cerebral infections may be accompanied by headache and are commonly associated with the development of either focal or generalized seizures. Fever may also be absent or intermittent in infectious cerebral disease, and clinicians should have a low threshold for considering these diagnoses in the appropriate context. Focal neurological findings in the setting of suspected or known infection constitute an emergency. This chapter focuses on focal cerebral infections in immunocompetent hosts. For a discussion of causes of fever and headache, see Chapter 39, Fever and Headache. For a discussion of central nervous system infections in the immunocompromised, see Chapter 42, Altered Mental Status in HIV-Infected Patients.

GENERAL DIFFERENTIAL DIAGNOSIS

Main Diagnoses to Consider

The most common serious causes of fever and focal neurological deficit are intracranial abscess from a local or hematogenous source, and focal encephalitis with herpes simplex virus.

Historical features suggestive of intracranial abscess include:

- recent dental work
- recent ear infection, mastoiditis, sinusitis, tooth abscess, or pneumonia
- recent trauma or neurological surgery
- history of valvular disease, congenital heart disease, or endocarditis
- history of chronic infection such as osteomyelitis
- recent travel to tropical environment
- recent intravenous drug abuse

Historical features suggestive of focal encephalitis include:

- history of insect bite
- history of vesicles/rash on lips or face
- recent upper respiratory infection (URI) or gastrointestinal (GI) prodrome

Other diagnoses to consider are shown in Table 40.1.

INTRACRANIAL ABSCESS

Epidemiology

A focus of infection within the cranial vault is due to trafficking of infection via one of three routes:

- local spread from adjacent infected site, such as the mastoid bone, frontal sinuses, or middle ear
- bloodborne infection from an intravascular source (endocarditis) or other remote site (dental abscess, lung infection, osteomyelitis)
- seeding through penetrating brain injury from trauma or a neurosurgical procedure

Intracranial abscesses affect persons of all ages, although specific etiologies are most common in certain risk groups. Intracranial abscesses due to contiguous infectious otitis are most common in children, whereas those secondary to sinusitis are found most often in young adults. Elderly and mildly immunocompromised patients (e.g., those with diabetes or chronic alcoholism) are at increased risk of brain abscesses from lung or other bloodborne sources of infection, as are young persons with cyanotic congenital heart disease. This condition has a mortality rate between 10% and 40% even in the current era of antibiotics and a high neurological morbidity rate in survivors of up to 60%. Because the risk of

Table 40.1 Differential Diagnosis of Fever and Focal Cerebral Dysfuction

- Exacerbation of chronic deficit in setting of systemic infection
- Bacterial or aseptic meningitis
- Lyme disease or neuroborreliosis
- West Nile virus encephalomyelitis
- Poliomyelitis or other enterovirus meningoencephalitis
- CNS Whipple's disease
- Inflammatory myopathy
- Acute intermittent porphyria
- Subarachnoid hemorrhage
- Oto-rhinocerebral infection
- Neoplasm

- Acute thiamine deficiency
- Paraneoplastic encephalitis
- Cerebral septic thrombophlebitis
- Mitochondrial myopathy, encephalopathy, lactic acidosis, and strokelike episodes (MELAS)
- Vasculitis of the nervous system
- Hemorrhagic leukoencephalitis
- Neuro-Behçet's disease

CNS, central nervous system.

Table 40.2 Intraparenchymal Brain Abscess: Etiological Organisms Based on Predisposing Condition

Sinusitis	*Streptococcus, Bacteroides, Fusobacterium, Haemophilus*
Dental Abscess	*Streptococcus, Bacteroides, Fusobacterium*
Ear Infection	*Enterobacteriaceae, Streptococcus, Staphylococcus, Pseudomonas, Bacteroides*
Lung Infection	*Streptococcus, Fusobacterium, Actinomyces, Nocardia*
Endocarditis	*Streptococcus viridans, Staphylococcus aureus*
Congenital Cardiac Disease	*Streptococcus, Haemophilus*
Penetrating Head Trauma or Postneurosurgery	*Staphylococcus aureus, Enterobacter, Clostridium, Streptococcus, Pseudomonas*

Table 40.3 Clinical Features: Intraparenchymal Brain Abscess

Abscess Development	• 1–3 days: focal cerebritis after local seeding • 4–9 days: necrosis of capsule core, angiogenesis around abscess • >10 days: collagen capsule formation around abscess, inflammation and edema
Signs and Symptoms	**Initial phase**: • May be neurologically asymptomatic or have progressive headache • If abscess due to dental, ear, sinus, or pulmonary infection, may have associated symptoms **Subacute phase**: • Progressively worsening headache (75%) • Focal neurological deficit (65%) • Symptoms of increased intracranial pressure (25%) • May or may not have signs of systemic infection (<50% in most series) • May progress to seizures (40%), sudden loss of consciousness with high fever if abscess ruptures into ventricle, or brain herniation and death
Laboratory and Radiologic Findings	• Peripheral white blood count is mildly elevated in two-thirds of patients • ESR is elevated in 60–90% of patients • CSF cultures are rarely diagnostic, lumbar puncture often contraindicated • Blood cultures positive in 15–30% of patients, most informative in those with systemic signs of infection • CT may demonstrate a hazy hypointense (dark) lesion that becomes surrounded by a bright ring of enhancement on the administration of contrast • MRI shows a distinctly hypointense lesion on T1 sequences, encircled by a ring of contrast after IV injection of gadolinium; extensive edema around the lesion is seen on T2 sequences; pyogenic abscesses appear bright on DWI sequences

CSF, cerebrospinal fluid; CT, computed tomography; DWI, diffusion-weighted imaging; ESR, erythrocyte sedimentation rate; MRI, magnetic resonance imaging.

neurological sequelae and death is directly correlated with time to diagnosis and treatment, early identification and management of this condition are essential.

Clinical Features

An intracranial abscess may be defined as an intraparenchymal brain abscess, a subdural empyema, or an intracranial epidural, also termed extradural abscess. Though all are rare, brain abscess is the most common, with 10,000 cases reported in the United States each year.

INTRAPARENCHYMAL BRAIN ABSCESS: CLINICAL PRESENTATION

Brain abscesses develop in the cerebral parenchyma, most commonly in the white matter of the brain, presumably due to the reduced blood supply of this region relative to the cerebral cortex. The most common means of infection is from extension of infection from adjoining tissues (Table 40.2). Contiguous infections lead to single abscesses in locations related to

the initial site of infection: otitis leads to temporal or cerebellar lesions, sinusitis usually to frontal or deep temporal lobe abscesses. These infections may be associated with septic venous thrombophlebitis, leading to cerebral infarction and metastatic infections.

Bloodborne infection may lead to single or multiple abscesses, with sources related to chronic lung disease, congenital heart disease with right-to-left shunting, pulmonary arteriovenous fistula, and rarely, bacterial endocarditis (brain abscess occurs in less than 1% of cases of infective endocarditis in most series). Streptococci (both aerobic and anaerobic), *Staphylococcus aureus*, and *Bacteroides* are the most common organisms isolated; anaerobic organisms are found in 50–90% and multiple organisms are found in 20% of brain abscesses. Specific typical causative organisms vary depending on the route and source of infection.

The classic presentation of a brain abscess includes rapid development over days of headache, focal neurological dysfunction, and fever (Table 40.3). However, the complete triad is rare, especially in the earliest stages of disease. Notably, a temperature greater than 38.5°C is present in only 20% to

57% of cases. Only approximately one quarter of patients with brain abscess exhibit signs of increased intracranial pressure, such as nausea and vomiting. Furthermore, signs and symptoms may be chronic, progressing over weeks. Often, an indolent, largely asymptomatic course is punctuated by the sudden onset of generalized or focal seizures (40%), leading to hospital presentation and diagnostic work-up.

Though the earliest stages of cerebritis and abscess capsule formation may be relatively asymptomatic, a mature abscess can cause symptoms by direct tissue compression or from the surrounding inflammatory reaction. As a result, the clinical presentation can be identical to that of malignant or inflammatory CNS lesions.

EPIDURAL BRAIN ABSCESS AND SUBDURAL EMPYEMA

Rarely, abscesses external to the brain but within the intracranial layers of the meninges can lead to focal neurological deficits. Intracranial epidural abscesses, by definition occurring in the space between the dura and the skull, are far less common than spinal epidural infections, parenchymal abscesses, and subdural empyema. They occur almost exclusively in the setting of underlying local infection such as mastoiditis, sinusitis, or otitis and often develop adjacent to a parenchymal or subdural pus collection, or in conjunction with septic venous thrombophlebitis. Their clinical presentation is characterized predominantly by headache. Focal neurological deficits are usually related to cortical structures local to the lesion and include disruptions of language, primary motor functions, or sensation.

Subdural empyema is an infectious collection occurring between the dura and the arachnoid, which most commonly occurs in the setting of infection in adjoining otic structures or sinuses (70–90% of cases), or along tracts created by trauma or surgery. Subdural empyema typically presents with fulminant headache, fever, and signs of increased intracranial pressure (ICP). The condition may progress rapidly over days and can be fatal if not promptly drained. The main means of differentiating between intraparenchymal brain abscess and epidural brain abscess or subdural empyema is via neuroimaging.

Differential Diagnosis

Because classic signs and symptoms of infection are often absent, a high index of suspicion is necessary to differentiate brain abscesses from other causes of focal neurological symptoms. An indolent brain abscess most often mimics the weeks- to months-long course of a primary or metastatic tumor, though occasionally the natural history is punctuated by sudden clinical worsening due to rupture into a ventricle or rapid expansion of the mass.

Key features that distinguish intracranial abscess from other conditions are:

- presence of infection at other sites including intravascular or local contiguous source
- focal neurological symptom and predominant headache in the setting of signs or symptoms of systemic infection

Other conditions to consider include:

- primary brain tumor
- epidural hematoma
- metastatic brain tumor

- ischemic or hemorrhagic stroke
- granulomatous disease (e.g., tuberculosis)
- demyelinating disease
- subdural hematoma

Laboratory and Radiographic Findings

Lumbar puncture is almost always contraindicated in the evaluation of a patient with suspected or confirmed brain abscess, because of the frequently associated mass effect and elevated ICP that increase the risk of cerebral herniation. In one series, 15% of patients who underwent lumbar puncture in the setting of brain abscess experienced brain herniation and death in the subsequent hours to days. In the same series, only 7% of cerebrospinal fluid (CSF) cultures obtained from these patients yielded an etiological organism found in the abscess cavity, whereas 11% of blood cultures were diagnostic. Based on the high risk of severe morbidity and the lack of information provided by CSF sampling, CSF analysis is not indicated in the evaluation of suspected brain abscess.

The gold standard for diagnosis of brain abscess is direct examination and culture of tissue obtained through a stereotactic biopsy or excision of the lesion. In early cerebritis, a computed tomographic (CT) scan may appear normal or show a hazy hypointense (dark) region that does not enhance following intravenous injection with contrast. The most typical CT findings of an established abscess are a hypointense lesion surrounded by a bright enhancing ring with the administration of contrast. An abscess or a malignant lesion may be surrounded by a large hypointense area of edema, which may be accompanied by mass effect and displacement of brain structures.

Magnetic resonance imaging (MRI) can be more helpful in differentiating an infectious abscess from a neoplastic lesion (Figure 40.1). In a T1-weighted MRI scan, abscesses demonstrate a hypointense core surrounded by a smooth ring of contrast when gadolinium is administered. T2-weighted MRI scans show a hyperintense lesion, a slightly hypointense surrounding rim, and extensive hyperintense surrounding signal representing edema. A diffusion-weighted imaging (DWI) sequence can be helpful in differentiating a noninfectious or inflammatory lesion from a pyogenic brain abscess.

Treatment and Prophylaxis

Management of brain abscess involves prompt hospitalization, close clinical monitoring, intravenous (IV) antibiotic therapy, and a plan for definitive diagnosis. Initial antibiotic therapy should be chosen based on the suspected route (hematogenous, local, or direct trauma or instrumentation) and source of infection (see Table 40.4). Dexamethasone at 8 to 12 mg IV (loading dose) followed by 4 to 6 mg every 6 hours may be an adjunct to antibiotic therapy in patients with life-threatening edema and mass effect. However, corticosteroids may decrease penetration of antibiotics, interfere with formation of an abscess capsule, and have long-term immunosuppressive effects; therefore they should be discontinued promptly once the mass effect is surgically or medically reduced.

In most cases, surgical intervention is required for effective treatment of brain abscesses, and it is the only means of definitive diagnosis. Though a proportion of brain abscesses remain cryptic in origin, up to 80% of cases of surgical drainage or

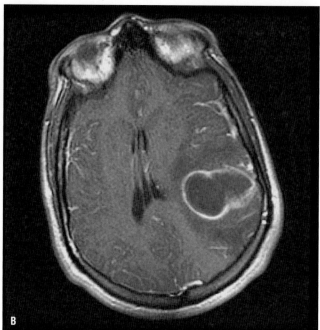

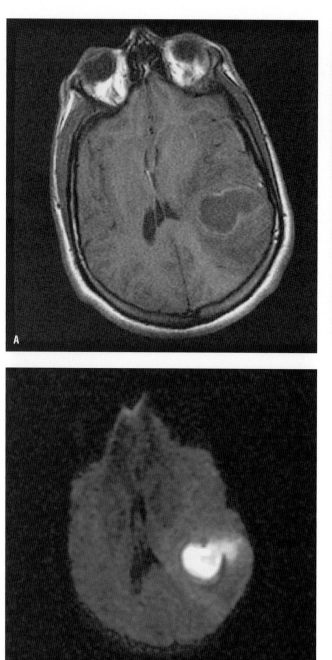

Figure 40.1   MRI images of a patient with a streptococcal brain abscess in the setting of congenital heart disease. T1-weighted image without contrast (A) shows a bi-lobed lesion with a hypointense (dark) core, surrounded by a brighter capsule, leading to significant local edema and mass effect upon the ventricles. After the administration of contrast, a typical outline of the lesion with contrast appears (B). The core of the lesion appears dramatically bright on diffusion weighted imaging (DWI), typical of a pyogenic brain abscess (C).

excision yield at least one causative organism, even in the setting of prior antibiotic therapy.

Duration of treatment with antibiotics is usually 6 to 8 weeks, although the clinical course and the appearance of lesions on neuroimaging should inform duration of therapy. Usually, neurological deficits improve promptly with reduction of mass effect by surgical intervention or antibiotic treatment, and signs of generalized infection, such as fever, improve in response to antibiotic treatment. Appearance of

edema on neuroimaging resolves within weeks of therapy, although vestigial enhancement around the abscess cavity can persist even in the setting of successful treatment.

In the setting of suspected or confirmed brain abscess, addition of prophylactic antiepileptic therapy is appropriate because of the high incidence (40%) of seizures in the course of the disease. As a result, neurologists often recommend prophylactic intravenous loading doses of phenytoin or phosphenytoin as soon as an infectious brain lesion is

Table 40.4 Intracranial Abscess: Initial Empiric Intravenous Antibiotic Therapy Based on Predisposing Route of Infection

Presumed Route of Infection	Therapy Recommendation (Same Doses for Each Drug for Each Indication)
Sinusitis, Dental Abscess, Ear Infection	metronidazole (15 mg/kg IV as a loading dose, followed by 7.5 mg/kg IV q6–8h) *plus* penicillin G (20 to 24 million units per day IV in six equally divided doses) *or* ceftriaxone (2 g IV q12h) *or* cefotaxime (2 g IV q4–6h).
Lung Infection or Congenital Cardiac Disease	nafcillin or oxacillin (2 g IV q4h) *or* vancomycin (15 mg/kg IV q12h) *plus* metronidazole (15 mg/kg IV as a loading dose, followed by 7.5 mg/kg IV q6–8h) Sulfadiazine and pyramethamine should be added if *Nocardia* is in consideration as etiological agent in pulmonary infection.
Endocarditis	nafcillin or oxacillin (2 g IV q4h) *or* vancomycin (15 mg/kg IV q12h)
Penetrating Head Trauma or Postneurosurgery	vancomycin (15 mg/kg IV q12h) *or* nafcillin (2 g IV q4h) *plus* ceftazidime (2 g IV q8h) *or* cefepime (2 g IV q8h)

suspected. Seizure therapy may eventually be discontinued in patients who have significant resolution with appropriate surgical or medical therapy, usually after several months and after further evaluation with electroencephalography.

Complications and Admission Criteria

All patients with suspected or confirmed brain abscess should be admitted for diagnosis, monitoring, and treatment. Potential complications include progressive loss of consciousness from increasing intracranial pressure, development of generalized seizures or status epilepticus, and sudden loss of consciousness and high fever in the setting of abscess rupture into the ventricles.

Infection Control

Transmission of underlying source infections, such as pulmonary tuberculosis, should be considered on an individual basis for determination of necessary infection control precautions. In general, however, standard precautions are adequate for patients with pyogenic brain abscesses.

Pearls and Pitfalls

1. Lumbar puncture is almost always contraindicated and CSF analysis is often uninformative in brain abscess.
2. Typical signs of infection (fever, elevated erythrocyte sedimentation rate [ESR] or markedly elevated peripheral

white blood cell count [WBC]) are absent in up to 50% of patients with brain abscess.
3. Diffusion-weighted imaging on MRI is sensitive and specific in differentiating brain tumors from pyogenic abscesses in the brain, subdural, and epidural space.

FOCAL ENCEPHALITIS

Epidemiology

Focal encephalitis is most commonly due to infection with the herpes simplex virus type 1 (HSV-1) and can rapidly lead to severe neurological dysfunction, coma, and death. Despite the availability of pathogen-specific antiviral treatment and supportive care, mortality from HSV-1 encephalitis remains at 30%. Early treatment decreases both morbidity and mortality, making early detection and antiviral intervention critical.

Approximately 4000 cases of HSV-1 encephalitis are identified in the United States each year. These infections occur in all age groups with a bimodal distribution: a third of infections affect children and young adults, but the peak incidence of disease is in the seventh decade. Although infants younger than 1 year old may be affected, the majority of cases of encephalitis are due to reactivation of prior infection rather than primary infection. There is no seasonal or geographic distribution to the incidence of encephalitis caused by HSV-1.

Clinical Features

Typically, HSV-1 encephalitis presents with a rapid clinical course over days, characterized by somnolence or disorientation, personality change, fever, headache, and focal or generalized seizures (Table 40.5). The classic focal findings of aphasia and hemiparesis indicate involvement of the temporal and frontal lobes and may be evident early in the course of disease or develop only after an initial period of seemingly diffuse encephalopathy. Any change in mentation in the setting of fever or other signs of infection should raise the possibility of HSV-1 encephalitis, even in the absence of more focal features, which may manifest later.

Differential Diagnosis

Although these patients occasionally present with focal seizures or language dysfunction that immediately suggests a focal encephalitis, they most commonly present with a nonspecific clinical picture that requires a high index of suspicion for encephalitis.

Key features that distinguish HSV-1 encephalitis from other conditions are:

- aphasia or hemiparesis, indicating focal involvement of the temporal and frontal lobes
- neuroimaging or electroencephalographic (EEG) findings that localize focal lesions to the temporal or frontal lobes
- hemorrhagic lesions on imaging or evidence of blood in CSF, suggestive of typical necrotic lesions of HSV
- changes in personality, behavior, and level of consciousness reflect involvement of the cerebral parenchyma rather than inflammation of the meninges that characterizes isolated meningitis

Table 40.5 Clinical Features: Herpes Simplex Encephalitis

Symptoms at Onset (Typically Days 1 Through 3)	• Reduced level of consciousness or confusion (97%) • Fever (90%) • Headache (80%) • Behavior change (70%) • Seizure (67%)
Symptoms at Presentation	• Fever (90%) • Behavior change (85%) • Aphasia (75%) • Hemiparesis (40%) • Continued seizures, may develop focal or generalized status epilepticus • Progressive confusion, somnolence, may progress to coma
Laboratory Findings	• CSF typically shows lymphocytic pleocytosis 10–500 cells/mm^3 • CSF may have xanthochromia or elevated red blood cells from hemorrhagic necrosis in cerebral lesions • Up to 10% of patients may have normal CSF cell count • CSF protein is elevated in 80% of cases • CSF glucose may be mildly reduced • Blood serologies and cultures are uninformative • CSF PCR for HSV-1 DNA is both >90% sensitive and specific before antibiotic therapy; sensitivity declines to 50% in first 2 weeks of therapy and <20% thereafter

PCR, polymerase chain reaction.

Other conditions to consider are:

- subarachnoid hemorrhage
- aseptic or bacterial meningitis
- early stage brain abscess
- non-herpes viral encephalitides (West Nile, St. Louis, alphavirus, enterovirus)
- varicella-zoster virus encephalitis
- human immunodeficiency virus (HIV)-1 encephalitis
- hemorrhagic leukoencephalitis
- acute disseminated encephalomyelitis (ADEM)
- paraneoplastic encephalitis
- human herpesvirus (HHV)-6 encephalitis
- noninfectious encephalopathy

Laboratory and Radiographic Findings

The gold standard for diagnosis of HSV-1 encephalitis is brain biopsy, though a highly sensitive and specific PCR assay for HSV-1 DNA from CSF has obviated this need in the majority of cases. If, however, a patient has seizures, focal neurological signs or symptoms, or an altered level of consciousness, neuroimaging should precede lumbar puncture to exclude a mass lesion that would place the patient at risk for herniation. CT should be obtained with and without contrast and will be negative in most patients early in the course of disease, although it may show hypointense lesions in the temporal lobes, indicating edema or necrosis. MRI is far more sensitive for the early abnormalities of HSV-1 encephalitis, but may also be normal in up to 10% of patients with evidence of disease by PCR. Typical findings on MRI are hypointense areas in the temporal and frontal lobes on T1 sequences that may hazily enhance with administration of gadolinium. Edema is especially evident on fluid attenuated inversion recovery (FLAIR) and T2 sequences (Figure 40.2), and

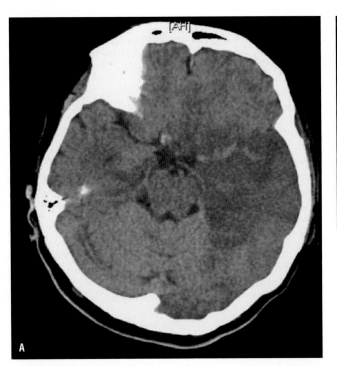

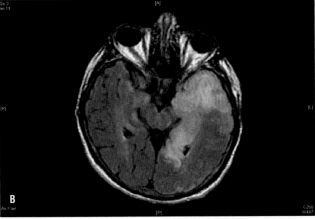

Figure 40.2   Brain images of a patient with HSV-1 encephalitis. CT scan (A) shows an area of hypodensity (darkness) in the temporal lobe on the right side of the image, suggesting edema and necrosis. Fluid attenuated inversion recovery (FLAIR) MRI image (B) better demonstrates extensive bright signal in the cortex of the temporal lobe on the same side, typical in location and appearance of HSV-1 encephalitis. Images courtesy of Dr. Steven K. Feske.

Table 40.6 Recommended Therapy for Focal Encephalitis

Acyclovir 10 mg/kg IV q6–8h × 14–21 days
Antiepileptic therapy such as IV phenytoin or phosphenytoin

gradient echo sequences may show evidence of petechial hemorrhage in the most necrotic areas of the lesions.

Once a mass lesion and severe cerebral edema are excluded, CSF should be sent for cell counts, protein and glucose, Gram stain, culture, and HSV-1/HSV-2 polymerase chain reaction (PCR). CSF HSV-1 PCR has diminishing sensitivity over the course of treatment, but also may be negative very early in the course. Herpes simplex rarely grows in culture from CSF, but if the diagnosis of HSV-1 encephalitis is incorrect, culture may yield the true etiological organism. Similarly, special CSF studies (fungal or mycobacterial cultures and stains, cryptococcal antigen, etc.) may be indicated, depending on the clinical suspicion for alternate entities.

Although temporal or frontal lobe focal involvement is thought to be a hallmark of HSV-1 encephalitis, other viruses (cytomegalovirus, Epstein-Barr virus, and varicella-zoster virus, as well as West Nile virus and a variety of enteroviruses) can cause focal signs and symptoms, though none of these has a particular predilection for the temporal lobes. Involvement of the temporal lobes is also typical in encephalitis due to HHV-6, and in the paraneoplastic limbic encephalitis classically associated with small-cell lung cancer. CSF analysis for detection of viral DNA or paraneoplastic antibodies should be considered on a case-by-case basis in conjunction with PCR testing for HSV-1.

Treatment and Prophylaxis

As soon as HSV-1 encephalitis is suspected, patients should be hospitalized for intensive supportive care and treated with IV acyclovir for 14–21 days (Table 40.6). Prompt initiation of antiviral therapy improves survival and clinical outcome. Although the yield of CSF HSV-1 PCR declines through the course of therapy, the effect has been noted over the first weeks of therapy rather than the first hours. Thus, treatment with IV acyclovir should be initiated in the emergency department when a diagnosis of HSV-1 encephalitis is being considered and may be started prior to neuroimaging and CSF collection if these tests are delayed.

Except when clearly contraindicated, such as in the setting of unstable heart failure, all patients should receive IV hydration during IV acyclovir therapy, to prevent crystalluria and acquired renal disease. There is no data to support the use of oral antiviral agents or adjunctive corticosteroids in the treatment of HSV-1 encephalitis.

When there is high clinical suspicion for HSV-1 encephalitis, antimicrobial therapy should continue even with negative HSV-1 PCR results, pending definitive brain biopsy.

Because many patients develop seizures during the natural history of HSV-1 encephalitis, even when treated with acyclovir, antiepileptic medications are recommended.

Complications and Admission Criteria

All patients with suspected encephalitis need to be admitted to the hospital for neurological monitoring and treatment.

Progressive involvement of temporal and orbitofrontal lobes may result in focal language difficulties, memory loss, agitation, hallucinations, and autonomic dysfunction that may evolve over days even after initiation of acyclovir. Patients who develop drowsiness and pupillary asymmetry should be transferred to an intensive care setting for monitoring of intracranial pressure. Patients who deteriorate to the level of coma should be evaluated emergently by a neurosurgeon for potential craniectomy and brain decompression. Typical complications related to treatment include renal impairment from acyclovir therapy and electrolyte disturbances from fluid and acyclovir administration.

Infection Control

Person-to-person transmission of HSV-1 encephalitis has not been documented. Therefore, standard precautions are considered adequate for patients with HSV-1 encephalitis. No isolation is required.

Pearls and Pitfalls

1. HSV-1 encephalitis should be considered in all patients who present with symptoms and signs of encephalitis.
2. Patients with a history of fever presenting with any focal signs or lesions on examination, neuroimaging, or electroencephalogram should be presumed to have HSV-1 encephalitis and treated with acyclovir.
3. CSF cell count may be normal in a small minority (<10%) of patients with HSV-1 encephalitis.

REFERENCES

Brock DG, Bleck TP. Extra-axial suppurations of the central nervous system. Semin Neurol 1992;12:263–72.

Carpenter J, Stapleton S, Holliman R. Retrospective analysis of 29 cases of brain abscess and review of the literature. Eur J Clin Microbiol Infect Dis 2007 Dec;26:1–11.

Chun CH, Johnson JD, Hofstetter M, Raff MJ. Brain abscess. A study of 45 consecutive cases. Medicine (Baltimore) 1986 Nov;65(6):415–31.

Kao PT, Tseng HK, Liu CP, et al. Brain abscess: clinical analysis of 53 cases. J Microbiol Immunol Infect 2003 Jun;36(2):129–36.

Kastrup O, Wanke I, Maschke M. Neuroimaging of infections. NeuroRx 2005 Apr;2:324–32.

Kennedy PG. Viral encephalitis: causes, differential diagnosis, and management. J Neurol Neurosurg Psychiatry 2004 Mar;75:i10–15.

McGrath N, Anderson NE, Croxson MC, Powell KF. Herpes simplex encephalitis treated with acyclovir: diagnosis and long term outcome. J Neurol Neurosurg Psychiatry 1997;63:321–6.

Tseng JH, Tseng MY. Brain abscess in 142 patients: factors influencing outcome and mortality. Surg Neurol 2006 Jun;65(6):557–62.

Whitley RJ, Soong SJ, Linnemann C, et al. Herpes simplex encephalitis: clinical assessment. JAMA 1982;247:317–20.

ADDITIONAL READINGS

Domingues RB, Tsanaclis AM, Pannuti CS, et al. Evaluation of range of clinical presentations of herpes simplex encephalitis by using polymerase chain reaction assay of cerebrospinal fluid samples. Clin Infect Dis 1997;25: 86–91.

Lakeman FD, Whitley RJ. National Institute of Allergy and Infectious Diseases Collaborative Antiviral Study Group. Diagnosis of herpes simplex encephalitis: application of polymerase chain reaction to cerebrospinal fluid from brain-biopsied patients and correlation with disease. J Infect Dis 1995;171:857–63.

Mathisen GE, Johnson JP. Brain abscess. Clin Infect Dis 1997 Oct;25(4):763–79.

Whitley RJ, Kimberlin DW, Roizman B. Herpes simplex viruses. Clin Infect Dis 1998;26:541–53.

41. Fever and Acute Weakness Localizing to the Spinal Cord

Alexander C. Flint

INTRODUCTION

Although the combination of an acute febrile illness and focal weakness should always raise the possibility of spinal epidural abscess, there are other critical diagnoses that may present similarly. The physical exam can often help localize a lesion to the brain, spinal cord, nerve root(s), peripheral nerve(s), neuromuscular junction, or muscles. While select laboratory testing may help stratify the risk of epidural abscess in a given patient, emergent imaging is indicated in any patient with signs, symptoms, and risk factors suggestive of the diagnosis.

EPIDEMIOLOGY

Spinal epidural abscess is a rare disorder, accounting for 0.2–20 per 10,000 hospital admissions. Reported risk factors include diabetes mellitus, intravenous (IV) drug use, prior spine surgery, trauma, and alcohol abuse. Spinal epidural abscess has been documented as a potential complication of epidural catheter placement and epidural injection of steroids or local anesthetics. As many as 5% of patients with epidural abscess may have a recent history of epidural anesthesia. More unusual risk factors include duodenolumbar fistula, bacterial endocarditis, and a recent history of tattooing.

Staphylococcus aureus is the most common causative organism in epidural spinal abscesses, reported in 65–73% of patients. Other important agents include *Streptococcus* species and *Escherichia coli*. Cases have been reported with a wide range of other bacterial species, and more unusual causes include *Nocardia*, *Brucella*, *Cryptococcus*, and *Aspergillus*. Specific agents may be associated with particular clinical settings. For example, in the postpartum setting, group B *Streptococcus* can cause an epidural abscess, and in the setting of endocarditis, an epidural abscess can develop from direct hematogenous spread.

CLINICAL FEATURES

The classic symptoms of an epidural abscess with spinal cord compression include neck or back pain, fever, leukocytosis, and focal motor deficit, though the entire constellation is present only in a minority of cases (Table 41.1). Back pain is present in 72–97% in various case series, while fever is reported in only 52–66%, leukocytosis in 60–78%, and a motor deficit in 56–60%. Symptoms of nerve root irritation, such as radicular pain or a positive straight leg raise test are reported in only 19–47%.

Epidural abscesses are more likely to occur around the spine than around the brain, likely because the cranial epidural space is a potential space and the spinal epidural space is a true space filled with fat and venous structures. Anatomically, spinal epidural abscesses are most often thoracic (35%) or lumbosacral (30%) and can be either anterior or posterior predominant. There can be isolated involvement of the epidural space, or additional involvement of neighboring vertebrae (osteomyelitis) and intervertebral disks ("diskitis"). Involvement of adjacent structures occurs in both bacterial and tuberculous epidural abscesses but is more frequent in tuberculous disease (Pott's disease).

Lesions causing extrinsic compression of the spinal cord produce dysfunction of the long tracts that control motor, sensory, bowel, and bladder function. Because extrinsic compressive lesions usually exert a mass effect on both sides of the cord, either anteriorly or posteriorly, they often produce bilateral symptoms. Sensory symptoms will usually, but not always, occur at the level of the lesion and below. In contrast, a lesion at any level of the cord can produce bowel or bladder dysfunction. This dysfunction may present as new or worsening nocturia, well before frank urinary incontinence develops. Because frank stool incontinence is a relatively late finding, the anal sphincter tone and anal wink reflexes are essential parts of the spinal cord neurological exam.

Lesions of the conus medullaris, the lowest portion of the spinal cord, have several distinguishing features. If the conus is impinged out of proportion to the roots of the cauda equina, the patient may have a selective "saddle anesthesia" without motor or sensory dysfunction in the legs. Because the conus contains the lower motor neurons controlling bowel, bladder, and sexual function, these functions may be profoundly affected. In isolated lesions of the conus medullaris, radicular pain may be absent.

Lesions of the cauda equina, instead, produce radicular pain as a rule and lead to motor and sensory dysfunction of many or all of the lumbar and sacral roots. Classically, there is motor dysfunction in both legs and a pattern of sensory loss in the legs and saddle area, with prominent bowel, bladder, and sexual dysfunction.

Table 41.1 "First-Pass Neurological Localization" Relevant to the Weak, Febrile Patient

Anatomical Location	Classic Signs and Symptoms
Brain	• Cortical signs (aphasia, neglect, higher cognitive dysfunction) • Hemiparesis (face, arm, and leg all contralateral to lesion but usually *not* equally affected) • Hemisensory loss (face, arm, and leg all contralateral to lesion but usually *not* equally affected)
Brainstem	• Cranial nerve symptoms (e.g., diplopia, dysarthria, dysphagia) • Cranial nerve signs (e.g., abnormal eye movements, decreased hemifacial sensation, facial droop, tongue deviation, or impaired pupillary, corneal, or gag reflexes) • Neurological deficit involving a hemifacial distribution and a contralateral extremity or extremities (e.g., lower motor neuron left facial paresis with right hemiparesis of the arm and leg)
Spinal Cord	• Weakness of both legs, or both legs and both arms • Sensory loss in a bilateral distribution, with a sensory level that approximates the level of the lesion • Hemicord (Brown-Sequard) pattern of symptoms (weakness and loss of position or vibration sense in one arm and leg, loss of pain or temperature sense in the other arm and leg) • Bladder and/or bowel symptoms • Hyperactive reflexes (variable, dependent on acuity) • Increased muscle tone (variable, dependent on acuity)
Conus Medullaris of Spinal Cord	• Little or no weakness • Sensory loss in "saddle" area or perineum • Bladder and/or bowel symptoms • Will have pain if roots involved by lesion as well
Nerve Roots (General)	• Pain • Weakness (distribution variable) • Sensory loss (distribution variable) • Hypoactive or absent reflexes • Decreased tone
Nerve Roots (Cauda Equina)	• Pain • Weakness in bilateral legs • Sensory loss including legs and "saddle" area and perineum • Hypoactive or absent reflexes • Decreased muscle tone • Bladder and/or bowel symptoms
Peripheral Nerves	• Weakness and sensory loss involving a distal > proximal distribution • Hypoactive or absent reflexes • Decreased muscle tone
Neuromuscular Junction	• Time-dependent weakness (worse or better over course of day or with repeated activity) • No sensory involvement
Muscle	• Proximal > distal weakness, often symmetric in the arms and legs • No sensory involvement • Muscle tenderness to palpation

It is important to note the distinction between the spinal cord level and vertebral body level, especially in the lower aspects of the spinal column. For example, an epidural abscess at the level of the T12 to L2 vertebral bodies would likely compress the conus, the cauda equina, or both, because the spinal cord ends at approximately the L1 vertebral body level. If a spinal sensory level is obtained on exam at approximately L1, this might correspond to a vertebral body level of T11. This anatomical distinction is of practical importance because focused MRI studies must usually be ordered as either thoracic or lumbosacral studies.

In addition, because the axons of the upper motor neurons controlling leg motor function and bladder control course from the medial surface of the cortex, a midline frontal lesion can cause bilateral leg weakness and bladder dysfunction, mimicking a spinal cord lesion. Such lesions will usually also cause signs and symptoms of higher cortical dysfunction such as cognitive dysfunction, perseveration, or abulia (loss or impairment of the ability to make decisions or act independently).

Because morbidity and mortality are increased by a delay in surgical decompression and antibiotic therapy, early diagnosis is critical. Unfortunately, a delay in diagnosis is common. In one series, 30% of patients were initially misdiagnosed and discharged from an emergency department (ED) or clinic setting. The variety and subtlety of presentations, the relative rarity of the diagnosis, and the serious consequences of missing it make a high degree of suspicion crucial.

DIFFERENTIAL DIAGNOSIS

Pott's disease, or spinal tuberculosis, unlike bacterial epidural abscess, usually involves multiple tissue compartments (Table 41.2). These include the vertebral bodies, intervening disk spaces, the epidural space, and the paravertebral soft tissues. The course of the disease is generally subacute to chronic, in contrast to bacterial epidural abscess. Because most patients presenting with Pott's disease do not have active pulmonary tuberculosis (TB), clinicians should consider TB as a cause of compressive myelopathy in all patients who have risk factors, come from endemic areas, or exhibit a more insidious course than would be expected for a bacterial epidural abscess.

Intrinsic lesions of the cord producing fever and weakness include viral myelitis, which can affect any area of the cord, and poliomyelitis, which is a selective infection of the anterior gray matter of the cord (the lower motor neurons). Paralytic poliomyelitis caused by poliovirus presents with fever, back pain, and rapidly progressive lower motor neuron weakness, with decreased muscle tone and eventual atrophy and fasciculations. Although poliomyelitis has not caused an outbreak of paralytic disease in the United States in many years as a result of widespread vaccination, a recent series of nonparalytic cases in a Amish community in Minnesota makes it clear that this disease could become more common in the absence of vaccination. Poliomyelitis is now regularly reported as a result of infection with West Nile virus, either as an isolated syndrome or together with encephalitis. Fungal and parasitic causes of myelitis are very rare, but should be considered in immunocompromised patients or in travelers to or residents of endemic areas. Intramedullary bacterial abscess is very rare and is clinically indistinguishable from epidural spinal abscess, but can be identified by magnetic resonance imaging (MRI).

Table 41.2 Distinguishing Features and Tests in the Differential of Fever with Focal Weakness

Differential Diagnosis	Distinguishing Features	Specific Testing
Spinal Epidural Abscess	• Fever and acute to subacute spinal syndrome • Elevated ESR	MRI WBC, ESR, CRP BCx
Pott's Disease (Spinal TB)	• Fever and subacute to chronic spinal syndrome • History of TB or exposure • Immunocompromised host	Plain films MRI WBC, ESR, CRP BCx, AFB PPD
Intramedullary Spinal Abscess	• Fever and acute to subacute spinal syndrome • Elevated ESR	Distinguished from epidural abscess by MRI
Viral Myelitis	• Acute to subacute spinal syndrome • Can be in setting of viral syndrome	MRI LP, including viral studies
Poliomyelitis	• Fever • Back pain • Rapidly progressive lower motor neuron syndrome	LP EMG/NC
Fungal or Parasitic Myelitis	• Acute to subacute spinal syndrome, compromised host or exposure to endemic area	MRI LP, including fungal studies, O&P, wet prep
CMV Radiculitis	• Almost always in setting of AIDS, painful progressive polyradiculopathy	EMG/NC LP
Vasculitic Neuropathy	• Mononeuritis multiplex	EMG/NC LP
Botulism	• Descending weakness, cranial neuropathies, exposure to source	EMG/NC LP Bedside respiratory testing
Tetanus	• Painful spasms (evoked and spontaneous), trismus, rigidity	EMG/NC Bedside respiratory testing
Myasthenic Crisis	• Descending weakness and cranial neuropathies, worse during day and with repetition	EMG/NC Edrophonium test (MG diagnosis) Bedside respiratory testing
Pyomyositis	• Proximal muscle weakness, swollen, warm, erythematous muscles	CT, MRI, or US of muscle
Brain Abscess	• Fever, acute to subacute cortical or subcortical syndrome, elevated ESR	MRI
Guillain-Barré Syndrome	• Febrile illness, then delayed onset of ascending weakness, areflexia	LP (elevated CSF protein) EMG/NC
Postinfectious Transverse Myelitis	• Febrile illness, then delayed acute to subacute spinal syndrome	MRI LP
Acute Disseminated Encephalomyelitis (ADEM)	• Febrile illness or vaccine, then delayed acute to subacute cortical or subcortical with or without spinal syndrome	MRI brain and spine LP
Lyme Radiculoneuropathy	• Subacute to chronic nerve root and peripheral nerve syndrome, rarely cord involvement	LP Lyme titers from blood and CSF MRI
Syphilis	• Chronic, slowly progressive spinal syndrome; usually history of primary or secondary syphilis	RPR LP with CSF VDRL MRI
HIV Myelopathy	• Slowly progressive posterior column syndrome	MRI EMG/NC
Leptomeningeal Carcinomatosis	• Slowly progressive radiculopathy or spinal syndrome	MRI with enhancement of leptomeninges LP for cytology

AFB, acid-fast bacilli; BCx, blood cultures; CRP, C-reactive protein; CSF, cerebrospinal fluid; EMG/NC, electromyography and nerve conduction studies; ESR, erythrocyte sedimentation rate; LP, lumbar puncture; MG, myasthenia gravis; O&P, ova and parasites; PPD, purified protein derivative; RPR, rapid plasma reagin; VDRL, venereal disease research laboratory; WBC, white blood (cell) count.

Botulism presents as a descending weakness starting with cranial nerve signs and symptoms progressing to respiratory weakness requiring mechanical ventilation. There is usually a documented exposure (home canning or intravenous drug use) to a potential source of *Clostridium botulinum*. Fever in botulism is variable. Tetanus is similarly easily to distinguish from spinal causes of fever and focal weakness, by the uniform presence of spasms induced by the toxins elaborated by *Clostridium tetani*. Tetanus can occur in local, cephalic, or generalized forms, but in all cases there is both tonic muscle contraction (rigidity) and superimposed painful muscle contractions, both stimulus-evoked and spontaneous.

Pyomyositis is a localized infection and abscess formation in proximal muscles and usually presents with fever and weakness. Pyomyositis, like spinal epidural abscess, is usually caused by *Staphylococcus aureus* and often requires surgical drainage in addition to antibiotic therapy. Clinically, pyomyositis should be easily distinguishable from spinal causes of fever and weakness by the presence of proximal muscle weakness with warm, erythematous, swollen, and tender muscles. Contrast computed tomography (CT), ultrasound, or MRI of the affected muscles confirms the diagnosis.

Syphilis, although often considered in neurological differential diagnoses as the "great mimicker," is a rare cause of progressive myelopathy in the modern era. Several features distinguish syphilitic myelopathy, due to either tabes dorsalis or gummatous myelopathy, from more acute causes of myelopathy with fever. Regardless of the subtype of syphilis, the course is indolent, and fever and signs of active systemic infection are almost always absent at the tertiary stage. Lyme radiculoneuropathy is a slowly progressive infectious or parainfectious process that usually diffusely involves the spinal roots and peripheral nerves and can involve the cervical cord as well (Lyme myeloradiculoneuropathy). Although Lyme disease is often entertained in a wide variety of neurological presentations, this condition is usually not acute enough to mimic epidural abscess. A brain abscess can have the appropriate timing of onset, but clinical features such as cortical dysfunction with hemiparesis or hemisensory loss distinguish this from a spinal process.

Human immunodeficiency virus (HIV) myelopathy is a common process in acquired immunodeficiency syndrome (AIDS) patients but is also slowly progressive and usually manifests as posterior column sensory deficits without fever, unless another opportunistic process is present. Cytomegalovirus (CMV) radiculitis presents almost exclusively in AIDS patients with very low CD4 counts as a rapidly progressive painful polyradiculopathy with ascending weakness in the legs.

Vasculitic neuropathy can be accompanied by fever and presents as a "mononeuritis multiplex" (focal and patchy involvement of multiple distinct peripheral nerves) or as a polyneuropathy (more diffuse, often symmetric and distal neuropathic picture). The neuropathy can be painful, but the neuropathic quality of the pain and lack of back pain should aid in distinguishing this entity from spinal causes of fever and weakness. The overall course is typically subacute and can be chronic, but the onset of each peripheral neuropathy in a mononeuritis multiplex is usually acute.

A myasthenic crisis is an acute exacerbation of myasthenia gravis, an autoimmune disorder that causes destruction and dysfunction of postsynaptic nicotinic acetylcholine receptors at the neuromuscular junction. A myasthenic crisis is commonly provoked by a febrile illness, so it is possible to see a febrile and acutely weak patient in the ED with the diagnosis of a myasthenic crisis. Although there is usually a history of myasthenia, an acute crisis in the setting of a febrile illness is not an uncommon first presentation of the disease. The diagnosis of this entity at first presentation relies on historic elements and physical findings of time- and use-dependent weakness, in addition to an edrophonium test, which can be performed in the ED with sufficient monitoring and rescue atropine at the bedside. The key in the management of patients with a suspected myasthenic crisis is to consider endotracheal intubation earlier than for other causes of respiratory deterioration. If the patient with myasthenia develops significant oxygen desaturation, he or she should have been intubated earlier. Other useful tests that can be easily done in the ED to assess the degree of neuromuscular respiratory weakness include measurement of vital capacity and peak inspiratory pressure, and the bedside "counting on one breath" test. Vital capacity of less than 20 mL/kg or a peak inspiratory pressure of less than 30 cm H_2O is generally accepted as a criterion for intubation. Having the patient take a deep breath and attempt to count as high as possible on breath is a crude but often useful tool to assess neuromuscular respiratory strength – the inability to count higher than 20 on a single breath is a cause for alarm and should at least indicate the need for urgent vital capacity and peak inspiratory pressure measurement.

Guillain-Barré syndrome is a subacute ascending weakness with areflexia caused by an autoimmune reaction against motor, more than sensory, peripheral nerves and roots. Signs and symptoms often develop 2–3 weeks following a febrile illness or, very rarely, following vaccinations. It is unusual for a patient with Guillain-Barré to still have signs of systemic illness by the time weakness develops. Postinfectious transverse myelitis and acute disseminated encephalomyelitis (ADEM) can both cause a fulminant myelopathy that may or may not be associated with a history of fever or infectious illness.

Leptomeningeal carcinomatosis (also known as carcinomatous meningitis) is metastatic cancer of the spinal subarachnoid space and is usually slowly progressive and without accompanying fever. In rare cases, fever is present and the disease can progress more rapidly. MRI should accurately distinguish between carcinomatosis and epidural abscess.

LABORATORY AND RADIOGRAPHIC FINDINGS

There are no signs, symptoms, or laboratory tests that reliably exclude a spinal epidural abscess. When a patient presents with concerning risk factors and objective findings, an emergent MRI is indicated (Figure 41.1), as early detection correlates with improved morbidity and mortality. MRI findings of central spinal canal narrowing by more than half, contrast enhancement of the abscess, and abnormal spinal cord signal are all associated with long-term weakness. Serial MRI scans may be useful to follow the clinical response to therapy.

Patients with viral myelitis may have a normal MRI acutely or may show a diffuse or patchy T2-prolongation of intrinsic cord signal, easily distinguished from extrinsic compressive infectious processes or even other intramedullary infectious processes. If imaging demonstrates the extensive bony and disk involvement typical of TB vertebral osteomyelitis, or an intramedullary lesion, a TB test and infectious disease consult are indicated.

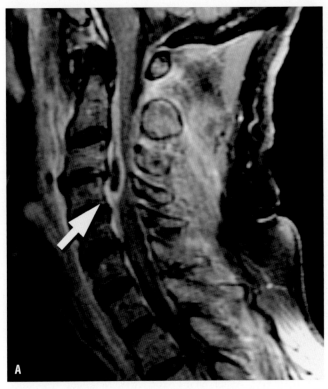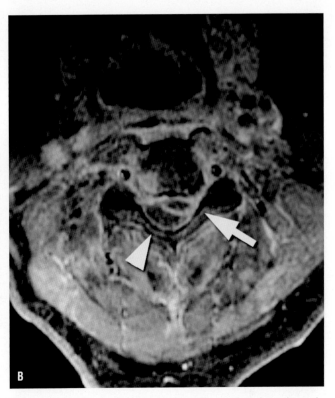

Figure 41.1 Magnetic resonance imaging (MRI) of a spinal epidural abscess. (A) Sagittal T1-weighted MRI after administration of gadolinium contrast shows abnormal enhancement anterior to the cervical spinal cord and posterior to the cervical vertebral bodies. In this case, there is a cystic, non-enhancing component with the abscess visible adjacent to the C3 and C4 vertebral bodies (arrow). (B) Axial view of the same abscess, showing the anterior and lateral position of the abscess (arrow) relative to the spinal cord (arrowhead), which is deviated laterally and posteriorly, with mass effect on the cord and effacement of the normal CSF space surrounding the cord.

When MRI is not available or is contraindicated, CT myelography is a useful alternate study. A CT myelogram is usually positive when a high degree of clinical suspicion is present. However, the sensitivity and specificity of CT myelography for epidural abscess have not been systematically compared to MRI, so results from CT-based imaging should be interpreted in light of the clinical scenario.

The erythrocyte sedimentation rate (ESR) is commonly elevated on presentation with a spinal epidural abscess and has been reported as greater than 20 mm/hr in 94–100% of patients, depending on the series. In a large meta-analysis, the average reported ESR in patients with confirmed epidural abscess was 77 mm/hr (range 2–150). By comparison, the average white blood cell (WBC) count was only 15,700/mm^3 (range 1,500–42,000).

Blood cultures are positive in more than half of patients with spinal epidural abscess and may be more likely to be positive if the causative organism is *Staphylococcus aureus*. Although the CSF is usually abnormal, with a pattern typically suggestive of bacterial infection, the CSF Gram stain and culture are rarely positive. Care should be taken with lumbar puncture to avoid seeding the subarachnoid space with a spinal needle that has traversed the abscess.

TREATMENT AND PROPHYLAXIS

Once the diagnosis is made, prompt neurosurgical decompression and antibiotic therapy remain the mainstay of therapy for an epidural spinal abscess causing a myelopathy. Although successful nonsurgical antibiotic therapy for epidural abscess without significant myelopathy has been reported,

the success rate of this approach is unclear from published series. Percutaneous CT-guided drainage in selected patients with little or no myelopathy has been reported, both by direct needle aspiration and by catheter placement. A minimally invasive surgical technique involving limited laminectomies and drainage catheter placement has also been reported.

Empiric antibiotics should begin as soon as possible in the ED after two sterile sets of blood cultures are obtained (Table 41.3). It is unlikely that a single dose of parenteral antibiotics will sterilize the surgical specimen culture. The optimal antibiotic choice depends on the local prevalence of methicillin-resistant *Staphylococcus aureus* (MRSA), the patient's general immune status, and the likely cause of the infection (i.e., related to prior surgery or instrumentation). Although vancomycin is often a reasonable choice to cover MRSA when the suspected organism is *S. aureus*, vancomycin alone may be insufficient therapy for serious MRSA infections. It is therefore appropriate to cover with both vancomycin and a third-generation cephalosporin until isolates and sensitivities are obtained. The addition of a third-generation cephalosporin or ciprofloxacin will also cover Enterobacteriaceae and gram-negative bacteria.

COMPLICATIONS AND ADMISSION CRITERIA

All patients diagnosed with epidural abscess should be admitted for monitoring and parenteral antibiotics. Those with myelopathic signs and symptoms require urgent neurosurgical decompression.

Table 41.3 Initial Antibiotic Therapy for Spinal Epidural Abscess

Patient Category	Therapy Recommendation
Adults	nafcillin 2 g IV q4h *or* oxacillin 2 g IV q4h *and* tobramycin 1.5–2 mg/kg IV q8h *or* third-generation cephalosporin (e.g., ceftriaxone 1 g IV q12h) *or* ciprofloxacin 400 mg IV q12h
Adults (Concern for MRSA)	vancomycin 1–1.5 g IV q12h *and* tobramycin 1.5–2 mg/kg IV q8h *or* third-generation cephalosporin (e.g., ceftriaxone 1 g IV q12h) *or* ciprofloxacin 400 mg IV q12h
Children	Consider infectious disease consultation – unusual in this group

Many other antibiotics and antibiotic combinations have been reported for empiric therapy of patients with a spinal epidural abscess. Therapy should be based on local resistance patterns and the most likely source for the abscess.

INFECTION CONTROL

Universal precautions should be observed. No isolation is required, except in cases of suspected concomitant pulmonary TB.

PEARLS AND PITFALLS

1. Because extrinsic compression lesions such as epidural abscesses usually exert a mass effect on both sides of the cord, there are often bilateral symptoms.
2. A lesion at any level of the cord can produce bowel or bladder dysfunction.
3. New or worsening nocturia may be the first sign of cord pathology, well before frank urinary incontinence develops.
4. A midline frontal lesion can cause bilateral leg weakness and bladder dysfunction, mimicking a spinal cord lesion.
5. Consider TB when the MRI shows involvement of multiple tissue compartments.
6. When neuromuscular disorders are in the differential, always assess respiratory function and consider early intubation.

REFERENCES

Bouchez B, Arnott G, Delfosse JM. Acute spinal epidural abscess. J Neurol 1985;231:343–4.

Brazis PW, Masdeu JC, Biller J. Localization in clinical neurology. New York: Lippincott Williams & Wilkins, 2001.

Bremer AA, Darouiche RO. Spinal epidural abscess presenting as intra-abdominal pathology: a case report and literature review. J Emerg Med 2004;26:51–6.

Brust JCM. The practice of neural science: from synapses to symptoms. New York: McGraw-Hill, 2000.

Centers for Disease Control and Prevention (CDC). Poliovirus infections in four unvaccinated children – Minnesota, August–October 2005. MMWR 2005;54(Dispatch):1–3.

Chowfin A, Potti A, Paul A, Carson P. Spinal epidural abscess after tattooing. Clin Infect Dis 1999;29:225–6.

Clark R, Carlisle JT, Valainis GT. *Streptococcus pneumoniae* endocarditis presenting as an epidural abscess. Rev Infect Dis 1989;11:338–40.

Cwikiel W. Percutaneous drainage of abscess in psoas compartment and epidural space. Case report and review of the literature. Acta Radiol 1991;32:159–61.

Darouiche RO, Hamill RJ, Greenberg SB, et al. Bacterial spinal epidural abscess. Review of 43 cases and literature survey. Medicine (Baltimore) 1992;71:369–85.

Fukui T, Ichikawa H, Kawate N, et al. Acute spinal epidural abscess and spinal leptomeningitis: report of 2 cases with comparative neuroradiological and autopsy study. Eur Neurol 1992;32:328–33.

Grewal S, Hocking G, Wildsmith JA. Epidural abscesses. Br J Anaesth 2006;96:292–302.

Gupta RK, Agarwal P, Rastogi H, et al. Problems in distinguishing spinal tuberculosis from neoplasia on MRI. Neuroradiology 1996;38(Suppl 1):S97–104.

Hanigan WC, Asner NG, Elwood PW. Magnetic resonance imaging and the nonoperative treatment of spinal epidural abscess. Surg Neurol 1990;34:408–13.

Hlavin ML, Kaminski HJ, Ross JS, Ganz E. Spinal epidural abscess: a ten-year perspective. Neurosurgery 1990;27:177–84.

Huang RC, Shapiro GS, Lim M, et al. Cervical epidural abscess after epidural steroid injection. Spine 2004;29:E7–9.

Jenkin G, Woolley IJ, Brown GV, Richards MJ. Postpartum epidural abscess due to group B *Streptococcus*. Clin Infect Dis 1997;25:1249.

Joshi SM, Hatfield RH, Martin J, Taylor W. Spinal epidural abscess: a diagnostic challenge. Br J Neurosurg 2003;17:160–3.

Khatib R, Riederer KM, Held M, Aljundi H. Protracted and recurrent methicillin-resistant *Staphylococcus aureus* bacteremia despite defervescence with vancomycin therapy. Scand J Infect Dis 1995;27:529–32.

Knight JW, Cordingley JJ, Palazzo MG. Epidural abscess following epidural steroid and local anaesthetic injection. Anaesthesia 1997;52:576–8.

Koppel BS, Tuchman AJ, Mangiardi JR, et al. Epidural spinal infection in intravenous drug abusers. Arch Neurol 1988;45:1331–7.

Latronico N, Tansini A, Gualandi GF, et al. Successful non-operative treatment of tuberculous spinal epidural abscess with cord compression: the role of magnetic resonance imaging. Eur Neurol 1993;33:177–80.

Lawn ND, Fletcher DD, Henderson RD, et al. Anticipating mechanical ventilation in Guillain-Barré syndrome. Arch Neurol 2001;58:893–8.

Leys D, Lesoin F, Viaud C, et al. Decreased morbidity from acute bacterial spinal epidural abscesses using computed tomography and nonsurgical treatment in selected patients. Ann Neurol 1985;17:350–5.

Li J, Loeb JA, Shy ME, et al. Asymmetric flaccid paralysis: a neuromuscular presentation of West Nile virus infection. Ann Neurol 2003;53:703–10.

Lyu RK, Chen CJ, Tang LM, Chen ST. Spinal epidural abscess successfully treated with percutaneous, computed tomography-guided, needle aspiration and parenteral antibiotic therapy: case report and review of the literature. Neurosurgery 2002;51:509–12; discussion 512.

Mampalam TJ, Rosegay H, Andrews BT, et al. Nonoperative treatment of spinal epidural infections. J Neurosurg 1989;71:208–10.

Numaguchi Y, Rigamonti D, Rothman MI, et al. Spinal epidural abscess: evaluation with gadolinium-enhanced MR imaging. Radiographics 1993;13:545–59; discussion 559–60.

Nussbaum ES, Rigamonti D, Standiford H, et al. Spinal epidural abscess: a report of 40 cases and review. Surg Neurol 1992;38:225–31.

Panagiotopoulos V, Konstantinou D, Solomou E, et al. Extended cervicolumbar spinal epidural abscess associated with paraparesis successfully decompressed using a minimally invasive technique. Spine 2004;29:E300–3.

Patten J. Neurological differential diagnosis. London: Springer-Verlag, 1996.

Pirofski L, Casadevall A. Mixed staphylococcal and cryptococcal epidural abscess in a patient with AIDS. Rev Infect Dis 1990;12:964–5.

Reihsaus E, Waldbaur H, Seeling W. Spinal epidural abscess: a meta-analysis of 915 patients. Neurosurg Rev 2000;23:175–204; discussion 205.

Rigamonti D, Liem L, Sampath P, et al. Spinal epidural abscess: contemporary trends in etiology, evaluation, and management. Surg Neurol 1999;52:189–96; discussion 197.

Sadato N, Numaguchi Y, Rigamonti D, et al. Spinal epidural abscess with gadolinium-enhanced MRI: Serial follow-up studies and clinical correlations. Neuroradiology 1994;36:44–8.

Sarubbi FA, Vasquez JE. Spinal epidural abscess associated with the use of temporary epidural catheters: report of two cases and review. Clin Infect Dis 1997;25:1155–8.

Shintani S, Tanaka H, Irifune A, et al. Iatrogenic acute spinal epidural abscess with septic meningitis: MR findings. Clin Neurol Neurosurg 1992;94:253–5.

Sillevis Smitt P, Tsafka A, van den Bent M, et al. Spinal epidural abscess complicating chronic epidural analgesia in 11 cancer patients: clinical findings and magnetic resonance imaging. J Neurol 1999;246:815–20.

Soehle M, Wallenfang T. Spinal epidural abscesses: clinical manifestations, prognostic factors, and outcomes. Neurosurgery 2002;51:79–85; discussion 86–7.

Solera J, Lozano E, Martinez-Alfaro E, et al. Brucellar spondylitis: review of 35 cases and literature survey. Clin Infect Dis 1999;29:1440–9.

Tabo E, Ohkuma Y, Kimura S, et al. Successful percutaneous drainage of epidural abscess with epidural needle and catheter. Anesthesiology 1994;80:1393–5.

Tessman PA, Preston DC, Shapiro BE. Spinal epidural abscess in an afebrile patient. Arch Neurol 2004;61:590–1.

Tung GA, Yim JW, Mermel LA, et al. Spinal epidural abscess: correlation between MRI findings and outcome. Neuroradiology 1999;41:904–9.

Walter RS, King JC Jr, Manley J, Rigamonti D. Spinal epidural abscess in infancy: successful percutaneous drainage in a nine-month-old and review of the literature. Pediatr Infect Dis J 1991;10:860–4.

Cheryl A. Jay

INTRODUCTION

Human immunodeficiency virus (HIV)–infected patients are vulnerable to developing altered mental status (AMS) for myriad reasons including the effects of HIV itself, the accompanying immune dysfunction, associated systemic illness, comorbid psychiatric disorders, and complicated medication regimens. Highly active antiretroviral therapy (HAART) has decreased the incidence of central nervous system (CNS) opportunistic infections (OIs) and HIV-associated dementia, but the benefits are not absolute. Moreover, patients with undiagnosed or untreated HIV infection may present with AMS. In addition to CNS OIs and complications of complex multisystem disease, immune reconstitution events developing in the early weeks and months after initiating HAART may affect the brain and cause AMS.

EPIDEMIOLOGY

Before HAART became the standard of HIV care in the developed world, approximately half of HIV-infected patients developed symptomatic central or peripheral nervous system disease, with neuropathology observed in nearly all individuals dying with HIV/acquired immunodeficiency syndrome (AIDS). Since the advent of HAART, the incidence of dementia, the major cerebral OIs (cryptococcal meningitis, toxoplasmosis, progressive multifocal leukoencephalopathy [PML]), and primary CNS lymphoma (PCNSL) has fallen. HIV-associated dementia is also less common and more indolent in patients on HAART. In the United States, fewer patients now develop the mutism, quadriparesis, and incontinence that were common with late-stage infection in the early years of the AIDS epidemic.

In approximately 25% of patients, the first weeks and months after initiation of HAART may be complicated by the immune reconstitution inflammatory syndrome (IRIS), with paradoxical worsening of previously diagnosed or subclinical OIs or the development of autoimmune disorders. IRIS affects most organ systems, including the brain. Patients with tuberculosis may be at particular risk of IRIS, and tuberculous meningitis and tuberculoma associated with initiation of HAART have been reported. Clinical exacerbation of cryptococcal meningitis, worsening PML, and rapidly progressive dementia in the setting of immune reconstitution have

also been described. The clinical spectrum of IRIS is not yet fully defined and should be considered when patients develop AMS in the first weeks and months after starting HAART.

Patients with HIV are at increased risk for substance abuse, affective disorders, and psychosis. Injection drug users with HIV remain at risk for the neurologic sequelae of endocarditis, including brain abscess, meningitis, ischemic stroke from septic embolism, and hemorrhagic stroke from mycotic aneurysm rupture. Patients coinfected with hepatitis C are at risk for hepatic encephalopathy with advanced liver disease or cognitive impairment, even in the absence of cirrhosis and portal hypertension. Additionally, HIV patients who use cocaine or methamphetamine are at risk for seizures and ischemic and hemorrhagic stroke.

Medications used to treat HIV disease or associated conditions may also contribute to AMS. Antiretroviral agents, particularly the non-nucleoside reverse transcriptase inhibitor efavirenz, can cause cerebral side effects, including psychiatric syndromes, as can the myriad other drugs used to treat HIV/AIDS and comorbid medical conditions.

Finally, as a multisystem illness, HIV infection can cause AMS even without primary neurologic, psychiatric, or medication-associated illness. For example, patients with HIV-associated nephropathy are subject to the neurologic complications of uremia, including encephalopathy. Septic patients may present with AMS in the absence of CNS infection.

CLINICAL FEATURES

As for any patient presenting to the emergency department (ED) with AMS, important elements of the history include: the temporal progression of symptoms, drug use (prescription, over-the-counter, illicit), trauma, and focal symptoms (aphasia, neglect, hemianopsia, hemiparesis, hemisensory loss), seizures, and symptoms suggesting increased intracranial pressure (ICP) (Tables 42.1 and 42.2). Additional important details in the HIV-infected patient include recent and nadir CD4 count, viral load and, for patients on HAART, the specific regimen and the duration of therapy. Regardless of treatment history, patients with CD4 counts below 200/mm^3 are at highest risk for cerebral OIs, primary CNS lymphoma, and HIV-associated dementia. Patients with prior cerebral

Table 42.1 Differential Diagnosis of AMS in the HIV High-Risk Population

IDU	• Drug intoxication or withdrawal • Endocarditis with septic encephalopathy • Ischemic stroke from septic embolism • Hemorrhagic stroke from mycotic aneurysm rupture • Brain abscess or meningitis, singly or in combination
Cocaine and Methamphetamine	• Seizure • Ischemic or hemorrhagic stroke
Medications	Prescription: • Efavirenz • Psychotropic drugs • Opiates and other analgesics Nonprescription: • Antihistamines • Ethanol (intoxication or withdrawal) Illicit: • Heroin • Stimulants • Other drugs of abuse
Multisystem Disease	• Uremic encephalopathy • Hepatic encephalopathy • Electrolyte abnormalities
Focal Cerebral Dysfunction	See Table 42.4
Diffuse Cerebral Dysfunction	See Table 42.5
IDU, injection drug user.	

Table 42.2 Key Elements of the History

- Temporal progression of symptoms
- Drug use (prescription, nonprescription, illicit)
- Trauma
- Focal symptoms (aphasia, neglect, hemianopsia, hemiparesis, hemisensory deficit)
- Seizures
- Symptoms suggesting increased ICP such as progressive or morning headache, nausea and vomiting, or deteriorating level of consciousness.

Additional important details in the HIV-infected patient include:
- Recent and nadir CD4 count
- Viral load
- Specific antiretroviral regimen and the duration of therapy

Table 42.3 Key Points in Recognizing Subtle CNS Infections in Advanced HIV Disease

- Absence of fever or headache does not exclude cerebral infections.
- Absence of meningismus does not exclude meningitis.
- Neurological exam should focus on identifying increased ICP and focal cerebral dysfunction.

disorders in immunocompetent individuals. In particular, the absence of fever or headache should not be used to exclude CNS infection, nor should the absence of meningismus be used to exclude meningitis (Table 42.3). Neurologic examination should focus on identifying evidence of increased ICP (anisocoria, papilledema) or focal cerebral dysfunction, such as visual field deficits, lateralized motor (pronator drift, hemiparesis, reflex asymmetry, unilateral Babinski sign) or sensory deficits, and, in patients alert enough to walk, gait disorder.

Whether the patient's AMS appears to be a manifestation of focal or diffuse cerebral dysfunction helps focus the long list of diagnostic considerations.

DIFFERENTIAL DIAGNOSIS

Focal Cerebral Dysfunction

Patients with signs or symptoms suggesting lateralized brain disturbance (Table 42.4) may have AMS by several mechanisms, more than one of which can coexist in a given patient. Brainstem or cerebellar lesions may impair level of alertness early. Patients with solitary hemispheric lesions are awake unless there is significant mass effect or concomitant meningitis or toxic-metabolic encephalopathy. Dominant hemisphere lesions cause aphasia (often with associated right homonymous hemianopsia, hemiparesis, or hemisensory loss) and nondominant hemisphere processes cause neglect or inattention with left-sided visual, motor, or sensory dysfunction. Patients with old focal brain lesions, such as prior trauma, stroke, tumor, or infection, may experience a worsening of stable focal deficits in the setting of drug intoxication, metabolic derangement, meningitis, or seizure. In general, CNS OIs and primary CNS lymphoma are more common in patients with CD4 below 200/mm^3, whereas cerebrovascular disease (which may complicate CNS infection, particularly tuberculosis [TB] or syphilitic meningitis) is more common in HIV-positive patients with focal cerebral deficit at higher CD4 counts.

Diffuse Cerebral Dysfunction

Patients with depressed level of alertness or milder cognitive or behavioral disturbances without aphasia, neglect or lateralizing motor, reflex, or sensory findings may have multiple brain lesions, meningitis, delirium, psychiatric decompensation or have had an unwitnessed seizure (Table 42.5). Dementia is a risk factor for delirium, but dementia alone does not cause depressed level of alertness (lethargy, obtundation, or stupor) except in its very advanced stages.

Additional considerations in patients with CNS infection or lymphoma who decompensate include medication effects and electrolyte disorder, particularly hyponatremia from the syndrome of inappropriate antidiuretic hormone secretion or cerebral salt wasting, or hypernatremia from diabetes insipidus.

toxoplasmosis or cryptococcal meningitis require secondary prophylaxis unless HAART increases CD4 counts above 200/mm^3 for 6 months, and clinicians should have a high index of suspicion for relapse in an altered patient with a history of cerebral OIs.

For patients recently started on HAART, additional diagnostic considerations include medication side effects (e.g., efavirenz) or IRIS. Patients with CD4 counts above 200/mm^3 may be at risk for major HIV-related brain disorders if treatment was begun within the past 6 months or if there is evidence of treatment failure, such as falling CD4 count, rising viral load, or both.

It is important to remember that the immune dysfunction that predisposes HIV-infected patients to cerebral infections also masks the symptoms and signs associated with similar

Table 42.4 Clinical Features: Focal Cerebral Dysfunction in HIV/AIDS

Common Etiologies (Usually CD4 <200/mm³)	
Cerebral toxoplasmosis	• Altered mental status, focal cerebral symptoms, or seizure, usually evolving over days to weeks, often with fever and headache • Reactivation of previously acquired, often asymptomatic, infection with the parasite *Toxoplasma gondii* • Unusual in patients on trimethoprim-sulfamethoxazole for *Pneumocystis* prophylaxis, because the drug also provides primary prophylaxis against toxoplasmosis
Progressive multifocal leukoencephalopathy (PML)	• Focal deficit, often homonymous hemianopsia or hemiparesis, steadily progressive over months without headache or fever • Reactivation of previously acquired, often asymptomatic, infection with the JC virus
Primary CNS lymphoma (PCNSL)	• Gradually progressive focal deficit or cognitive dysfunction, sometimes with headache, evolving over months • Almost always associated with EBV in tumor cells in HIV-positive patients
Less Common Infectious Etiologies	
CMV ventriculoencephalitis	• CD4 <100/mm³ • Cognitive impairment with brainstem findings (cranial neuropathies, ataxia) • Sometimes associated with polyradiculitis (cauda equina syndrome with paraparesis, incontinence, and hyporeflexia) evolving over days to weeks • CSF profile may resemble bacterial meningitis with elevated protein, polymorphonuclear pleocytosis, and low or normal glucose
Brain abscess (bacterial or fungal)	• Progressive focal cerebral deficit, with or without headache • Consider in patients with proven or suspected bacteremia (injection drug use, indwelling line, chronic skin infection, prosthetic heart valve) or craniofacial infection • Consider angioinvasive fungi (*Mucor* or *Aspergillus*, discussed below) in patients with CD4 <50/mm³ and associated sinus infection
Tuberculoma	• Presentation similar to brain abscess • Rare, but may develop as immune reconstitution inflammatory syndrome in patients on anti-tuberculous therapy for systemic TB (or tuberculous meningitis) in the first weeks to months of HAART
Stroke	
Meningovascular syphilis	• Occurs with or after secondary syphilis as ischemic stroke(s) with or without clinically manifested meningitis
Angioinvasive fungi (*Aspergillus, Mucor*)	• CD4 <50/mm³, associated sinus infection or palatal lesion or brain abscess, in addition to hemorrhagic or ischemic stroke(s)
VZV vasculopathy	• Multiple small-vessel strokes with recent or remote history of shingles
Bacterial endocarditis	• Septic embolism (infarction, abscess, or both), mycotic aneurysm rupture, bacterial meningitis

CSF, cerebrospinal fluid; CMV, cytomegalovirus; EBV, Epstein-Barr virus; VZV, varicella-zoster virus.

Table 42.5 Clinical Features: Diffuse Cerebral Dysfunction in HIV/AIDS

Common Etiologies (Usually CD4 <200/mm³)	
HIV-associated dementia	• Cognitive, behavioral, and motor slowing over months with hyperreflexia and, in more advanced disease, gait disturbance • More common in patients with untreated HIV disease. • Alertness is typically preserved except in end-stage dementia or if there is a coexisting cause for altered mental status
Cryptococcal meningitis	• Most common complaint is mild to moderate headache • Some patients present with symptomatic increased intracranial pressure, including coma • Severe headache with prominent meningismus is unusual, except as a manifestation of immune reconstitution inflammatory syndrome
Other Causes of Meningitis	
Tuberculous meningitis	• Usually presents as chronic meningitis with typical symptoms (headache, meningismus, altered mental status, cranial neuropathies), sometimes with small-vessel ischemic stroke • Risk of extrapulmonary disease, including meningitis or tuberculoma, is increased in HIV-positive patients • May present as immune reconstitution event in patients with systemic TB or as exacerbation of TB meningitis (in the first weeks to months of HAART)
Syphilitic meningitis	• Occurs weeks to years after primary infection, usually as an aseptic or chronic meningitis with or without cranial neuropathies • May be complicated by ischemic stroke (meningovascular syphilis), seizures, or hydrocephalus
Lymphomatous meningitis	• Presents as headache, altered mental status, cranial neuropathies, or cauda equina syndrome, individually or in combination • Usually with history of systemic lymphoma, although may occasionally be presenting feature
Bacterial meningitis	• Consider *Listeria monocytogenes*, in addition to pneumococcus and meningococcus
Other Etiologies	
Multifocal brain disease	• Toxoplasmosis and PCNSL may occasionally present as diffuse brain dysfunction
Drug ingestion	• Prescription: efavirenz, psychotropic drugs, opiates and other analgesics, among many others • Nonprescription: antihistamines, ethanol • Illicit: heroin, stimulants, and other drugs of abuse
Metabolic encephalopathies	• Renal or hepatic failure, electrolyte abnormalities (in particular sodium, calcium), hypo- or hyperglycemia, hypothyroidism, B₁₂ deficiency

LABORATORY AND RADIOGRAPHIC FINDINGS

Initial evaluation proceeds as for any patient with AMS, with particular attention to evidence of increased ICP, first-time seizure, trauma, or focal cerebral deficit. Appropriate laboratory studies include electrolytes, blood urea nitrogen (BUN) and creatinine, liver function tests, complete blood count (CBC), prothrombin time, and toxicology screen.

Although magnetic resonance imaging (MRI) is more sensitive for many HIV-related cerebral disorders, multidetector computed tomographic (CT) scanners are preferable for agitated and otherwise unstable patients. If there are contraindications to iodinated contrast, noncontrast CT can identify hydrocephalus, hemorrhage, or large mass lesions that would contraindicate lumbar puncture (Table 42.6).

Studies of the yield of noncontrast CT in HIV-infected patients presenting to the ED with neurologic dysfunction indicate that AMS was significantly associated with abnormal findings on CT. For patients with CD4 count less than $200/mm^3$, who are at highest risk for HIV-related cerebral complications, CT with and without contrast can sometimes obviate the need for lumbar puncture (LP) if the findings suggest toxoplasmosis (Figure 42.1), primary CNS lymphoma (Figure 42.2), or PML (Figure 42.3).

Whereas neuroradiologic findings in PML are relatively distinct, toxoplasmosis and primary CNS lymphoma can be difficult to distinguish definitively, even by MRI. In patients with meningitis, CT may reveal complications such as edema, infarction, or obstructive or communicating hydrocephalus. Patients with mass lesions should have serum *Toxoplasma* IgG antibodies sent, because a negative serology significantly decreases the likelihood that mass lesions are due to *Toxoplasma gondii*.

If laboratory studies have not revealed the cause of the patient's AMS and CT reveals no contraindication to LP, cerebrospinal fluid (CSF) examination should be performed. Once the opening pressure is determined, CSF should be withdrawn and sent for protein, glucose, cell count, cryptococcal antigen, and VDRL, as well as for bacterial, fungal, and acid-fast bacillus (AFB) smears and cultures. Most laboratories require around 10ml of CSF for AFB analysis. If possible, additional CSF should be obtained and held in the laboratory for possible polymerase chain reaction (PCR) testing for JC virus (PML), EBV (primary CNS lymphoma), or herpesviruses (cytomegalovirus [CMV], varicella-zoster virus [VZV], herpes simplex virus).

The CSF opening pressure is critical for the management of cryptococcal meningitis, because increased ICP (>200 mm H₂O) contributes independently to the morbidity and mortality associated with the infection. Markedly elevated ICP may require serial LPs, lumbar drainage, or ventriculoperitoneal shunting; measurement of initial opening pressure at the time of admission is very helpful in guiding subsequent management. Acetazolamide and steroids do not have a role in ICP management in HIV-associated cryptococcal meningitis.

CSF cryptococcal antigen is very informative because the sensitivity exceeds 95%. India ink smear is specific, but not sensitive, and cultures may take weeks or months to grow the organism. Testing has similarly limited yield in tuberculous meningitis; hence a negative CSF AFB smear or prior negative CSF culture does not exclude the diagnosis. Typical CSF findings of chronic meningitis (markedly elevated protein, normal or low glucose, and lymphocytic pleocytosis) are not always seen in cryptococcal meningitis in the setting of HIV disease. Routine CSF studies (protein, glucose, cell count) may occasionally be entirely normal in cryptococcal meningitis, highlighting the importance of the cryptococcal antigen as a diagnostic test. In patients who refuse LP or have other

Table 42.6 Selected HIV-Related Brain Disorders: Neuroimaging, CSF

Cerebral Toxoplasmosis	• Toxoplasma IgG positive: serologic screening is part of routine HIV care, so results may be available in patients with established HIV diagnosis • CT/MRI (Figure 42.1): Ring-enhancing lesions with marked surrounding edema in basal ganglia or cortical/subcortical junction • Enhancing lesions with negative *Toxoplasma* serology are more likely to be other infectious cause or PCNSL • LP may be contraindicated, depending on imaging results: elevated protein, normal glucose, lymphocytic/monocytic pleocytosis; *Toxoplasma* serologies usually not done routinely in CSF
Primary CNS Lymphoma (PCNSL)	• CT/MRI (Figure 42.2): Homogeneously enhancing lesion or lesions in periventricular regions or corpus callosum, with mild to moderate surrounding edema • LP may be contraindicated, depending on imaging results: elevated protein, normal glucose (unless associated lymphomatous meningitis, in which case glucose may be low), lymphocytic pleocytosis, sometimes with positive EBV PCR or more rarely cytology
Progressive Multifocal Leukoen-cephalopathy (PML)	• CT/MRI (Figure 42.3): Nonenhancing, asymmetric white matter lesion or lesions, often in parietal or occipital white matter, without surrounding edema in most patients. May be confused with ischemic stroke – sparing of gray matter in PML is a helpful clue • Patients who have just started HAART and have IRIS may have atypical imaging findings of enhancement and mass effect • LP: elevated protein, normal glucose, mild lymphocytic pleocytosis, positive JC virus PCR
Cryptococcal Meningitis	• CT/MRI: normal (or generalized atrophy) or may show hydrocephalus or cerebral edema. • LP: elevated opening pressure, normal or elevated protein, normal or low glucose, lymphocytic pleocytosis, positive cryptococcal antigen
HIV-Associated Dementia	• CT/MRI: generalized atrophy with mild, symmetric periventricular white matter abnormalities especially bifrontally • LP: normal opening pressure, normal or elevated protein (<100 mg/dL), normal glucose, mild lymphocytic pleocytosis
Tuberculous Meningitis	• CT/MRI: normal or basilar enhancement, hydrocephalus or small-vessel infarctions • LP: elevated opening pressure, elevated protein, low glucose, lymphocytic pleocytosis; negative AFB smear does not exclude diagnosis and cultures are not always positive
Syphilitic Meningitis	• CT/MRI: normal or basilar enhancement, sometimes with infarction (meningovascular syphilis) • LP: normal or elevated opening pressure, elevated protein, normal or low glucose, lymphocytic pleocytosis; CSF VDRL is ≤70% sensitive, so diagnosis may depend on positive serum serology with compatible CSF profile and overall clinical picture
CMV Ventricu-loencephalitis	• CT/MRI: normal or periventricular enhancement, with or without hydrocephalus • LP: may resemble bacterial meningitis with elevated protein, polymorphonuclear pleocytosis, and low or normal glucose, positive CMV PCR

Patients whose altered mental status remains unexplained after blood work, CT, and CSF examination may require electroencephalogram (EEG) to exclude nonconvulsive status epilepticus.

Left   **Center**   **Right**

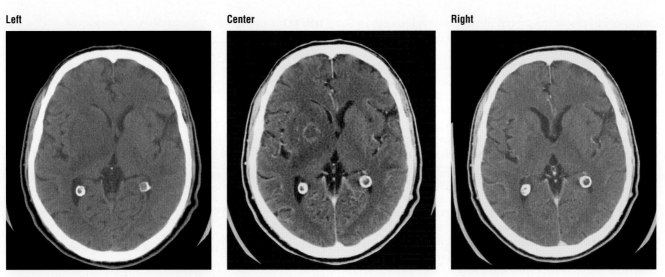

Figure 42.1   Cerebral toxoplasmosis. Head CT pre- (left) and post-contrast (center) from a patient who presented with headache, speech difficulty, and left arm weakness demonstrated a ring-enhancing lesion with surrounding edema in the right globus pallidus (and a smaller lesion in the left temporal lobe not seen on this image). HIV serology came back positive, with positive *Toxoplasma* IgG. The patient's headache and focal deficits resolved with empiric therapy for toxoplasmosis. Repeat post-contrast head CT 2 months later (right) showed decreased edema and resolution of abnormal enhancement.

Left   **Right**

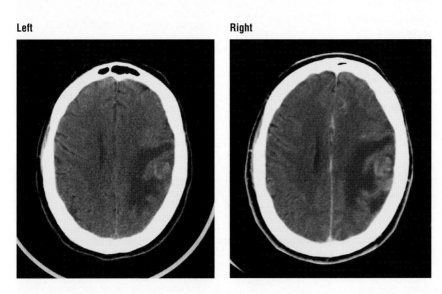

Figure 42.2   Primary CNS lymphoma. Head CT pre- (left) and post- (right) contrast from an untreated AIDS patient who presented with a generalized seizure after a week of dysarthria and right-sided weakness and numbness demonstrated an intrinsically hyperdense left frontoparietal lesion with mass effect and slight homogeneous enhancement. Toxoplasma serology was negative, and brain biopsy revealed primary CNS lymphoma.

Left   **Right**

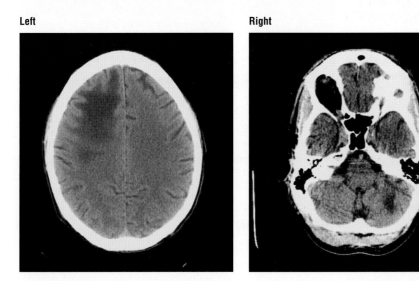

Figure 42.3   Progressive multifocal leukoencephalopathy. Noncontrast head CT from an AIDS patient with left-sided weakness showed a right frontal white matter lesion without mass effect (left) and a clinically silent lesion in the left cerebellar white matter (right). The lesions were not enhanced on gadolinium MRI (not shown). Brain biopsy confirmed the presumptive diagnosis of PML.

contraindications to the procedure, serum cryptococcal antigen can be useful because it is only rarely negative in cryptococcal meningitis.

One challenge in interpreting CSF results from patients with HIV infection is the high prevalence of mild protein elevation (<100 mg/dL) and lymphocytic pleocytosis (<50/mm^3). More marked abnormalities in CSF protein or cell count, low glucose, or polymorphonuclear pleocytosis at any CD4 count warrants investigation for causes other than HIV itself, as does pleocytosis in patients with CD4 count below 50/mm^3 or whose HIV disease is well controlled on HAART. If the CSF profile resembles bacterial meningitis, with elevated protein, polymorphonuclear pleocytosis, and low or normal glucose, an additional diagnostic consideration, particularly in patients with CD4 counts less than 50/mm^3, is CMV ventriculoencephalitis. In such patients, CT may be normal or reveal mild hydrocephalus, periventricular enhancement, or both. CSF polymerase chain reaction for CMV nucleic acids can establish the diagnosis.

COMPLICATIONS AND ADMISSION CRITERIA

Except for patients with a secure diagnosis of a rapidly reversible and definitively treatable toxic-metabolic encephalopathy, such as hypoglycemia or opiate overdose, or seizure with full recovery (and negative work-up), most patients with AMS and HIV disease require admission. Patients with focal CNS infection, meningitis, or primary CNS lymphoma are at risk for seizures and increased ICP, though antiepileptic drugs (AEDs) are not given as routine prophylaxis without a documented seizure. Elevated ICP may develop as a consequence of focal or generalized cerebral edema, hydrocephalus, or both. Patients with meningitis may develop cranial neuropathies, and ischemic stroke may complicate syphilitic, tuberculous, or acute bacterial meningitis.

TREATMENT AND PROPHYLAXIS

Therapy may not always be started in the acute care setting for HIV-related cerebral OIs if there is significant diagnostic uncertainty and no indication of neurologic emergency (i.e., no increased ICP, seizure, bacterial meningitis, or acute stroke) (Table 42.7).

Increased ICP is managed in the usual fashion, as is status epilepticus. The recurrence risk for seizures in patients with HIV disease appears to be higher than in seronegative patients; hence it is reasonable to consider AED therapy for a single seizure, in the absence of an obvious reversible toxic-metabolic precipitant such as withdrawal, cocaine or methamphetamine use, hypoglycemia, hyponatremia, or hypocalcemia. That decision is particularly complicated in patients on HAART, because first-line AEDs such as phenytoin and carbamazepine, as hepatic enzyme inducers, have adverse drug-drug interactions with most HAART regimens. Failure of antiretroviral therapy has been reported in this context, highlighting the importance of prescribing very carefully in patients on HAART.

In the absence of other contraindications, it would be reasonable to treat HIV-positive patients with community-acquired bacterial meningitis with dexamethasone before or with the first dose of antibiotics. In patients with IRIS, HAART

Table 42.7 Initial Treatment of Selected CNS Infections in HIV/AIDS

Cerebral Toxoplasmosis	• Pyrimethamine 200 mg PO loading dose then 50 mg (<60 kg) or 75 mg PO daily, sulfadiazine 1 g (<60 kg) or 1.5 g PO q6h, folinic acid 10–20 mg PO daily • Consult infectious diseases specialist for patients with antibiotic allergies or who cannot take oral medications
Cryptococcal Meningitis	• Amphotericin B 0.7 mg/kg IV daily with flucytosine 25 mg/kg PO q6h (caution if significant marrow failure) • Consult infectious disease specialist for patients with renal insufficiency, for consideration of liposomal amphotericin • Consider high-dose oral fluconazole 400–800 mg PO daily, with flucytosine 25 mg/kg PO q6h (caution if significant marrow failure) for patients without intravenous access or who decline admission
PML	• None (HAART in treatment-naïve patients)
Tuberculous Meningitis	• Four-drug therapy; consult infectious disease specialist due to complex drug-drug interactions between many antituberculous drugs, particularly rifampin, and many HAART regimens • Consider adjunctive dexamethasone (may be started after antituberculous drugs begun)
Neurosyphilis	• Penicillin G 18–24 million units per day (3–4 million units IV q4h or continuous infusion) *or* • Procaine penicillin 2.4 million units IM once daily plus probenecid 500 mg PO qid (if adherence with daily injections and oral probenecid can be assured for 10–14 days)
VZV Encephalitis	• Acyclovir 10 mg/kg IV q8h
CMV Encephalitis	• Ganciclovir with or without foscarnet; consult infectious disease specialist
Bacterial Meningitis (Community-acquired)	• Consider adjunctive dexamethasone, 10–20 minutes prior to or at the same time as initial dose of antibiotics, 0.15 mg/kg q6h for 2–4 days for proven or suspected pneumococcal meningitis • Cover for *Listeria monocytogenes* (ampicillin or penicillin), in addition to meningococcus and pneumococcus (ceftriaxone and vancomycin): vancomycin 30–45 mg/kg/day IV divided q8–12h + ceftriaxone 4 g/day IV divided q12h (or once daily) + ampicillin 2 g IV q4h. In penicillin-allergic patients, ampicillin should be substituted with trimethoprim-sulfamethoxazole 10–20 mg/kg trimethoprim component divided every q6–12h

is usually continued; steroids are sometimes administered to attenuate the inflammatory response, although controlled data are lacking.

INFECTION CONTROL

Other than usual universal precautions and consideration of respiratory isolation in patients with proven or suspected TB, no additional infection control measures are required in HIV-positive patients with AMS.

PEARLS AND PITFALLS

1. Key elements of the history in HIV-infected patients with AMS include recent and nadir CD4 count, recent viral load, prior neurologic or psychiatric disorders, and detailed medication history, including antibiotic use and allergies, illicit and other nonprescribed drugs, and composition and duration of HAART regimen.
2. AMS in the first weeks to months of HAART may be medication-related if efavirenz is one of the prescribed drugs, or may be due to an immune reconstitution of tuberculous or cryptococcal meningitis or PML.
3. For patients experiencing AMS from efavirenz, modifications to HAART should be discussed with the patient's HIV provider or HIV or an infectious disease consultant.
4. The risk of major cerebral opportunistic infections and malignancies is highest for patients with CD4 $<200/mm^3$. The absence of headache, fever or meningismus should not be used to exclude these diagnoses.
5. Noncontrast head CT is indicated in the evaluation of AMS in HIV-positive patients; contrast-enhanced CT should be considered in patients with CD4 $<200/mm^3$ or symptoms or signs of focal cerebral dysfunction.
6. Cerebral toxoplasmosis is a common cause of fever and focal cerebral dysfunction in patients with AIDS and ring-enhancing lesions on neuroimaging studies; *Toxoplasma* IgG serology is usually positive.
7. AIDS patients with headache may have cryptococcal meningitis, even with normal mental status, nonfocal examination, and normal neuroimaging
8. Serum cryptococcal antigen can help suggest or exclude the diagnosis in patients who refuse or have other contraindications to lumbar puncture.
9. Medications should be prescribed carefully for patients on HAART, because of complex drug-drug interactions, particularly for hepatic enzyme-inducing agents such as older antiepileptic drugs and rifampin.

REFERENCES

Bhigjee AI, Rosemberg S. Optimizing therapy of seizures in patients with HIV and cysticercosis. Neurology 2006;67 (Suppl 4):S19–22.
Centers for Disease Control and Prevention (CDC). Treating opportunistic infections among HIV-infected adults and adolescents: recommendations from CDC, the National Institutes of Health, and the HIV Medicine Association/Infectious Disease Society of America. MMWR 2004;53(No. RR-15):1–112. Available at: http://www.cdc.gov/mmwr/preview/mmwrhtml/rr5315a1.htm. Accessed December 12, 2007.
Liedtke MD, Lockhart SM, Rathbun RC. Anticonvulsant and antiretroviral interactions. Ann Pharmacother 2004;38:482.
Manji H, Miller R. The neurology of HIV infection. J Neurol Neurosurg Psychiatry 2004;75(Suppl 1):i29–i35.
McNicholl IR, Peiperl L, eds. HIVInSite Database of Antiretroviral Drug Interactions. Available at: http://hivinsite.ucsf.edu/arvdb? page = ar-0002. Accessed December 12, 2007.
Murdoch DM, Venter WDF, Van Rie A, Feldman C. Immune reconstitution inflammatory syndrome (IRIS): review of common infectious manifestations and treatment options. AIDS Res Ther 2007;4:9. Available at: http://www.aidsrestherapy.com/content/4/1/9. Accessed December 12, 2007.
Portegies P, Solod L, Cinque P, et al. Guidelines for the diagnosis and management of neurological complications of HIV infection. Eur J Neurol 2004;11:297–304.
Quagliariello V. Adjunctive steroids for tuberculous meningitis – more evidence, more questions. N Engl J Med 2004;351:1792–4.
Rothman RE, Keyl PM, McArthur JC, et al. A decision guideline for emergency department utilization of noncontrast head computerized tomography in HIV-infected patients. Acad Emerg Med 1999; 6:1010–9.
Saag MS, Graybill RJ, Larsen RA, et al. Practice guidelines for the management of cryptococcal disease. Clin Infect Dis 2000;30:710–8.
Shelburne III SA, Hamill RJ. The immune reconstitution inflammatory syndrome. AIDS Rev 2003;5:67–79.
Snider WD, Simpson DM, Nielsen S, et al. Neurological complications of acquired immune deficiency syndrome: analysis of 50 patients. Ann Neurol 1983;14:403–18.
Spudich SS, Nilsson AC, Lollo ND, et al. Cerebrospinal fluid HIV infection and pleocytosis: relation to systemic infection and antiretroviral treatment. BMC Infect Dis 2005;5:98.
Treisman GJ, Kaplin AI. Neurologic and psychiatric complications of antiretroviral agents. AIDS 2002;16:1201–15.
Tunkel AR, Hartman BJ, Kaplan SL, et al. Practice guidelines for the management of bacterial meningitis. Clin Infect Dis 2004; 39:1201–15.
Tso EL, Todd WC, Groleau GA, Hooper FJ. Cranial computed tomography in the emergency department evaluation of HIV-infected patients with neurologic complaints. Ann Emerg Med 1993;27:1169–76.
Venkataramana A, Pardo CA, McArthur JC, et al. Immune reconstitution inflammatory syndrome in the CNS of HIV-infected patients. Neurology 2006;67:383–8.

43. Bacterial Skin and Soft-Tissue Infections

Teri A. Reynolds and Bradley W. Frazee

Outline   Introduction
              Epidemiology
              Clinical Features
              Differential Diagnosis
              Laboratory and Radiographic Findings
              Treatment and Prophylaxis
              Complications and Admission Criteria
              Infection Control
              Pearls and Pitfalls
              References
              Additional Readings

INTRODUCTION

Skin and soft-tissue infections, comprising abscess, cellulitis, and necrotizing soft-tissue infection (NSTI), account for 1.8 million annual emergency department (ED) visits in the United States alone (Table 43.1). There has been a recent dramatic shift in bacteriology, with a rise in the prevalence of staphylococcal infection and of community-acquired methicillin-resistant *Staphylococcus aureus* (CA-MRSA), requiring new empiric antibiotic strategies. Emergency physicians are often in a position to make the first diagnosis and treatment of skin and soft-tissue infections. In the case of potentially lethal NSTI, highly time-dependent morbidity and mortality require familiarity with diverse presentations and the limitations of diagnostic tests.

EPIDEMIOLOGY

Abscess

Risk factors for abscess formation include injection drug use (IDU), shaving, and known colonization or infection with CA-MRSA. *Staphylococcus aureus* is implicated in 19–71% of abscess cases. It is highly prevalent, colonizing approximately 30% of the general population and an even higher propor-

tion of injection drug users, diabetics, and health care workers. The rising prevalence of CA-MRSA in the United States has manifested largely as a rise in spontaneous skin and soft-tissue infections. Nearly all *S. aureus* strains secrete exotoxins (including hemolysins, nucleases, proteases, lipases, hyaluronidase, and collagenase) that convert host tissues into nutrients required for bacterial growth. Additionally, some methicillin-sensitive *S. aureus* (MSSA) and the majority of CA-MRSA strains carry genes for Panton-Valentine leukocidin (PVL), a cytotoxin causing leukocyte destruction, tissue necrosis, and enhanced abscess formation.

Abscesses frequently contain a mix of anaerobes and aerobes. Oral flora (including *Streptococcus milleri*, *Eikenella*, and *Peptostreptococcus*) are commonly found in abscesses associated with IDU. Gut flora such as *E. coli* and *Bacteroides fragilis* are uncommon except in abscesses occurring around the groin and anal area.

Cellulitis

Risk factors for cellulitis include processes that disrupt the skin barrier, such as wounds, bites, surgical procedures, injection drug use, body piercing, and dermatophytoses, as well as conditions that render local immune defenses less effective, such as peripheral edema. Rarely, cellulitis can be due to subjacent primary infection such as osteomyelitis, or due to hematogenous spread in the setting of bacteremia. Most cases are caused by streptococcal species. Staphylococcal cellulitis is less common, unless there is associated abscess or penetrating trauma. There are a few notable risk factors for cellulitis associated with other organisms (Table 43.2).

NSTI

Although NSTI can develop after minor wounds or trauma, most cases are associated with at least one of the following risk factors: IDU, diabetic foot ulcers, surgery, trauma, peripheral vascular disease, malnutrition, or alcoholism (Table 43.3). IDU is by far the most common risk factor in community-acquired NSTI.

Depending on the study, approximately one-third to two-thirds of NSTIs are polymicrobial. Staphylococcal species (*aureus* and *epidermidis*) are the most common isolates, and

Table 43.1 Skin and Soft-Tissue Infections: Definitions

Abscess	Subcutaneous collection of pus
Furuncle ("Boil")	An infection originating in a hair follicle that produces a localized subcutaneous abscess
Carbuncle	Coalescence of multiple furuncles, typically involving the deep subcutaneous tissues of the neck and upper back
Cellulitis	Acute spreading infection of the dermis and subcutaneous tissue
NSTI (Includes Necrotizing Fasciitis and Myonecrosis)	Characterized by necrosis of deep structures such as fascia and muscle Fulminant course with eventual development of systemic manifestations

Table 43.2 Risk Factors and Pathogens Associated with Severe Forms of Cellulitis

Clinical Presentation	Likely Organisms
Diabetic foot ulcer	Gram-positive cocci, gram-negative rods, (including *Pseudomonas*) and anaerobes (including *Bacteroides*)
Cat bite	*Pasteurella multocida*
Human bite	*Eikenella corrodens*, anaerobes
Fresh water exposure	*Aeromonas hydrophila*
Salt water exposure	*Vibrio vulnificus*
Fish tank owner or fish handler	*Erysipelothrix rhusiopathiae*

Table 43.3 Necrotizing Soft-Tissue Infections

Type I	Associated with devitalized tissue: ● Postop setting ● Battlefield injuries ● Injection drug use ● Decubitus or diabetic foot ulcer Polymicrobial synergistic infection often involving anaerobes such as clostridial species Includes gas gangrene, Fournier's gangrene, Ludwig's angina
Type II	Caused by group A *Streptococcus*, usually monomicrobial Trivial or occult injury in most cases Synonymous with streptococcal toxic shock syndrome and "flesh-eating bacteria"

CA-MRSA NSTI has been reported. Oral and bowel flora such as non-group-A streptococcal species, gram-negative rods, and non-clostridial anaerobes are common in polymicrobial infections. Clostridial species (*perfringens, novyi*) are associated with myonecrosis (gas gangrene) and fatal NSTI in injection drug users. Group A *Streptococcus* causes a distinct monomicrobial form of NSTI that is often associated with only trivial or occult injury. The pathophysiology of these often fulminant infections involves bacterial exotoxins, like those produced by *C. perfringens* and group A *Streptococcus*, and release of cytokines such as tumor necrosis factor.

CLINICAL FEATURES

The initial diagnostic approach (Figure 43.1) to acute cutaneous erythema, warmth, and tenderness should be to look for evidence of a purulent fluid collection, as evidenced by fluctuance on exam or a hypoechoic fluid pocket on bedside ultrasound (Figure 43.2). Blind needle aspiration in the absence of these findings is generally not recommended. The presence of pus mandates immediate drainage and often obviates the need for antibiotics. In the absence of pus, diagnostic possibilities include both simple cellulitis and NSTI.

Abscess

Abscess usually presents as a localized, circular area of erythema, warmth, and tenderness. Palpable fluctuance is a critical sign that can be subtle, and a deep abscess can easily be missed. Abscesses may be accompanied by a significant surrounding cellulitis. However, a uniform rim of reactive erythema and dense induration is often present around an uncomplicated abscess, and does not necessarily signify an infectious cellulitis. Overlying necrosis and drainage may

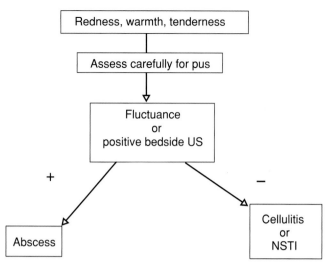

Figure 43.1 General approach to undifferentiated skin and soft-tissue infections.

be present in a mature abscess. Fever can occur, and large abscesses accompanied by fever are associated with up to a 20% incidence of bacteremia. In contrast, bacteremia appears to be uncommon in afebrile patients with abscesses, either before or immediately after drainage.

Hidradenitis suppurativa is a disease defined by multiple and recurrent abscesses involving the apocrine glands of the axilla and inguinal region. There is usually a personal and/or family history of multiple abscesses. Although incision and drainage of individual abscesses is frequently necessary, it is rarely sufficient for cure. More aggressive treatments include extensive debridement of the affected areas with skin grafts. Topical clindamycin and long-term (3 months) tetracycline therapy have been shown to be effective.

Cellulitis

Cellulitis also presents with erythema, warmth, and tenderness, though cellulitic erythema often has an irregular margin or blotchy appearance. Unlike an abscess, cellulitis lacks a frank pus pocket, is not walled off, and spreads laterally. Unlike a necrotizing soft-tissue infection, it can be cured with antibiotics alone and does not require debridement. Areas of

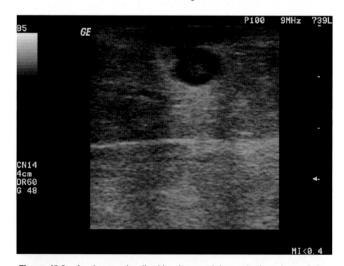

Figure 43.2 An abscess visualized by ultrasound demonstrating a hypoechoic fluid pocket with farfield enhancement.

superficial hemorrhagic transformation or skin necrosis can be seen in severe cellulitis, but such findings should always raise concern for a necrotizing infection requiring urgent surgical intervention. Lymphangitis and fever may be present and are considered markers of severity. A portal of entry, such as a recent site of drug injection or fungal infection of the feet, may or may not be evident.

Erysipelas is a specific form of cellulitis caused by group A *Streptococcus*. It is characterized by bright erythema with a sharp, raised margin and peau d'orange appearance caused by subcutaneous edema around hair follicles. It typically occurs on the face or on the lower extremities in the setting of preexisting edema.

NSTI

Recognition of NSTI can be difficult because the initial clinical features are nonspecific. On average, the diagnosis of NSTI is made 3–4 days from onset of symptoms. Pain out of proportion to skin signs is common, but by no means universal. Erythema and induration are the most common findings, and a characteristic woody edema extending beyond the border of erythema may be apparent. Classic findings that are frequently absent include bullae, crepitus, skin sloughing, hemorrhage, necrosis, and cutaneous sensory deficit. These findings usually appear late in the course of necrotizing infections, if at all. Fever is present in 30–80% of cases of NSTI, and leukocytosis in about 85%, whereas hypotension occurs in only 0–40% of cases.

A number of types of community-acquired NSTI deserve special mention. NSTI associated with group A *Streptococcus* infection and toxic shock syndrome classically follows varicella infection in children but is actually more common in adults, often without risk factors or an obvious portal of entry. Clustered outbreaks in both children and adults have been described. IDU-related NSTI is common in the western United States, usually related to nonintravenous injection (skin popping, muscling) of black tar heroin. Outbreaks have been described in the United Kingdom and the United States, implicating contaminated batches of drugs or paraphernalia. IDU-associated NSTI may present with massive swelling of the extremity where recent injection has occurred, often with spread to the trunk. Case mortality exceeds 25%. Other classic presentations of NSTI include:

- diabetic foot ulcer with proximal swelling or signs of systemic inflammation
- any significant skin infection of the perineum (Fournier's gangrene)
- odontogenic infection in which symptoms or edema extend into the floor of the mouth or the neck (Ludwig's angina)

Given the nonspecific and variable nature of presenting signs and symptoms, and the limitations of imaging, maintaining a high index of suspicion for NSTI is imperative. Illustrating the difficulty of making this diagnosis, in one series of 15 cases of group A streptococcal necrotizing fasciitis missed on initial outpatient presentation, the leading incorrect diagnoses were musculoskeletal pain, influenza, gastroenteritis, and first-degree burn.

DIFFERENTIAL DIAGNOSIS

As described above, when faced with tender skin erythema and edema concerning for bacterial infection, the crucial initial distinction is among abscess, cellulitis, and NSTI. Other superficial skin infections with a distinctive appearance, such as impetigo and fungal infections, are easily diagnosed in most cases. Impetigo is a staphylococcal or streptococcal infection common in young children and characterized by discrete pustules or bullae on the face and extremities that rupture and give rise to a lacquer-like crust. Fungal infections typically give rise to round, plaquelike lesions with discrete borders.

Other conditions that are sometimes difficult to differentiate from cellulitis include reactive viral exanthems, autoimmune rashes, dermatitis, allergic reactions to insect bites and stings, gout, deep venous thrombosis (DVT), and chronic changes associated with edema and venous stasis. Dermatitis and autoimmune rashes typically produce lesions with a distinctive appearance, or pattern, such as target lesions, serum-filled bullae, scales, and plaques. Of note, dermatitis and infection often coexist, as many chronic inflammatory skin conditions are prone to bacterial superinfection. Local allergic reactions to insect envenomation, particularly bee stings, can closely mimic cellulitis, and the temptation to treat for superinfection is great. A large area of erythema, with marked warmth and a peau d'orange appearance may mimic cellulitis, but tenderness is minimal and pruritis is intense. Allergic reactions usually appear within several hours of envenomation, typically earlier than superinfection.

LABORATORY AND RADIOGRAPHIC FINDINGS

The Infectious Diseases Society of America recommends that all patients with soft-tissue infection accompanied by signs and symptoms of systemic toxicity (including fever or hypothermia, heart rate greater than 100 beats/min, or systolic blood pressure less than 90 mm Hg or 20 mm Hg below baseline) have blood drawn for studies, including culture, complete blood count (CBC) with differential, creatinine, bicarbonate, creatine phosphokinase (CPK), and C-reactive protein (CRP) (although routine use of CRP has yet to be integrated into U.S. emergency practice). Many experts also recommend obtaining lactate levels in all cases manifesting systemic inflammation.

Abscess

Computed tomographic (CT) scan likely represents the gold standard for diagnosis of deep subcutaneous or intramuscular abscesses, although it is rarely indicated. Bedside ultrasound, by contrast, has emerged as a useful adjunct to the physical exam when fluctuance is not obvious (Figure 43.2). Abscess cavities usually appear as hypo- or anechoic on ultrasound, and acoustic enhancement may be seen farfield of the collection. Traditionally, culturing of abscesses has not been recommended. However, with the emergence of CA-MRSA, some experts now recommend cultures, especially if the prevalence of CA-MRSA in the community is unclear, or if treatment with a beta-lactam antibiotic alone is planned.

Cellulitis

The main role of imaging in suspected cellulitis is to rule out an occult abscess or necrotizing infection. Studies of the etiology of cellulitis have relied on needle aspiration of the infected area or punch biopsies, though there is no role for these tests in routine care. Blood cultures prior to admission for cellulitis are no longer recommended in most immunocompetent patients, as the yield is around 5% and even positive cultures rarely change management. Cultures are indicated in patients with lymphangitis, rigors, or high fever suggesting bacteremia; in immunosuppressed patients, including those with human immunodeficiency virus (HIV), severe renal disease, diabetes mellitus (DM), or neutropenia; and in all cases of cellulitis associated with animal bites, or with salt or fresh water immersion.

NSTI

All patients suspected of having NSTI should have a CBC, metabolic panel, CPK, lactate, and blood cultures sent. Unfortunately, there is no sensitive laboratory or imaging finding that can be used to rule out NSTI. Leukocytosis is neither sensitive nor specific for the diagnosis, but a markedly elevated white blood cell count (WBC) ($>20,000/mm^3$) is frequently seen and should raise concern for NSTI. There are some data suggesting that NSTI is distinguished by the combination of leukocytosis and hyponatremia. An elevated anion gap or lactate may be present. Azotemia and other signs of organ failure usually are not evident on initial presentation.

Plain soft-tissue x-rays reveal subcutaneous gas in 20–60% of cases, typically in a stippled pattern that follows tissue planes. CT and MRI can delineate the extent of inflammation and identify small gas pockets and fluid along the fascial planes, but sensitive and specific diagnostic criteria have yet to be defined for these modalities. Moreover, CT and MRI are time-consuming, costly, and dangerous for unstable patients. No patient with a suspected diagnosis of NSTI should have surgical care delayed for an imaging study, as these infections progress on the order of minutes to hours. Use of bedside ultrasound to diagnose necrotizing fasciitis has been described by one group. A significant fluid stripe adjacent to the deep fascia was reported to be diagnostic, although these findings have yet to be validated.

Ultimately, the rapid diagnosis of NSTI requires a high index of suspicion on the part of the emergency physician, immediate surgical consultation, and a low threshold for surgical exploration. Surgical exploration remains the gold standard for diagnosis, and swollen fascia with easily separable tissue planes is diagnostic of necrotizing fasciitis. All patients should have surgical specimen cultures sent, although the yield is surprisingly low.

TREATMENT AND PROPHYLAXIS

Abscess

In most cases of abscess, the host defense has successfully walled off infection to the extent that simple drainage is curative. Abscesses should undergo immediate drainage in almost all cases, as antibiotics alone are unlikely to result in cure. Aspiration with a large-bore needle is sufficient for very small and superficial abscess, although in most cases, scalpel incision is required. Thorough evacuation of pus from the abscess

Table 43.4 Initial Treatment for Abscess and Cellulitis*

Incision and drainage required for abscess (often sufficient for cure without antibiotics)
Antibiotics (for cellulitis, and abscess complicated by surrounding cellulitis or in immunocompromised hosts):
Oral antibiotics:
cephalexin 500 mg PO qid
plus
TMP-SMX one DS tab PO bid
or
clindamycin 300–450 mg tid, alone

IV antibiotics:
clindamycin 600–900 mg q8h
plus
vancomycin 1 g q12h

*Always consider local and institutional susceptibility patterns.
DS, double strength.

cavity often requires blunt dissection of loculations. Use of wall suction is advised for large abscesses. Packing is mandatory after incision and drainage, to prevent closure of the opening and reaccumulation of purulent fluid. Sterile or iodinated packing strips or woven gauze (such as Kerlex) can be used. Tight packing may be required for initial hemostasis, but subsequent packing should be loose. Removal of the packing and inspection of the wound by medical personnel is recommended at 12–48 hours, and subsequent daily or twice daily packing changes can be done by the patient.

Local anesthesia is sufficient for incision and drainage in many cases; other options include regional anesthesia, such as peripheral nerve block. Adjunctive narcotic analgesia is often used, and procedural sedation, such as with propofol and fentanyl, may be required.

Adjunctive Antibiotics

Predrainage parenteral antibiotics should be considered in patients at high risk for infectious endocarditis, including those with congenital heart disease, major valvular abnormalities, or a history of endocarditis. Postdrainage antibiotics are unnecessary in most cases, and two prospective, placebo-controlled trials in the 1970s and 1980s failed to demonstrate any benefit of antibiotics after successful simple abscess drainage. Antibiotics are indicated in abscesses complicated by surrounding cellulitis or host immunosuppression (Table 43.4). Many experts recommend that all patients with an abscess accompanied by fever receive antibiotics, because, as discussed earlier, a significant minority of them will prove to be bacteremic. Selection of empiric antibiotics should be guided by the local prevalence of MRSA; if it is high, an antibiotic with appropriate activity, such as trimethoprim-sulfamethoxazole (TMP-SMX), should be included. There is limited recent evidence that empirical therapy for CA-MRSA may lead to better outcomes in skin or soft-tissue infection (SSTI).

Cellulitis

Most cases of cellulitis can be treated with oral therapy if close follow-up is available. For uncomplicated cellulitis, empirical therapy must cover *Streptococcus* and should cover

Table 43.5 Initial Therapy for Necrotizing Fasciitis

Prompt surgical debridement
Aggressive fluid resuscitation
piperacillin-tazobactam 3.375 g IV q6h
plus
clindamycin 900 mg IV q6h
plus
vancomycin 1 g IV q12h
(Alternative for penicillin-allergic patients: vancomycin plus ciprofloxacin plus clindamycin)

Staphylococcus aureus except in classic erysipelas. Antistaphylococcal penicillins or first-generation cephalosporins are first-line agents. Macrolides are no longer recommended for penicillin-allergic patients because of rising resistance in group A *Streptococcus* isolates. Adjunctive therapies include elevation of the infected area and treatment of any underlying predisposing condition such as fungal dermatitis or eczema.

NSTI

Any suspicion of NSTI should prompt immediate surgical consultation without delay for laboratory or imaging results. The surgical approach to diagnosis has been likened to the traditional approach to appendicitis, where more patients should be taken to surgery and explored than actually have the disease. Underscoring the importance of early surgical intervention, numerous studies have found that delay to surgery is the major determinant of mortality. Delay of greater than 12–24 hours quadruples mortality rates. Diagnostic delay has been correlated with admission to a medical service and "negative" blind needle aspiration.

Surgical intervention with wide debridement of the affected area is the major therapeutic modality. Initial empiric antibiotic therapy should be extremely broad-spectrum (see Table 43.5) and must cover *Staphylococcus aureus* (likely including MRSA depending on local prevalence) and group A *Streptococcus*, as well as gram negatives and anaerobes. Vancomycin is recommended for its MRSA activity, whereas high-dose clindamycin is recommended both for its activity against Streptococcal species and anaerobes and because it suppresses toxin production. An advanced penicillin plus beta-lactamase inhibitor, such as ampicillin sulbactam or piperacillin-tazobactam, is generally recommended as these offer gram-negative, gram-positive, and anaerobic activity. Additional measures include aggressive fluid resuscitation, hemodynamic monitoring, vasopressors as needed, and ample analgesia.

COMPLICATIONS AND ADMISSION CRITERIA

The Infectious Diseases Society of America recommends admission for all patients with skin and soft-tissue infections accompanied by hypotension, elevated creatinine, low serum bicarbonate, creatine phosphokinase at 2–3 times the upper limit of normal, marked left shift. Additionally, a lactate level above 4 mmol/L mandates admission. Immunosuppressed states such as diabetes or social factors such as homelessness, which might prevent elevation of an infected limb, should lower the threshold for hospitalization.

Abscess

When incision and drainage of abscess is successful, the need for admission is rare. Exceptions include:

- abscesses requiring drainage in the operating room
- significant surrounding cellulitis requiring parenteral antibiotics
- evidence of a systemic inflammatory response suggesting bacteremia
- immunocompromised patients (diabetes, HIV, end-stage renal disease [ESRD])

Cellulitis

Patients with cellulitis should be admitted in the following cases:

- failure of outpatient therapy
- fever or extreme leukocytosis
- cellulitis of the hand after a bite
- cellulitis in the setting of fresh or salt water exposure
- concern for compliance with outpatient therapy
- immunocompromised states (diabetes, HIV, ESRD)

NSTI

All patients suspected to have NSTI should be treated empirically, taken emergently for surgical exploration, and subsequently admitted to a monitored setting.

INFECTION CONTROL

Other than universal precautions, no additional infection control measures are required.

PEARLS AND PITFALLS

1. In an undifferentiated skin and soft-tissue infection, a pus pocket is present more often than not.
2. Bedside ultrasound can reveal and localize an unsuspected abscess.
3. The emergence of CA-MRSA has made the need for drainage and debridement even more common and reintroduced the need for abscess cultures.
4. In the evaluation of cellulitis, always consider risk factors (such as animal bites or water exposure) that are associated with esoteric pathogens and severe cellulitis, as well as the possibility of a necrotizing infection.
5. In NSTI, time to surgical debridement significantly affects morbidity and mortality. Request an immediate surgical consult as soon as the diagnosis is suspected. Do not delay for laboratory or imaging studies.
6. NSTIs are usually accompanied by a systemic inflammatory response at the time of presentation. Aggressive IV fluid resuscitation is required. For hypotension or elevated lactate, begin early goal-directed therapy for sepsis. Consider adrenal replacement therapy for persistent hypotension.

REFERENCES

Bobrow BJ, Pollack CV Jr, Gamble S, Seligson RA. Incision and drainage of cutaneous abscesses is not associated with bacteremia in afebrile adults. Ann Emerg Med 1997 Mar;29(3):404–8.

Chen JL, Fullerton KE, Flynn NM. Necrotizing fasciitis associated with injection drug use. Clin Infect Dis 2001 Jul 1;33(1):6–15.

Kaul R, McGeer A, Low DE, et al. Population-based surveillance for group A streptococcal necrotizing fasciitis: clinical features, prognostic indicators, and microbiologic analysis of seventy-seven cases. Ontario Group A Streptococcal Study. Am J Med 1997 Jul;103(1):18–24.

Meislin HW, Lerner SA, Graves MH, et al. Cutaneous abscesses. Anaerobic and aerobic bacteriology and outpatient management. Ann Intern Med 1977 Aug;87(2):145–9.

Moran GJ, Krishnadasan A, Gorwitz RJ, et al. Methicillin-resistant *S. aureus* infections among patients in the emergency department. N Engl J Med 2006;355:666–7.

Perl B, Gottehrer NP, Raveh D, et al. Cost-effectiveness of blood cultures for adult patients with cellulitis. Clin Infect Dis 1999 Dec;29(6):1483–8.

Rutherford WH, Hart D, Calderwood JW, Merrett JD. Antibiotics in surgical treatment of septic lesions. Lancet 1970 May 23;1(7656):1077–80.

Squire BT, Fox JC, Anderson C. ABSCESS: applied bedside sonography for convenient evaluation of superficial soft tissue infections. Acad Emerg Med 2005 Jul;12(7):601–6.

ADDITIONAL READINGS

Stevens DL, Bisno AL, Chambers HF, et al. Practice guidelines for the diagnosis and management of skin and soft tissue infections (IDSA Guidelines). Clin Infect Dis 2005;41:1373–1406.

PART II

Pediatrics

44. Fever and Rash in the Pediatric Population

Catherine A. Marco, Janel Kittredge-Sterling, and Rachel L. Chin

INTRODUCTION

The combination of fever and rash is common in the pediatric population. Systemic etiologies, including meningococcal disease, rickettsial infections, viral infections such as measles and rubella, and drug hypersensitivity reactions are discussed in Chapter 4, Systemic Diseases Causing Fever and Rash. This chapter will discuss several additional etiologies specific to pediatric patients, including nonspecific viral exanthems, roseola infantum, erythema infectiosum, varicella-zoster infection, staphylococcal scalded skin syndrome, and Kawasaki disease.

A careful description of the timing of fever and appearance of skin lesions may be sufficient to narrow the diagnosis. Key elements of the history and physical are listed in Table 44.1.

EPIDEMIOLOGY

The large majority of cases of pediatric fever and rash, more than 70% in one study, are caused by viruses, and only approximately 20% are caused by bacteria. Viral exanthems are usually reactive and may be caused by enteroviruses, adenoviruses, echovirus, and numerous others. Infections with enteroviruses often peak in summer and autumn months.

Nonspecific Viral Exanthems

A variety of enteroviruses may cause a symptom complex including fever, malaise, gastrointestinal complaints, meningitis, and rash (Table 44.2). The enterovirus exanthem is typically maculopapular, although petechiae mimicking meningococcal infection may be seen. Petechiae have also been reported with coxsackievirus A9, echovirus 9, coxsackievirus A4, B2–5, and echovirus 3, 4, and 7 infections.

Roseola Infantum

Roseola infantum is thought to be caused by human herpes virus-6, though rotavirus and human herpes virus-7 have also been implicated as possible etiologies (Table 44.3). The incubation period is 1–2 weeks and most cases occur in spring and early fall. Children between 6 months and 3 years of age are most commonly affected.

Fever often precedes the exanthem, and the febrile child usually appears well and is playful. Cervical lymphadenopathy, pharyngeal erythema with or without exudates, and otitis media may occur. The exanthem typically appears after fever resolution (hence the term "roseola subitum"), beginning on the trunk and spreading upward to the neck and proximal extremities. The exanthem is often pink and may be macular, papular, or maculopapular (Figure 44.1). Berliner's sign may be seen, with palpebral and periorbital edema, resulting in the appearance of "heavy eyelids."

The diagnosis is made clinically. Therapy is supportive and should include antipyretics and oral hydration.

Erythema Infectiosum

Erythema infectiosum was first recognized in 1889 and was termed *fifth disease* because it was first described after four other common childhood exanthems (measles, scarlet fever, rubella, and Dukes' disease). Caused by the virus parvovirus B19, erythema infectiosum is common in childhood, with peak rates between the ages of 5 and 14 years. Transmission of the virus occurs via respiratory droplets.

Many cases are asymptomatic. Following an incubation period of 5–14 days, a prodromal phase may include low-grade fever, headache, pharyngitis, myalgias, nausea, diarrhea, and joint pain (Table 44.4). Skin findings include erythema of cheeks, the result of coalescent erythematous papules that produce the "slapped cheek" appearance (Figure 44.2). Approximately 2 days after the onset of the facial erythema, the typical lacy reticular extremity rash appears and

Table 44.1 Key Elements of the History and Physical in Pediatric Fever and Rash

History
- Duration of symptoms
- Associated symptoms (such as fever, headache, gastrointestinal symptoms, pruritus)
- Evolution of lesions
- Distribution
- History of animal or arthropod bites
- Exacerbating and relieving factors (such as environmental exposures, foods, medications)
- Medical history, occupational history, sexual history, medications, illicit drug history, travel, and allergies may be relevant

Physical Examination

Type of lesions, size, color, secondary findings (such as scale, excoriations), and distribution. Primary lesions should be identified and may include the following:
- *Macules* are flat lesions defined by an area of changed color (i.e., a blanchable erythema).
- *Papules* are raised, solid lesions <5 mm in diameter.
- *Plaques* are lesions >5 mm in diameter with a flat, plateaulike surface.
- *Nodules* are lesions >5 mm in diameter with a more rounded configuration.
- *Wheals* (urticaria, hives) are papules or plaques that are pale pink and may appear annular (ringlike) as they enlarge; classic (nonvasculitic) wheals are transient, lasting only 24 to 48 hours in any defined area.
- *Vesicles* (<5 mm) and *bullae* (>5 mm) are circumscribed, elevated lesions containing fluid.
- *Pustules* are raised lesions containing purulent exudates. Vesicular processes such as varicella or herpes simplex may evolve to pustules.
- *Nonpalpable purpura* is a flat lesion that is due to bleeding into the skin. If <3 mm in diameter the purpuric lesions are termed *petechiae*. If >3 mm, they are termed *ecchymoses*. *Palpable purpura* is a raised lesion that is due to inflammation of the vessel wall (vasculitis) with subsequent hemorrhage.
- An *ulcer* is a defect in the skin extending at least into the upper layer of the dermis.
- *Eschar* is a necrotic lesion covered with a black crust.

Secondary lesions may include:
- Scale
- Crust
- Fissure
- Erosions
- Ulcer
- Scar
- Excoriation
- Infection
- Pigment changes
- Lichenification

Color may be:
- Normal
- Erythematous
- Violaceous
- Hyperpigmented
- Hypopigmented

Patterns of lesions should be established as:
- Single
- Grouped
- Scattered
- Linear
- Annular
- Symmetric
- Dermatomal
- Central or peripheral
- Along Blaschko's lines (linear skin patterns thought to be of embryonic origin, usually forming a "V" shape over the spine and "S" shapes over the chest, stomach, and sides)

Table 44.2 Clinical Features: Nonspecific Viral Exanthems

Organisms	Enterovirus 3, 4, 7, and 9; coxsackievirus A9, A4, B2–5; adenovirus; RSV; parainfluenza 1, 2, and 3; influenza A, B; cytomegalovirus; Epstein-Barr; parvovirus B19
Signs and Symptoms	- Fever - Nonspecific maculopapular eruption - Petechiae - Nausea, vomiting, diarrhea - Malaise
Laboratory Findings	No laboratory testing necessary
Treatment	- Hydration (oral or intravenous) - Antipyretic agents - Antipruritic agents - Instructions for caregivers, including warning signs of severe infection

RSV, respiratory syncytial virus.

patients with hemoglobinopathies. Among immunocompromised patients, including those with human immunodeficiency virus (HIV) infection, congenital immunodeficiencies, acute leukemia, organ transplants, and lupus erythematosus, or in infants younger than 1 year old, parvovirus B19 may cause a serious prolonged chronic anemia resulting from persistent lysis of red-blood-cell (RBC) precursors. Administration of intravenous immune globulin (IVIG), which contains pooled, neutralizing anti-B19 antibody, has been used successfully in these patients.

Parvovirus B19 infection during pregnancy may result in vertical transmission to the fetus, causing infection of erythroid precursors and extensive hemolysis, leading to severe anemia, tissue hypoxia, high-output heart failure, and generalized edema (hydrops fetalis). Most reported fetal losses secondary to parvovirus B19 have occurred in the first trimester of pregnancy (see Chapter 53, Fever in Pregnancy).

Table 44.3 Clinical Features: Roseola Infantum

Organisms	Likely human herpesvirus-6 (HHV-7), though rotavirus and HHV-7 have also been suggested
Incubation Period	1–2 weeks
Signs and Symptoms	- Febrile child usually appears well and is playful. - Cervical lymphadenopathy, pharyngeal erythema with or without exudates, and otitis media may occur. - The exanthem appears after fever resolution. - The rash typically begins on the trunk and spreads upward to the neck and proximal extremities. - The exanthema is often pink and may be macular, papular, or maculopapular. - Palpebral and periorbital edema (Berliner's sign) is common.
Laboratory Findings	Not recommended. Clinical diagnosis.
Treatment	Therapy is supportive and should include antipyretics and oral hydration.

usually fades in 6–14 days. An enanthema may also be seen, with erythema of the tongue and pharynx, and macules on the buccal mucosa and palate. Arthralgias or arthritis may be seen in 10% of affected children, typically involving large joints.

Significant complications of parvovirus B19 infection may occur in the immunocompromised, the fetus, and

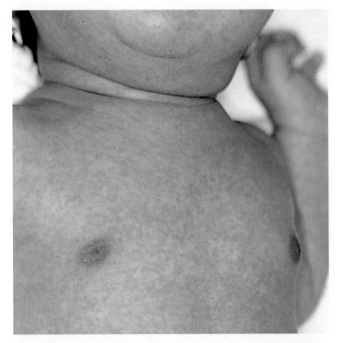

Figure 44.1 Roseola. Photograph source: www.derm101.com, with permission.

Table 44.4 Clinical Features: Erythema Infectiosum

Organism	Parvovirus B19
Incubation Period	Defined by days prior to appearance of rash; ranges from 5 to 14 days
Signs and Symptoms	• **Skin**: erythema infectiosum (fifth disease): facial erythema ("slapped cheek"), circumoral pallor (18 days after infection); reticular rash (trunk and limbs) • **Bone marrow**: transient aplasia (patients with thalassemia, hemolytic anemia); chronic pure red cell aplasia (immunosuppressed, especially HIV, transplant, sickle cell); hemophagocytic syndrome (immunocompromised) • **Fetus**: Hydrops fetalis (risk ~1.6% for acute infection during pregnancy; highest between 11 and 23 weeks gestation); anemia; thrombocytopenia • **Other**: CNS (encephalopathy); liver (hepatitis); heart (myocarditis)
Laboratory Findings	• Laboratory testing not indicated in uncomplicated cases. • IgM (85%+ with erythema infectiosum or aplastic crisis; turns negative within 3 months); IgG (2 weeks postinfection; lifelong); PCR most sensitive (*not* diagnostic alone). Giant pronormoblasts visible on microscopy of blood or bone marrow aspirate suggest the diagnosis.
Treatment	• In uncomplicated cases: supportive care (hydration, antipyretics) • NSAIDs for arthropathy; blood products for transient aplasia; weekly US for infected pregnant women; cordicentesis and intrauterine transfusions for hydrops fetalis **Immunosuppressed treatment regimen**: • Chronic pure red cell aplasia: IVIG 0.4 g/kg/day for 5 days or 1 g/kg/day for 2–3 days; may need to repeat monthly

CNS, central nervous system; NSAID, nonsteroidal anti-inflammatory drug; PCR, polymerase chain reaction; US, ultrasound.

In patients with chronic hemolytic anemias, transient aplastic crisis manifested by anemia, reticulocytopenia, and RBC aplasia may result. Aplastic crisis may also be seen in patients with hereditary spherocytosis, sickle-cell disease, glucose-6-phosphate dehydrogenase (G6PD) deficiency, pyruvate-kinase deficiency, iron deficiency, and the thalassemias.

Management of patients with erythema infectiosum includes supportive care with antipyretics, oral hydration, and antipruritic agents, if needed. There are no published timing recommendations for returning to school or day care, though the onset of the facial rash corresponds with a decrease in contagion.

Additional therapies may be indicated for complicated cases. Patients with chronic hemolytic anemias who develop transient aplastic crisis (pallor, weakness, and lethargy) may require blood transfusion. Pregnant women with signs or symptoms suggestive of B19 infection or known recent exposure to infected contacts should have serum B19 IgM and IgG titers drawn. If acute maternal infection is identified by positive IgM titiers, serial fetal ultrasounds should be performed to evaluate for hydrops fetalis.

Varicella Zoster

Varicella zoster (chickenpox) is a clinical disease caused by the varicella-zoster virus (VZV), a double-stranded DNA virus and a member of the Herpesviridae family. VZV is the agent that causes both varicella (chickenpox) and subsequently, the dermatomal reactivation rash of herpes zoster (shingles). Varicella infections are more prevalent in temperate climates and are common during March, April, and May. Although children rarely develop shingles, it may be seen in children who are immunosuppressed, such as those with HIV infection, immunosuppressive drugs, or cancer. Varicella is contagious, with an estimated 80–90% transmission rate among household contacts. Transmission occurs by respiratory inoculation via airborne droplet, or by direct contact with infected vesicular fluid.

Acute varicella among young, healthy, nonpregnant patients typically follows a benign, self-limiting disease course. Prior to the appearance of the rash, a 1- to 2-day prodrome may occur, with headache, malaise, and fever (Table 44.5). Children may present with the rash and fever simultaneously. The typical exanthem of varicella begins on

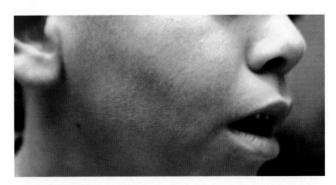

Figure 44.2 Erythema infectiosum. Photograph source: Centers for Disease Control Public Health Image Library, http://www.phil.cdc.gov/phil/home.asp.

Table 44.5 Clinical Features: Varicella Zoster

Organism	Varicella-zoster virus
Incubation period	10–21 days
Signs and Symptoms	• Prodrome: fever, malaise • 1–2 days later: rash • Three phases: macules, papules, vesicles • Lesions crust and scab • Lesions appear in crops; often all three phases are seen simultaneously in the same patient
Laboratory Findings	Not indicated. Clinical diagnosis.
Treatment	Therapy is supportive and should include antipyretics, antipruritics, and oral hydration.

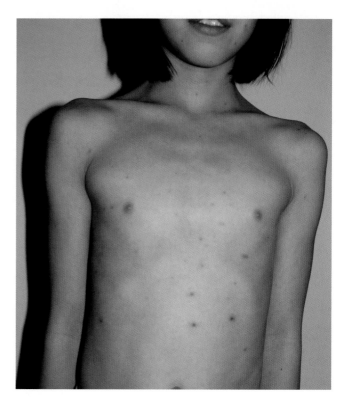

Figure 44.3 Varicella-zoster infection.

the head, spreads centripetally, extending to the extremities. The rash typically occurs in three stages, beginning with macules, evolving to papules, and then to vesicles on an erythematous base, commonly described as "dewdrop on a rose petal" (Figure 44.3). After the vesicles have formed, they may develop to pustules that later crust and scab. New crops of vesicles may form during the ensuing days. Complications of varicella may include skin bacterial superinfection, neurologic complications, pneumonia, encephalitis, asymptomatic transient hepatitis, thrombocytopenia, ophthalmologic keratitis, anterior uveitis, and death.

After the resolution of primary varicella, the latent virus lies dormant in ganglia, most commonly the thoracic and trigeminal ganglia. The reactivation of VZV appears in one or more ganglia as herpes zoster (shingles). A prodrome of burning, pain, itching, or tingling may precede the skin lesions. The vesicles are distributed along a dermatome and may persist for up to 4 weeks. Significant morbidity may occur in elderly patients, including postherpetic neuralgia, with persistent pain and dysesthesia. The disease course may be more severe in immunocompromised patients, with involvement of multiple nerve roots or, rarely, disseminated visceral disease. Ocular manifestations of VZV may include herpes zoster ophthalmicus, affecting the areas distributed by the ophthalmic division of the trigeminal nerve. Herpes zoster virus (HZV) ophthalmicus may result in chronic ocular inflammation, visual loss, tissue scarring, and debilitating pain. Ocular manifestations should be considered if Hutchinson's sign is present, with skin involvement of the tip of the nose (see Chapter 30, Conjunctival and Corneal Infections). Herpes zoster oticus may present with devastating otalgia, associated with vesicular involvement of the external ear canal and pinna. Ramsey Hunt syndrome occurs when herpes zoster oticus produces a facial paralysis (VII) (see Chapter 6, Otitis Externa). The onset of pain in and around the ear, mouth, and face may precede the rash for hours to days.

The varicella vaccine, a live attenuated vaccine, was approved in 1995 for use in the United States. The administration of this vaccine has reduced the incidence of primary varicella as well as the incidence of varicella-related hospitalizations. The efficacy of the vaccine is estimated to be 70–90%. The vaccine is administered between 12 and 15 months of age. Controversy exists regarding the vaccine's lifetime immunity and a booster is recommended at ages 4–6 years.

Treatment of primary varicella is generally supportive and should include antipruritics, skin hygiene, antipyretics, and adequate oral hydration. The use of antiviral agents (acyclovir, famciclovir, valacyclovir) has not been proven to decrease the complication rate in healthy young children. Therefore, the use of these agents is typically reserved for primary disease in newborns and preterm infants, and for primary or reactivation disease in individuals older than 13 years of age. If antiviral therapy is used in primary disease, it should be initiated within 24 to 48 hours from the onset of the rash. Intravenous acyclovir is recommended for immunocompromised patients to reduce the incidence of dissemination and shorten the disease course. Antiviral agents should also be administered for all patients who present with reactivation herpes zoster within 3 days of the appearance of the skin lesions. Steroids may reduce the incidence of postherpetic neuralgia, if administered within 72 hours of the appearance of lesions.

Staphylococcal Scalded-Skin Syndrome

The staphylococcal scalded-skin syndrome (SSSS; Ritter's disease) is a generalized form of bullous impetigo and is caused by the organism *Staphylococcus aureus*. In infants this disease entity is termed "pemphigus neonatorum." SSSS is most common in patients under 2 years of age. Mortality is typically less than 5%.

Patients often have fever, irritability, and skin tenderness (Table 44.6). Cutaneous findings include diffuse erythema, flaccid blisters, and superficial skin sloughing (Figure 44.4). Nikolsky's sign (the superficial layers of skin slipping free from the lower layers with slight pressure) is positive.

The diagnosis is usually made clinically, and may be confirmed by a positive staphylococcal culture. SSSS may appear clinically very similar to toxic epidermal necrolysis and may require skin biopsy to differentiate.

Table 44.6 Clinical Features: StaphylococcalScalded Skin Syndrome

Organisms	*Staphylococcus aureus*
Incubation Period	Unknown
Signs and Symptoms	• Fever: >38.9°C. Hypotension: SBP < 90 in adults or orthostatic hypotension. • Rash: diffuse macular erythroderma. Desquamation: palms and soles usually involved, 1–2 weeks after onset of illness.
Laboratory Findings	• None indicated • Blood cultures and skin biopsy may be performed in cases of uncertain diagnosis
Treatment	nafcillin 12.5 to 25 mg/kg IV q6h for newborns >2 kg and 25 to 50 mg/kg for older children is given until improvement is noted *followed by* oral cloxacillin 12.5 mg/kg q6h (for infants and children weighing ≤20 kg) and 250–500 mg q6h (for older children). **Alternative treatment:** clindamycin 900 mg IV q8h *plus* oxacillin 2 g IV q4h for methicillin-sensitive *S. aureus* *or* clindamycin 900 mg IV q8h *plus* vancomycin 1 g IV q12h for MRSA. Some favor linezolid instead of vancomycin if MRSA is a concern, mainly because of protein synthesis inhibition. Consider IVIG: 2 g/kg IV × 1, repeat in 48 hours if patient remains unstable Supportive case or ICU monitoring

SBP, systolic blood pressure.

Management should include an intravenous antistaphylococcal antibiotic, such as nafcillin or dicloxacillin. Alternatives may include clindamycin plus oxacillin, or vancomycin, if methicillin-resistant *S. aureus* (MRSA) is suspected and/or prevalent in the community. Supportive care should include aggressive hydration, skin care, and temperature regulation.

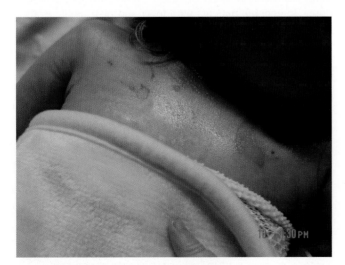

Figure 44.4 SSSS. Photograph courtesy of Dr. David C. Brancati.

Supportive care, wound care, and burn unit or intensive care unit (ICU) admission may be indicated.

Kawasaki Disease – Mucocutaneous Lymph Node Syndrome

Kawasaki disease (mucocutaneous lymph node syndrome) is an acute febrile vasculitis of small- and medium-sized blood vessels throughout the body including the coronary arteries. It typically occurs in winter and spring, with a peak incidence at 1–2 years old. Eighty percent of cases occur in children younger than 4 years of age and Kawasaki disease is uncommon after the age of 8. It is more common in boys than girls, and although cases of Kawasaki disease have been reported in children of all ethnic origins, the highest incidence remains in children of Asian, especially Japanese, descent. Annually, 3500 children are hospitalized for Kawasaki disease in the United States.

Clinical features are characterized by three phases (Table 44.7). The acute febrile period (phase I) is characterized by the abrupt onset of fever lasting approximately 12 days, typically poorly responsive to antipyretics. Symptoms of diarrhea, arthritis, and photophobia may be present. During phase I, erythematous skin changes are first noted on the palms and soles and typically appear 1–3 days after the onset of the fever. Within 2 days, the blotchy, erythematous, macular lesions spread to the extremities and trunk. Nonexudative injected conjunctivae may be present for 1–3 weeks (Figure 44.5). Diffuse oropharyngeal erythema with "strawberry" tongue is often present.

In the subacute phase (phase II), as the exanthem resolves, desquamation is apparent on the fingertips, toes, palms, and soles and may be accompanied by thrombocytosis, arthritis, arthralgias, and carditis. This phase may last 30 days. There is a significant risk for sudden death during this phase of the illness in untreated patients. Overall, 20–25% of patients who are untreated or treated only with aspirin will develop coronary artery aneurysms by day 13, and approximately 2% will die. The rate of aneurysm among patients among fully treated patients is less than 5%, and the mortality less than 1%.

During the convalescent phase (phase III), which occurs within 8–10 weeks after the onset of the illness, most signs of the illness have resolved; mortality drops significantly during this phase.

The diagnosis is typically made based on clinical findings, though it is associated with several laboratory abnormalities. Liver function tests may be elevated, and leukocytosis and thrombocytosis may be seen. The erythrocyte sedimentation rate (ESR) is elevated during phase II and returns to normal in phase III. Pyuria may be seen on urinalysis. Electrocardiography (ECG) may show PR and QT prolongation or acute ST/T wave changes. Coronary aneurysms may be diagnosed by echocardiography or coronary angiography.

Management of Kawasaki disease includes hospital admission, high dose intravenously administered immunoglobulin (IVIG) (2 g/kg single dose) therapy, and aspirin therapy (80–100 mg/kg/day) (Table 44.8). Steroids have not been shown to improve outcomes. Early cardiology evaluation is important to identify and treat possible coronary artery involvement, and children who have coronary involvement require follow-up echocardiography.

Table 44.7 Clinical Features: Kawasaki Disease

Acute Stage (Days 1–11)	• Sudden onset of fever that lasts for 1 week or longer and does not respond to antibiotic treatment • An extremely irritable child • Red eyes (bilateral conjunctival injection) • Dry, red, and cracked lips • Strawberry tongue • Hands and feet that are red and swollen, so much so that child refuses to walk • Rashes that involve the trunk, arms, and legs, usually within 5 days after onset of fever. The rashes may appear in several forms and can be pruritis, especially in the groin. • Enlarged lymph glands • Abnormal liver function test • Heart complications in the first stage may include myocarditis, pericarditis, and coronary artery dilatation that may later progress to frank aneurysm
Subacute Stage (Days 11–21)	• Fever, rash and enlarged lymph nodes have usually resolved by this stage. A persistent fever may result in a less favorable outcome because of greater risk of heart complications. • Persistent irritability, poor appetite, and conjunctival injection (red eyes) • Peeling of skin of the fingertips and toes • Thrombocytosis may develop, with the platelet count topping 1 million (normal range 150–400/mm^3) • Arthritis and arthralgia • Coronary aneurysms develop by day 13 in 20–25% of patients who are untreated or treated only with aspirin, and less than 5% of patients treated with aspirin and IVIG
Convalescent Stage (Days 21–60)	• Clinical signs begin to disappear and laboratory test results return to normal • Most significant clinical finding that persists through this stage is that coronary artery aneurysms continue to enlarge, and this may lead to rupture of the blood vessels
Late Effects/Chronic Stage	• During the first year or two after the illness, coronary aneurysms heal and the amount of coronary artery dilation can become less • Vessel walls will never return to normal as thickening of these walls occurs during the healing process • Aneurysms formed during an episode of Kawasaki disease are of lifetime significance

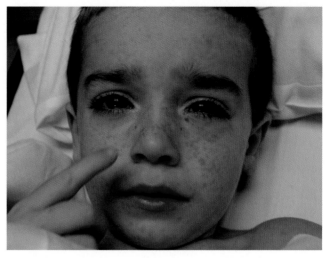

Figure 44.5 Kawasaki disease. Photograph courtesy of Dr. David C. Brancati.

- Viral infections:
  - varicella-zoster infection
  - measles
  - rubella
  - nonspecific viral exanthema
  - roseola
  - erythema infectiosum
  - pityriasis rosea
  - infectious mononucleosis
- Drug hypersensitivity reactions
- Systemic and connective tissue disorders:
  - erythema multiforme
  - toxic epidermal necrolysis
  - erythema nodosum
  - systemic lupus erythematosus
  - Kawasaki disease
  - juvenile rheumatoid arthritis
  - Schönlein-Henoch purpura
  - malignancies

LABORATORY AND RADIOGRAPHIC FINDINGS

Many laboratory tests are discussed above with specific diagnoses. In general, patients with fever and rash can be evaluated with a thorough physical examination alone. In selected cases, complete blood count, platelet count, serologic tests,

Table 44.8 Kawasaki Disease: Treatment

Treatment	**Acute phase:** IVIG, 2 g/kg, as a single infusion over 10 to 12 hours *plus* acetylsalicylic acid (aspirin), 80–100 mg/kg/day orally in four divided doses until the patient has been afebrile for several days* **Subacute and convalescent phases:** aspirin, 3–5 mg/kg orally once daily for as long as 6–8 weeks†

*Some clinicians recommend the use of high-dose aspirin therapy until day 14 of illness.
†Aspirin can be discontinued after 6–8 weeks if all echocardiograms show no evidence of coronary artery abnormalities. If coronary artery abnormalities are detected, low-dose aspirin therapy should be continued indefinitely.

DIFFERENTIAL DIAGNOSIS

The differential diagnosis of fever and rash in the pediatric population is broad. Some of the potential diagnoses that should be considered include:

- Bacterial and rickettsial infections:
  - meningococcal disease
  - SSSS
  - Rocky Mountain spotted fever
  - scarlet fever
  - toxic shock syndrome

Table 47.3 Clinical Features: Acute Hematogenous Osteomyelitis in Children

Organism	*Staphylococcus aureus* most common
Signs and Symptoms	• Fever • Localized pain, swelling, erythema, warmth • Limited use of extremity • Lower extremity long bone at metaphysis • Single site (multiple sites in neonates) • Concomitant septic arthritis
Laboratory and Radiographic Findings	• WBC, ESR, CRP elevated (90%) • Blood culture positive (30–60%) • X-ray: changes appear at 48 hours • MRI • Bone scan • Bone aspiration
Treatment	• Empiric IV antibiotics, usually 3 weeks, followed by PO antibiotics • Neonates (covers group B *Streptococcus*, *S. aureus*, gram-negative rods): cefotaxime 150 mg/kg/day in divided doses q6–8h *or* oxacillin 100–150 mg/kg/day in divided doses q6–8h and gentamicin 2.5 mg/kg • Infants and children (covers *S. aureus*): oxacillin 100–200 mg/kg/day in divided doses q6–8h • For MRSA: vancomycin 15 mg/kg/dose q8h (target trough 5–15 mg/L)

CRP, C-reactive protein; ESR, erythrocyte sedimentation rate; MRI, magnetic resonance imaging; WBC, white blood (cell) count.

Epidemiology

In the United States, osteomyelitis in children is relatively uncommon. The annual incidence is estimated to be 1 in 5000 in children younger than 13 years old. Most cases occur during the first decade of life, with half of cases in children younger than 5 years old. *Staphylococcus aureus* is the causative organism in up to 90% of cases, followed by *Streptococcus* species. The widespread implementation of the *Haemophilus influenzae* type B vaccine has led to a marked decline in gram-negative infections. High-risk groups include children with sickle cell anemia (*Salmonella*) and human immunodeficiency virus (HIV)-positive and asplenic children (*Streptococcus pneumoniae*).

Clinical Features

Unexplained bone pain accompanied by fever should be considered osteomyelitis until proven otherwise. The physical signs and symptoms are nonspecific. Most children present acutely and are often systemically ill. There may be swelling, redness, warmth, and pain of the affected limb (Table 47.3). The most frequent clinical findings are fever, localized pain, and limited use of the extremity. Acute hematogenous osteomyelitis is usually localized to a single site, with the long bones of the lower extremities most commonly involved. Most patients have been symptomatic for less than 2 weeks prior to presentation. A history of preceding infection or trauma can be elicited in approximately one-third of patients.

Differential Diagnosis

The clinical presentation of osteomyelitis is highly variable and nonspecific. A wide range of conditions must be considered, including trauma, systemic disease, and local inflammation. Other conditions to consider are:

• soft-tissue infection (cellulitis, myositis)
• fracture/nonaccidental trauma
• overuse syndromes
• acute rheumatic fever
• Legg-Calvé-Perthes disease (idiopathic osteonecrosis of the femoral head)
• juvenile rheumatoid arthritis (and other inflammatory arthritides)
• bone tumor or malignancy
• sickle cell associated pain crisis

Laboratory and Radiographic Findings

A leukocytosis may be present, and the erythrocyte sedimentation rate (ESR) and C-reactive protein (CRP) are elevated in over 90% of cases of osteomyelitis. Blood cultures should be drawn with reported yields ranging from 30% to 60%.

Plain radiographs should be performed on every patient. The first appreciable sign is soft-tissue swelling, which appears within 48 hours of infection, followed by new periosteal bone formation within 5–7 days and osteolysis at 10–14 days. Compared with plain radiographs, magnetic resonance imaging (MRI) with gadolinium contrast offers superior visualization of the bone marrow cavity and adjacent soft tissues. Technetium-99 bone scan is highly sensitive starting 24–48 hours after onset of symptoms.

Bone aspiration should be considered early in the work-up. An 18-gauge spinal needle easily penetrates the thin metaphyseal bone. Although aspiration through an abscess should be avoided, overlying cellulitis should not be considered a contraindication to bone aspiration. The needle should be used to aspirate the extraperiosteal, subperiosteal, and intraosseous spaces. Local infiltration with lidocaine combined with intravenous agents should provide effective analgesia. Direct culture yields an organism in 48–85% of specimens.

Treatment and Prophylaxis

Treatment is largely nonoperative. An initial course of intravenous antibiotics is usually transitioned to oral medication as the patient responds clinically. The ESR and CRP are expected to decrease over the course of treatment and can be followed serially. Empiric treatment is often necessary because of low culture yields and should cover *S. aureus*. Traditionally, intravenous antibiotics are administered for 3 weeks, followed by oral treatment, although the duration of intravenous therapy is ultimately decided by the clinical response and downward-trending CRP. The indications for surgical debridement are the subject of debate but include presence of an abscess on aspiration, chronic infection with sequestrum formation, septic arthritis, and failure to respond to antibiotics within 36 hours.

In general, outcomes are good. Complications are usually the result of late recognition or inadequate treatment. Worse outcomes have been noted in children who have concomitant septic arthritis.

Special Considerations

NEONATAL OSTEOMYELITIS

Neonatal osteomyelitis should be considered separately because of the significant morbidity and poor outcomes associated with the disease in this high-risk population. Affected infants are usually systemically ill. Presentation may be subtle and include pseudoparalysis, anorexia, irritability, or lethargy. The incidence is estimated to be 1 to 3 of every 1000 neonatal intensive care unit admissions. Because of their immature immune systems, neonates are vulnerable to infections caused by group B *Streptococcus* and gram-negative rods with involvement at multiple sites. Temperature and WBC may remain normal, causing a delay in diagnosis, and ESR and CRP are similarly unreliable.

SUBACUTE HEMATOGENOUS OSTEOMYELITIS

Subacute hematogenous osteomyelitis is marked by a relatively benign presentation of little pain, no fever, and normal laboratory results. Plain radiographs demonstrate abnormalities such as lucency or cortical bone loss, which may be confused for tumor, notably Ewing's sarcoma. Debridement is indicated if there is a sequestrum causing a chronic infection.

Pearls and Pitfalls

1. Plain radiographic changes may not be evident until 7 to 10 days after onset of infection.
2. MRI is the gold standard in the detection of osteomyelitis. Nuclear medicine bone scan may be helpful if localization is unclear.
3. Initial antibiotic therapy is empiric, and should target *Staphylococcus* and *Streptococcus*.
4. Because the metaphyseal region of the proximal humerus, proximal femur, distal tibia, and distal humerus is intraarticular, monitor for signs and symptoms of septic arthritis in the shoulder, hip, ankle, and elbow. Between 10% and 16% of cases of septic arthritis are secondary to bacterial osteomyelitis, and the presence of septic arthritis in the setting of osteomyelitis is associated with worse outcomes.

SEPTIC ARTHRITIS IN CHILDREN

Introduction

Septic arthritis in a child is a true clinical emergency requiring prompt antibiotics and drainage. Although any joint can be affected, it most commonly occurs in the hip in neonates and infants, and the knee in older children. An associated osteomyelitis may also be present. Complications from inadequately treated septic arthritis can be devastating and include osteonecrosis, growth arrest, and sepsis. Poor outcomes have been reported in as many as 40% of cases when the hip is involved.

Epidemiology

Although the exact incidence of septic arthritis in children is difficult to estimate, it is thought to be roughly twice that of osteomyelitis, or 1 in 2500. Peak incidence is during the early years of the first decade of life. Neonates (<28 days old) are most commonly infected by group B *Streptococcus*. In infants and children up to 3 years, the organism is usually *Staphylococcus aureus*. Infection with *Haemophilus influenzae* has declined

because of widespread vaccination but has been replaced by a rise in cases involving *Kingella kingae*, a gram-negative organism. *Neisseria gonorrhoeae* can cause septic arthritis in newborns infected via the birth canal, as well as in sexually active teenagers or younger children who have been victims of sexual abuse.

Clinical Features

Children with septic arthritis typically present with acute-onset fever, irritability, and anorexia (Table 47.4). Passive range of motion of the affected joint will cause severe pain. With lower extremity involvement, the child may present with a limp or refusal to bear weight. If the hip is involved, the child may hold it in a flexed, externally rotated, and abducted position for comfort as this relieves intracapsular pressure. Signs in neonates may be more subtle, such as decreased movement of the affected limb (pseudoparalysis).

Differential Diagnosis

Key features that distinguish septic arthritis from other conditions are:

Table 47.4 Clinical Features: Pediatric Septic Arthritis

Organisms	• *Staphylococcus aureus* most common • Group B *Streptococcus* in neonates • *Kingella kingae* • *Neisseria gonorrhoeae* in at-risk populations
Signs and Symptoms	• Fever • Severe pain with passive range of motion • Limp or refusal to bear weight • Pseudoparalysis, anorexia, irritability, lethargy in neonates

Laboratory and Diagnostic Findings	• WBC, ESR, CRP elevated
	• Blood culture positive
	• X-ray: capsular distension and joint space widening
	• Ultrasound for hip
	• Joint aspiration:
	  ○ WBC count (>50,000/mm^3 positive for infection)
	  ○ Gram stain
	  ○ Culture

Treatment	• Intravenous antibiotics immediately after joint aspiration • Neonates: oxacillin 100–150 mg/kg/day IV in divided doses q6–8h *or* cefotaxime 150 mg/kg/day IV in divided doses q6–8h; for high-risk neonate *add* gentamicin 2.5 mg/kg/dose q8h • Infants and children: cefazolin 50 mg/kg/dose IV q8h *or* ceftriaxone 50 mg/kg once daily *or* (if allergic to penicillin) clindamycin 500 mg/kg/day in three divided doses • Children (gonococcal arthritis): ceftriaxone 50–100 mg/kg/day IV in divided doses q12–24h • Emergent surgical incision and drainage • Serial daily aspiration with close monitoring may be attempted in a superficial joint

skin biopsy, or cultures of blood or skin lesions may be ordered.

COMPLICATIONS AND ADMISSION CRITERIA

Many pediatric patients with fever and rash can be safely discharged home, following appropriate physical and laboratory evaluation.

Those who should be managed as inpatients include patients with immunosuppression, systemic bacterial infections, Kawasaki disease, sepsis, unstable vital signs, and those lacking appropriate home resources or medical follow-up.

INFECTION CONTROL

Pediatric patients with fever and rash often do not have a definitive diagnosis made while in the emergency department. Thus, patients presenting with fever and rash should be considered contagious. Standard precautions should be used when treating patients with fever and rash.

Close contacts of possible cases of meningococcal disease (including household contacts, child care contacts, and health care providers) should undergo prophylactic treatment with rifampin (600 mg by mouth [PO] bid for four doses), ceftriaxone (250 mg intramuscular [IM]), or ciprofloxacin (500 mg PO).

PEARLS AND PITFALLS

1. Consider life-threatening infections, especially meningococcal infection, in pediatric patients presenting with fever and rash.
2. Administer antibiotics early, even if the definitive diagnosis is not established.
3. Administer IVIG in all patients with Kawasaki disease to reduce the rate of coronary complications.
4. Admit patients with possible life-threatening conditions or uncertain diagnosis.

REFERENCES

American Heart Association Committee on Rheumatic Fever, Endocarditis, and Kawasaki Disease. Diagnostic guidelines for Kawasaki disease. Am J Dis Child 1990;144:1218–9.

Burns JC. The riddle of Kawasaki disease. N Engl J Med 2007;356:659–61.

Centers for Disease Control and Prevention (CDC). Chickenpox vaccine – what you need to know. Available at: http://www.cdc.gov/vaccines/pubs/vis/downloads/vis-varicella.pdf. Accessed February 11, 2008.

Chen MT. Clinical manifestations of varicella-zoster virus infection. Dermatol Clin 2002 Apr; 20(2):267–82.

Cunha BA. Rocky Mountain spotted fever revisited. Arch Intern Med 2004;164:221–3.

Dajani AS, Taubert KA, Takahashi M, et al. Guidelines for long-term management of patients with Kawasaki disease. Report from the Committee on Rheumatic Fever, Endo-

carditis, and Kawasaki Disease, Council on Cardiovascular Disease in the Young, American Heart Association. Circulation 1994;89:916–22.

Diaz PS. The epidemiology and control of invasive meningococcal disease. Pediatr Infect Dis J 1999 Jul;18:633–4.

Duke T, Mgone CS. Measles: not just another viral exanthem. Lancet 2003 Mar 1;36(9359):763–73.

Frickhofen N, Abkowitz JL, Safford M, et al. Persistent B19 parvovirus infection in patients infected with human immunodeficiency virus type 1: a treatable cause of anemia in AIDS. Ann Intern Med 1990;113:926–33.

Gardner P. Clinical practice: prevention of meningococcal disease. N Engl J Med 2006;355:1466–73.

Goodyear HM, Laidler PW, Price EH, et al. Acute infectious erythemas in children: a clinico-microbiological study. Br J Dermatol 1991;124:433–8.

Heegaard ED, Brown KE. Human parvovirus B19. Clin Microbiol Rev 2002;15(3):485–505.

Hoey J. Varicella vaccine update: need for a booster? Can Med Assoc J 2003 Mar 4;168(5):589.

Metry D, Katta, R. New and emerging pediatric infections. Dermatol Clin 2003;21(2):269–76

Newburger JW, Sleeper LA, McCrindle BW, et al. Randomized trial of pulsed corticosteroid therapy for primary treatment of Kawasaki disease. N Engl J Med 2007;356:663–76.

Norbeck O, Papadogiannakis N, Petersson K, et al. Revised clinical presentation of parvovirus B19-associated intrauterine fetal death. Clin Infect Dis 2002;35(9):1032–8.

Patel GK, Finlay AY. Staphylococcal scalded skin syndrome: diagnosis and management. Am J Clin Dermatol 2003;4:165–75.

Pollard AJ, Britto J, Nadel S, et al. Emergency management of meningococcal disease. Arch Dis Child 1999;80:290–6.

Rotbart HA, McCracken GH, Whitley RJ, et al. Clinical significance of enteroviruses in serious summer febrile illnesses of children. Pediatr Infect Dis J 1999;18:869–74.

Stanley JR, Amagai M. Pemphigus, bullous impetigo, and the staphylococcal scalded-skin syndrome. N Engl J Med 2006;355:1800–10.

Thomas SL, Hall AJ. What does epidemiology tell us about risk factors for herpes zoster? Lancet Infect Dis 2004 Jan;4(1):26–33.

Young N, Brown K. Mechanisms of disease: parvovirus B19. N Engl J Med 2004;350:586–97.

ADDITIONAL READINGS

Centers for Disease Control and Prevention (CDC). Prevention and control of meningococcal disease. MMWR 2005;54 (RR07):1–21.

Cherry JD: Viral exanthems. Curr Probl Pediatr 1983;13:1.

McCann DJ, Nadel ES, Brown DF. Rash and fever. J Emerg Med 2006;31:293–7.

Shulman ST, De Inocencio J, Hirsch R. Kawasaki disease. Pediatr Clin North Am 1995;42:1205–22.

Mancinci A. Exanthems in childhood: an update. Pediatr Ann 1998;27:163–70.

45. Work-Up of Newborn Fever

Maureen McCollough

INTRODUCTION

The neonate is defined as a newborn infant younger than 4 weeks old, and fever as a temperature greater than 100.4°F or 38°C. Because clinical exam is limited and because of the high risk of serious bacterial infection in this age group, all febrile neonates must be admitted for a sepsis workup and empiric antibiotic therapy.

Neonatal infections are unique, in that transmission of organisms can occur transplacentally during gestation and can present early on or be delayed by months or longer. Vertical transmission can occur in utero or during delivery. The newborn immune system is immature, increasing the susceptibility to infection. Other disease processes such as hyaline membrane disease may complicate infectious presentations. Finally, the presentation of infectious diseases in neonates is variable, often with subtle signs and symptoms.

EPIDEMIOLOGY

Neonates who are less than 2 weeks old who present to the ED have a particularly high incidence of serious illness with 10–33% requiring hospital admission. The most common diagnoses in admitted neonates include respiratory infections, sepsis, dehydration, congenital heart disease, bowel obstruction, hypoglycemia, and seizures.

Group B *Streptococcus* is the most common bacterial cause of neonatal sepsis in the United States. *Listeria monocytogenes*, *Escherichia coli*, *Klebsiella*, enterococcus, non-group D alpha hemolytic strep, and nontypeable *Haemophilus influenzae* are other bacterial causes. Viral causes include herpes simplex virus (sometimes with no symptoms in the mother), enterovirus (coxsackie and echoviruses), and adenovirus (typically with liver and CNS involvement).

CLINICAL FEATURES

Fever in the newborn period is defined as greater than 100.4°F or 38°C. Any ill-appearing young infant should be considered septic until proven otherwise. "Early onset" sepsis occurs within hours or a few days of birth and is often associated with perinatal risk factors. "Late onset" sepsis usually occurs after 1 week of age, develops more gradually, and is more commonly associated with community-acquired organisms.

Undressing the baby to look for signs of poor perfusion or petechiae is important, though the clinical signs of sepsis may be subtle. Lethargy, irritability, or decreased oral intake is common. Other clinical features include apnea, tachypnea, cyanosis, respiratory distress, tachycardia, bradycardia, jaundice, pallor, vomiting, diarrhea, temperature instability (high or low), abdominal distension, or ileus. It is not uncommon for septic newborns to be unable to mount a febrile response.

Well-appearing febrile neonates are common. Most neonatal visits to the acute care setting will be an otherwise healthy-appearing newborn with fever. Despite a non-toxic appearance, fever in the neonatal period must be taken seriously and a thorough work-up for a source is still indicated.

The past medical history for a neonate is obviously limited but must include both prenatal and postnatal risk factors. The mother may have had serological screens for *Treponema pallidum*, rubella, and hepatitis B virus. Cultures may have been taken for group B streptococci, herpes simplex, *Neisseria gonorrhoeae*, or *Chlamydia*. Prenatal infections that can be transmitted transplacentally include syphilis, rubella, cytomegalovirus (CMV), parvovirus B19, human immunodeficiency virus (HIV), varicella zoster, *Listeria monocytogenes*, *Borrelia burgdorferi*, and toxoplasmosis (see Chapter 53, Fever in Pregnancy). Vertically transmitted organisms (colonizing the birth canal) include group B streptococci, gonococci, *Listeria monocytogenes*, *E. coli*, *Chlamydia*, genital *Mycoplasma*, and herpes and enteroviruses. The evaluation of a neonate who appears critically ill requires a physical examination looking for sources of infection such as herpes lesions or omphalitis (Table 45.1). Herpes may present as a disseminated infection involving multiple organ systems, or encephalitis with or without a rash, or less commonly as a disease localized to the skin, eyes, or mouth. If lesions are found, they will usually appear on the birth "presenting" portion of the baby. If the child was delivered head-first, thoroughly examine the scalp for lesions, especially where a fetal scalp electrode may have been inserted. The fontanelle of a newborn should be flat. A depressed fontanelle can indicate dehydration; a full fontanelle can suggest meningitis. The umbilical area should be examined for signs of omphalitis, a true medical emergency. Redness at the area of the umbilical cord should be considered an early sign of omphalitis. Omphalitis, a mixed gram-positive and gram-negative infection, can spread hematogenously or directly into the peritoneum.

Table 45.1 Clinical Features: Neonatal Fever

	Organisms	Signs and Symptoms	Laboratory and Radiologic Findings
Meningitis	**Bacterial:** • Group B *Streptococcus* • *Listeria* • *Escherichia coli* • *Klebsiella* • *Enterococcus* • Non-group D alpha-hemolytic strep • *Haemophilus influenzae* **Viral:** • Herpes simplex • Enterovirus • Adenovirus	• Fever • Apnea, tachypnea, cyanosis, respiratory distress • Tachycardia, bradycardia • Jaundice, pallor • Vomiting, diarrhea, abdominal distension, or ileus • Hyper- or hypothermia	• CSF Gram stain – bacteria • CSF WBC <20/mm³ normal • CSF protein 20–170 mg/dL normal • CSF glucose 34–119 mg/dL normal • Consider herpes if CSF shows pleocytosis, predominance of RBCs or high protein; PCR is >95% sensitive for herpes in CSF; may also be isolated by viral culture
Bacteremia	• Group B *Streptococcus* • *Listeria* • *Escherichia coli* • *Klebsiella* • *Enterococcus* • Non-group D alpha-hemolytic strep • *Haemophilus influenzae*	• Fever • Irritability • Apnea, tachypnea, cyanosis, respiratory distress • Tachycardia, bradycardia • Jaundice, pallor • Vomiting, diarrhea, abdominal distension, or ileus • Hyper- or hypothermia	• Positive blood culture • Serum markers are too insensitive to rule out bacteremia
Otitis Media	• *Escherichia coli* • *Klebsiella pneumoniae* • *Pseudomonas aeruginosa* • group B streptococcus	• Tympanic membranes can be difficult to visualize	• No laboratory or radiographs
Pneumonia	**At birth:** • Group B *Streptococcus* • Herpes simplex virus • CMV • Adenovirus • *Treponema pallidum* • *Listeria* • *Mycobacterium tuberculosis* • *Chlamydia* trachomatis **After birth (>24 hours later):** • Group B *Streptococcus* • *Escherichia coli* • *Klebsiella pneumoniae* • *Ureaplasma urealyticum* **After 7 days:** • RSV • *Streptococcus pneumoniae* • *Staphylococcus aureus* • *Haemophilus influenzae* type B and nontypeable • *Bordetella pertussis*	• Fever • Apnea • Tachypnea, grunting, rales, wheezing, cyanosis, respiratory distress or overt failure • Hypotension, sepsis, meningitis, especially Group B streptococcus • Feeding difficulty, irritability • *Chlamydia* often presents with an afebrile well-appearing infant with cough; conjunctivitis may be present • Pertussis – often no catarrhal stage of sneezing and congestion; often no paroxysmal cough or whoop; more often tachypnea, apnea, cyanosis, gagging, feeding difficulty, post-tussive vomiting; rarely ventricular fibrillation, seizures, subarachnoid hemorrhage, rectal prolapse, hernias, dehydration • RSV – apnea, wheezing, tachypnea, difficulty feeding; more severe in premature or infants with underlying cardiac or pulmonary disease	• Chest x-ray: usually diffuse bilateral granular or patchy infiltrates • RSV may show hyperinflation, peribronchial cuffing, interstitial infiltrates, or atelectasis *Chlamydia* may show bilateral interstitial infiltrates with hyperinflation • Pertussis may show perihilar infiltrates and atelectasis; possible pneumothorax and pneumomediastinum • Laboratory tests are generally unhelpful for the diagnosis of pneumonia • Rapid RSV or pertussis nasopharyngeal testing can be useful • Pertussis does not commonly produce lymphocytosis
Omphalitis	• Mixed gram-positive, and gram-negative	• Redness surrounding the umbilical cord	• No laboratory or radiographs
Urinary Tract Infection	• *Escherichia coli* • Other gram-negative bacilli • *Enterococcus* sp.	• Fever • Irritability • Apnea, tachypnea, cyanosis, respiratory distress • Tachycardia, bradycardia • Jaundice, pallor • Vomiting, diarrhea, abdominal distension, or ileus • Hyper- or hypothermia	• Urinalysis alone is insufficient to rule out a UTI
Rash/Lesions	• Herpes simplex virus	• May be disseminated and present as encephalitis with or without lesions	• Tzanck smear of lesion may show multinucleated giant cells • Direct fluorescent antibody testing of air-dried smear may be more sensitive

CSF, cerebrospinal fluid; PCR, polymerase chain reaction; RBC, red blood cell; WBC, white blood (cell) count.

Table 45.2 Differential Diagnosis for the Critically Ill-Appearing Neonate in the Emergency Department: S-S-I-C-C-C-F-I-T mnemonic

S – Sepsis S – Seizures I – Inborn errors of metabolism or other metabolic disorders C – CNS bleed C – Congenital adrenal hyperplasia C – Congenital heart disease F – Formula mixups I – Intestinal disasters, e.g., volvulus, incarcerated hernia T – Toxins, including any herbs, teas, or powders such as baking soda given to infants for ailments such as colic, spitting up, or constipation
CNS, central nervous system.

Table 45.3 Work-Up of Febrile Neonates in the Emergency Department

CBC (other serum markers such as CRP may be included but are not diagnostic) Blood culture Urinalysis Urine culture Stool culture if applicable CSF for cell count, glucose, protein, Gram stain and culture Chest x-ray if indicated RSV swab if indicated Pertussis swab if indicated Rapid influenza A test (not yet accepted as standard practice to rule out the need for a full work-up in a febrile neonate)
CBC, complete blood count; CRP, C-reactive protein; CSF, cerebrospinal fluid.

In a male infant who has been circumcised, the penis should be examined for signs of infection. Male infants are at greater risk for urinary tract infections (UTIs) than are females in the neonatal period. Neonatal UTI often presents with nonspecific signs and symptoms, such as vomiting, diarrhea, irritability, or jaundice.

Respiratory infections are a significant cause of fever or illness in neonates. Pneumonia in the first week of life (less than 7 days since birth) is most commonly due to group B *Streptococcus*, but may also be caused by *Escherichia coli*, *Listeria monocytogenes*, or *Klebsiella pneumoniae*. If pneumonia is accompanied by eye discharge, *Chlamydia* testing is imperative. Other organisms causing pneumonia in young neonates, include herpes simplex virus, cytomegalovirus, adenovirus, treponema pallidum, and *Mycobacterium tuberculosis*. Pneumonia in neonates older than 7 days may also be caused by respiratory syncytial virus (RSV), *Streptococcus pneumoniae*, *Staphylococcus aureus*, or type B and nontypeable *Haemophilus influenzae*.

Signs of neonatal pneumonia include tachypnea, retractions, grunting, rales, wheezing, cyanosis, and respiratory distress or overt respiratory failure. Other associated symptoms include fever, feeding difficulty, or irritability. RSV can cause bronchiolitis and may present with apnea. *Chlamydia* often presents in a nonfebrile well-appearing infant. Neonatal pertussis commonly presents with apnea, cyanosis, and posttussive vomiting. Serious sequelae such as ventricular fibrillation or seizures may develop.

Otitis media is another febrile illness that can be difficult to diagnose in neonates because the tympanic membranes are difficult to visualize. In up to one-third of infants in the first month diagnosed with otitis media, the etiological organisms are *Escherichia coli*, *Klebsiella pneumoniae*, *Pseudomonas aeruginosa*, and group B *Streptococcus*.

DIFFERENTIAL DIAGNOSIS

The most common sources of bacterial infections in neonates are meningitis, bacteremia, urinary tract infections, and pneumonia, though the noninfectious differential of an ill-appearing neonate is broad and includes some disease processes unique to the neonatal period. The mnemonic S-S-I-C-C-C-F-I-T describes possible etiologies of critical illness in the neonate (Table 45.2).

Neonatal seizures will often present with tonic or clonic movements or autonomic repetitive movements such as blinking, lip smacking or bicycling. Inborn errors of metabolism

and congenital adrenal hyperplasia present with altered mental status, vomiting and dehydration. Congenital adrenal hyperplasia will produce electrolyte imbalances including hyponatremia and hyperkalemia. Neonates with central nervous system (CNS) bleeds often exhibit altered mental status, vomiting, and bulging fontanelles. Congenital heart disease presenting emergently in the neonatal period is often due to closure of the ductus arteriosus. Infants with structural lesions requiring a patent ductus arteriosus for blood flow will develop sudden cyanosis or shock. Prostaglandin E1, a potent vasodilator, is vital to their survival. Toxin ingestion may be accidental or intentional (such as mistaking other powders for formula, or giving baking soda to alleviate colic). Volvulus occurs secondary to congenital malrotation of the intestine and is a surgical emergency. Volvulus may present rather benignly with vomiting and irritability but will soon progress to altered mental status and shock as the bowel infarcts. Surgery is the only treatment.

LABORATORY AND RADIOGRAPHIC FINDINGS

The work-up of a febrile neonate in the ED (Table 45.3) includes evaluation of blood, urine, cerebrospinal fluid (CSF), and stool if indicated by symptoms. Recent studies have attempted to establish whether a viral process (such as RSV bronchiolitis or influenza A diagnosed by rapid bedside test) can explain the fever in a well-appearing neonate and obviate the need for a complete workup for bacterial infection. For example, in one recent study, in infants younger than 28 days with fever and positive RSV testing, there were no cases of meningitis, though the difference in the rate of meningitis between the RSV-positive and RSV-negative groups was not statistically significant. In addition, the overall rate of serious bacterial infections (or SBI, including UTI, bacterial enteritis, bacteremia, and bacterial meningitis) in infants younger than 28 days was high at 13%, and still significant at 10% in the RSV-postive group. If rapid viral diagnostic tests such as RSV or influenza are to be used in the ED, the particular sensitivity and positive predictive value of these tests and the overall prevalence of SBI in the relevant age group must be taken into account. Further studies are needed to determine whether positive, rapid bedside viral tests can mitigate the need for a complete septic work-up in a febrile neonate.

More recently, serum markers have been evaluated as early indicators of neonatal sepsis. Unfortunately, they all lack the sensitivity and specificity to rule out sepsis in the febrile neonate in the ED. For neonatal sepsis, an abnormal C-reactive protein (CRP), the most readily available of the newer serum markers, is 75% sensitive and 86% specific; while an immature neutrophil (band) to total neutrophil ratio above 0.2 is 60–90% sensitive and 70–80% specific for diagnosing neonatal sepsis. An elevated interleukin-6 level (100 or 135 pg/mL cutoff) is 81–93% sensitive and 86–96% specific; a procalcitonin level above 0.5 µg/L is 93–100% sensitive and 92–98% specific; and an elevated tumor necrosis factor alpha is 72–95% sensitive and 43–78% specific for diagnosing neonatal sepsis in very limited studies. Given the lack of predictive value of serum markers, they should not be used to decide on cessation of a septic work-up of a febrile neonate, patient admission, or administration of antibiotics.

A lumbar puncture is indicated not only in a septic or ill appearing infant but also in well-appearing febrile neonates. The infant should be placed in a sitting or lateral non-flexed position to minimize the development of hypoxia during the LP. If the infant is critically ill the risk of apnea increases, and it may be better to delay the LP, obtain blood cultures, administer antibiotics, and then examine the CSF at a later time when the infant is more clinically stable. If the CSF has many white blood cells (WBCs) or a predominance of red blood cells without organisms on Gram stain, herpes meningitis should be considered. A polymerase chain reaction (PCR) assay on CSF for herpes simplex virus is more than 95% sensitive.

A urinalysis is insufficient to rule out a UTI in very young infants. Young infants often cannot mount an inflammatory response in the bladder. Testing for a positive bacterial nitrite response is not sensitive as it requires the urine to be held within the bladder for a period of time; in general, this does not occur in neonates. For these reasons, a culture must be sent along with a urinalysis. Because a bag specimen can often result in false-positive growth, a catheterized specimen is recommended. Urine latex agglutination testing for group B *Streptococcus* is available but has limited sensitivity.

For newborns with signs of lower respiratory tract disease or complaints of apnea or an apparent life-threatening event (ALTE), a nasopharyngeal swab should be sent for RSV by immunoassay or PCR, and for pertussis by direct fluorescent antibody (DFA) test or enzyme-linked immunoassay (ELISA) test. If conjunctivitis with discharge is present in a newborn with pneumonia, the eye secretions should be tested for *Chlamydia trachomatis* using DFA, ELISA, or culture. Blood cultures are positive in minority of neonates with bacterial pneumonia but are often positive in neonates with urinary tract infections.

Chest radiographs may show diffuse bilateral granular or patchy infiltrates. RSV often causes hyperinflation, peribronchial cuffing, interstitial infiltrates, or atelectasis on x-ray. *Chlamydia trachomatis* typically causes bilateral interstitial infiltrates with hyperinflation, and *Bordetella pertussis* infection may result in perihilar infiltrates, atelectasis, pneumothorax, and pneumomediastinum.

TREATMENT AND PROPHYLAXIS

The evaluation of a critically ill-appearing neonate who presents to the ED begins with placement of a cardiac monitor, pulse oximeter, assessment of vital signs including blood pressure, and bedside testing for blood glucose. Blood pressure is often a forgotten vital sign in very ill-appearing young infants. A systolic blood pressure below 60 mm Hg is considered abnormal. Neonates may be hypothermic or hyperthermic when septic. The temperature of the undressed neonate should be rechecked periodically because young infants have difficulty maintaining their temperature as a result of their large body surfaces. For this reason, consider radiant warming for hypothermic and even normothermic neonates.

Intubation may be necessary if a high-flow oxygen mask is not sufficient to reverse hypoxia. The infant's work of breathing must also be considered when deciding whether or not to intubate. Uncuffed endotracheal tubes are recommended for neonates. Intravenous lines are often hard to establish in young infants, especially when they are ill, dehydrated, or in extremis. Scalp veins can be used to deliver both fluid boluses and medications. An intraosseous (IO) line or an umbilical vein line can be used if no intravenous lines can be established. Young infants have a limited ability to maintain normal glucose; therefore, frequent bedside measurement of serum glucose is mandatory. Blood glucose concentrations below 40 mg/dL are considered abnormal in neonates, whereas a blood glucose concentration between 40 and 50 mg/dL can be normal or abnormal. Bedside glucose tests can be inaccurate, and therefore levels below 50 mg/dL mandate intervention consisting of 5 mL/kg of intravenous D10.

If saline boluses are required, begin with 10–20 mL/kg at a time and reassess. For premature neonates, and neonates with asphyxia or suspected cardiac disorders, limit fluid boluses to 10 mL/kg at a time. Maintenance fluids can be sustained with D5$\frac{1}{4}$NS at 4 mL per kg per hour while in the ED. Packed red blood cells, platelets, or fresh frozen plasma should be administered in 10 mL/kg dosages. Communication with a neonatal or pediatric intensive care unit early is important to expedite the transfer of the critically ill neonate. Ampicillin 50 mg/kg per dose IV q6h (covering *Streptococcus*, *Listeria*, some *Enterococcus*) plus gentamicin (which provides synergism and broad gram-negative coverage) are recommended in the treatment of neonatal fever and sepsis. Gentamicin is nephrotoxic and ototoxic with prolonged administration, and doses should be adjusted for gestational age and weight.

If the CSF is positive or suspicious for bacterial infection, ampicillin plus cefotaxime should be administered; this regimen will cover *Listeria*, group B *Streptococcus*, and enteric gram-negative rods. If herpes simplex meningitis is suspected, acyclovir should be initiated. A high suspicion for herpes meningitis is warranted if (a) CSF has high WBC or high protein or predominance of red blood cells (RBCs) but no organisms, or (b) CSF pleocytosis is present with vesicular rash on infant, seizures, focal neurological signs, pneumonitis or hepatitis, or a maternal history of genital herpes.

Admit all neonates with evidence of lower respiratory tract infection or wheezing consistent with bronchiolitis, as the risk of apnea is significant. Evaluation should focus on work of breathing and oxygen requirement of the infant. Supportive care includes suctioning, oxygen, and possibly intubation. Neither inhaled beta-agonists nor epinephrine or systemic steroids have been shown to be useful, except in infants with a strong family history of atopic disease or asthma.

Ampicillin plus either gentamicin or cefotaxime is indicated for neonatal pneumonia. *Chlamydia* can be treated with a macrolide. Pertussis treatment with macrolides or trimethoprim-sulfamethoxazole may be effective only during the coryza stage.

COMPLICATIONS AND ADMISSION CRITERIA

All febrile neonates should be admitted to the hospital regardless of appearance. Correct hypothermia, hypovolemia, hypoglycemia, and other electrolyte abnormalities early. If the child is ill-appearing or if a bacterial source for the fever has been established, antibiotics should be administered in the ED. Emergency physicians should also have a low threshold for administering empiric antibiotics to febrile neonates.

PEARLS AND PITFALLS

1. All emergency departments should be prepared to care for all critically ill infants and children, which includes having the correct pediatric equipment.
2. Emergency physicians should have knowledge of the normal findings of a newborn including the physical exam, vital signs, and serum parameters, which will allow for identification of neonates at risk for serious illness.
3. Emergency physicians should be aware that infants are at risk for both perinatal and community-acquired infections during the first month of life.
4. Febrile neonates are at high risk for meningitis, bacteremia, and UTIs and therefore a complete septic work-up is indicated.
5. Septic young infants may present with very subtle signs such as tachypnea or decreased feeding.
6. Admission to the hospital with intravenous antibiotics is strongly advised for any neonate presenting with a fever.

REFERENCES

American Academy of Pediatrics, Subcommittee on Diagnosis and Management of Bronchiolitis. Diagnosis and management of bronchiolitis. Pediatrics 2006 Oct;118(4):1774–93.

Bonsu BK, Harper MB. Utility of the peripheral blood white blood cell count for identifying sick young infants who need lumbar puncture. Ann Emerg Med 2003 Feb;41(2):206–14.

Gerdes JS. Diagnosis and management of bacterial infections in the neonate. Pediatr Clin North Am 2004;51:939–59.

Griffin MP, Lake DE, Moorman JR. Heart rate characteristics and laboratory tests in neonatal sepsis. Pediatrics 2005;115(4):937–41.

Grijalva CG, Poehling KA, Edwards KM, et al. Accuracy and interpretation of rapid influenza tests in children. Pediatrics 2007 Jan;119(1):e6–11.1.

Hoppe JE. Neonatal pertussis. Pediatr Infect Dis J 2000;19:244–7.

Hsiao AL, Chen L, Baker MD. Incidence and predictors of serious bacterial infections among 57- to 180-day-old infants. Pediatrics 2006 May;117(5):1695–701.

Levine DA, Platt SL, Dayan PS, et al. Risk of serious bacterial infection in young febrile infants with respiratory syncytial virus infections. Pediatrics 2004 Jun;113(6):1728–34.

Malk A, Hui CPS, Pennie RA, Kirpalani H. Beyond the complete blood cell count and C-reactive protein. Arch Pediatr Adolesc Med 2003;57:511–6.

Poland R, Watterberg K. Sepsis in the newborn. Pediatr Rev 1993;14(7):262–3.

Sadow KB, Derr R, Teach SJ. Bacterial infections in infants 60 days and younger. Arch Pediatr Adolesc Med 1999;153:611–4.

Scarfone RJ. Controversies in the treatment of bronchiolitis. Curr Opin Pediatr 2005 Feb;17(1):62–6.

Smitherman HF, Caviness AC, Macias CG. Retrospective review of serious bacterial infections in infants who are 0 to 36 months of age and have influenza A infection. Pediatrics 2005 Mar;115(3):710–8.

Tipple MA, Beem MO, Saxon EM. Clinical characteristics of the afebrile pneumonia associated with *Chlamydia trachomatis* infection in infants less than 6 months of age. Pediatrics 1979;63:192–7.

Willwerth BM, Harper MB, Greenes DS. Identifying hospitalized infants who have bronchiolitis and are at high risk for apnea. Ann Emerg Med 2006 Oct;48(4):441–7.

ADDITIONAL READINGS

American College of Emergency Physicians (ACEP) Pediatric Committee. Clinical policy for children younger than three years presenting to the emergency department with fever. Ann Emerg Med 2003 Oct;42(4):530–45.

American Heart Association (AHA). 2005 guidelines for cardiopulmonary resuscitation (CPR) and emergency cardiovascular care (ECC) of pediatric and neonatal patients: pediatric advanced life support. Pediatrics 2006 May;117(5):e1005–28.

Millar KR, Gloor JE, Wellington N, Joubert G. Early neonatal presentations to the pediatric emergency department. Pediatr Emerg Care 2000;16:145–52.

46. The Febrile Child

Paul Ishimine

INTRODUCTION

The challenge for the emergency physician faced with a febrile child is to identify the patient at high risk for serious underlying infection, while limiting unnecessary testing and treatment. Because immune function, likely pathogens, and exam findings vary significantly from birth to early childhood, the risk of serious bacterial illness in febrile children is usually stratified by age.

EPIDEMIOLOGY

Neonates (birth to 1 month) are at particularly high risk for serious bacterial infection (SBI), including bacteremia, meningitis, pneumonia, urinary tract infections (UTIs), bacterial gastroenteritis, and osteomyelitis (see Chapter 45, Work-Up of Newborn Fever). About 12% of all febrile neonates presenting to a pediatric emergency department (ED) have SBI. The most common types of bacterial infection in this age group are UTIs and bacteremia, and the predominant bacterial pathogen overall is *Escherichia coli*. Neonates are typically infected by more virulent bacteria (e.g., group B streptococci) than older children. Only a small percentage of neonates are infected with other streptococcal species, such as *Streptococcus pneumoniae*, and there has been an overall decline in invasive pneumococcal disease since the introduction of the heptavalent pneumococcal conjugate vaccine (PCV7), even in this unvaccinated age group. In addition, neonates are more likely than older children to develop serious sequelae from viral infections (e.g., herpes simplex virus meningitis).

The predominant bacterial pathogen in the 2-month to 6-month age range is also *Escherichia coli*, which causes most UTIs, but notably, 10 different pathogens caused 45 bacterial infections in one study. In a PCV7 era study of febrile children (>37.9°C) 2–6 months old, 0.9% of patients had bacteremia (one pneumococcal), 9.7% had UTIs, and 39% had positive viral cultures (predominantly respiratory syncytial virus [RSV] and influenza A). Only 4.9% with positive viral testing had concomitant bacterial infection, compared to a 13.5% rate of SBI in the group with negative viral testing.

The epidemiologic landscape for children 6 months and older has changed dramatically since the introduction of PCV7. With the near-elimination of *Haemophilus influenza* type B as a significant pathogen in the early 1990s, *S. pneumoniae* emerged as a dominant bacterial pathogen in young children. The overall prevalence of occult bacteremia in febrile children presenting to EDs in the mid-1990s was 1.6–1.9%, and *S. pneumoniae* represented 83–92% of positive blood cultures. Since the introduction of the heptavalent pneumococcal conjugate vaccine, however, there has been a decline in invasive pneumococcal disease for vaccine-covered serotypes, with a decline of 94% and 91% in children younger than 1 year of age and 2 years of age, respectively. There has also been a 25% decrease in invasive pneumococcal disease in people older than 5 years (suggesting herd immunity, as this age group was not immunized). Although the overall rate of pneumococcal bacteremia has declined, however, some studies have shown an increased prevalence of nonvaccine serotype infections.

Though pneumococcus is still the predominant cause of bacteremia in febrile children aged 3–36 months, *E. coli* bacteremia is very common as well and is more common than pneumococcus in children younger than 12 months. *E. coli* bacteremia is almost always associated with a concomitant UTI. *Salmonella* bacteremia has been found in 1–7% of children in this age group with fever and no obvious source, and the relative contribution of *Salmonella* as a cause of bacteremia is believed to be increasing as pneumococcal disease becomes less common. Although the majority of patients with *Salmonella* bacteremia had gastroenteritis in one study, 5% had occult bacteremia.

Meningococcal infections are infrequent but are associated with high rates of morbidity and mortality. Usually, these patients are overtly sick, though 12–16% of patients with meningococcal disease have unsuspected infection.

CLINICAL FEATURES

The most commonly accepted definition of fever is a temperature of 38.0°C (100.4°F). Rectal thermometry is the current reference standard for outpatient temperature measurement because this method most accurately reflects core body temperature. Bundling of infants may raise the skin temperature but does not raise core temperature.

There is some evidence that suggests children with hyperpyrexia have higher rates of serious bacterial infection. Of children less than 3 months of age with temperatures greater than or equal to 40.0°C, 38% had serious bacterial infection. A response (or lack thereof) to antipyretic medications, however, does not predict etiology. Additional important data include localizing signs and symptoms, underlying medical conditions, exposure to ill contacts, and immunization status.

An assessment of the child's overall appearance is crucial. If a child looks toxic (e.g., irritable or lethargic, or poorly interactive with his/her environment), an aggressive work-up including antibiotic treatment and hospitalization is indicated, regardless of age or risk factors. The physical examination may reveal a focal infection, and decrease the need for additional testing. Febrile patients with clinically recognizable viral conditions (e.g., croup, varicella, and stomatitis) or viral infections confirmed by laboratory testing (e.g., influenza A or RSV infection) have lower rates of bacteremia than patients with no obvious source of infection. Of note, however, febrile children with otitis media appear to have the same rate of bacteremia as febrile children without otitis media. Although the physical examination can be informative, it is also important to recognize its limitations, especially in neonates and young infants.

In febrile children between 2 or 3 months and 24 months, a temperature of 39.0°C is commonly used as the threshold temperature for initiating further evaluation. This higher temperature cutoff has been used because of the increasing likelihood of pneumococcal bacteremia with increasing temperatures. The history is often helpful in this age group. Patients are more likely to be able to communicate complaints and the physical examination is more informative. Well appearance does not completely exclude bacteremia, but children who are toxic-appearing are much more likely to have serious illness when compared to merely ill- or well-appearing children (92% vs. 26% vs. 3%).

Urinary tract infections are common sources of fever in young children. In older children, classical features such as dysuria, urinary frequency, and abdominal and flank pain may suggest UTIs, but in young children, symptoms are usually nonspecific. A validated clinical decision rule for girls less than 24 months old recommends urine testing if two or more of the following risk factors are present:

- age less than 12 months
- fever for 2 or more days
- temperature of 39.0°C or higher
- Caucasian race
- no alternative source of fever

This rule has a sensitivity of 95–99% and a false-positive rate 69–90% in detecting girls with UTI. No similar clinical decision rules exist for boys, but because the prevalence in boys younger than 6 months is 2.7%, urine should be collected in all boys in this age group. The prevalence of UTIs in uncircumcised boys is 8–9 times higher than in circumcised boys, and so uncircumcised boys less than 12 months old should also undergo urine testing.

DIFFERENTIAL DIAGNOSIS

The complete differential in the febrile child is extremely broad and includes viral and mycobacterial infections, as well as bacteremia and localized bacterial infections. The latter include infections of the ears, eyes, sinuses, pharynx, and surrounding tissues; of the brain and meninges; of the cardiac,

pulmonary, gastrointestinal, and urogenital systems; and of the musculoskeletal, dermatological, and lymphatic systems. Noninfectious causes of fever in a child must also be considered and include autoimmune disease (including rheumatoid arthritis, systemic lupus erythematosus, Kawasaki disease, serum sickness, and inflammatory bowel disease); neoplastic disease (leukemia and lymphoma); brain (usually hypothalamic) lesions and seizures; and thyroid dysfunction. Exogenous etiologies of fever include vaccine reactions, environmental heat exposure, and toxic ingestions (e.g., amphetamines, anticholinergics, cocaine, and salicylates).

LABORATORY AND RADIOGRAPHIC FINDINGS

The younger the febrile child, the less reliable the history and physical for detecting serious bacterial infection, and the more extensive the initial work-up needs to be.

In febrile neonates, a full sepsis work-up is indicated, including blood cultures, urine analysis and culture, and cerebrospinal fluid (CSF) analysis. A peripheral white blood cell count (WBC) is often ordered, but is neither sensitive nor specific for bacterial infection. Although various options for rapid testing for UTIs exist (e.g., urine dipstick, standard urinalysis, enhanced urinalysis), no rapid test detects all cases of UTI, and urine cultures must be sent in all of these patients. Urine should be collected by bladder catheterization or, if necessary, suprapubic aspiration, because bag urine specimens are associated with unacceptably high rates of contamination. Chest x-rays are indicated only in the presence of respiratory symptoms, and stool analyses are indicated only in the presence of diarrhea. In neonates, the presence of signs suggestive of viral illness does not negate the need for a full diagnostic evaluation. Unlike older children, in whom documented RSV infections decrease the likelihood of serious bacterial illness, RSV infected neonates have the same rate of SBI when compared to RSV negative neonates.

The approach to febrile young children out of the neonatal period is more controversial. There is general consensus that a febrile infant 1–2 months of age needs a full sepsis evaluation, consisting of a complete blood count, blood culture, urinalysis, urine culture, and CSF analysis. Some authors advocate performing a full sepsis evaluation in children up until 3 months of age; others advocate selective testing in a child older than 2 months. Symptom-directed testing in this 1- to 3-month-old group should include fecal leukocytes and stool cultures for diarrhea, and chest x-rays for signs of pulmonary disease (e.g., tachypnea >50 breaths/minute, rales, rhonchi, retractions, wheezing, coryza, grunting, nasal flaring, or cough).

The utility of the peripheral WBC is limited, and although some fever management algorithms incorporate the WBC, the WBC is neither particularly sensitive nor specific for bacterial infection in older children. However, in most studies of febrile young children aged 1 to 2 or 3 months, an abnormal WBC generally resulted in treatment with antibiotics and hospital admission. The WBC is considered abnormal if the count is above 15,000/mm^3 or below 5000/mm^3 and the band-to-neutrophil ratio is above 0.2. The urine is considered abnormal if the urine dipstick is positive for nitrite or leukocyte esterase, if there are five or more WBCs per high-power field (hpf) on microscopy, or if there are organisms seen on Gram stain of unspun urine. Rapid viral testing may also be helpful in risk stratification. The presence of a documented viral infection lowers, but does not eliminate, the likelihood of serious bacterial infection in this age group.

The diagnosis of pneumonia in young children can be difficult. The role of pulse oximetry in detecting pneumonia is unclear, and although the chest x-ray is often thought of as the gold standard, there is well-documented variability in the interpretation of x-rays among pediatric radiologists. In addition, radiographic findings cannot be used to reliably distinguish between bacterial and nonbacterial causes of pneumonia. Although no clinical finding alone is specific for pneumonia, tachypnea and crackles increase the likelihood of radiographic pneumonia. In addition, whereas clinically occult pneumonia is very rare in children younger than 3 months of age, some studies suggest that a significant percentage of febrile children older than 3 months with no clinically evident pulmonary disease will have pneumonia on chest x-ray. The American College of Emergency Physicians recommends a chest x-ray in children older than 3 months with:

1. a temperature greater than 39°C
   and
2. a white blood cell count greater than 20,000/mm³ (if a WBC is obtained)

A chest x-ray is *not* indicated in febrile children younger than 3 months with no clinical evidence of pulmonary disease, or in those older than 3 months with a temperature less than 39°C, WBC below 20,000/mm³, and no clinical evidence of pulmonary disease.

TREATMENT AND PROPHYLAXIS

The treatment of the febrile child depends largely on the age of the patient. Because of the high rates of serious bacterial infections in neonates, all febrile neonates should receive antibiotics (Table 46.1). Typically, these patients are treated with a third-generation cephalosporin (though ceftriaxone is not recommended for neonates with jaundice because of the concern for inducing unconjugated hyperbilirubinemia) and ampicillin to cover *Listeria monocytogenes*, though the incidence of *Listeria* infection is quite low.

For 1- to 3-month-old infants who have abnormal tests or who look ill, antibiotic therapy and hospitalization is warranted. Ceftriaxone is commonly used for these patients in the ED. Additional antibiotics should be considered in select circumstances. Patients with findings suspicious for meningitis should get higher doses of ceftriaxone, and vancomycin should be considered. Although some studies suggest that patients in this age group with UTIs may be treated on an outpatient basis, there are no large prospective studies that address this question.

The use of ceftriaxone prior to discharge for full-term, well-appearing 1- to 3-month-old infants with no laboratory abnormalities is acceptable, as is withholding antibiotics in these low-risk patients. Patients who did not undergo LP in the ED, however, should not receive antibiotics, as this will confound the evaluation for meningitis if the patient is still febrile on follow-up examination. Close follow-up must be ensured prior to discharge.

For children 2 months old and older, antibiotics are generally reserved for treatment of clinically apparent or documented infections. UTIs are the most common serious bacterial infections. Empiric antibiotic therapy should be tailored to

Table 46.1 Antibiotic Treatment

	Therapy Recommendation
Empiric Antibiotic Therapy	Neonates: ampicillin 50 mg/kg IV q6–8h and cefotaxime 50 mg/kg IV q6–8h Young infants (if given): ceftriaxone 50 mg/kg IV or IM qd Older infants: empiric antibiotic therapy generally not indicated
Otitis Media	Amoxicillin: 80–90 mg/kg/day PO in two divided doses for 7–10 days *or* Amoxicillin-clavulanate: 90 mg/kg/day PO of amoxicillin with 6.4 mg/kg/day of clavulanate in two divided doses
Pneumonia	Amoxicillin: 80–90 mg/kg/day PO in three divided doses for 7–10 days *or* Azithromycin: 10 mg/kg PO on first treatment day, then 5 mg/kg/day for 4 more days
UTI	Cefixime: 16 mg/kg PO twice on first day, then 8 mg/kg/day PO qd for 7–14 days *or* Cephalexin: 25–100 mg/kg/day PO in four divided doses for 7–14 days
CNS	Ceftriaxone or cefotaxime: 100 mg/kg IV Vancomycin: 10–15 mg/kg IV Acyclovir: 20 mg/kg IV (if HSV encephalitis suspected)

CNS, central nervous system; HSV, herpes simplex virus.

local bacterial epidemiology, but reasonable outpatient medications include cefixime or cephalexin. Duration of therapy should be from 7 to 14 days.

Although many children with pneumonia have viral pneumonia, the underlying microbiologic etiology is difficult to determine based on laboratory and radiographic studies. Therefore most patients with infiltrates on chest radiographs are treated with antibiotics. Both amoxicillin and macrolide antibiotics are acceptable. Treatment duration is usually from 7 to 10 days (with the exception of azithromycin), but no definitive evidence supports a specific duration of therapy. These recommendations may change with declining rates of pneumococcal pneumonia.

COMPLICATIONS AND ADMISSION CRITERIA

All febrile neonates, regardless of test results, should be hospitalized. For infants between 1 and 2 months or 3 months who undergo full sepsis evaluations, those with CSF or WBC abnormalities should be hospitalized. Traditionally, most infants with UTIs in this age range have been admitted to the hospital.

Patients who return with positive blood cultures should be reexamined and, when ill-appearing, need repeat blood cultures, LP, intravenous antibiotics, and hospital admission. Patients with pneumococcal bacteremia who are afebrile on repeat evaluation can be followed on an outpatient basis after repeat blood cultures and antibiotics. Children with pneumococcal bacteremia who are persistently febrile need repeat blood cultures and generally should undergo LP and be admitted. The treatment and disposition for well-appearing children with *Salmonella* bacteremia is less clear, but patients with meningococcal bacteremia should be hospitalized for parenteral antibiotics pending results of repeat blood cultures.

INFECTION CONTROL

Universal precautions should be maintained. No isolation is required.

PEARLS AND PITFALLS

1. All febrile neonates need a full sepsis evaluation, parenteral antibiotics, and hospital admission.
2. Febrile young infants (1–2 months) need a full sepsis evaluation. If this is normal, the child looks well, and close follow-up can be ensured, these children may be discharged. Parenteral antibiotics are optional prior to discharge.
3. Older children (>2–24 months) who look otherwise well require only selective testing. Generally, boys younger than 6 months of age (uncircumcised boys <12 months) and girls younger than 2 years old who have fever without source require urinalysis and urine cultures.
4. A response (or lack thereof) to antipyretic medications does not predict whether the underlying etiology is bacterial or viral.

REFERENCES

Alpern ER, Alessandrini EA, Bell LM, et al. Occult bacteremia from a pediatric emergency department: current prevalence, time to detection, and outcome. Pediatrics 2000;106(3):505–11.

American College of Emergency Physicians. Clinical policy for children younger than three years presenting to the emergency department with fever. Ann Emerg Med 2003;42(4):530–45.

Baker MD, Avner JR, Bell LM. Failure of infant observation scales in detecting serious illness in febrile, 4- to 8-week-old infants. Pediatrics 1990;85(6):1040–3.

Baker MD, Bell LM, Avner JR. Outpatient management without antibiotics of fever in selected infants. N Engl J Med 1993;329(20):1437–41.

Baker MD, Bell LM, Avner JR. The efficacy of routine outpatient management without antibiotics of fever in selected infants. Pediatrics 1999;103(3):627–31.

Baskin MN, O'Rourke EJ, Fleisher GR. Outpatient treatment of febrile infants 28 to 89 days of age with intramuscular administration of ceftriaxone. J Pediatr 1992;120(1):22–7.

Black S, Shinefield H, Fireman B, et al. Efficacy, safety and immunogenicity of heptavalent pneumococcal conjugate vaccine in children. Northern California Kaiser Perma-

nente Vaccine Study Center Group. Pediatr Infect Dis J 2000;19(3):187–95.

Bonsu BK, Harper MB. Utility of the peripheral blood white blood cell count for identifying sick young infants who need lumbar puncture. Ann Emerg Med 2003;41(2):206–14.

Byington CL, Enriquez FR, Hoff C, et al. Serious bacterial infections in febrile infants 1 to 90 days old with and without viral infections. Pediatrics 2004;113(6):1662–6.

Gorelick MH, Shaw KN. Clinical decision rule to identify febrile young girls at risk for urinary tract infection. Arch Pediatr Adolesc Med 2000;154(4):386–90.

Herz AM, Greenhow TL, Alcantara J, et al. Changing epidemiology of outpatient bacteremia in 3- to 36-month-old children after the introduction of the heptavalent-conjugated pneumococcal vaccine. Pediatr Infect Dis J 2006;25(4):293–300.

Hsiao AL, Chen L, Baker MD. Incidence and predictors of serious bacterial infections among 57- to 180-day-old infants. Pediatrics 2006;117(5):1695–701.

Kuppermann N, Malley R, Inkelis SH, Fleisher GR. Clinical and hematologic features do not reliably identify children with unsuspected meningococcal disease. Pediatrics 1999;103(2):E20.

Lee GM, Harper MB. Risk of bacteremia for febrile young children in the post-*Haemophilus influenzae* type b era. Arch Pediatr Adolesc Med 1998;152(7):624–8.

Levine DA, Platt SL, Dayan PS, et al. Risk of serious bacterial infection in young febrile infants with respiratory syncytial virus infections. Pediatrics 2004;113(6):1728–34.

Poehling KA, Talbot TR, Griffin MR, et al. Invasive pneumococcal disease among infants before and after introduction of pneumococcal conjugate vaccine. JAMA 2006;295(14):1668–74.

Shaw KN, McGowan KL, Gorelick MH, Schwartz JS. Screening for urinary tract infection in infants in the emergency department: which test is best? Pediatrics 1998;101(6):E1.

ADDITIONAL READINGS

Alpern E, Henretig F. Fever. In: Fleisher G, Ludwig S, Henretig F, et al., eds. Textbook of pediatric emergency medicine, 5th ed. Philadelphia: Lippincott Williams & Wilkins, 2006:295–306.

Bachur R, Perry H, Harper MB. Occult pneumonias: empiric chest radiographs in febrile children with leukocytosis. Ann Emerg Med 1999;33(2):166–73.

Baraff L. Management of fever without source in infants and children. Ann Emerg Med 2000;36(6):602–14.

Baraff LJ. Editorial: Clinical policy for children younger than three years presenting to the emergency department with fever. Ann Emerg Med 2003;42(4):546–9.

Kuppermann N. The evaluation of young febrile children for occult bacteremia: time to reevaluate our approach? Arch Pediatr Adolesc Med 2002;156(9):855–7.

47. Pediatric Orthopedic Infections

James M. Mok and Paul D. Choi

OPEN FRACTURE IN CHILDREN

Introduction

Motor vehicle accidents and falls from height account for the majority of open fractures in children. They differ from open fractures in adults in that children have greater potential for healing due to the thicker periosteum. Infection rates are also lower in children compared to adults. Open fractures in children with closed physes should receive the same treatment as in adults.

Epidemiology

Open fractures have been reported to account for 9% of fractures treated at a pediatric tertiary trauma center. Most studies show a preponderance of boys. The tibia and forearm are the areas most frequently involved.

Clinical Features

The modified Gustilo classification system is used to classify open fractures in children (Table 47.1). The overall rate of infection following open fracture in children is reported as 3%. By type, infection occurs in 2% of type I, 2% of type II, and 8% of type III fractures.

Although community-acquired methicillin-resistant *Staphylococcus aureus* (MRSA) is of increasing concern, no studies have been published demonstrating superior efficacy of vancomycin, clindamycin, or other antibiotics over cefazolin for open fracture. Indiscriminate use of second-tier agents may lead to increased resistance. Therefore, in the absence of a cephalosporin allergy, cefazolin is recommended as first-line prophylaxis.

Table 47.2 summarizes important clinical features of open fractures in children.

Treatment

Initial treatment consists of management of the trauma ABCs (airway, breathing, circulation) and appropriate cervical spine stabilization. Further evaluation and treatment should follow the Pediatric Advanced Life Support (PALS) and Advanced Trauma Life Support (ATLS) protocols. Intravenous antibiotics should be administered immediately on recognition of the open fracture. Tetanus prophylaxis should be administered if immunization status is not up-to-date or is unknown. Routine cultures of the wound are not indicated.

Plain radiographs consisting of at least two orthogonal views should be obtained of the fracture site, the joint above, and the joint below. A thorough neurologic examination should be performed of all extremities. In the child who is too young, frightened, or otherwise unable to cooperate, the examination may depend on observing spontaneous movement and reaction to stimuli. Portions that could not be performed should be noted and the parents informed of the limitations of the initial exam. The vascular examination includes evaluation of capillary refill and of distal pulses by palpation and Doppler as needed. The compartments should be carefully assessed for compartment syndrome.

Following assessment and irrigation of the wound, the wound should be covered with a sterile dressing. Repeat wound examinations should be avoided to reduce the risk of further contamination. A gentle reduction and splinting should be performed to correct any gross deformity of the extremity.

Although the traditional teaching is that open fractures should undergo surgery within 6–8 hours of injury, the current literature suggests that operative treatment up to 24 hours after injury in children does not increase the risk of infection if antibiotics are administered early. If a child is undergoing anesthesia for irrigation and debridement, however, fixation adds little more risk while producing substantial benefit. The operative treatment of type I fractures is controversial given that the risk of infection is so low. However, because of the potentially serious sequelae, patients with type I

Table 47.1 Gustilo Classification of Open Fractures

Fracture Type	Soft-Tissue Injury	Bone Injury	Antibiotics*†
Type I	<1-cm skin opening, minimal soft-tissue damage	Simple transverse or short oblique fracture	cefazolin 100 mg/kg/day divided into three doses (max 2 g q8h)
Type II	>1-cm skin opening, moderate to severe soft-tissue damage but adequate bone coverage	Transverse and oblique fractures, minimal comminution	cefazolin 100 mg/kg/day divided into three doses (max 2 g q8h) *plus* gentamicin 5–7.5 mg/kg/day divided into three doses*
Type III: >10-cm skin break with extensive soft-tissue injury, often with a severe crushing component and fracture pattern consistent with a high-energy mechanism			
Type IIIA	Limited periosteal stripping, bone coverage usually adequate	Segmental fractures, highly comminuted fractures	cefazolin 100 mg/kg/day divided into three doses (max 2 g q8h) *plus* gentamicin 5–7.5 mg/kg/day divided into three doses*
Type IIIB	Extensive periosteal and muscle stripping from bone, usually severe contamination	Segmental fractures, highly comminuted fractures	cefazolin 100 mg/kg/day divided into three doses (max 2 g q8h) *plus* gentamicin 5–7.5 mg/kg/day divided into three doses*
Type IIIC	Any open fracture associated with vascular injury requiring surgical repair	Variable	cefazolin 100 mg/kg/day divided into three doses (max 2 g q8h) *plus* gentamicin 5–7.5 mg/kg/day divided into three doses*

*Penicillin 150,000 units/kg/day divided into 4 doses (max 24,000,000 units daily) should be added for highly contaminated wounds (e.g., barnyard injuries) to cover *Clostridium perfringens*.
†If penicillin-allergic: replace cefazolin with clindamycin 15–40 mg/kg/day divided into 3–4 doses (max 2.7 g daily).

Table 47.2 Clinical Features: Open Fractures in Children

Signs and Symptoms	See Table 47.1
Laboratory and Diagnostic Tests	• X-rays • Preoperative laboratory exams
Treatment	• Trauma evaluation per PALS and ATLS protocols • Immediate antibiotics, continued 48 hours (see Table 47.1) • Tetanus prophylaxis • Irrigation, reduction, sterile dressing, splinting • Urgent operative irrigation and debridement

ATLS, Advanced Trauma Life Support; PALS, Pediatric Advanced Life Support.

fractures should undergo irrigation in either the operating room or the emergency department and be admitted for intravenous antibiotics and observation for 48 hours.

Complications and Admission Criteria

Complications include:

- unrecognized fractures
- compartment syndrome
- vascular injury
- osteomyelitis

All patients with open fractures should be admitted for surgical irrigation, debridement, and intravenous antibiotics.

Pearls and Pitfalls

1. Any visible bleeding in the setting of a fracture should lead to suspicion for an open fracture.
2. Intravenous antibiotics should be administered immediately on recognition of an open fracture.
3. A thorough neurovascular examination and assessment for compartment syndrome should be performed.
4. Open fractures in children should undergo urgent operative debridement and stabilization.
5. The need for operative treatment because of type I open fractures in children is controversial.

ACUTE HEMATOGENOUS OSTEOMYELITIS IN CHILDREN

Introduction

Osteomyelitis is an inflammation of the bone usually caused by bacterial infection. In children, acute osteomyelitis is primarily hematogenous in origin. Historically, acute osteomyelitis in children was associated with high mortality rates of 20–50%. Heightened awareness and advances in treatment have considerably improved outcomes. Failure to promptly recognize this condition, however, may result in significant morbidity, including recurrent infection, chronic osteomyelitis, pathologic fracture, and growth disturbance.

Table 47.3 Clinical Features: Acute Hematogenous Osteomyelitis in Children

Organism	*Staphylococcus aureus* most common
Signs and Symptoms	• Fever • Localized pain, swelling, erythema, warmth • Limited use of extremity • Lower extremity long bone at metaphysis • Single site (multiple sites in neonates) • Concomitant septic arthritis
Laboratory and Radiographic Findings	• WBC, ESR, CRP elevated (90%) • Blood culture positive (30–60%) • X-ray: changes appear at 48 hours • MRI • Bone scan • Bone aspiration

Treatment	• Empiric IV antibiotics, usually 3 weeks, followed by PO antibiotics
	• Neonates (covers group B *Streptococcus*, *S. aureus*, gram-negative rods): cefotaxime 150 mg/kg/day in divided doses q6–8h
	  or
	  oxacillin 100–150 mg/kg/day in divided doses q6–8h and gentamicin 2.5 mg/kg
	• Infants and children (covers *S. aureus*): oxacillin 100–200 mg/kg/day in divided doses q6–8h
	• For MRSA: vancomycin 15 mg/kg/dose q8h (target trough 5–15 mg/L)

CRP, C-reactive protein; ESR, erythrocyte sedimentation rate; MRI, magnetic resonance imaging; WBC, white blood (cell) count.

Epidemiology

In the United States, osteomyelitis in children is relatively uncommon. The annual incidence is estimated to be 1 in 5000 in children younger than 13 years old. Most cases occur during the first decade of life, with half of cases in children younger than 5 years old. *Staphylococcus aureus* is the causative organism in up to 90% of cases, followed by *Streptococcus* species. The widespread implementation of the *Haemophilus influenzae* type B vaccine has led to a marked decline in gram-negative infections. High-risk groups include children with sickle cell anemia (*Salmonella*) and human immunodeficiency virus (HIV)-positive and asplenic children (*Streptococcus pneumoniae*).

Clinical Features

Unexplained bone pain accompanied by fever should be considered osteomyelitis until proven otherwise. The physical signs and symptoms are nonspecific. Most children present acutely and are often systemically ill. There may be swelling, redness, warmth, and pain of the affected limb (Table 47.3). The most frequent clinical findings are fever, localized pain, and limited use of the extremity. Acute hematogenous osteomyelitis is usually localized to a single site, with the long bones of the lower extremities most commonly involved. Most patients have been symptomatic for less than 2 weeks prior to presentation. A history of preceding infection or trauma can be elicited in approximately one-third of patients.

Differential Diagnosis

The clinical presentation of osteomyelitis is highly variable and nonspecific. A wide range of conditions must be considered, including trauma, systemic disease, and local inflammation. Other conditions to consider are:

• soft-tissue infection (cellulitis, myositis)
• fracture/nonaccidental trauma
• overuse syndromes
• acute rheumatic fever
• Legg-Calvé-Perthes disease (idiopathic osteonecrosis of the femoral head)
• juvenile rheumatoid arthritis (and other inflammatory arthritides)
• bone tumor or malignancy
• sickle cell associated pain crisis

Laboratory and Radiographic Findings

A leukocytosis may be present, and the erythrocyte sedimentation rate (ESR) and C-reactive protein (CRP) are elevated in over 90% of cases of osteomyelitis. Blood cultures should be drawn with reported yields ranging from 30% to 60%.

Plain radiographs should be performed on every patient. The first appreciable sign is soft-tissue swelling, which appears within 48 hours of infection, followed by new periosteal bone formation within 5–7 days and osteolysis at 10–14 days. Compared with plain radiographs, magnetic resonance imaging (MRI) with gadolinium contrast offers superior visualization of the bone marrow cavity and adjacent soft tissues. Technetium-99 bone scan is highly sensitive starting 24–48 hours after onset of symptoms.

Bone aspiration should be considered early in the work-up. An 18-gauge spinal needle easily penetrates the thin metaphyseal bone. Although aspiration through an abscess should be avoided, overlying cellulitis should not be considered a contraindication to bone aspiration. The needle should be used to aspirate the extraperiosteal, subperiosteal, and intraosseous spaces. Local infiltration with lidocaine combined with intravenous agents should provide effective analgesia. Direct culture yields an organism in 48–85% of specimens.

Treatment and Prophylaxis

Treatment is largely nonoperative. An initial course of intravenous antibiotics is usually transitioned to oral medication as the patient responds clinically. The ESR and CRP are expected to decrease over the course of treatment and can be followed serially. Empiric treatment is often necessary because of low culture yields and should cover *S. aureus*. Traditionally, intravenous antibiotics are administered for 3 weeks, followed by oral treatment, although the duration of intravenous therapy is ultimately decided by the clinical response and downward-trending CRP. The indications for surgical debridement are the subject of debate but include presence of an abscess on aspiration, chronic infection with sequestrum formation, septic arthritis, and failure to respond to antibiotics within 36 hours.

In general, outcomes are good. Complications are usually the result of late recognition or inadequate treatment. Worse outcomes have been noted in children who have concomitant septic arthritis.

Special Considerations

NEONATAL OSTEOMYELITIS

Neonatal osteomyelitis should be considered separately because of the significant morbidity and poor outcomes associated with the disease in this high-risk population. Affected infants are usually systemically ill. Presentation may be subtle and include pseudoparalysis, anorexia, irritability, or lethargy. The incidence is estimated to be 1 to 3 of every 1000 neonatal intensive care unit admissions. Because of their immature immune systems, neonates are vulnerable to infections caused by group B *Streptococcus* and gram-negative rods with involvement at multiple sites. Temperature and WBC may remain normal, causing a delay in diagnosis, and ESR and CRP are similarly unreliable.

SUBACUTE HEMATOGENOUS OSTEOMYELITIS

Subacute hematogenous osteomyelitis is marked by a relatively benign presentation of little pain, no fever, and normal laboratory results. Plain radiographs demonstrate abnormalities such as lucency or cortical bone loss, which may be confused for tumor, notably Ewing's sarcoma. Debridement is indicated if there is a sequestrum causing a chronic infection.

Pearls and Pitfalls

1. Plain radiographic changes may not be evident until 7 to 10 days after onset of infection.
2. MRI is the gold standard in the detection of osteomyelitis. Nuclear medicine bone scan may be helpful if localization is unclear.
3. Initial antibiotic therapy is empiric, and should target *Staphylococcus* and *Streptococcus*.
4. Because the metaphyseal region of the proximal humerus, proximal femur, distal tibia, and distal humerus is intraarticular, monitor for signs and symptoms of septic arthritis in the shoulder, hip, ankle, and elbow. Between 10% and 16% of cases of septic arthritis are secondary to bacterial osteomyelitis, and the presence of septic arthritis in the setting of osteomyelitis is associated with worse outcomes.

SEPTIC ARTHRITIS IN CHILDREN

Introduction

Septic arthritis in a child is a true clinical emergency requiring prompt antibiotics and drainage. Although any joint can be affected, it most commonly occurs in the hip in neonates and infants, and the knee in older children. An associated osteomyelitis may also be present. Complications from inadequately treated septic arthritis can be devastating and include osteonecrosis, growth arrest, and sepsis. Poor outcomes have been reported in as many as 40% of cases when the hip is involved.

Epidemiology

Although the exact incidence of septic arthritis in children is difficult to estimate, it is thought to be roughly twice that of osteomyelitis, or 1 in 2500. Peak incidence is during the early years of the first decade of life. Neonates (<28 days old) are most commonly infected by group B *Streptococcus*. In infants and children up to 3 years, the organism is usually *Staphylococcus aureus*. Infection with *Haemophilus influenzae* has declined

Table 47.4 Clinical Features: Pediatric Septic Arthritis

Organisms	• *Staphylococcus aureus* most common • Group B *Streptococcus* in neonates • *Kingella kingae* • *Neisseria gonorrhoeae* in at-risk populations
Signs and Symptoms	• Fever • Severe pain with passive range of motion • Limp or refusal to bear weight • Pseudoparalysis, anorexia, irritability, lethargy in neonates

Laboratory and Diagnostic Findings	• WBC, ESR, CRP elevated
	• Blood culture positive
	• X-ray: capsular distension and joint space widening
	• Ultrasound for hip
	• Joint aspiration:
	  ○ WBC count (>50,000/mm³ positive for infection)
	  ○ Gram stain
	  ○ Culture

Treatment	• Intravenous antibiotics immediately after joint aspiration
	• Neonates:
	  oxacillin 100–150 mg/kg/day IV in divided doses q6–8h
	  or
	  cefotaxime 150 mg/kg/day IV in divided doses q6–8h; for high-risk neonate *add* gentamicin 2.5 mg/kg/dose q8h
	• Infants and children:
	  cefazolin 50 mg/kg/dose IV q8h
	  or
	  ceftriaxone 50 mg/kg once daily
	  or
	  (if allergic to penicillin) clindamycin 500 mg/kg/day in three divided doses
	• Children (gonococcal arthritis):
	  ceftriaxone 50–100 mg/kg/day IV in divided doses q12–24h
	• Emergent surgical incision and drainage
	• Serial daily aspiration with close monitoring may be attempted in a superficial joint

because of widespread vaccination but has been replaced by a rise in cases involving *Kingella kingae*, a gram-negative organism. *Neisseria gonorrhoeae* can cause septic arthritis in newborns infected via the birth canal, as well as in sexually active teenagers or younger children who have been victims of sexual abuse.

Clinical Features

Children with septic arthritis typically present with acute-onset fever, irritability, and anorexia (Table 47.4). Passive range of motion of the affected joint will cause severe pain. With lower extremity involvement, the child may present with a limp or refusal to bear weight. If the hip is involved, the child may hold it in a flexed, externally rotated, and abducted position for comfort as this relieves intracapsular pressure. Signs in neonates may be more subtle, such as decreased movement of the affected limb (pseudoparalysis).

Differential Diagnosis

Key features that distinguish septic arthritis from other conditions are:

- severe joint pain with passive range of motion
- elevated inflammatory laboratory markers (WBC, ESR, CRP)
- rash, tenosynovitis, and migratory polyarthralgia in gonococcal arthritis
- episodic mono- or poly-articular involvement with asymptomatic intervals in Lyme arthritis

Other conditions to consider:

- transient synovitis (also called toxic synovitis)
- slipped capital femoral epiphysis
- Legg-Calvé-Perthes disease
- fracture
- inflammatory arthritis
- soft-tissue infection (cellulitis, myositis)

In particular, it may be difficult to differentiate septic arthritis from transient synovitis of the hip in children. Distinguishing the two diagnoses is critical, however, as treatment and prognostic implications differ vastly. Transient synovitis is a common inflammatory condition that is self-limiting and treated supportively with nonsteroidal anti-inflammatory drugs (NSAIDs). Septic arthritis requires urgent intervention with surgical drainage and intravenous antibiotics to avoid serious complications.

Laboratory and Radiographic Findings

The WBC, ESR, and CRP are all usually elevated. Blood cultures will be positive in 30–50% of cases. Four useful clinical criteria for evaluation of the painful hip are:

- inability to bear weight
- ESR greater than 40 mm/hour
- presence of fever
- WBC above 12,000/mm^3

According to one study, the presence of four factors had a positive predictive value for septic arthritis of 90% and three factors had a predictive value of 70%.

Findings on plain radiographs may be subtle, including capsular distension and joint space widening. Ultrasound is highly sensitive for detecting a joint effusion, particularly in the hip, and may also guide needle aspiration.

Joint aspiration is an essential part of the evaluation and should be performed before antibiotics are administered. A WBC in synovial fluid higher than 50,000/mm^3 with a differential containing 75% neutrophils is considered positive for infection. The Gram stain is positive in only 30–50%, but synovial fluid culture will yield an organism in 50–80%.

Treatment and Prophylaxis

Septic arthritis is a surgical emergency requiring incision and drainage of the deep joints to prevent destruction of articular cartilage. Serial needle aspirations performed at least once daily may be attempted in accessible joints such as the knee, but surgery is indicated for any signs of worsening.

Broad-spectrum intravenous antibiotics should be initiated immediately following aspiration and subsequently tailored to culture results. Following adequate drainage, significant improvement is expected within 24 hours. The CRP should decrease and can be followed serially. If the clinical response is delayed, osteomyelitis should be suspected.

After significant improvement, intravenous antibiotics can be transitioned to oral agents. No firm guidelines for duration of antibiotics have been published, although typically a total course of 3 weeks is administered in uncomplicated cases. Poor outcomes are associated with history of premature birth, age younger than 6 months, delay of more than 4 days from onset of symptoms to diagnosis, concurrent osteomyelitis, and septic dislocation if the hip is involved.

Pearls and Pitfalls

1. Joint aspiration is essential for the diagnosis of septic arthritis.
2. Prompt surgical drainage and debridement are indicated to avoid sequelae.
3. Signs and symptoms of septic hip arthritis in children include fever, inability to bear weight, and elevated ESR, WBC, and CRP.

CHILDHOOD DISKITIS

Introduction

Although historically there has been debate among clinicians about the true etiology of childhood diskitis, it is now generally accepted as an infection of the intervertebral disk and adjacent end plates requiring treatment with intravenous antibiotics. The unique vascular anatomy of the immature cartilaginous plates makes the disk prone to infection by septic emboli, whereas the vertebral body is relatively spared because of collateral circulation.

Epidemiology

Childhood diskitis is rare, occurring with an estimated incidence of 0.3 to 0.6 per 10,000. There is a slight male predominance. Affected children are usually younger than 5 years, and the lumbar spine is most frequently involved. *Staphylococcus aureus* is most commonly isolated.

Table 47.5 Clinical Features: Pediatric Diskitis

Organism	*Staphylococcus aureus* most common
Signs and Symptoms	• Low-grade fever • Back pain variable • Limp or refusal to bear weight • Vague abdominal pain

Laboratory and Diagnostic Findings	• WBC, ESR, CRP usually elevated
	• X-ray: changes appear after 1 week:
	  ○ disk space narrowing
	  ○ scalloping of end plates
	  ○ permanent loss of disk height or block vertebrae in resolved infection
	• Bone scan if unable to localize

Treatment	• Immobilization with brace and empiric antibiotics for 6–8 weeks • Children (>3 years): oxacillin 100–200 mg/kg/day in four to six divided doses

Clinical Features

Because young children may be unable to verbalize the location of their pain, diagnosis can be challenging (Table 47.5). Duration of symptoms is highly variable, from hours to weeks, and symptoms can progress to the point where the child is only comfortable when lying supine. Low-grade fever may be present but most children do not appear acutely ill. Classically, the child sits with the spine extended or lies with hands behind the trunk for support. They may indicate abdominal pain or refuse to bear weight; the spine should be examined in all limping children. A history of preceding infection is common and any prior or current otitis media, urinary tract infection, or respiratory infection should be noted. On physical examination, the back may be rigid and stiff during ambulation and be tender to palpation. There are usually no abnormal neurologic findings.

Differential Diagnosis

Other conditions to consider are:

- metastatic tumor or leukemia
- Scheuermann's kyphosis in adolescents
- eosinophilic granuloma, osteoid osteoma, osteoblastoma
- sacroiliitis

Key features that distinguish childhood diskitis from other conditions are:

- acutely ill presentation or neurologic signs should raise suspicion for epidural or soft-tissue abscess
- severe irritability with movement suggests a septic arthritis
- back pain in an adolescent with Schmorl's nodes (protrusions of disk cartilage into the vertebral body) on plain radiographs suggests Scheuermann's kyphosis

Laboratory and Radiographic Findings

Both ESR and CRP are usually elevated in diskitis. Blood cultures may help narrow therapy and should be drawn prior to the administration of antibiotics. The characteristic radiographic finding of disk space narrowing appears 1 week after onset (Figure 47.1), and by 3–5 weeks, "sawtooth" erosions of the vertebral end plates may be appreciated. Pott's disease, or spinal tuberculosis, may cause similar radiographic findings, and a purified protein derivative (PPD) test should be ordered. MRI offers potentially higher sensitivity but may require general anesthesia in young children and rarely changes treatment. Its use is reserved for those uncommon cases when the child presents with a deformity or fails to show improvement after 2–3 days of treatment. A bone scan may be positive in 3–5 days after onset of symptoms and can be useful when the source of the child's discomfort is unclear. Given the potential morbidity and need for anesthesia, routine biopsy is not recommended unless symptoms do not resolve with initial empiric treatment.

Treatment and Prophylaxis

Treatment consists of immobilization and empiric antistaphylococcal antibiotics. A thoracolumbosacral orthosis (TLSO) brace is recommended in the presence of significant pain,

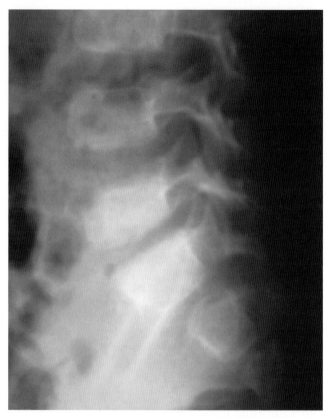

Figure 47.1 Four-year-old boy with plain radiograph showing disk space narrowing consistent with L5-S1 diskitis. Biopsy revealed *Staphylococcus aureus*. Courtesy of Dr. Charles A. Gooding.

deformity, or extensive bony destruction and soft-tissue involvement. Although in the past some have advocated holding antibiotics for immunocompetent children, most authors recommend initiating intravenous antibiotics until clinical signs of improvement appear. The risks of delayed treatment include prolonged hospitalization, worsening infection, or recurrent symptoms. A typical course of antibiotics is 1–2 weeks of intravenous therapy followed by 4–6 weeks of oral agents. Surgery is rarely necessary and is indicated for abscess in the setting of systemic illness, progressive neurologic deficit, or progressive deformity.

Complications and Admission Criteria

Complications and admission criteria include:

- osteomyelitis
- autofusion and spinal deformity
- neurologic compromise (rare)

Because the diagnosis is often unclear, patients suspected of having childhood diskitis should be admitted for administration of antibiotics, monitoring of response, and further evaluation, if necessary.

Pearls and Pitfalls

1. Back pain is a presenting complaint in only 50% of children with diskitis. Younger children (younger than 3 years) may present with a limp or refusal to bear weight on the lower extremities.

2. Biopsy or direct culture is rarely necessary, because *Staphylococcus aureus* is the most commonly isolated organism.

3. Empiric therapy directed against *Staphylococcus aureus* is usually successful.

4. As the presenting symptoms are vague and nonspecific, consider a broad differential diagnosis in a child with irritability and back pain, including septic arthritis of the sacroiliac joint, osteomyelitis, paraspinal or epidural abscess, and noninfectious etiologies, such as metastatic tumor, leukemia, osteoid osteoma, and osteoblastoma.

REFERENCES

Early SD, Kay RM, Tolo VT. Childhood diskitis. J Am Acad Orthop Surg 2003 Nov-Dec;11(6):413–20.

Kocher MS, Mandiga R, Murphy JM, et al. A clinical practice guideline for treatment of septic arthritis in children: efficacy in improving process of care and effect on outcome of septic arthritis of the hip. J Bone Joint Surg Am 2003 Jun;85-A(6):994–9.

Kocher MS, Zurakowski D, Kasser JR. Differentiating between septic arthritis and transient synovitis of the hip in children: an evidence-based clinical prediction algorithm. J Bone Joint Surg Am 1999 Dec;81(12):1662–70.

McCarthy JJ, Dormans JP, Kozin SH, Pizzutillo PD. Musculoskeletal infections in children: basic treatment principles and recent advancements. Instr Course Lect 2005;54:515–28.

Song KM, Sloboda JF. Acute hematogenous osteomyelitis in children. J Am Acad Orthop Surg 2001 May–Jun;9(3):166–75.

Stewart DG Jr, Kay RM, Skaggs DL. Open fractures in children. Principles of evaluation and management. J Bone Joint Surg Am 2005 Dec;87(12):2784–98.

ADDITIONAL READINGS

Chapman MW. Chapman's orthopaedic surgery, 3rd ed. Chapter 176: Bone and joint infections in children. Philadelphia: Lippincott Williams & Wilkins, 2001.

Herring JA. Tachdjian's pediatric orthopaedics, 3rd ed. Chapter 34: Bone and joint infection. Philadelphia: Saunders: Philadelphia, 2002.

48. Pediatric Urinary Tract Infection

Laura W. Kates

INTRODUCTION

Urinary tract infections (UTIs) are a common problem among pediatric patients and an important cause of acute and chronic morbidity, including hypertension and renal scarring. It is often difficult to differentiate between cystitis and pyelonephritis in children.

It is estimated that 75% of children younger than 5 years old with febrile UTI have signs of pyelonephritis by renal nuclear scans. Of children with pyelonephritis, an estimated 27–64% will develop renal scarring, putting them at risk for renal insufficiency and hypertension as adults and adolescents. The risk of long-term renal damage is highest in infants and small children (<2 years old) and the diagnosis of UTI in this population can help identify patients with urinary system obstructive anomalies or vesicoureteral reflux (VUR).

EPIDEMIOLOGY

Ascending infections predominate among pediatric UTI, with *Escherichia coli* causing 60–80% of cases. In neonates, group B *Streptococcus* should be considered if mothers are colonized. Other pathogens include *Proteus* (more commonly in boys and children with renal stones), *Klebsiella*, *Enterococcus*, and coagulase-negative *Staphylococcus*.

At all ages, girls are more likely to have UTIs than boys, with 3% of girls and 1% of boys being diagnosed with UTI before puberty. The prevalence of urinary tract infection in febrile young children aged 2 months to 2 years without a clinically apparent source is approximately 3–7% (Table 48.1).

Table 48.1 UTI Prevalence in Pediatric Population

• Circumcised male >1 year	1%
• Circumcised male <1 year	2–8%
• Uncircumcised male <2 years	8%
• Caucasian females <2 years	8%
• Females 1–2 years	16%
• Sexually active teenage females	4–8%

Specific risk factors for UTI include age younger than 1 year, Caucasian race, temperature above 39°C, fever for more than 2 days, and absence of other source of fever on physical exam. Breastfed infants are at lower risk because of the protective effects of maternal IgA. Children with diabetes mellitus and immunocompromised children have higher rates of UTI. Of note, bathing and wiping patterns have not proven to increase or decrease risk for UTI.

CLINICAL FEATURES

The American Academy of Pediatrics recommends consideration of urinary tract infection in all febrile children 2 months to 2 years of age, particularly in the toxic-appearing patient. Fever may be the *only* symptom in young children, so consideration of UTI must be part of every work-up of pediatric fever. The age of the child greatly affects the clinical presentation (Table 48.2). In general, older children may articulate symptoms of urinary complaints, whereas infants and small children will present in a myriad of ways.

DIFFERENTIAL DIAGNOSIS

Infants and Small Children Younger Than 2 Years

Differential diagnosis in febrile infants and toddlers (to 36 months) is broad and includes:

- occult bacteremia
- bacterial or viral meningitis
- acute gastroenteritis
- viral syndromes
- otitis media

In children who have received vaccinations for *Haemophilus influenzae* and *Streptococcus pneumoniae*, the likelihood of UTI is higher than other sources. Other important diagnoses that should be considered include:

- vaginitis
- vaginal foreign body
- sexually transmitted diseases

Table 48.2 Clinical Features: Urinary Tract Infection – Pediatric

Organisms	• *Escherichia coli* • Group B *Streptococcus* • *Klebsiella* • *Enterococcus* • Coagulase-negative *Staphylococcus*
Signs and Symptoms	**Young children** >2 years: • Fever • Vomiting • Diarrhea • Irritability • Poor feeding • Foul-smelling urine • Change in voiding pattern • Conjugated hyperbilirubinemia **Children** >2 years: • Fever • Crying with urination • Dysuria • Urinary frequency • Vomiting • Hypertension
Laboratory and Radiographic Findings	• Urine dipstick: Positive nitrite, positive leukocyte esterase • Urine microscopy: pyuria and bacteriuria • Urine culture: Depending on collection method: Catheterization: >10^3 Clean catch: >10^4 Suprapubic aspirate: any number CFU
Treatment	**Parenteral therapy:** for infants 1–3 months old with fever >38°C and positive urinalysis: ceftriaxone 50 mg/kg IM × 1 **Oral therapy:** amoxicillin 20–40 mg/kg/day PO tid *or* trimethoprim-sulfamethoxazole 6–12 mg/kg/day of TMP PO bid *or* cephalexin 50–100 mg/kg/day PO qid

Radiography and other renal imaging modalities can be helpful to define urinary tract anatomy and diagnose vesicoureteral reflux.
CFU, colony-forming units; TMP, trimethoprim.

Table 48.3 Definitions of Bacteriuria by Urine Culture and Mode of Specimen Collection

Adults and children >2 years, clean catch	>10^5 CFU/mL	**Positive**
Children <2 years, any collection technique	>50,000 CFU/mL	**Positive**
Children any age, clean catch	10–50,000 CFU/mL	**Equivocal** – send second culture and treat if grows >10,000 CFU/mL
Catheter	>10,000 CFU/mL	**Positive**
Suprapubic aspiration	Any number of colonies of gram-negative bacilli; >2000 CFU/mL for gram-positive cocci	**Positive**

CFU, colony-forming units.

Older Children

Because older children are better able to differentiate urinary symptoms, the differential includes:

- vaginitis
- vaginal foreign body
- urethritis including sexually transmitted diseases
- ureteral calculi
- dysfunctional elimination.
- vulvar ulcerative disease (herpes infections, Behçet's disease)

Children with appendicitis, group A streptococcal disease, and Kawasaki disease can present with fever, pyuria, and abdominal pain. Dysuria may also accompany other more occult sources of fever including malignancy and autoimmune disease.

LABORATORY DIAGNOSIS

Urinalysis and urine culture remain the mainstay of diagnosis of UTI. Leukocytes on dipstick or microscopic urine analysis are suggestive of the diagnosis. Transurethral catheterization and suprapubic aspiration are the preferred methods of urine specimen collection. Suprapubic aspiration is recommended when catheterization is not feasible (e.g., a child with phimosis) or the results of a catheterized specimen are inconclusive.

Bag-collected specimens generally have unacceptable rates of contamination, and urine culture from a bag-collected specimen has a false-positive rate of up to 85%. The only situation in which a bag-collected specimen may be helpful is in circumcised male infants older than 1 year, but too young to cooperate with a clean catch. A negative urine analysis in this situation has a high negative predictive value and can spare the patients a more invasive method of specimen collection.

Laboratory urinalysis with microscopy is more sensitive than dipstick alone but still has a false negative rate of between 10% and 50%, and urine cultures should be sent and follow-up arranged for all pediatric patients with suspected UTI (Table 48.3). The decision to perform imaging studies can usually be deferred to the primary pediatrician, as renal imaging will not change clinical management in a febrile child with a primary UTI. The American Academy of Pediatrics recommends ultrasound and urethrogram in any child 2 months to 2 years of age with UTI. Others recommend imaging in all girls younger than 3 years of age and all boys with UTI.

TREATMENT AND PROPHYLAXIS

Empiric treatment pending culture results is recommended for febrile patients for whom clinical suspicion is high, regardless of urinalysis results, as the false negative rate is significant. Afebrile patients with negative urinalysis may follow up with their primary pediatrician for treatment pending urine cultures.

Amoxicillin is the mainstay of antibiotic therapy for pediatric UTI (Table 48.4). The *E. coli* resistance to amoxicillin common in adults has not been seen in pediatric populations.

Table 48.4 Oral Antibiotic Therapy

Cefixime (Suprax)	16 mg/kg divided bid on 1st day, followed by 8 mg/kg qd (max dose 200 mg)
Cefpodoxime (Vantin)	10 mg/kg divided bid (max dose 400 mg)
Amoxicillin*	20–40 mg/kg divided tid (max dose 500 mg)
Trimethoprim-sulfamethoxazole* (TMP-SMX) (Bactrim, Septra)	6–12 mg/kg TMP/30–60 mg/kg SMX divided bid (max dose 160 mg TMP/800 mg SMX)
Cephalexin* (Keflex)	25–50 mg/kg divided qid (max dose 1 g)
Nitrofurantion (Macrodantin)	5–7 mg/kg divided qid (max dose 100 mg)
Loracarbef (Lorabid)	15–30 mg/kg divided bid (max dose 400 mg)

*Associated with increasing rates of resistance. Choice of antibiotic therapy should be guided by local resistance patterns.

Rates of microbiologic cure and clinical improvement do not vary significantly between oral and parenteral antibiotic routes, though parental therapy might be preferred in a vomiting child. Short-course therapy (3 to 5 days) may be as effective as a longer (7- to 14-day) course therapy and has been a subject of debate among pediatricians. Generally, patients with UTI should be started on antibiotic therapy and followed-up within 72 hours for reevaluation and culture results.

A first parenteral dose in the ED of ceftriaxone 50 mg/kg intramuscular (IM)/intravenous (IV) is indicated for infants 1–3 months old with fever above 38°C and a positive urine dipstick for nitrite or leukocyte esterase, positive urine Gram stain, or a white blood cell count (WBC) over 15,000/mm^3. A first parenteral dose may be indicated in children 3 months to 36 months with fever above 39°C and positive urine dipstick.

COMPLICATIONS AND ADMISSION CRITERIA

Complications of urinary tract infection can include perinephric and retroperitoneal abscesses, pyonephrosis (collection of purulent material in the urinary collecting system), and urinary calculi secondary to stasis or urease-splitting bacteria. Long-term complications include recurrent infection, renal scarring, hypertension, and renal damage. Morbidity appears to be additive and associated with earlier age of infection.

Admission is indicated for all toxic-appearing children in whom sepsis is a concern. Other indications for admission include:

- persistently high fevers (>38°C)
- dehydration requiring intravenous rehydration
- excessive vomiting precluding oral antibiotic therapy
- poor social situation or other barriers to close follow-up

PEARLS AND PITFALLS

1. Consider urinary tract infection in all febrile children.
2. Bag urine specimens are usually contaminated and will only slow disposition of children in whom UTI is suspected.
3. Send all urine specimens for culture.
4. When clinical suspicion for UTI is high, treat despite negative urinalysis, as there is a high false negative rate.
5. Urine culture is the gold standard for diagnosis of pediatric UTI, and should be sent on all urine specimens.
6. Ensure follow-up within 72 hours.
7. Consider a single dose of ceftriaxone 50–100 mg/kg IM/IV prior to discharge in selected patients.

REFERENCES

Alper BS, Curry SH. Urinary tract infection in children. Am Fam Physician 2005;72(12):2483–8.

Hoberman A, Charron M, Hickey RW, et al. Imaging studies after a first febrile urinary tract infection in young children. N Engl J Med 2003;348:2195–202.

Layton KL. Diagnosis and management of pediatric urinary tract infections. Clin Fam Med 2003;5(2):367–83.

Ma JF, Dairiki Shortliffe JM. Urinary tract infection in children: etiology and epidemiology. Urol Clin North Am 2004;31:517–26.

Shaw KN, Gorelick M, McGowan KL, et al. Prevalence of urinary tract infection in febrile young children in the emergency department. Pediatrics 1998;102:e16.

ADDITIONAL READINGS

American Academy of Pediatrics. Practice parameter: the diagnosis, treatment, and evaluation of the initial urinary tract infection in febrile infants and young children. Committee on Quality Improvement, Subcommittee on Urinary Tract Infection. Pediatrics 1999;103:4.

Ishimine P. Fever without source in children 0 to 36 months of age. Pediatr Clin North Am 2006;53:167–94.

49. Pediatric Respiratory Infections

Seema Shah and Ghazala Q. Sharieff

INTRODUCTION – AGENTS

Respiratory failure is the most common cause of cardiopulmonary arrest in infants and children. Because morbidity may be time-dependent and appropriate treatment may vary significantly depending on etiology, prompt assessment and management of pediatric respiratory disease is essential. This chapter will discuss the most common respiratory diseases in children focusing on epiglottitis, bacterial tracheitis, croup, retropharyngeal abscess, pertussis, bronchiolitis, and pneumonia.

EPIGLOTTITIS

Epidemiology

Epiglottitis or supraglottitis is a serious, life-threatening infection of the epiglottis and constitutes an airway emergency (see Chapter 8 for a discussion of supraglottitis). It is more common in the winter but can occur throughout the year. Peak incidence is in children between 2 and 8 years of age, but epiglottitis also occurs in infants and adults. Since widespread vaccination against *Haemophilus influenzae* type B, previously the most common cause, the incidence has decreased from 41 to 4.1 cases per 100,000, and the typical age of presentation is increasing. The most common identified organisms causing epiglottitis are now group A beta-hemolytic *Streptococcus*, *Streptococcus pneumoniae*, *Klebsiella*, *Pseudomonas*, and *Candida*.

Clinical Features

Epiglottitis usually presents abruptly within 6–24 hours of a prodromal viral illness. Patients with epiglottitis classically have high fever, irritability, and throat pain that may manifest as unwillingness to eat or drink (Table 49.1). They may also present with symptoms of impending airway obstruction such as drooling, stridor, cyanosis, marked anxiety, and a toxic appearance. Characteristic voice changes include hoarseness and a muffled voice. These children usually prefer to rest in the tripod position, a sitting position with their jaws thrust forward. As the supraglottic edema worsens, it becomes difficult

Table 49.1 Clinical Features: Epiglottitis

Organisms	• Group A beta-hemolytic *Streptococcus* • *Streptococcus pneumoniae* • *Klebsiella* • *Pseudomonas* • *Candida*
Signs and Symptoms	• Abrupt presentation within 6–24 hours of illness • High fever, irritability, throat pain • "4 Ds" of epiglottitis: drooling, dyspnea, dysphonia, and dysphagia • Symptoms of impending airway obstruction: drooling, stridor, and cyanosis • Tripod positioning
Laboratory and Radiographic Findings	• Routine laboratory tests are not indicated • Lateral neck radiograph* has classic "thumbprint" sign (may be absent in up to 20% of cases) • Blood and supraglottic cultures and sensitivities
Treatment	ceftriaxone 100 mg/kg/day IV in one dose *or* cefotaxime 200 mg/kg/day in four divided doses *or* ampicillin-sulbactam 450 mg/kg/day in four divided doses Steroids are not routinely recommended

*Radiographs are helpful in ruling out croup, retropharyngeal abscess, and foreign bodies.

for the patient to swallow saliva, and drooling is a common complaint. High fevers (e.g., 104°F or 40.0°C) and tachycardia may be present.

Differential Diagnosis

The differential diagnosis of epiglottitis includes:

- croup
- bacterial tracheitis
- retropharyngeal abscess
- peritonsillar abscess
- vocal cord paralysis
- pharyngitis
- anaphylaxis
- inhaled foreign body

Key features that may help to distinguish epiglottitis are:

- sore throat with odynophagia and fever
- four D's – drooling, dyspnea, dysphonia, and dysphagia
- these children *do not* cough
- classic "thumbprint sign" on lateral neck radiograph (absent in ~20%)

Laboratory and Radiographic Findings

Routine laboratory tests are not indicated, particularly because agitation of the child prior to definitive airway management is contraindicated. Gentle visualization of the oropharynx may be performed, but without the use of a tongue depressor, because manipulation may result in complete obstruction of the airway. Occasionally, an erythematous epiglottis may be seen protruding at the base of the tongue. Radiographs are helpful in ruling out croup, retropharyngeal abscess, or foreign body. The lateral neck radiograph, especially in hyperextension during inspiration, is the imaging study of choice. The classic finding is the "thumbprint sign," indicative of a round and thick epiglottis (Figure 49.1). However, this finding may be absent in up to 20% of cases. Once the airway has been secured, cultures and sensitivities should be obtained from both the blood and supraglottic region.

Treatment and Prophylaxis

When a diagnosis of epiglottitis is made by history and physical exam, every effort should be made to avoid any anxiety-provoking procedures, including phlebotomy or intraoral examination. It is imperative to allow the patient to sit in the most comfortable position possible. The confirmatory diagnosis of epiglottitis is made by direct visualization with a laryngoscope, usually during intubation. The mucosa will appear erythematous and pooling of secretions may be present. The supraglottic structures, including the epiglottis, arytenoids, and aryepiglottic folds, may appear cherry red and edematous. Unless there is severe airway compromise requiring immediate emergency department management, laryngoscopy should be performed under sedation, in a controlled setting with an intubation team and surgical personnel present. Broad-spectrum antibiotics such as third-generation cephalosporins should be started as soon as possible, but again, painful procedures such as phlebotomy or

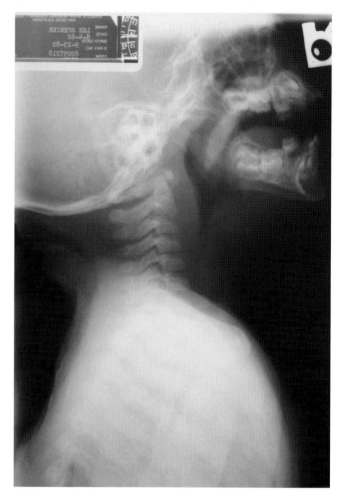

Figure 49.1 Epiglottis. Courtesy of Children's Hospital, San Diego Department of Radiology.

intramuscular injection are contraindicated until the airway is secured. Steroids are not routinely indicated.

Complications and Admission Criteria

Airway obstruction is the most serious complication of this disease. A surgical airway is necessary if the patient cannot be endotracheally intubated. All children with suspected epiglottitis should be admitted to the intensive care unit (ICU).

Infection Control

Universal precautions should be maintained. No isolation is required.

Pearls and Pitfalls

1. Once epiglottis is suspected, minimize patient anxiety.
2. If the patient is in extremis, immediate orotracheal intubation should be performed, preferably with the help of an anesthesiologist or otolaryngologist.
3. If the patient is stable, then the preferred examination and intervention area is the operating room.
4. Starting an intravenous (IV) line or obtaining blood cultures may exacerbate the patient's condition, and these tests should not be performed in the initial stages of evaluation and treatment.
5. Treatment should not be delayed for radiographs.

CROUP

Epidemiology

Croup, or laryngotracheobronchitis, is the most common cause of infectious airway obstruction in children. The most commonly affected age group is 6 months to 4 years, with a peak incidence of 60 per 1000 children 1 to 2 years old. Croup has a peak incidence in early fall and winter, but occasionally may be seen throughout the year. The most common causative organism is parainfluenza virus type I however, other organisms such as parainfluenza types II and III, *Mycoplasma pneumoniae*, respiratory syncytial virus (RSV), influenza A and B, and adenovirus have been implicated.

Clinical Features

A 1- to 2-day prodrome of nasal congestion, rhinorrhea, and cough is followed by the onset of a harsh, barky cough often described as sounding similar to a seal. The patient may also have stridor, which is typically inspiratory but may also be biphasic. Biphasic stridor, as well as nasal flaring, suprasternal and intercostal retraction, tachypnea, and hypoxia, are indications of severe respiratory compromise. Typical symptom duration is less than 1 week with a peak of 1–2 days (Table 49.2).

Differential Diagnosis

The differential for croup includes:

- foreign body aspiration
- spasmodic croup
- epiglottitis
- bacterial tracheitis
- retropharyngeal abscess

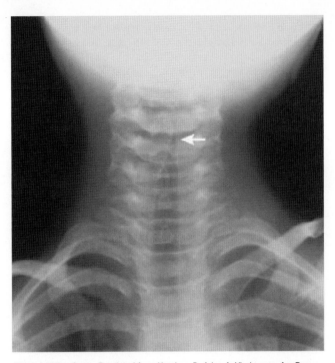

Figure 49.2 Croup. Reprinted from Knudson D, Aring A. Viral croup. Am Fam Physician 2004;40:541–2, with permission.

- subglottic stenosis after prolonged endotracheal (ET) tube placement
- laryngeal web
- anaphylaxis with angioedema of the subglottic area
- hemangioma
- neoplasm
- laryngomalacia
- vascular ring
- burn or thermal injuries
- laryngeal papillomatosis

Key features that may help distinguish croup from other respiratory infections are:

- harsh, barky cough
- inspiratory stridor
- classic steeple sign on anteroposterior (AP) neck radiograph (absent in ~50%)

Laboratory and Radiographic Findings

The diagnosis of croup is a clinical one, as complete blood counts (CBCs) tend to be normal. Radiographs may be helpful in differentiation of other disease entities such as epiglottitis, retropharyngeal abscess, congenital abnormalities, foreign body, or hemangioma. The classic radiographic finding in a patient with croup is the "steeple sign" (Figure 49.2) representing subglottic edema. However, the absence of this finding does not rule out croup, because almost half of patients with croup have normal radiographs.

Treatment and Prophylaxis

The management of croup, usually a self-limited disease, is dependent on the severity of respiratory symptoms.

Table 49.2 Clinical Features: Croup

Organisms	• Parainfluenza virus type I • Parainfluenza type II and III • *Mycoplasma pneumoniae* • RSV • Influenza A and B • Adenovirus
Signs and Symptoms	• Viral prodrome (cough, rhinorrhea, fever) • Harsh, barky cough • Inspiratory stridor more common • Tachypnea, hypoxia, and biphasic stridor concerning for respiratory compromise
Laboratory and Radiographic Findings	• Classic "steeple sign" • X-ray can help rule out retropharyngeal abscess, epiglottitis, foreign body, congenital abnormalities
Treatment	• Oral or IM dexamethasone 0.6 mg/kg (maximum 16 mg) • Racemic epinephrine at 0.25 mL to 0.5 mL in NS *or* nebulized budesonide 2 mg or 4 mg

NS, normal saline.

Traditionally, patients with croup have been treated with humidified air believed to soothe inflamed mucosa and thus decrease coughing. Several studies have shown that mist therapy is not effective in improving clinical symptoms in children presenting to the ED with moderate croup. Because these treatments are harmless, however, many practitioners still use them, particularly in patients who are being held for observation.

Glucocorticoids are used to treat moderate to severe croup because oral or intramuscular dexamethasone decreases hospitalization rates. Patients with mild croup also benefit from dexamethasone with faster resolution of symptoms. Although the standard dose of dexamethasone is 0.6 mg/kg, lower doses of 0.15 mg/kg and 0.3 mg/kg have showed similar efficacy in patients with moderate croup. Because the half-life of dexamethasone is 36–52 hours, it is the preferred agent for croup therapy; there is no need to discharge the patient with additional doses of steroids.

Nebulized budesonide dosed at both 2 mg and 4 mg has also shown efficacy in mild to moderate croup as single-dose therapy. Nebulized racemic epinephrine contains both levo (L) and dextro (D) epinephrine isomers and is the mainstay of treatment for moderate to severe croup. Although racemic epinephrine does not alter the natural course of croup, it may reduce the need for emergent airway management. The preferred dose is 0.25 to 0.5 mL with 3 mL of saline. Patients who receive nebulized epinephrine should also receive dexamethasone. Patients who receive corticosteroids and demonstrate a sustained response to racemic epinephrine 3 hours after treatment are generally safe for discharge. If racemic epinephrine is not available, epinephrine can be used in its place. The administration of a mixture of helium and oxygen (heliox) can improve oxygenation in patients with severe croup.

In patients with severe croup that is unresponsive to nebulized epinephrine, corticosteroids, and heliox, endotracheal intubation and ventilation may be necessary. If intubation is necessary, an endotracheal tube with a diameter smaller than recommended for age and size should be used.

Complications and Admission Criteria

Patients who have persistent tachypnea, hypoxia, or inability to tolerate oral fluids or who require more than two treatments of racemic epinephrine should be admitted. Fortunately, fewer than 10% of children with croup are hospitalized. Complications include airway compromise and respiratory arrest.

Infection Control

Universal precautions should be maintained. No isolation is required.

Pearls and Pitfalls

1. Consider anatomical abnormalities in patients with recurrent croup.
2. Always administer concurrent steroids to patients ill enough to require nebulized epinephrine.
3. Observe all children receiving nebulized epinephrine for at least three hours.

Table 49.3 Clinical Features: Bacterial Tracheitis

Organisms	• *Staphylococcus aureus* (most common) • *Streptococcus viridans* • *Haemophilus influenzae* • *Moraxella catarrhalis* • *Streptococcus pneumoniae*
Signs and Symptoms	• Prodromal low-grade fever, cough, and stridor (similar to croup) • Rapid onset of high fevers and respiratory distress; child appears toxic • May or may not have tripod positioning
Laboratory and Radiographic Findings	• Routine laboratory test are not indicated • CBC may show marked leukocytosis • Blood cultures are typically negative • X-ray is usually normal. AP neck radiograph* may show "steeple sign" or irregularity of the proximal mucosa • Diagnosis is made endoscopically by visualizing normal supraglottic structures with prominent subglottic edema, ulcerations, and copious purulent secretions. • Culture secretions
Treatment	• Intubation is often required for 3–7 days. • Additional endoscopy may be needed to remove pseudomembrane • Vancomycin 10 mg/kg IV every 6 hours *plus* ceftriaxone 50 mg/kg/day IV qd

*Radiograph in bacterial tracheitis is very similar to that in viral croup, with the marked subglottic narrowing known as the "steeple sign."

BACTERIAL TRACHEITIS

Epidemiology

Bacterial tracheitis, also known as laryngotracheobronchitis, pseudomembranous croup, or bacterial croup, is an entity that was first described in 1979. Although it is an uncommon disease, it may be life-threatening. The peak incidence is in the fall and winter in children between 6 months and 8 years of age. Marked subglottic edema and thick mucopurulent (membranous) secretions characterize the illness. The organisms most commonly implicated include *Staphylococcus aureus* and, to a lesser extent, *Streptococcus viridans*, *Haemophilus influenzae*, *Moraxella catarrhalis*, and *Streptococcus pneumoniae*.

Clinical Features

The clinical presentation of bacterial tracheitis has features of both epiglottitis and viral croup. Typically, the child may have prodromal viral upper respiratory symptoms such as low-grade fever, cough, and stridor, similar to patients with croup. However, the patient then develops the rapid onset of high fever, respiratory distress, and a toxic appearance. Unlike patients with epiglottitis, these children typically do have a cough, are comfortable lying flat, and do not drool (Table 49.3).

Differential Diagnosis

Similar to croup, the differential diagnoses to consider include:

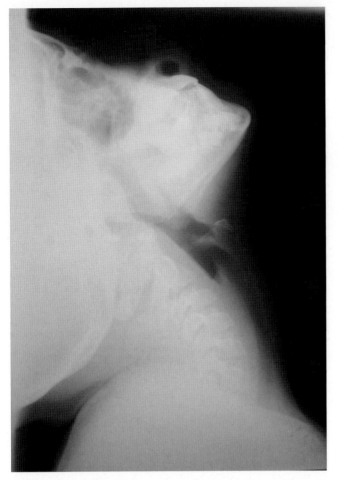

Figure 49.3 Bacterial Tracheitis. Courtsey of Dr. Lee Harvey.

- croup
- epiglottis
- foreign body aspiration
- retropharyngeal or peritonsillar abscess

Key features that distinguish bacterial tracheitis from epiglottitis and viral croup are:

- comfortable lying flat
- no drooling
- presence of cough

Laboratory and Radiographic Findings

Routine laboratory data are not indicated; however, a complete blood count may show marked leukocytosis. Blood cultures are typically negative. Radiographically, bacterial tracheitis is similar to croup in that the marked subglottic narrowing known as the "steeple sign" may be present on AP neck films. Occasionally, a slight irregularity of the proximal tracheal mucosa, representing pseudomembranous detachment, may also be seen (Figure 49.3). If found, these radiographic findings may aid in the diagnosis of bacterial tracheitis; however, their absence does not rule it out. Diagnosis is made endoscopically, by visualizing normal supraglottic structures with prominent subglottic edema, ulcerations, and copious purulent secretions. These secretions should be sent for Gram stain and culture.

Treatment and Prophylaxis

When possible, patients in severe respiratory distress should be managed in the operating suite for both the endoscopic diagnosis and intubation. Copious purulent secretions can be suctioned from the endotracheal tube and should be sent for culture. If endotracheal intubation is unsuccessful, a tracheostomy may be necessary. In the acute setting, needle cricothyrotomy is the appropriate emergency intervention if endotracheal intubation is unsuccessful. Occasionally, repeat endoscopy may be required to remove pseudomembranous material. Intubation is often required for 3–7 days, until the patient is afebrile, there is a decrease in the quantity and viscosity of secretions, and an air leak is present (i.e., there is passage of air around the endotracheal tube indicating decreased edema). Antibiotics should be initiated early with an initial regimen of vancomycin and a third-generation cephalosporin such as ceftriaxone.

Complications and Admission Criteria

Complications include airway obstruction, pneumothorax, formation of pseudomembranes, and toxic shock syndrome. These patients frequently have concurrent pneumonia. All patients with bacterial tracheitis should be admitted to the ICU for close monitoring.

Pearls and Pitfalls

1. Bacterial tracheitis should be considered in an ill-appearing child with high fever and with crouplike symptoms that are refractory to conventional treatment with racemic epinephrine and corticosteroids.
2. Intubate promptly.
3. An endotracheal tube size smaller than estimated for patient size should be used and suction should be readily available.

RETROPHARYNGEAL ABSCESS

Epidemiology

The retropharyngeal space is a potential area located between the anterior border of the cervical vertebrae and the posterior wall of the esophagus; the space contains connective tissues and lymph nodes that receive lymphatic drainage from adjacent structures. A retropharyngeal abscess (RPA) is a life-threatening deep infection of this area (see Chapter 10, Deep Neck Space Infections). Fifty percent of cases occur in patients between 6 months and 12 months of age and 96% of all cases occur in children less than 6 years of age, because the nodes of Ruvier that drain the retropharyngeal space typically atrophy after this age. There is also a male predominance, in some studies up to 3:1. The most common causative organisms are *Streptococcus pyogenes*, anaerobic organisms, and *Staphylococcus aureus*.

Clinical Features

The initial clinical picture of retropharyngeal abscess is similar to that of other illnesses such as croup, epiglottitis, tracheitis, and peritonsillar abscess. Patients frequently present with symptoms of an upper respiratory infection, fever, sore throat, neck stiffness, and poor oral intake (Table 49.4). As purulent

Table 49.4 Clinical Features: Retropharyngeal Abscess

Organisms	• *Streptococcus pyogenes* • Anaerobic organisms • *Staphylococcus aureus*
Signs and Symptoms	• Initially may have an upper respiratory infection, fever, sore throat • As mass enlarges, drooling, stridor, neck stiffness and poor intake
Laboratory and Radiographic Findings	• Routine laboratory test are not indicated • Radiograph* reveals widening of the retropharyngeal space
Treatment	• Supportive care, ABCs (airway, breathing, circulation) • Clindamycin 30 mg/kg/day IV in four divided doses *or* cefazolin 100 mg/kg/day IV in four divided doses

*Radiographs are helpful in ruling out croup, retropharyngeal abscess, and foreign bodies.

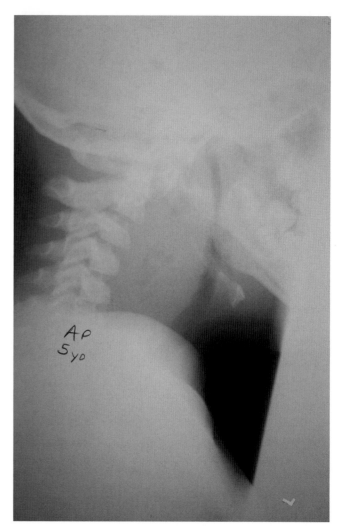

Figure 49.4 Retropharyngeal abscess. Courtesy of Children's Hospital, San Diego Department of Radiology.

material collects, a fluctuant mass may begin to cause airway compromise, and patients may develop drooling, stridor, and respiratory distress. Physical examination may reveal an oropharyngeal mass, though this is only present in half of all children with retropharyngeal abscess. Patients often present with a stiff neck and may be misdiagnosed with meningitis.

Differential Diagnosis

The differential diagnosis of retropharyngeal abscess includes:

- foreign body ingestion
- tonsillitis
- peritonsillar abscess
- meningitis
- nasopharyngeal mass

Key features that may help distinguish retropharyngeal abscess are:

- neck stiffness
- sore throat
- stridor

Laboratory and Radiographic Findings

Routine laboratory testing is not useful in the diagnosis of a retropharyngeal abscess. The lateral neck radiograph is very useful in the initial diagnosis of retropharyngeal abscesses. In children, the normal soft tissue should measure no more than 7 mm at the level of the second cervical vertebrae, less than 5 mm anterior to the third and fourth cervical vertebrae (or less than 40% of the AP diameter of the vertebral body), and 14 mm at the sixth cervical vertebrae on a film done with proper neck extension (Figure 49.4). Retropharyngeal thickening is seen on lateral neck radiograph in 88% to 100% of RPA cases. In clinically stable patients, a computed tomographic (CT) scan of the neck is helpful to delineate whether there is

a retropharyngeal cellulitis rather than a true abscess. Ultrasound may also be useful in this differentiation as well.

Treatment and Prophylaxis

Previously, the standard of care for management of RPA was surgical drainage. This has since become controversial in the setting of data showing that antibiotic therapy alone is successful in treating up to 37% of RPA diagnosed by CT scan. For patients with signs of airway obstruction, endotracheal intubation followed by surgical drainage is still the treatment of choice. When visualizing the airway for endotracheal intubation, care must be taken to avoid abscess rupture. Antibiotic therapy should be initiated in all patients; clindamycin is an appropriate first choice, and cefazolin, a suitable alternative.

Complications and Admission Criteria

Because retropharyngeal abscess is a life-threatening airway illness, all patients should be admitted and closely monitored. Complications include airway compromise, abscess rupture leading to asphyxiation or aspiration pneumonia, or spread of infection to adjacent structures in the neck including infection of carotid artery sheath, osteomyelitis of the cervical spine, or infection of the structures of the mediastinum.

Infection Control

Universal precautions should be maintained. No isolation is required.

Pearls and Pitfalls

1. Palpation of the abscess is not recommended because rupture may occur.
2. Retropharyngeal abscesses may mimic croup, epiglottitis, tracheitis, and peritonsillar abscess.
3. Peripheral white blood cell count is neither sensitive nor specific in the diagnosis of RPA.
4. Ensure correct positioning of the child for the lateral neck radiograph. Flexion or persistent crying can give the illusion of a large retropharyngeal space.

PERTUSSIS

Epidemiology

Pertussis, or whooping cough, is an acute infection of the respiratory tract caused by *Bordetella pertussis*. There are other organisms that may cause a similar clinical syndrome, such as *Bordetella parapertussis*, adenovirus, or *Chlamydia* species. Following the introduction of immunization in the mid-1940s, pertussis incidence declined more than 99% by 1970 and to an all-time low of 1010 cases by 1976. However, since then, an increase in disease incidence has been documented, with nearly 26,000 cases reported in 2004, 40% in children less than 11 years old.

Clinical Features

Pertussis can be divided into three phases; the first phase (catarrhal) usually is characterized by mild cough, conjunctivitis, and coryza and may last 1 to 2 weeks (Table 49.5). The second phase, the paroxysmal phase, is characterized by a worsening cough for 2 to 4 weeks. The classic description of the cough in this phase is after a spasmodic cough, the sudden inflow of air produces a "whoop." In infants, the cough is usually a staccato cough with no whoop, and they may present with apneic episodes. Post-tussive emesis is also very common. Fever is rare. Conjunctival hemorrhages and facial petechiae may be caused by harsh coughing. The third phase, the convalescent phase, is characterized by a chronic cough that may last several weeks.

Differential Diagnosis

The differential diagnosis for pertussis is extensive, including:

- asthma
- acute sinusitis with postnasal drip
- gastroesophageal reflux
- foreign body aspiration
- pneumonia
- bronchiolitis
- tuberculosis
- cystic fibrosis
- other viral illnesses (rhinovirus, adenovirus, RSV, etc.)

Table 49.5 Clinical Features: Pertussis

Organisms	• *Bordetella pertussis* • *Bordetella parapertussis*, adenovirus, or *Chlamydia* causes a similar clinical syndrome
Signs and Symptoms	• Catarrhal phase: cough, coryza, conjunctivitis • Paroxysmal phase: spasmodic cough, infants may have a staccato cough with apnea • Convalescent phase: chronic cough
Laboratory and Radiographic Findings	• Positive PCR of nasopharyngeal swabs • Chest radiograph may show a shaggy right heart border • Leukocytosis may be present on CBC
Treatment and Chemoprophylaxis	azithromycin,* 10 mg/kg day 1, then 5 mg/kg for 4 days *or* clarithromycin,[†] 15 mg/kg PO in two divided doses (max 1 g/day) for 7 days *or* erythromycin ethyl succinate,[‡] 40–50 mg/kg/day in four divided doses (max 2 g/day) for 14 days **Macrolide allergy:** trimethoprim-sulfamethoxazole,[§] 8 mg/kg/day PO in two divided doses for 14 days

*For infants less than 6 months of age, use 10 mg/kg qd for 5 days.
[†]Not recommended for use in infants less than 6 months of age.
[‡]Linked to infantile hypertrophic pyloric stenosis in infants less than 1 month of age.
[§]Contraindicated in infants less than 2 months of age.

Key clinical questions that help to distinguish pertussis include:

- Was the coughing spell prolonged?
- Did the infant have tachypnea?
- Was there a preceding viral illness?
- Is the patient vaccinated?

Laboratory and Radiographic Findings

Bordetella pertussis is a gram-negative, pleomorphic bacterium that can be cultured, though culture is gradually being replaced by polymerase chain reaction (PCR) testing of nasopharyngeal specimens. The chest radiograph in a patient with pertussis is of minimal benefit as it is usually normal, though it may infrequently show a shaggy right heart border. In one study, 75% of unvaccinated patients with pertussis have a lymphocytosis on complete blood count. The leukocytosis may reach 20,000 to 50,000/mm^3, however, this finding is not often seen in children less than 6 months of age. In infants, lymphocytic leukocytosis with pulmonary infiltrates is associated with poor prognosis.

Treatment and Prophylaxis

By the time the paroxysmal phase has begun, treatment has little effect on the clinical course of pertussis. However, treatment should be started in all patients presenting within 3–4 weeks of symptom onset to prevent disease spread. Treatment options are erythromycin, azithromycin, or clarithromycin. Trimethoprim-sulfamethoxazole (TMP-SMX) may be used for patients with an allergy to macrolides. Erythromycin use has been associated with a risk of pyloric stenosis when used in infants less than 1 month of age.

Chemoprophylaxis recommendations for adults are erythromycin 200–250 mg by mouth (PO) four times a day for 2 weeks, TMP-SMX double strength PO twice a day for 14 days, or azithromycin 500 mg PO once a day for 5 days.

Complications and Admission Criteria

Major complications of pertussis infection include pneumonia (20%), encephalopathy and seizures (1%), failure to thrive, and death (0.3%). Pneumonia accounts for 90% of deaths from pertussis. Secondary complications of severe coughing and increased intrathoracic pressure include intracranial hemorrhage, diaphragmatic rupture, pneumothorax, and rectal prolapse. Patients less than 6 months of age with severe symptoms of pertussis generally warrant hospital admission.

Infection Control

Patients with pertussis should be placed in respiratory isolation to prevent transmission. Prophylaxis is recommended for household contacts. Exposed children less than 7 years of age who are unimmunized or have received fewer than four doses of the pertussis vaccine should be evaluated for vaccine initiation or boosting.

Pearls and Pitfalls

1. Pertussis should be suspected in infants presenting with apnea or cyanosis after episodes of prolonged coughing
2. Always treat household contacts who have been exposed to pertussis.

BRONCHIOLITIS

Epidemiology

Bronchiolitis is an infection of the upper and lower respiratory tract causing marked inflammation and obstruction of the smaller airways. Although it may occur in all age groups, incidence decreases with age, as the larger airways of older children and adults better accommodate mucosal edema. Severe symptoms are usually seen in children under the age of 2 years. There are approximately 125,000 hospitalizations per year with 80% of admissions occurring in children less than 1 year of age. The most common cause of bronchiolitis is RSV, isolated in 75% of the children less than 2 years of age who are hospitalized for bronchiolitis. Other causes include parainfluenza virus types 1 and 3, influenza B, adenovirus type 1, 2 and 5, *Mycoplasma*, rhinovirus, enterovirus, and herpes simplex virus. In temperate climates, RSV epidemics begin in winter and last until late spring, whereas parainfluenza occurs in the fall.

Clinical Features

Patients with bronchiolitis initially develop mild rhinorrhea, cough, and low-grade fever over the course of 2–3 days (Table 49.6). The illness progresses to an increased cough,

Table 49.6 Clinical Features: Bronchiolitis

Organisms	• Most common cause is RSV • Parainfluenza virus types 1 and 3, influenza B, adenovirus type 1, 2 and 5, *Mycoplasma*, rhinovirus, enterovirus, herpes simplex virus
Signs and Symptoms	• Initially, mild rhinorrhea, cough, and low-grade fever • Progresses to increased cough • Develops post-tussive emesis, respiratory distress, poor feeding • Respiratory distress with tachypnea
Laboratory and Radiographic Findings	• If necessary, may do a rapid ELISA to test for RSV • Chest radiographs may help rule out complications (atelectasis, pneumonia, hyperinflation) • Consider UA and culture for RSV in infants <60 days old
Treatment	• Mostly supportive care with oxygen, hydration, and nasal suctioning • Consider beta-agonists, racemic epinephrine, and steroids in select patients
UA, urinalysis.	

which is often paroxysmal, post-tussive emesis, respiratory distress, poor feeding, and increased fussiness. Respiratory distress in these children manifests as tachypnea with respiratory rates as high as 80 to 100 breaths per minute, nasal flaring, intercostal and supraclavicular retractions, apnea, grunting, and cyanosis. Hypoxia may be due to ventilation-perfusion mismatch. Other associated findings are tachycardia and dehydration. The natural course of the illness is about 7–10 days but can last several weeks to a month, and reinfection is possible.

Differential Diagnosis

The differential diagnosis of tachypnea and wheezing with preceding upper respiratory symptoms in a child less than 1 year of age must include:

- pneumonia
- asthma
- congestive heart failure

Key features that distinguish bronchiolitis from other respiratory problems are:

- upper respiratory tract symptoms
- wheezing
- respiratory distress

Laboratory and Radiographic Findings

The diagnosis of bronchiolitis in the acute care setting is a clinical one, so routine testing for RSV is not necessary, because it does not change treatment in most cases. In infants or children at high risk for complications, the work-up may include a nasopharyngeal swab for a rapid ELISA to test for RSV. Although a routine chest radiograph is not necessary, it often

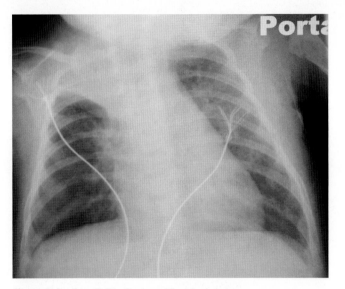

Figure 49.5 Bronchiolitis. Courtesy of Dr. John A. Amberg.

shows hyperinflation with flattening of the diaphragm and may be helpful in ruling out complications such as atelectasis, hyperinflation, or pneumonia (Figure 49.5).

Importantly, positive RSV testing in very young febrile infants does not mitigate the need for full evaluation of other causes of fever. It has been shown, for example, that the prevalence of urinary tract infection (UTI) in febrile RSV-positive patients less than 60 days of age is around 2–5%, and therefore urinalysis and/or culture is warranted in all such patients.

Treatment and Prophylaxis

The mainstay of treatment of bronchiolitis is supportive care including hydration, oxygenation, nasal suction, and even endotracheal intubation and ventilation for children with respiratory failure. Many therapies have been studied including epinephrine, beta2 agonist bronchodilators, corticosteroids, and ribavirin, but little evidence supports a routine role in management. However, in actual hospital practice, beta2-agonists are used in 53% to 73% of cases in various studies.

Deep airway suctioning is extremely helpful in infants who present with acute distress. Thick secretions compromise the infant's airway, and this simple therapy can provide immediate relief. Patients with respiratory distress are often quite dehydrated because of insensible losses, and therefore hydration status should be addressed.

Respiratory failure and apnea occur more frequently in children that have underlying conditions such as bronchopulmonary dysplasia, chronic lung disease, congenital heart disease, or immunodeficiencies. These are a subset of high-risk children that receive palivizumab (Synagis), a monoclonal antibody that has proven effective in preventing severe bronchiolitis. Palivizumab is given as a monthly IM injection through the RSV season. The American Academy of Pediatrics (AAP) has established guidelines for administration of palivizumab, but in general, it is given to children under the age of 24 months with comorbidities such as prematurity less than 28 weeks, congenital heart disease, severe immune deficiencies, severe neuromuscular disease, or congenital airway abnormalities.

Complications and Admission Criteria

Complications include apnea, respiratory failure, or pneumonia. Patients with persistent hypoxia, respiratory distress, or inability to tolerate fluids, and patients in whom close follow-up cannot be ensured should be admitted. Admission should also be strongly considered in patients less than 2 months of age and premature infants because of the risk of apnea.

Infection Control

Universal precautions should be maintained. No isolation is required.

Pearls and Pitfalls

1. Deep suctioning can help in the immediate management of infants with bronchiolitis.
2. Insensible losses contribute significantly to dehydration in infants and small children with respiratory distress.
3. Infants less than 2 months of age are at risk for apnea in the setting of bronchiolitis.

PNEUMONIA

Epidemiology

Community-acquired pneumonia in childhood is a serious infection, leading to significant mortality and morbidity in the United States. The annual incidence in Europe and North America is 34 to 40 cases per 1000 children under 5 years of age. Pneumonia is usually defined by fever, acute respiratory symptoms, or both, plus evidence of parenchymal infiltrates on chest radiograph. The most common causative organisms include respiratory viruses and bacteria such as *Mycoplasma, Chlamydia trachomatis, Streptococcus pneumoniae, Staphylococcus aureus,* and *Haemophilus influenzae,* including nontypable strains. The relative frequency of these organisms varies greatly with age and is different for infants, toddlers, and school-age children.

Clinical Features

The clinical features of pneumonia depend on the causative organism, the age of the patient, and the presence of immunosuppression or comorbid disease. Bacterial pneumonia generally has an abrupt onset with fever and chills, productive cough, and chest pain. Frequently, respiratory rate and work of breathing are increased, and have been studied as clinical predictors of pneumonia. Upper-lobe pneumonias may evoke suspicion for meningitis as pain may radiate to the neck (Figure 49.6). The presence of vague abdominal pain and fever should also raise the suspicion for pneumonia. Wheezing is typically associated with viral, *Mycoplasma,* or chlamydial pneumonias (Table 49.7).

Differential Diagnosis

Included in the differential are:

- airway foreign body
- aspiration syndromes
- bronchiectasis
- bronchitis

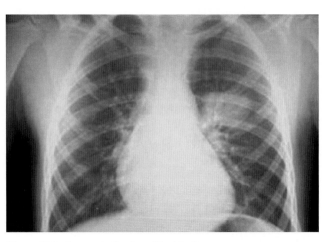

Figure 49.6 Pneumonia. Courtesy of Dr. John Kanegaye.

Table 49.7 Clinical Features: Pneumonias

Organisms	• Viruses (e.g., influenza, parainfluenza, RSV) • *Mycoplasma* • *Chlamydia trachomatis* • *Streptococcus pneumoniae* • *Staphylococcus aureus* • *Haemophilus influenzae*
Signs and Symptoms	• Fever, chills, productive cough, chest pain (especially bacterial pneumonia) • Tachypnea, increased work of breathing • Wheezing • Abdominal pain and fever • Radiating pain to neck (especially upper lobe pneumonias)
Laboratory and Radiographic Findings	• CBC may show leukocytosis • CXR infiltrates • Mycoplasma IGM

- reflux
- Goodpasture's syndrome
- hemosiderosis
- congestive heart failure
- pertussis
- pulmonary sequestration
- cystic fibrosis

Key features that may help to distinguish pneumonia are:

- fever
- cough
- tachypnea

Laboratory and Radiographic Findings

A peripheral complete blood count may show leukocytosis; however, a normal white blood cell count does not exclude the possibility of bacterial pneumonia. Decubitus chest radiographs are helpful in the evaluation of pleural effusions. Children who are dehydrated may not have an infiltrate on initial radiography, and repeat radiography after hydration may be necessary. Serologic tests (e.g., *Mycoplasma* IgM assay) may be helpful in children less than 3 years of age who present with pneumonias not responsive to amoxicillin.

Table 49.8 Pneumonia Treatment Based on Age and Type

	Organisms	Treatment	
Birth to 4 Weeks	• Group B *Streptococcus* • Gram-negative enteric bacteria • Cytomegalovirus • *Listeria monocytogenes*	Preferred	cefotaxime 50 mg/kg IV q8h *and* ampicillin 50 mg/kg IV q6h
		Outpatient	Requires inpatient therapy
4 to 8 Weeks	• *Chlamydia trachomatis* • RSV • Parainfluenza 3 • *Streptococcus pneumoniae* • *Bordetella pertussis* • *Staphylococcus aureus*	Preferred	ceftriaxone 50 mg/kg IV q4h
		Outpatient	High-dose amoxicillin 100 to 120 mg/kg PO in three divided doses
8 Weeks to 3 Years	• RSV • Parainfluenza viruses • Influenza virus • Adenovirus • Rhinovirus • *Streptococcus pneumoniae* • *Haemophilus influenza* (non-B type) • *Mycoplasma pneumoniae*	Preferred	ceftriaxone 50 mg/kg IV q24h
		Outpatient	High-dose amoxicillin 100 to 120 mg/kg PO in three divided doses *or* azithromycin 10 mg/kg 1st day then 5 mg/kg PO qd for 4 days* *or* Augmentin 40 mg/kg PO in three divided doses

*Erythromycin or clarithromycin are acceptable alternatives.

Treatment and Prophylaxis

Management is based on identification of the presumed causative agent (Table 49.8). For all pneumonia, supportive care should be initiated with hydration, oxygenation, and continuous cardiorespiratory monitoring for ill-appearing children. Children with large pleural effusions who are ill-appearing or immunocompromised should undergo thoracentesis and chest tube placement. For infants less than 2 months of age, blood, urine, and cerebrospinal fluid cultures should be obtained. Otherwise, blood cultures are rarely positive in pediatric pneumonia. Bronchodilators and steroids should be considered in patients with wheezing or a history of reactive airway disease. An arterial or venous blood gas should be obtained in ill-appearing children and infants in respiratory distress. Endotracheal intubation followed by mechanical ventilation should be initiated in children with respiratory failure.

Complications and Admission Criteria

Infants less than 3 months of age with peumonia should be admitted for intravenous antibiotics because of their high risk for associated sepsis and meningitis. Other criteria for admission include persistent hypoxia, inability to tolerate fluids, outpatient antibiotic failure, or any difficulty ensuring close follow-up. Complications include bacteremia, with associated meningitis, pericarditis, epiglottitis, or septic arthritis.

Infection Control

Universal precautions should be maintained. A patient should be placed in respiratory isolation in a negative-pressure room if tuberculosis is suspected.

Pearls and Pitfalls

1. Early pulse oximetry is crucial.
2. Chest radiograph may help rule out other causes of respiratory distress, such as foreign body ingestions, cardiac disease, and pneumothorax.
3. Maintain a high index of suspicion for pneumonia in a child with abdominal or neck pain.
4. Ensure adequate hydration because insensible losses are significant in infants and children with respiratory distress.
5. Ensure next-day follow up for patients who are discharged.

REFERENCES

Bachur R, Perry H, Harper MB. Occult pneumonias: empiric chest radiographs in febrile children with leukocytosis. Ann Emerg Med 1999;33(2):166–73.

Blackstock P, Adderhey RJ, Steward DJ. Epiglottitis in young infants. Anesthesiology 1987;67:97–100.

Bordley WC, Viswanathan M, King VJ, et al. Diagnosis and testing in bronchiolitis: a systematic review. Arch Pediatr Adolesc Med 2004;158(2):119–26.

Broughton RA. Nonsurgical management of deep neck infections in children. Pediatr Infect Dis J 1992;11(1):14–8.

Centers for Disease Control and Prevention (CDC). Pertussis. Epidemiology and prevention of vaccine-preventable diseases (The Pink Book) course textbook, 79–96.

Centers for Disease Control and Prevention (CDC). Progress toward eliminating *Haemophilus influenzae* type b disease among infants and children – United States, 1987–1997. MMRW 1998;47(46):993–8.

Cooper WO, Griffin MR, Arbogast P, et al. Very early exposure to erythromycin and infantile hypertrophic pyloric stenosis. Arch Pediatr Adolesc Med 2002 Jul;156(7):647–50.

Coulthard M, Isaacs D. Retropharyngeal abscess. Arch Dis Child 1991;66:1227–30.

Craig FW, Schunk JE. Retropharyngeal abscess in children: clinical presentation, utility of imaging, and current management. Pediatrics 2003;111:1394–8.

Cunningham MJ. The old and new of acute laryngotracheal infection. Clin Pediatr 1992;31(1):56–64.

Denny FW, Murphy TF, Clyde WA Jr, et al. Croup: an 11-year study in a pediatric practice. Pediatrics 1983;71(6):871–6.

Donaldson D, Poleski D, Knipple E, et al. Intramuscular versus oral dexamethasone for the treatment of moderate-to-severe croup: a randomized, double blind trial. Acad Emerg Med 2003;10(1):16–21.

Donaldson JD, Mathby CC. Bacterial tracheitis in children. J Otolaryngol 1989;18(3);48:101–4.

Duncan NO, Sprecher RC. Infections of the airway. In Cummings CW, ed, Otolaryngology – head and neck surgery, 3rd ed. St. Louis, MO: Mosby, 1998:388–400.

Geelhoed GC, Macdonald WB. Oral dexamethasone in the treatment of croup: 0.15 mg/kg versus 0.3 mg/kg versus 0.6 mg/kg. Pediatr Pulmonol 1995 Dec;20(6):362–8.

Geelhoed GC, Turner J, Macdonald WB. Efficacy of a small single dose of oral dexamethasone for outpatient croup: a double blind placebo controlled clinical trial. BMJ 1996;313(7050):140–2.

Greenberg DP, von Konig CH, Heininger U. Health burden of pertussis in infants and children. Pediatr Infect Dis J 2005;24(5Supp):S39–43.

Gupta VK, Cheifitz IM. Heliox administration in the pediatric intensive care unit: an evidence-based review. Pediatr Crit Care Med 2005;6(2):204–11.

Heininger U, Klich K, Stehr K, Cherry JD. Clinical findings in *Bordetella pertussis* infections: results of a prospective multicenter surveillance study. Pediatrics 1997;100(6):E10.

Johnson DW, Jacobson S, Edney PC, et al. A comparison of nebulized budesonide, intramuscular dexamethasone, and placebo for moderately severe croup. N Engl J Med 1998;339(8):498–503.

Jones R, Santos JI, Overall JC Jr. Bacterial tracheitis. JAMA 1979;242(8):721–6.

Kelley PB, Simon JE. Racemic epinephrine use in croup and disposition. Am J Emerg Med 1992;10(3):181–3.

King VJ, Viswanathan M, Bordley WC, et al. Pharmacologic treatment of bronchiolitis in infants and children: a systematic review. Arch Pediatr Adolesc Med 2004;158(2):127–37.

Klassen TP, Craig WR, Moher D, et al. Nebulized budesonide and oral dexamethasone for treatment of croup: a randomized control trial. JAMA 1998;279(20):1629–32.

Ledwith C, Shea L. The use of nebulized racemic epinephrine in the outpatient treatment of croup. Pediatr Emerg Care 1993;9:318.

Loos GD. Pharyngitis, croup and epiglottitis. Prim Care 1990;17(2):335–45.

Mansbach JM, Edmond JA, Camargo CA. Bronchiolitis in U.S. emergency departments 1992 to 2000: epidemiology and practice variation. Pediatr Emerg Care 2005;21:242–7.

Mauro RD, Poole SR, Lockhart CH. Differentiation of epiglottitis from laryngotracheitis in the child with stridor. Am J Dis Child 1988 Jun;142(6):679–82.

McIntosh K. Community-acquired pneumonia in children. N Engl J Med 2002;346(6):429–37.

Melendez E, Harper MB. Utility of sepsis evaluation in infants 90 days of age or younger with fever and clinical bronchiolitis. Pediatr Infect Dis J 2003;22(12):1053–6.

Morrison JE, Pashley NRT: Retropharyngeal abscesses in children: A 10-year review. Pediatr Emerg Care 1988;4:9–11.

Plint AC, Johnson DW, Wiebe N. Practice variation among pediatric emergency departments in the treatment of bronchiolitis. Acad Emerg Med 2004;11:353–60.

Rothrock SG, Green SM, Fanella JM, et al. Do published guidelines predict pneumonia in children presenting to an urban ED? Pediatr Emerg Care 2001;17(4):240–3.

Scolnik D, Coates AL. Controlled delivery of high vs. low humidity vs. mist therapy for croup in emergency departments: a randomized controlled trial. JAMA 2006 Mar 15;295(11):1274–80.

Shah SS, Alpern ER, Zwerling L, et al. Risk of bacteremia in young children with pneumonia treated as outpatients. Arch Pediatr Adolesc Med 2003 Apr;157(4):389–92.

Shroeder LL, Knapp JF. Recognition and Emergency management of infectious causes of upper airway obstruction. Semin Respir Infect 1995;10(1):21–30.

Skolnik NS. Treatment of croup: a critical review. Am J Dis Child 1989;143(9):1045–9.

Toikka P, Virkki R, Mertsola J, et al. Bacteremic pneumococcal pneumonia in children. Clin Infect Dis 1999;29:568–72.

Zorc JJ, Levine DA, Platt SL, et al. Multicenter RSV-SBI Study Group of the Pediatric Emergency Medicine Collaborative Research Committee of the American Academy of Pediatrics. Pediatrics 2005;116(3):644–8.

Special Populations

50. Bites

Sukhjit S. Takhar and Gregory J. Moran

Outline   Introduction
Epidemiology
Clinical Features
Microbiology
Initial Evaluation
Treatment of Noninfected Wounds
Treatment of Infected Wounds
Pearls and Pitfalls
References

INTRODUCTION

Animal and human bites are a common problem in the United States, and approximately half of all Americans will be bitten by an animal or another human during their lifetime. Caring for patients with animal or human bites focuses on treating the acute traumatic injuries and preventing the potential infectious complications.

EPIDEMIOLOGY

Dog bites account for 80–90% of all bites seen in emergency departments. Accurate statistics on dog bite injuries are difficult to obtain because the majority of victims do not seek medical attention. Dog bites account for 0.3–1.1% of all emergency visits. A Centers for Disease Control and Prevention (CDC) analysis of the National Electronic Injury Surveillance System (NEISS) estimates that in 2001 there were 368,245 people who were treated in U.S. emergency departments for dog-bite related injuries – a rate of 129.3 per 100,000. Of the victims, 42% were younger than 14 years, with the highest injury rate seen in boys between the ages of 5 and 9 years. There are approximately 20 deaths each year in the United States as a result of dog attacks.

Dog bites occur more often during the summer, on weekends, and in the afternoon. Most dog bites are committed by younger dogs and larger breeds such as Rottweilers, pit bulls, Huskies, and German shepherds. The victim often knows the animal and the majority of attacks are provoked.

Cat bites account for an estimated 5–15% of all bite injuries (up to 25% in some studies). In contrast to dog bite victims, cat bite victims tend to be women over the age of 20. It is estimated that approximately 400,000 people are bitten by cats each year.

Human bites are the third most frequent form of bite injuries seen by physicians, accounting for 2–3% of all bite wounds. Human bite wounds can occur in a variety of ways and in all age groups. They are especially common in young children and are a leading cause of injuries at day care. Most serious bite wounds are the result of aggressive behavior. The "fight-bite" clenched-fist injury occurs over the metacarpophalangeal joint when the patient punches another person in the mouth (see Chapter 22, Hand Infections: Fight Bite, Purulent Tenosynovitis, Felon, and Paronychia). Bites can also occur during sexual and sporting activities or can be self-inflicted in the psychiatric population. Human bite wounds are frequently associated with severe infections and serious complications, which may be partly due to selection bias in patients who delay seeking medical attention.

CLINICAL FEATURES

The majority of dog bites do not require medical attention. However, some dogs have powerful jaws and can inflict serious or even fatal injuries. Dog bites can produce a variety of tissue injury patterns such as avulsions, lacerations, and crush injuries. A dog's bite can penetrate body cavities, puncture the skull, and break bones. The most likely type of injury varies by age. Children younger than 4 years are more susceptible to bites to the head and neck. In contrast, more than 80% of injuries in patients over the age of 15 are to the extremities. Approximately 5–15% of dog bites become infected. The infection rate for hand bites is higher.

Cats have slender, sharper teeth that usually cause puncture wounds. Most cat bites are to the dominant hand of the victim, and up to 80% of cat bites become infected. Wounds that may appear minor can extend into deeper structures such as tendons, joints, vessels, and bones.

Human bites can be punctures, lacerations, or avulsions. Bites often involve the hands and arms in men and the breasts and genitals of females. Bite wounds in most locations have only a slightly higher rate of infection than traumatic lacerations in the same areas. In contrast, bites to the hand have a much higher infection rate than other hand injuries. The clenched-fist injury is the most serious and infection prone. This mechanism can involve considerable force and may cause injury to deeper structures, including fractures, joint penetration, and tendon damage. Infections related to clenched-fist injuries can range from a simple cellulitis to severe deep-space infection of the hand that requires amputation. Patients presenting with a fight bite often present with an established infection rather than immediately after the injury.

Bites from children appear as semicircular erythematous or bruised areas, often over the face, upper extremities, or trunk. The intercanine distance for a child bite is less than 2.5 cm. If it is more than 3 cm, then the bite is likely from an adult and child abuse should be considered.

Patients presenting soon after an injury are usually concerned about wound repair or the need for rabies prophylaxis.

In contrast, patients presenting later are more likely to have an established infection. They will often have signs of localized cellulitis, pain, edema, and purulent discharge. Infections related to animal and human bites often develop rapidly, within 12–24 hours of the injury, and puncture wounds are more prone to infection than others. Fortunately, it is uncommon for facial wounds to get infected.

Patients with pain out of proportion to the exam findings may have a deeper, more serious infection such as septic arthritis, osteomyelitis, or necrotizing fasciitis (see Chapter 21, Adult Septic Arthritis; Chapter 23, Osteomyelitis; and Chapter 43, Bacterial Skin and Soft-Tissue Infections). Immunocompromised patients can present with fulminant sepsis after a bite wound.

MICROBIOLOGY

Much has been learned about the microbiology of infected dog, cat, and human bites (Tables 50.1 and 50.2). Unlike typical cellulitis in which the organism is usually group A *Streptococcus* or *Staphylococcus aureus*, bite wounds tend to have a more complex microbiology derived from the oral flora of the biting animal. These infections tend to be polymicrobial with various streptococci, *Staphylococcus* spp., gram-negative species, and oral anaerobes. The average infection yields five species of bacteria. Abscesses tend to have more organisms isolated than purulent wounds.

Pasteurella species are the most common pathogens in dog and cat bites. They are found in approximately 75% of cat bites and 50% of dog bites. *Pasteurella* species are found in the oral cavity and gastrointestinal tract of many animals and cause a rapid-onset infection. The most common infections due to *Pasteurella* are soft-tissue infections, but endocarditis, meningitis, septicemia, and pneumonia have been reported.

Streptococci and staphylococci were found in approximately 40% of bite infections from both dogs and cats. Anaerobic bacteria such as *Bacteroides* spp., *Fusobacterium* spp., *Prevotella* spp., and *Peptostreptococcus* spp. are often present in mixed infections and foul-smelling wounds. *Capnocytophaga canimorsus* has been associated with severe infections, especially in patients with comorbid conditions such as asplenia, and those on corticosteroids or with liver disease. *Capnocytophaga* sp. is involved in approximately 5% of dog and cat bite infections.

Infected human bite wounds tend to be polymicrobial. In the largest case series, an average of four organisms were found in infected human bite wounds. The most common organism found was *Streptococcus anginosus*. This organism is a *viridans*-like organism with a tendency to form abscesses. *Staphylococcus aureus* was the next most common organism. Anaerobic bacteria are present in about 50% of human bites, and the anaerobic organisms in human bites have a higher tendency to produce beta-lactamase. A major difference in the microbiology of human bite wounds and those of dogs and cats is the presence of *Eikenella corrodens* and the absence of *Pasteurella multocida*. *Eikenella* is a slow-growing gram-negative rod that is often found in combination with other isolates. Much like *Pasteurella*, *Eikenella* is often sensitive to penicillin and second- or third-generation cephalosporins while being resistant to first-generation cephalosporins, clindamycin, and oxacillin. Transmission of herpes simplex, hepatitis B and C, and human immunodeficiency virus (HIV) has been reported from human bites. The rare reports in the medical literature in which HIV appeared to have been transmitted by a bite were associated with significant injury and the presence of blood. The risk is probably less than that of a contaminated needle-stick injury.

Our knowledge of the organisms involved in exotic animal bites is based on case reports and anecdotal data. Many of these reports suggest that other animals have oral flora that includes staphylococci, streptococci, and anaerobes, similar to domestic animals. Rodents can transmit a variety of diseases including rat-bite fever. This rare infection, manifested by fever and a rash, is caused by either *Streptobacillus moniliformis* or *Spirillum minus*. Bites from adult macaque monkeys have been known to transmit the potentially lethal virus herpesvirus simiae ("B virus").

INITIAL EVALUATION

The physician must deal with life- and limb-threatening injuries accordingly. In the majority of cases, serious injuries can quickly be ruled out. A careful history of the circumstances of the bite should be taken (Table 50.3). This includes the ownership of the animal and what led to the bite. History should also include the patient's comorbid conditions and vaccination status. A careful physical exam must be performed and documented. Joints should be examined through a full range of motion. The wound should be visualized under proper lighting to assess for teeth fragments, underlying

Table 50.1 Dog and Cat Bites: Selected Microbiology

Pasteurella **species**:
- Gram-negative coccobacillus
- Most common cause of dog and cat bite infections
- Can be difficult to culture
- Rapid development of an intense inflammatory response
- Resistant to many antibiotics that are commonly used to treat cellulitis

Streptococcus **species**:
- Usually of the *viridans* group
- Normal oral flora of animal

Capnocytophaga canimorsus:
- Fastidious gram-negative rod
- Can cause fatal infections in immunocompromised hosts (asplenia, chronic steroids or liver disease) characterized by shock, purpuric lesions, DIC, and gangrene at the bite site
- Often found in the normal flora of canines and occasionally in other animals

Anaerobes:
- *Fusobacterium, Bacteroides, Porphyromonas, Prevotella, Propionibacterium, Peptostreptococcus* are commonly isolated from bite wounds
- Found in approximately 50% of bite wounds from dogs and 65% of wounds from cats
- Usually part of mixed infections with aerobic organisms
- Variably produce penicillinase
- Foul-smelling wounds

DIC, disseminated intravascular coagulation.

Table 50.2 Rare Systemic Infections in Human Bites

HIV
Hepatitis B and C
Syphilis
Tetanus
Herpes simplex virus

Table 50.3 Initial Evaluation of Bites

History:
- Type of animal and behavior and vaccination history of animal
- Circumstances leading to the injury
- Time elapsed since the bite
- Existence of antimicrobial allergies
- Tetanus immunization status
- Associated medical conditions (liver disease, splenectomy, immunosuppressive medications, HIV, lymphedema, diabetes)

Physical examination:
- Temperature
- Skin exam for edema, tenderness, erythema, and lymphangitis
- Record a diagram of the wound noting depth and location
- Careful vascular and neurologic exam
- Range of motion of joint and musculoskeletal exam for tendon, muscle, bone, or intra-articular injury

Studies:
- Anaerobic and aerobic culture of wound if infected
- Radiographs of site if suspected fracture or joint involvement, or to rule out foreign body

Table 50.4 Management of Early Noninfected Bites

Wound care:
- Irrigation of wound with large amounts of normal saline
- Careful debridement of devitalized tissue
- Attention to deeper structures and consultation with a specialist if needed
- Wound cultures are not indicated in uninfected wounds

Antibiotic prophylaxis – consider for:
- Hand bites
- Immunocompromised patients
- Proximity to joint, tendon, or other deep structures
- Wounds with devitalized tissue
- Wounds closed primarily, or prior to delayed primary closure
- Cat bites
- Human bites

Wound closure:
- Consider risk/benefit balance for the individual wound
- Selected facial wounds and those of cosmetic importance could be primarily closed

Systemic diseases:
- Tetanus immunization if necessary
- Rabies prophylaxis if necessary
- Consider possible hepatitis or HIV exposure for human bites

Discharge instructions:
- Stress importance of elevating wound
- Return early if any signs of infection
- Return in 3–4 days for consideration of delayed primary closure

fractures, lacerated tendons, vessels, or nerves. Wounds on the hands or feet may require a tourniquet to adequately visualize the important structures. It is particularly important to realize that teeth can penetrate bones and joints, leading to osteomyelitis and septic arthritis. A search for signs of infection such as edema, fever, erythema, pain, and purulent discharge is vital.

Plain radiographs may be used to identify fractures and foreign bodies. Head injuries in children will often need a computed tomographic (CT) scan to further characterize injuries. Vascular injuries will need appropriate work-up (e.g., Doppler ultrasound or angiography) and urgent consultation with a qualified surgeon.

Infected purulent wounds should be cultured (anaerobic and aerobic). Gram stain of infected wounds is not generally useful because the infections are often polymicrobial. Culturing fresh wounds or noninfected wounds is of little benefit. Blood cultures should be obtained in patients who display systemic symptoms such as fever or rigors.

TREATMENT OF NONINFECTED WOUNDS

The location and type of wound, the species of the biting animal, and the medical condition of the patient are factors associated with the probability of developing an infection. Bite wounds tend to have multiple bacteria in high numbers. The bacterial count usually increases dramatically several hours after the injury. Infections are more common in the very young, the elderly, and the immunocompromised.

The wound should be irrigated with a large amount of saline at high pressure; this is the most important factor in decreasing the bacterial load.

This can be accomplished by using a 12-mL or larger syringe attached to an 18-gauge catheter. All visible foreign material should be removed. Approximately 150–300 mL or 50–100 mL/cm has been suggested. Devitalized tissue should be debrided.

The decisions about primary wound closure and "prophylactic" antibiotics are the two most problematic and controversial issues in dealing with bite wounds (Table 50.4). Multiple small studies have evaluated the utility of primary closure in bite wounds, but unfortunately, there are no reliable prospec-

tive data to support standardized guidelines on primary closure. These studies do support the practice of primary closure in selected wounds after careful wound preparation. Facial wounds have a lower overall risk of infection than other locations, and cosmetic result is more critical. Primary closure is not appropriate for most puncture wounds or for other high-risk wounds, such as those involving the hand, and should be considered only in special circumstances.

The decision about primary closure of bite wounds should be based on a risk-benefit analysis of the characteristics of the individual wound. Potential advantages of primary closure include a better cosmetic result, less need for repeat visits, and better protection of underlying structures. Wounds that heal by secondary intention tend to undergo more scarring and contraction than those that are approximated with sutures. In addition, for some areas such as the scalp or pretibial area, the surrounding skin is sometimes unable to completely close the defect. Exposed tendons, vessels, and bone can desiccate in an open wound. The main disadvantage is that primary closure of contaminated wounds can increase the risk of infection. Because of the recognized risk of complications related to bite wounds, it is prudent to document a discussion with the patient about the potential risks and benefits of wound closure.

After careful inspection and cleansing, "clean" wounds can be closed. Another option is delayed primary closure, in which the wound is cleansed and debrided, left open, and then reevaluated 3–4 days later for suturing. Closure at that time is possible if the wound remains clean and uninfected. Wound edges may sometimes need to be sharply debrided. Delayed primary closure may give a better cosmetic result than closure by secondary intention.

The role of antibiotic prophylaxis is still controversial. In general, prophylactic antibiotics would be appropriate for patients who suffer higher risk wounds such as deep punctures, those that are primarily closed, and hand injuries (Table 50.5). Cat and human bites tend to be associated with more infections. The treatment for lower

Table 50.5 Conditions Predisposing for a Wound Infection

Host factors:
- Age <2 and >50
- Comorbid medical conditions

Location:
- Wrist, hand, and foot wounds
- Scalp wounds in infants and small children (risk of skull injury)
- Adjacent to tendon, joint, bone, or other deep structures

Wound type:
- Crush injuries
- Puncture wounds

Biting animal:
- Human bite
- Cat bite

---

risk wounds remains controversial. When antibiotic prophylaxis is used, the regimen should be active against *P. multocida* (*Eikenella* in human bites), staphylococci, streptococci, and anaerobes (Table 50.6). Oral amoxicillin-clavulanic acid is commonly used. Alternative agents for penicillin-allergic patients should also be active against these same organisms. First-generation cephalosporins, antistaphylococcal penicillins, and clindamycin show poor in vitro activity against *Pasteurella* and *Eikenella* and have led to clinical failures in bite wounds; they should be avoided as single agents.

Table 50.6 Antimicrobial Treatment and Prophylaxis for Dog, Cat, or Human Bites

Prophylaxis or treatment of mild infection: Adult or child with No PCN allergy	amoxicillin-clavulanate 875 mg PO bid (20 mg/kg PO bid)
Prophylaxis or treatment of mild infection: Adult with PCN allergy	moxifloxacin 400 mg PO daily *or* ciprofloxacin 500 mg PO bid *plus* clindamycin 450 mg PO qid
Prophylaxis or treatment of mild infection: Child with PCN allergy	clindamycin (10 mg/kg) PO qid *plus* trimethoprim-sulfamethoxazole (5 mg/kg of TMP PO q12h)
Treatment: Adult or child with No PCN allergy	ampicillin-sulbactam 3 g (50 mg/kg) IV q6h *or* ertapenem 1 g q24h
Treatment: Adult with PCN allergy	clindamycin 600 mg IV q8h *plus* ciprofloxacin 400 mg IV q12h *or* ceftriaxone 1 g q24h (if non-life-threatening PCN allergy) *plus* metronidazole 500 mg PO/IV q6h
Treatment: Child with PCN allergy	clindamycin (15 mg/kg IV q8h) *plus* trimethoprim-sulfamethoxazole (5 mg/kg of TMP q12h IV)
Treatment: Pregnant with PCN allergy	azithromycin 500 mg IV daily *plus* clindamycin 600 mg IV q8h

PCN, penicillin; TMP, trimethoprim.

For patients with a penicillin allergy, moxifloxacin has activity against the likely organisms, or combination therapy with ciprofloxacin and clindamycin could be used. A long course of antibiotics is not necessary for prophylaxis; 3 to 5 days is usually adequate. If an infection has not developed in that time frame, then it becomes unlikely.

Antimicrobial treatment for bites by other mammals is similar, providing activity against anaerobes, streptococci, staphylococci, and gram-negative organisms (e.g., amoxicillin-clavulanate). Penicillin remains the drug of choice for treatment of rat bite fever, but giving routine prophylaxis is probably not necessary, as rat bites have a low risk of infection. The best way to prevent herpesvirus simiae is by aggressive local wound lavage. In at-risk patients (such as those who were bitten by a sick monkey), acyclovir should be given.

Animal bites should be considered tetanus-prone wounds. Patients who have not received their booster in the past 5 years should be reimmunized. Those who have never completed a primary tetanus series of three doses should be given immune globulin (see Chapter 63, Tetanus). The possibility of rabies exposure should also be considered. The epidemiology of animal rabies varies by geographic area. In many areas, some types of animal bites are reportable to the local health department, which can usually assist with decisions regarding rabies prophylaxis (see Chapter 60, Rabies). For a possible hepatitis B exposure related to a human bite, hepatitis B immunoglobulin and immunization may be appropriate. Postexposure prophylaxis for HIV may be indicated if the assailant is known to be positive or there is a high likelihood. A baseline HIV test should be drawn and then repeated in 3–6 months.

Patients with bite wounds should be carefully instructed on return precautions and on the importance of elevating the affected extremity.

TREATMENT OF INFECTED WOUNDS

Many patients with bite wounds present with an established infection. It is important to differentiate the normal inflammatory response of wound healing from an overt infection. Any abscess or fluctuance must be drained. A surgeon may be needed for drainage of a large abscess or those in proximity to deeper structures. The infected fluid or tissue should be cultured to direct future antibiotic therapy. Sutures in closed wounds that have become infected should be removed. Radiographs may be useful to evaluate for foreign body or for osteomyelitis.

Again, antimicrobial agents should be directed at *Pasteurella* spp., streptococci, staphylococci, and anaerobic organisms (Table 50.6). If a patient was taking prophylactic antibiotics, switching to a broader spectrum agent in another antimicrobial class should be considered. Unless the infection is minor, the first dose should be admitted intravenously. Intravenous (IV) ampicillin-sulbactam 3 g- is an appropriate choice. It is unclear whether methicillin-resistant *Staphylococcus aureus* (MRSA) will become a likely causative agent in bite infections. If the incidence of MRSA is high in the community, it is reasonable to add vancomycin or another drug with MRSA activity (e.g., linezolid or daptomycin) for initial empiric treatment for life- or limb-threatening infections. A treatment course of 7–14 days is appropriate for most bite-related infections. Deeper infections may require longer treatment; osteomyelitis will likely need 4 to 6 weeks or more of intravenous therapy.

PEARLS AND PITFALLS

1. Prophylactic antibiotics are appropriate for high-risk bites.
2. Stress the importance of elevating the wound and of follow-up care.
3. Good documentation is important, as these high-risk cases may be associated with bad outcomes resulting in legal action.
4. Do not miss joint penetration or tendon or bone damage in clenched-fist injury.

REFERENCES

Abrahamian FM. Dog bites: bacteriology, management, and prevention. Curr Infect Dis Rep 2000;2;446–52.

Bartholomew CF, Jones AM. Human bites: a rare risk factor for HIV transmission. AIDS 2006;20:631–2.

Centers for Disease Control and Prevention (CDC). Nonfatal dog bite–related injuries treated in hospital emergency departments – United States, 2001. MMWR 2003;52;605–10.

Chen E, Horing S, Shepherd SM, et al. Primary closure of mammalian bites. Acad Emerg Med 2000;7:157–61.

Cummings P. Antibiotics to prevent infection in patients with dog bite wounds: a meta-analysis of randomized trials. Ann Emerg Med 1994;23:535–40.

Goldstein EJC. Bite wounds and infections. Clin Infect Dis 1992; 14:633–40.

Goldstein EJC, Citron DM, Finegold SM. Dog bite wounds and infection: a prospective clinical study. Ann Emerg Med 1980;9:508–12.

Griego RD, Rosen T, Orengo IF. Dog, cat, and human bites: a review. J Am Acad Dermatol 1995;33(6):1019–29.

Steele MT, Ma OJ, Nakase J, et al. Epidemiology of animal exposures presenting to emergency departments. Acad Emerg Med 2007;14: 398–403.

Talan DA, Abrahamian FM, Moran GJ, et al. Clinical presentations and bacteriological analysis of infected human bites presenting to Emergency Departments. Clin Infect Dis 2003;37:1481–9.

Talan DA, Citron DM, Abrahamian FM, et al. Bacteriologic analysis of infected dog and cat bites. N Engl J Med 1999;340:85–92.

Weiss HB, Freidman DJ, Cohen JH. Incidence of dog bite injuries treated in emergency departments. JAMA 1998;279:51–3.

51. Infections in Oncology Patients

Erik R. Dubberke

Outline   Introduction
Epidemiology
Clinical Features
Differential Diagnosis
Laboratory and Radiographic Findings
Treatment and Prophylaxis
Pearls and Pitfalls
References

INTRODUCTION

Multiple risk factors contribute to making infection a leading cause of morbidity and mortality in oncology patients: both neoplastic disease and treatment regimens may cause disruption of mucocutaneous barriers, altered immunity, and/or viscus obstruction. The approach to a febrile oncology patient must take into consideration the nature and stage of the underlying disease, past and present treatments, any recent instrumentation or hospitalization, and any recent antibiotic exposures.

EPIDEMIOLOGY

Solid malignancies can increase the risk of infection by various means. Obstruction of natural passages leads to inadequate drainage of body fluids, stasis, and increased risk of bacterial colonization and infection. In this setting, infections are typically due to organisms that are a part of the normal flora (e.g., upper respiratory tract flora causing postobstructive pneumonia, gastrointestinal flora causing postobstructive cholangitis). Solid malignancies can invade across tissue planes, leading to conduits between normally sterile areas and the external environment (e.g., rectovesicular fistulas). Central nervous system malignancies can lead to aspiration and subsequent respiratory tract infection by compromising the cough and/or swallow reflex. In addition to these secondary effects, necrotic tissue within a solid tumor itself can also be a nidus for infection.

Although hematologic malignancies (lymphomas, leukemias, and plasma cell dyscrasias) are rarely associated with obstruction or with the invasion of tissue planes, they are often associated with innate, cellular and/or humoral immune system dysfunction. Lymphomas and T-cell leukemias are associated with T-cell dysfunction that can persist even after complete remission. Diminished T-cell function predisposes to a wide variety of atypical bacteria infections (mycobacterial, *Listeria*, *Nocardia*), viral infections (varicella-zoster virus [VZV], cytomegalovirus [CMV], Epstein-Barr virus [EBV], respiratory syncytial virus [RSV], adenovirus), fungal infections (*Cryptococcus*, *Histoplasma*, *Coccidioides*, *Blastomyces*, *Pneumocystis*), and parasitic infections (*Toxoplasma*, *Giardia*, *Cryptosporidium*, *Strongyloides*). Plasma cell dyscrasias and B-cell leukemias are associated with impaired antibody production, which can lead to sinopulmonary infections due to decreased IgA-mediated mucosal immunity and to increased susceptibility to encapsulated organisms (*Streptococcus pneumoniae*, *Haemophilus influenzae*, *Pseudomonas aeruginosa*, *Cryptococcus*). Anatomic or functional splenectomy, common in hematologic malignancy, increases susceptibility to encapsulated organisms, as well as to the *Capnocytophaga* species, babesiosis, and malaria.

Beyond the direct effects of a neoplastic process, chemotherapeutic agents used in the treatment of both hematologic and solid malignancies may lead to neutropenia. Overall, oncology patients are most likely to develop infections when they are neutropenic. The risk of developing an infection is related to both the severity and the duration of neutropenia. Up to 80% of patients who are neutropenic for at least 1 week develop a fever, and up to 60% of these patients will have a clinically or microbiologically documented infection. Because chemotherapy for hematologic malignancies is typically associated with more profound neutropenia and more severe mucositis than chemotherapy for solid malignancies, patients being treated for hematologic malignancies are more likely to develop an infection while neutropenic. Approximately 40% of febrile neutropenic patients with solid malignancies will have a documented source of infection and about 30% of these patients will have bacteremia. In contrast, up to 60% of febrile neutropenic patients with hematologic malignancies will have a documented source of infection, and half of these will be bacteremic. Whereas gram-negative infections during the neutropenic period predominated two decades ago, gram-positive bacteria now account for approximately 60% of microbiologically documented infections. This shift is likely related to increased utilization of central venous catheters and prophylactic antibiotics. Although gram-positive infections predominate, coverage for gram-negative bacteria, and in particular *Pseudomonas aeruginosa*, is still essential in the febrile neutropenic patient. Patients with prolonged neutropenia are also at risk for infections due to environmental molds, such as *Aspergillus*.

Several chemotherapeutic agents can also impair the cellular and humoral immune systems and predispose to opportunistic infections. Corticosteroids inhibit T-cell activation and immunoglobulin production. Purine analogues, such as fludarabine and cladribine, are directly lymphotoxic, particularly to CD4 T-cells. Methotrexate, an inhibitor of dihydrofolate reductase, is highly immunosuppressive to T-cells as well. The immunosuppression due to these medications can last for months after completion of therapy. Alemtuzumab is a monoclonal antibody directed against CD52, a protein expressed on the surface of lymphocytes, natural killer cells, and monocytes. CD4 T-cell counts can remain suppressed for over 12 months after administration of alemtuzumab. Rituximab is another monoclonal antibody, directed against CD20, a protein expressed on B-cells.

Recent exposure to health care settings and prophylactic antibiotics increase the risk of developing infections due to antibiotic-resistant organisms. Knowledge of common resistance patterns in your health care setting and community are important when selecting empiric therapy for oncology patients with infections.

CLINICAL FEATURES

Because of the blunted inflammatory response due to their immunocompromised state, oncology patients may not present with typical features of infection. Infection should be suspected in any oncology patient presenting with the systemic inflammatory response syndrome or onset of new end-organ dysfunction without an obvious cause. On exam, special attention should be given to areas where bacteria are commonly able to evade compromised mucocutaneous defenses: central venous catheter sites, areas of recent invasive procedures, oropharynx and periodontium, lung, perineum, and perianal areas. Whenever possible, clinical specimens should be obtained to microbiologically confirm the diagnosis and direct therapy.

Clinical Features of Bacteremia and Fungemia

A sudden onset of fever, often with tachycardia and chills, is associated with a high rate of positive blood cultures (Table 51.1). Although patients with solid malignancies are likely to have a documented site of infection at the time of bacteremia, 50% of infected patients with hematologic malignancies will have a primary bacteremia. It is thought that the vast majority of early-onset (within 7 days after the onset of neutropenia) febrile episodes in neutropenic patients are due to translocation of intestinal flora across the gut mucosa; however, the presence of central venous catheters is associ-

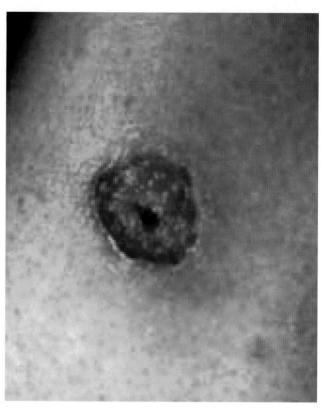

Figure 51.1 Ecthyma gangrenosum in a neutropenic patient with *Pseudomonas aeruginosa* bacteremia. Image courtesy of Dr. Nigar Kirmani.

ated with a higher risk of gram-positive bacteremia. Hypotension is most frequently seen with gram-negative and *Staphylococcus aureus* bacteremia. Patients with severe mucositis are at increased risk for bacteremia from oral flora. A syndrome of high spiking fevers ($\geq 40°$C), refractory hypotension, and adult respiratory distress syndrome has been associated with *Streptococcus mitis* bacteremia. Ecthyma gangrenosum is classically associated with *Pseudomonas aeruginosa* bacteremia (Figure 51.1); however, it has also been described with bacteremia due to *Aeromonas* and mold infections of the skin.

Approximately 10% of bloodstream infections in oncology patients are due to *Candida* species. The syndrome is clinically indistinguishable from bacterial bloodstream infections; however, onset is typically later than bacterial bloodstream infections in patients on broad-spectrum antibiotics. About 10% of patients with candidal fungemia will develop pinkish subcutaneous nodules. Patients with a history of candidal fungemia are at risk for developing hepatosplenic candidiasis, which becomes clinically evident when their neutropenia resolves.

Clinical Features of Oropharyngeal Infections

Infections of the oropharynx occur in 15–25% of neutropenic oncology patients with a documented source of infection. Loss of oral mucosal integrity due to chemotherapy provides a portal of entry for oral flora (Table 51.2). Bacterial infections tend to be polymicrobial and can present as gingivostomatitis, pharyngitis, Ludwig's angina, or retropharyngeal abscesses. In addition, oral mucositis predisposes to reactivation of latent herpes simplex virus (HSV) and candidal infections. Reactivated HSV can be severe and can arise in patients without a known history of oral herpes. Thrush is the most common

Table 51.1 Clinical Features: Bacteremia and Fungemia

Signs and Symptoms	• May present with sudden onset of fever or evidence of end-organ dysfunction (e.g., mental status changes) • Tachycardia and chills • Hypotension frequently seen with gram-negative and *Staphylococcus aureus* bacteremia • Syndrome of high fevers ($\geq 40°$C), refractory hypotension, and ARDS has been associated with *Streptococcus mitis* bacteremia • Ecthyma gangrenosum is classically associated with *Pseudomonas aeruginosa* bacteremia • 10% of patients with candidal fungemia will develop pinkish subcutaneous nodules
Laboratory Findings	• 10% of bloodstream infections in oncology patients are due to *Candida* species • Local patterns of bloodstream infection isolates are important when choosing empiric therapy
Treatment	• Start empiric treatment for neutropenic fever (see sections on treatment and prophylaxis of low- and high-risk patients)

ARDS, acute respiratory distress syndrome.

Table 51.2 Clinical Features: Oropharyngeal Infection

Signs and Symptoms	• Usually polymicrobial due to loss of oral mucosal integrity • May present as gingivostomatitis, pharyngitis, Ludwig's angina, or retropharyngeal abscesses • Oral mucositis predisposes to reactivation of latent HSV and candidal infections • Thrush is the most common candidal infection of the oropharynx, but invasive disease can occur
Laboratory Findings	• CT scan of head and neck can be used to identify patients who require surgical intervention
Treatment	• If neutropenic, start empiric treatment for neutropenic fever (refer to text) • If ceftazidime or cefepime chosen for initial coverage, add metronidazole 500 mg IV q8h for additional anaerobic coverage • If oral ulcerations are present, add acyclovir 5 mg/kg IV q8h • If thrush is present, add an echinocandin or an amphotericin product

CT, computed tomography.

candidal infection of the oropharynx, and invasive disease can occur.

Clinical Features of Skin and Soft-Tissue Infections

Infections of the skin and soft tissues account for 10–20% of neutropenic oncology patients with a documented source of infection. Areas of the skin that have been disrupted (e.g., post–venous puncture) and areas that tend to be moist with high bacterial counts (e.g., axilla, perianal area) are predisposed to infection (Table 51.3). Patients initially complain of tenderness with minimal erythema. If left untreated, these infections can rapidly progress and lead to abscess formation, necrosis, and gangrene. The causative organisms are typically local skin flora. *Cryptococcus* can cause a cellulitis in patients on corticosteroids or with impaired T-cell function. As mentioned above, skin lesions may also be the manifestation of a disseminated infection, such as ecthyma gangrenosum in *Pseudomonas* bacteremia or as skin nodules from disseminated candidiasis or fusariosis.

Table 51.3 Clinical Features: Skin and Soft-Tissue Infection

Signs and Symptoms	• Often found in areas of skin disruption (e.g., post–venous puncture) and areas that are moist with high bacterial counts (e.g., axilla, perianal area) • VZV is the leading viral cause of skin infections in one or two dermatomes (patients with impaired T-cell function are at increased risk for disseminated disease)
Treatment	• If neutropenic, start empiric treatment for neutropenic fever (refer to text); add vancomycin 1 g IV q12h • If infection is in an area commonly colonized with anaerobes (e.g., neck, oropharynx, axilla, perianal area) and ceftazidime or cefepime is chosen for initial coverage, add metronidazole, 500 mg IV q8h, for additional anaerobic coverage • If concern for VZV, add acyclovir 10 mg/kg and place patient in a negative-pressure room

The leading viral cause of skin infections in this population is VZV. Patients typically present with vesicular lesions on an erythematous base limited to one or two dermatomes; patients with impaired T-cell function are at increased risk for disseminated disease.

Clinical Features of Respiratory Tract Infections

Ten to fifteen percent of neutropenic oncology patients will develop a respiratory tract infection, although infections of the upper respiratory tract (e.g., otitis, sinusitis) are uncommon, accounting for only 1% of episodes. Because of the impaired inflammatory response, only about half to two-thirds of oncology patients with radiographic or culture-positive pneumonia will present with typical clinical features (fever, cough, dyspnea, chest pain, sputum production, discrete infiltrates). Neutropenic patients rarely produce sputum (Table 51.4). *Pneumocystis jiroveci* pneumonia (formerly *Pneumocystis carinii*) presents more acutely in oncology patients than in patients with AIDS, and signs and symptoms often begin after discontinuation of corticosteroid therapy. Fungal pneumonias typically have an insidious onset with nodular or cavitating disease on chest x-ray (CXR) or chest computed tomography (CT) (Figure 51.2).

Patients at greatest risk for fungal pneumonia due to environmental molds (e.g., *Aspergillus* species) include patients with prolonged neutropenia (≥3 weeks) and corticosteroid therapy. Patients on corticosteroids are at risk for *Nocardia* infections. They have a similar presentation to mold infections and only culture and/or histopathology can differentiate between the two.

Table 51.4 Clinical Features: Respiratory Tract Infection

Signs and Symptoms	• Neutropenic patients rarely produce sputum • Only half to two-thirds of oncology patients with radiographic or culture-positive pneumonia will present with typical clinical features (fever, cough, dyspnea, chest pain, sputum production, infiltrates) • PCP presents more acutely in oncology patients than in patients with AIDS • Fungal pneumonias typically have an insidious onset with nodular or cavitating disease on CXR or chest CT • Patients on corticosteroids are at risk for environmental (e.g., *Aspergillus* species) and *Nocardia* infections
Laboratory Findings	• Nodular or cavitating disease on CXR or chest CT are concerning for a mold infection • Interstitial infiltrates can be seen with atypical bacterial, viral, and PCP
Treatment	• If neutropenic, start empiric treatment for neutropenic fever (refer to text) • If there is concern for aspiration or postobstructive pneumonia and ceftazidime or cefepime is chosen for initial coverage, add metronidazole, 500 mg IV q8h, for additional anaerobic coverage • If there is concern for PCP, start trimethoprim/sulfamethoxazole 5 mg/kg trimethoprim component IV q8h • If there are nodules or cavitary lesions, start an antifungal with activity against molds (e.g., amphotericin product, echinocandin, voriconazole, posaconazole)

AIDS, acquired immunodeficiency syndrome; PCP, *Pneumocystis* pneumonia.

Special Populations

317

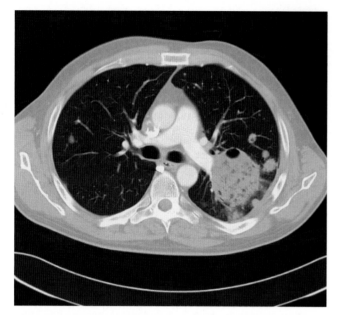

Figure 51.2 Chest CT of a patient with acute lymphoblastic leukemia who had received alemtuzumab 4 months before presentation. The patient presented with 1 week of cough, malaise, and mild left-sided chest pain. The patient's white blood cell count (WBC) was 7.0 with 85% neutrophils. *Aspergillus fumigatus* grew from a bronchial washing.

Clinical Features of Gastrointestinal Tract Infections

The gastrointestinal tract is the source of infection in 4–8% of oncology patients with a documented infection. The most common manifestations in the neutropenic patient are esophagitis and enterocolitis (Table 51.5). Patients receiving chemotherapy and/or with impaired T-cell function are at increased risk for esophagitis due to HSV or *Candida*. These patients typically present with odynophagia as their primary complaint. The etiological agent can be presumed if the patient has oral herpetic lesions or thrush; however, HSV and *Candida* esophagitis can occur in the absence of oral lesions.

Table 51.5 Clinical Features: Gastrointestinal Tract Infections

Signs and Symptoms	• Most common manifestations in the neutropenic patient are esophagitis and enterocolitis • Odynophagia • HSV and *Candida* esophagitis can occur in the absence of oral lesions • Diarrhea, nausea, vomiting, abdominal pain, abdominal distension, and fever commonly occur with colitis • Neutropenic leukemic patients are at risk for developing neutropenic enterocolitis, also known as typhlitis
Laboratory and Radiographic Findings	• *Clostridium difficile* toxin testing should be performed if there is concern for colitis • CT scan of abdomen should be obtained in patients with abdominal pain
Treatment	• If patient is neutropenic, start empiric treatment for neutropenic fever (refer to text) • If ceftazidime or cefepime is chosen for initial coverage, add metronidazole, 500 mg IV q8h, for additional anaerobic coverage • If concern for *Clostridium difficile*, consider empiric metronidazole while tests are pending

Table 51.6 Clinical Features: Central Nervous System Infections

Signs and Symptoms	• Often subtle findings such as headache, confusion, or more remarkable findings such as seizures, meningismus, changes in behavior, or focal neurological findings
Laboratory Findings	• Send CSF for cell count and differential, glucose, protein, bacterial counts, cryptococcal antigen and culture, and HSV PCR[*] • If neutropenic, neutrophils may not be present in the CSF
Treatment	• If neutropenic and there is concern for bacterial meningitis, treat with cefepime 2 g q8h, vancomycin 1 g q12h, and ampicillin 2 g q4h • If cryptococcal antigen positive, start amphotericin-containing product

[*]Because of the increased risk for mass lesions, a CT scan of the brain should be obtained before a lumbar puncture is attempted in oncology patients. CSF, cerebrospinal fluid; PCR, polymerase chain reaction.

Clostridium difficile is the most common infectious cause of colitis. Presenting complaints commonly include diarrhea, nausea, vomiting, abdominal pain, abdominal distension, and fever. Patients with severe colitis may have ileus and thus not have diarrhea. Neutropenic leukemic patients are at risk for developing neutropenic enterocolitis, also known as typhlitis, which can mimic an acute appendicitis. Because of chemotherapy-induced neutropenia and mucosal disruption, intestinal flora are able to invade the gut wall and can cause a life-threatening necrotizing colitis.

Clinical Features of Urinary Tract Infections

Urinary tract infections should be considered but are an uncommon source of infection in oncology patients, accounting for only 1–3% of infections. Symptoms are typically minimal, and pyuria is rare because of generalized neutropenia.

Clinical Features of Central Nervous System Infection

Although central nervous system infections are an uncommon source of infection in oncology patients, patients with impaired T-cell and splenic function are at increased risk for central nervous system infections due to *S. pneumoniae, Listeria, Cryptococcus, Toxoplasma, Nocardia*, and *Aspergillus*. Signs and symptoms of central nervous symptom infections can be subtle in immunocompromised patients, and many agents are associated with indolent infections (Table 51.6). Patients may present with headache, confusion, seizures, meningismus, changes in behavior, or focal neurological findings, though the absence of meningismus cannot be used to exclude CNS infection in this population. Because of the increased risk for mass lesions, a CT scan of the brain should be obtained before a lumbar puncture is attempted in oncology patients.

DIFFERENTIAL DIAGNOSIS

Potential Causes of Fever in Oncology Patients

The differential diagnosis of suspected infections in oncology patients is quite broad as oncology patients are also at high risk for complications that can mimic infectious

Table 51.7 Differential Diagnosis: Persistent Neutropenic Fever of Unknown Origin in the Oncology Patient*

CMV
EBV
Tuberculosis
Histoplasmosis
Blastomycosis
Coccidioidomycosis
Tumor fever: • Primary or secondary brain tumor • Primary or secondary liver tumor • Hypernephroma • Hematologic malignancies
Acute or delayed transfusion reaction
Drug fever
*The source of fever in patients with persistent neutropenic fever will never be identified in the vast majority of cases, particularly if they are otherwise clinically stable. Evaluation of persistent neutropenic fever of unknown origin should be based on risk factors present and other signs and symptoms.

Table 51.8 Differential Diagnosis: Sepsis Syndrome in the Oncology Patient

Gram-negative infection
Staphylococcus aureus infection
Streptococcus mitis bacteremia
Candidemia
Drug reaction
Thrombotic thrombocytopenic purpura: • Mitomycin C
Tumor lysis syndrome: • Tamoxifen • Bleomycin • Cytosine arabinoside • Daunomycin
Acute or delayed transfusion reaction
Anaphylaxis

Table 51.9 Differential Diagnosis: Oropharyngeal infection in the Oncology Patient

Polymicrobial bacterial infection (oral flora)
HSV
Candida
Cryptococcus
Histoplasmosis
Mucositis

Table 51.10 Differential Diagnosis: Skin and Soft-Tissue Infection in the Oncology Patient

Cellulitis: • Bacterial (local flora) • Deep venous thrombosis • *Cryptococcus* • Atypical mycobacteria
Disseminated rash: • Drug reaction • CMV • EBV • Disseminated bacterial infection
Nodular lesion: • Disseminated bacterial infection • *Cryptococcus* • *Nocardia* • Atypical mycobacteria • Sweet's syndrome
Ulcerative lesion: • HSV • VZV • Ecthyma gangrenosum • Pyoderma gangrenosum • Environmental mold

processes, including drug and tumor fevers, and transfusion reactions. Most patients with an undocumented source of fever will defervesce within 5 days after initiation of antibiotics. Patients with a documented source of infection typically take longer to respond to antibiotics. Tables 51.7 through 51.13 list potential causes of fever based on the clinical syndrome.

LABORATORY AND RADIOGRAPHIC FINDINGS

Two sets of blood cultures should be drawn on all oncology patients with suspected infection. If possible, both sets of blood cultures should be drawn from peripheral veins. Initial diagnostic tests should include a complete blood count with differential, serum electrolytes including creatinine, liver function tests, urinalysis, urine culture, and a chest radiograph (Table 51.14).

Additional evaluation will depend on the presenting complaint. Patients with diarrhea should have stool tested for *C. difficile* toxin. A CT of the abdomen and pelvis or abdominal ultrasound should be obtained in patients with abdominal tenderness. A CT of the head followed by a lumbar puncture should be obtained in patients with suspected central nervous system infection. Cerebrospinal fluid (CSF) should be sent for cell count and differential, glucose, protein, bacterial culture, cryptococcal antigen and culture, and HSV polymerase chain reaction (PCR). Unless contraindications exist (e.g., thrombocytopenia), samples should be obtained for Gram stain and culture from areas where infection is suspected. Chronic skin lesions should also be tested for fungi and mycobacteria, and necrotic skin lesions should be tested for fungi. Early bronchoscopy with alveolar lavage and transbronchial biopsy should be considered in patients with suspected or documented pneumonia.

Table 51.11 Differential Diagnosis: Respiratory Tract Infections in the Oncology Patient

Sinusitis:
- Polymicrobial bacterial
- Environmental mold
- Allergy

Focal pulmonary consolidation:
- *Streptococcus pneumoniae*
- *Haemophilus influenzae*
- Gram negative
- Postobstructive pneumonia
- *Cryptococcus*
- Pulmonary embolism
- Pulmonary hemorrhage

Interstitial infiltrates:
- Respiratory virus
- *Mycoplasma pneumoniae*
- *Chlamydia pneumoniae*
- *Pneumocystis jiroveci*
- Adult respiratory distress syndrome
- Congestive heart failure
- Pericardial effusion
- Drug reaction:
  azacitidine
  bleomycin
  busulfan
  chlorambucil
  cyclophosphamide
  cytosine arabinoside
  fludarabine
  melphalan
  methotrexate
  mitomycin
  nitrosoureas
  procarbazine
- Radiation pneumonitis
- Lymphangitic spread of malignancy

Nodules/cavities:
- Malignancy
- Environmental mold
- Histoplasmosis
- Blastomycosis
- Coccidioidomycosis
- Tuberculosis
- *Nocardia*

Table 51.12 Differential Diagnosis: Gastrointestinal Infection in the Oncology Patient

Esophagitis:
- HSV
- *Candida*
- Radiation esophagitis
- Mucositis
- Bacterial esophagitis
- Malignancy

Enterocolitis:
- *Clostridium difficile*
- Typhlitis
- Mucositis
- Radiation poisoning
- Radiation enterocolitis
- Viral gastroenteritis
- *Giardia*
- *Cryptosporidium*

Table 51.13 Differential Diagnosis: Central Nervous System Infection in the Oncology Patient

Streptococcus pneumoniae

Listeria monocytogenes

Haemophilus influenzae

Cryptococcus

Carcinomatous meningitis

Brain abscess

HSV

Radiation toxicity

Chemotherapy toxicity:
- Cytosine arabinoside
- Methotrexate
- Ifosfamide

Environmental mold

Sedatives/narcotics

Hemorrhage

Diabetes mellitus

Hypercalcemia

Malignancy

Table 51.14 Baseline Laboratory Assessment of Febrile Neutropenic Oncology Patients

Two sets of blood cultures (venipuncture if possible)

Complete blood count with differential

Serum electrolytes

Serum creatinine

Liver function tests

Urinalysis

Urine culture

CXR

TREATMENT AND PROPHYLAXIS

The Infectious Disease Society of America guidelines define febrile neutropenia as a single temperature at or above 38.3°C or a temperature of 38.0°C to 38.2°C for 1 hour or longer in patients with a neutrophil count below 500 polymorphonuclear neutrophil leukocytes (PMNs)/mL, or at of below 1000 PMNs/mL with an expected drop to below 500. All neutropenic patients with suspected infection should receive prompt empiric antibiotics. The institution of recommendations for broad gram-negative (in particular, antipseudomonal) coverage at the onset of fever in the neutropenic patient has been the single most effective advance in supportive care of oncology patients in the past 30 years.

Table 51.15 Scoring Index for Identification of Low-Risk Patients Presenting with Neutropenic Fever*

Characteristic	Score
Extent of illness (choose one): • No symptoms • Mild symptoms • Moderate symptoms	5 5 3
No hypotension	5
No chronic obstructive pulmonary disease	4
Solid tumor or no fungal infection	4
No dehydration	3
Outpatient at onset of fever	3
Age 17–60	2

*Highest score is 26. Patients with a score between 21 and 26 indicate the patient is at low risk for complications. Adapted from Hughes et al. (2002) and Klastersky et al. (2000).

Risk Assessment

In the past, all febrile neutropenic patients were started on intravenous broad-spectrum antibiotics and admitted to the hospital. Subsequently, a group of low-risk patients have been identified that may be treated as outpatients with oral antibiotics.

Factors associated with a low risk of adverse outcomes:

- anticipated duration of neutropenia less than 7 days
- solid malignancy, lymphoma, or myeloma in remission
- no obvious site of infection
- absence of comorbidities

Factors associated with a high risk of complications:

- anticipated duration of neutropenia greater than 10 days
- acute leukemia
- temperature at or above 39°C
- rigors
- severe sepsis
- an identified site of infection
- end-organ dysfunction
- presence of comorbidities

Based on these factors, a scoring system was developed and validated prospectively by the Multinational Association for Supportive Care in Cancer (Table 51.15). A high score from 21 to 26 identified patients with a less than 5% risk of developing severe complications with a positive predictive value of 91%, specificity of 68%, and sensitivity of 71%. Other factors to consider when deciding whether or not to treat a low-risk patient with oral antibiotics include:

- patient adherence
- patient's ability to swallow
- gut motility and absorption
- use of antibiotic prophylaxis

Once oncology has been consulted, patients who meet low-risk criteria are appropriate candidates for oral outpatient therapy if they will have continuous and rapid access to high-level inpatient care.

Treatment of Low-Risk Patients

Oral combination therapy with ciprofloxacin 500 mg tid and amoxicillin/clavulanate 500 mg tid was found to be just as efficacious as intravenous antibiotics in two studies of low-risk patients. This regimen has good coverage of both gram-negative and gram-positive bacteria. However, widespread use of oral fluoroquinolones as prophylaxis may soon limit the efficacy of this regimen. Ciprofloxacin and levofloxacin are the only orally available antibiotics that have adequate activity against *Pseudomonas*, and patients who develop microbiologically proven infections while on fluoroquinolones are more likely to have a fluoroquinolone-resistant organism. Therefore patients on fluoroquinolone prophylaxis will require initial treatment with intravenous antibiotics regardless of risk stratification. Other factors to consider include the prevalence of antibiotic-resistant organisms in the community (such as community-associated methicillin-resistant *S. aureus* or fluoroquinolone-resistant *E. coli*), and whether the patient has recently been hospitalized.

Treatment of High-Risk Patients

All high-risk neutropenic patients should be started on broad-spectrum intravenous antibiotics and admitted to the hospital. Choices of empiric intravenous antibiotics include monotherapy with:

- ceftazidime: 2 g intravenous (IV) q8h
- cefepime: 1–2 mg IV q8h (FDA approved dose is 2 g)
- imipenem: 500 mg IV q6h
- meropenem: 1 g IV q8h or 500 mg q6h
- piperacillin-tazobactam: 4.5 g IV q6h

Ceftazidime has poor gram-positive coverage, but the other agents provide excellent coverage against streptococci and beta-lactam sensitive staphylococci. Choice of agent depends on local sensitivity patterns, formulary availability, and suspected site of infection. Fluoroquinolone monotherapy has not always performed favorably in trials of treatment of neutropenic fever and should be avoided in the absence of severe drug allergies. As mentioned earlier, fluoroquinolones should also be avoided in patients on fluoroquinolone prophylaxis.

Addition of an Aminoglycoside

Although studies of beta-lactam monotherapy versus beta-lactam plus an aminoglycoside have not demonstrated a benefit of combination therapy, combination therapy may be considered in a select group of patients. When possible, aminoglycosides should be avoided in patients at increased risk for adverse events, including the elderly and patients with renal insufficiency, heart failure, or moderate to severe liver disease, as well as patients on other nephrotoxic drugs. Gentamicin or tobramycin 5 mg/kg IV q24h, when indicated, should be considered for patients with:

- severe sepsis
- risk factors for infections due to resistant gram-negative bacteria

Once-daily dosing is likely just as efficacious as traditional dosing, but with a lower incidence of nephrotoxicity.

Addition of Vancomycin

Routine empirical use of vancomycin 1 g q12h has not been associated with improved patient outcomes. However, there are several settings when empiric vancomycin use should be considered. These include:

- temperature of 40°C or above
- severe sepsis
- high rates of penicillin-resistant streptococci
- high local rates of methicillin-resistant *S. aureus*
- catheter exit-site infections
- severe mucositis
- recent fluoroquinolone prophylaxis

Other Considerations

- Atypical pneumonia pathogen coverage (macrolide or respiratory fluoroquinolone) for patients with interstitial infiltrates
- *Pneumocystis jiroveci* pneumonia (PCP) coverage for patients with impaired T-cell function or who are on (or have recently discontinued) corticosteroids
- Antifungal coverage for patients with thrush and esophagitis or nodular/cavitating lesions on CXR
- Anaerobic coverage for patients with oropharyngeal or intra-abdominal infections
- Antiviral coverage for patients with oral herpes and esophagitis
- Ampicillin for patients with meningitis (to cover *Listeria monocytogenes*)
- Oral metronidazole or vancomycin for patients with suspected *C. difficile*-associated disease

PEARLS AND PITFALLS

1. Broad-spectrum antibiotics must be started as soon as possible in febrile neutropenic patients.
2. Consulting with the patient's oncologist is imperative to learn about disease status, recent antimicrobial use, and prior infections.
3. Patients with a history of invasive fungal infections are at increased risk for reactivation while neutropenic.
4. *Pneumocystis jiroveci* is more difficult to diagnose in non-AIDS patients and may require bronchoscopy and transbronchial biopsy to confirm the diagnosis.
5. Neutropenic patients with bacterial pneumonia rarely produce sputum.
6. Fungal pneumonia typically has an insidious onset with chest nodules or cavitating lesions on imaging.

7. Skin lesions can be a manifestation of disseminated infection, such as ecthyma gangrenosum due to *Pseudomonas* bacteremia or skin nodules from disseminated candidiasis or fusariosis.
8. VZV is the leading viral cause of skin infections.
9. *Clostridium difficile* is the most common infectious cause of colitis.
10. Because they have a high rate of infection with resistant organisms, patients on fluoroquinolone prophylaxis often require admission and intravenous antibiotics regardless of risk stratification.

REFERENCES

Behre G, Link H, Maschmeyer G, et al. Meropenem monotherapy versus combination therapy with ceftazidime and amikacin for empirical treatment of febrile neutropenic patients. Ann Hematol 1998;76(2):73–80.

Bodey GP, Buckley M, Sathe YS, Freireich EJ. Quantitative relationships between circulating leukocytes and infection in patients with acute leukemia. Ann Intern Med 1966;64(2):328–40.

Cometta A, Calandra T, Gaya H, et al. Monotherapy with meropenem versus combination therapy with ceftazidime plus amikacin as empiric therapy for fever in granulocytopenic patients with cancer. The International Antimicrobial Therapy Cooperative Group of the European Organization for Research and Treatment of Cancer and the Gruppo Italiano Malattie Ematologiche Maligne dell'Adulto Infection Program. Antimicrob Agents Chemother 1996;40(5):1108–15.

Cometta A, Kern WV, de Bock R, et al. Vancomycin versus placebo for treating persistent fever in patients with neutropenic cancer receiving piperacillin-tazobactam monotherapy. Clin Infect Dis 2003;37(3):382–9.

Cox AL, Thompson SA, Jones JL, et al. Lymphocyte homeostasis following therapeutic lymphocyte depletion in multiple sclerosis. Eur J Immunol 2005;35(11):3332–42.

Dubberke ER, Augustine K, Olsen MA, et al. Epidemiology of bloodstream infections on a hematopoietic stem cell transplant unit. Infect Dis Soc Am 2004;Abstract number 648.

Freifeld A, Marchigiani D, Walsh T, et al. A double-blind comparison of empirical oral and intravenous antibiotic therapy for low-risk febrile patients with neutropenia during cancer chemotherapy. N Engl J Med 1999;341(5):305–11.

Hasbun R, Abrahams J, Jekel J, Quagliarello VJ. Computed tomography of the head before lumbar puncture in adults with suspected meningitis. N Engl J Med 2001;345(24):1727–33.

Hughes WT, Armstrong D, Bodey GP, et al. 2002 guidelines for the use of antimicrobial agents in neutropenic patients with cancer. Clin Infect Dis 2002;34(6):730–51.

Kern WV, Cometta A, de Bock R, et al. Oral versus intravenous empirical antimicrobial therapy for fever in patients with granulocytopenia who are receiving cancer chemotherapy. International Antimicrobial Therapy Cooperative Group of the European Organization for Research and Treatment of Cancer. N Engl J Med 1999;341(5):312–8.

Klastersky J, Paesmans M, Rubenstein EB, et al. The Multinational Association for Supportive Care in Cancer risk index: a multinational scoring system for identifying low-risk febrile neutropenic cancer patients. J Clin Oncol 2000;18(16):3038–51.

Neuburger S, Maschmeyer G. Update on management of infections in cancer and stem cell transplant patients. Ann Hematol 2006;85(6):345–56.

Sickles EA, Greene WH, Wiernik PH. Clinical presentation of infection in granulocytopenic patients. Arch Intern Med 1975;135(5):715–9.

Suster S, Rosen LB. Intradermal bullous dermatitis due to candidiasis in an immunocompromised patient. JAMA 1987;258(15):2106–7.

Tamura K, Matsuoka H, Tsukada J, et al. Cefepime or carbapenem treatment for febrile neutropenia as a single agent is as effective as a combination of 4th-generation cephalosporin + aminoglycosides: comparative study. Am J Hematol 2002;71(4):248–55.

52. Ectoparasites

Jan M. Shoenberger, William Mallon, and Matthew Lewin

INTRODUCTION

Ectoparasitosis includes all infestations where parasites live in or on human skin. Most human ectoparasites are arthropods, primarily insects and arachnids, including ticks. Many ectoparasite infestations result in significant morbidity and yet go unrecognized in the acute care setting. Failure to treat affected patients leads to spread of ectoparasites through vulnerable populations both inside and outside the hospital. Recognition and treatment of ectoparasitosis (including resistant strains of pediculosis and scabies) is particularly important because these infestations are increasing geographically and within traditionally less vulnerable populations.

GENERAL ECTOPARASITE EPIDEMIOLOGY

Ectoparisitoses are most prevalent in resource-poor populations, including the homeless, immigrants, refugees, the incarcerated, the malnourished, and those who are underinsured and uninsured. The worldwide prevalence of scabies has been estimated at 300 million cases and is expanding. Crusted (or Norwegian) scabies are now an important nosocomial disease resulting in a large number of bed closures in intensive care units (ICUs) and wards across the United States. Head lice result in the loss of 12 to 24 million school days for U.S. children annually. Emerging resistance makes control more difficult, and incidence is also increasing due to the expanded use of steroids for asthma, arthritis, lupus, and other inflammatory diseases. (See Table 52.1.)

SCABIES

Clinical Features

Scabies is a common ectoparasitic infestation caused by the mite *Sarcoptes scabiei*. They are also known as "human itch mites." In general, the infestation causes an intensely pruritic rash as the pregnant female mite burrows into the skin and deposits eggs in a burrow. Larvae hatch in 3–10 days and migrate to the skin surface while maturing into adults. The pruritic rash of scabies is a result of both the infestation itself and the host's hypersensitivity reaction to the mite and its feces. Superinfections with staphylococci and streptococci are common, and complications such poststreptococcal glomerulonephritis, although rare, have been reported.

For a primary infestation, the incubation period before symptoms is usually between 3 and 6 weeks (Table 52.2). Transmission can be direct (person to person) or indirect (through infested bedding or clothing, which can remain infectious for up to several days). Transmission between members of the same household and among institutionalized people is common.

The itching caused by scabies is typically worse at night. The rash is most commonly found on the hands (particularly the webbing between the fingers) and the flexor surfaces of the wrists, elbows, and knees, as well as on the genitalia and breasts of women. The rash usually spares the face, scalp, and head in adults but can affect those areas in infants. Itching may be reported in areas of the body where no mites are detectable. It is very common to see secondary excoriations, eczematous skin changes, and superinfection (impetigo). In patients who have had a prior scabies infestation, a papular "scabies rash" can be seen on the buttocks, scapular region, and abdomen and is thought to be cause by a delayed hypersensitivity reaction.

There are also "atypical" forms of scabies, such as crusted or Norwegian scabies, which cause a psoriatic hyperkeratotic dermatitis of the hands and feet (with nail involvement) and an erythematous, scaly eruption on the face, neck, scalp, and trunk. These lesions are highly contagious because of a high concentration of mites and usually affect immunocompromised and bed-bound patients.

Table 52.1 Major Ectoparasites of the World

Category of Ectoparasite	Scientific/Common Name	Comments
Scabies	*Sarcoptes scabiei*, classic scabies, crusted (Norwegian) scabies	Crusted scabies seen in bed-ridden, malnourished, immunosuppressed
Mites	Bedbugs, dust mites, chiggers	More than 30,000 species
Ticks (and Tick-Borne Illnesses)	Many diseases transmitted	Important vectors for many viral and bacterial diseases
Tungiasis	Sand-flea disease	Presents as a slow-growing, sometimes painful nodule from which the parasite must be extracted. Endemic to the West Indies, Africa, India, Latin America. In the United States, a rare disease in returning travelers or immigrants from endemic regions.
Bedbugs (Cimicidae)	Bedbugs	Worldwide. Nearly eradicated in United States 50 years ago. Outbreaks reported in all 50 U.S. states during 2007. Not considered a major vector of disease, but bites can be numerous and also become secondarily infected.
Human Louse (Pediculosis)	Head louse, body louse, pubic louse	Worldwide. Head lice have greatest impact on children.
Cutaneous Larva Migrans	Hookworm larvae, "clam-digger's itch"	Disease of travelers who stepped on feces of dogs/cat. Most common travel-associated skin disease.
Myiasis	Flies and maggots (larval stages)	Most are not invasive in the United States

Table 52.2 Clinical Features: Scabies

Incubation Period	3–6 weeks for primary infestation, 1–3 days for reinfestation
Transmission	• Direct (person to person) *or* • Indirect (through infested bedding or clothing)
Scabies Signs and Symptoms	• Pruritis typically worse at night • Rash commonly found on the hands, flexor surface of wrists, elbows, knees, genitalia, and breasts • Rash usually spares the face, scalp, and head in adults but can affect those areas in infants
Crusted or Norwegian Scabies	• Psoriatic hyperkeratotic dermatitis of the hands and feet (with nail involvement) • Erythematous, scaly rash on face, neck, scalp, and trunk • Highly contagious because of the large number of mites involved • Common among immunocompromised patients
Diagnosis	• Clinical diagnosis *or* • Direct visualization under a light microscope • Skin biopsy

Laboratory and Radiographic Findings

The diagnosis of scabies is primarily a clinical one, because definitive diagnosis requires microscopic visualization of the mite, eggs, or feces of the mite in skin scrapings from areas with burrows. Samples should be obtained by scraping laterally across the skin with a scalpel blade. Alternatively, strong adhesive tape can be applied over the burrow areas, peeled off, and viewed under the microscope. Under low power, the mites will appear translucent with brown legs and are 0.2–0.5 mm long. One challenge to diagnosis is that in classic scabies (the most common form), the mite burden is low and the detection by microscopy is tissue sample and operator dependent. Failure to find mites is common and does not rule out the diagnosis. Diagnosis is sometimes made by skin biopsy.

In areas of high prevalence, the presence of diffuse itching and visible lesions associated with either at least two typical locations of scabies or a household member with itching can have nearly 100% sensitivity and specificity for the diagnosis.

Treatment and Prophylaxis

Index patients and all close contacts need to be treated to achieve eradication. First-line treatment is 5% permethrin cream given as a single overnight application. Lindane is no longer a first-line therapy because of reports of neurotoxicity and seizures in children. Though effective, topical therapy has some disadvantages: It is messy, difficult to apply for some, and can burn or sting on excoriated areas. An alternative therapy is oral ivermectin, an arthropod neurotoxin. The only major adverse event reported from ivermectin is a transient, mild increase in itching that occurs after drug ingestion and is thought to be a result of an enhanced hypersensitivity reaction to dead mites. The dose is 200 µg/kg, and the cost is generally higher than for topical agents. A combination of topical and oral therapy is recommended for crusted scabies.

Differential Diagnosis

The differential diagnosis of pruritic rashes is vast and includes infestation by fleas (Siphonaptera), bedbugs (Cimicidae), lice, and other mites. Flea and bedbug bites tend to be punctate, and flea bites tend toward the extremities, whereas bedbug bites tend toward areas of exposed skin such as the neck and face. Repeated failed treatment of scabies suggests infestation by free-living arthropods, such as bedbugs and fleas.

Table 52.3 Treatment of Scabies

Drug Name	Dose	Side Effects	Comments
Permethrin (Elimite)	5% cream applied to entire body and rinsed off in 8–14 hours	May burn or sting	First-line topical therapy. Should reapply 1 week after initial application.
Lindane (Kwell)	1% lotion or 30 g cream applied to entire body and rinsed off after 8–10 hours	Seizures, muscle spasm, aplastic anemia. Not to be used in infants or lactating mothers.	Second-line topical therapy
Crotamiton (Eurax)	100% cream applied for 24 hours, rinsed and reapplied for 24 hours	Seizures (rare)	Second- or third-line topical therapy
Ivermectin (Mectizan, Stromectol)	200 μg/kg orally single dose. Repeat on days 15 and 24 for persistent symptoms.	Increased itching initially	Literature to support this drug is emerging. May be more expensive than topical agents.

Oral ivermectin can also be used alone as a single dose, and repeated on days 15 and 24 if symptoms persist. Table 52.3 summarizes treatment options for scabies.

In addition to pharmacologic treatment, environmental control measures are crucial. All bedding, clothes, and towels used by the patient in the 48 hours prior to treatment should be washed in hot water (125 °F) and dried in a hot drier.

OTHER MITES

Besides scabies, there are many other mites that result in ectoparasitosis and other medical conditions in humans. Mites have complex symbiotic associations with larger organisms, both plant and animal. The vast majority are very small (fractions of a millimeter) and are visible only under magnification.

Clinical Features

Medical conditions associated with mites include allergic rhinitis, asthma, childhood eczema, dermatitis, and superinfection of lesions due to excoriation (Table 52.4).

- **Dust and bedmite:** *Dermatophagoides* species survive best in warm, humid locations, particularly in high-traffic areas, upholstered furniture, and especially beds, where they feed on skin flakes, mold, fungus, and household detritus. Both dust and bed mites can become airborne with bed making, cleaning, and vacuuming, causing allergic and dermatologic problems. These mites do not bite, sting, or transmit any disease-causing pathogens.
- **Harvest mite:** *Trombicula autumnalis* will move from plants to people (and dogs, cats, and reptiles) in the six-legged larval stage, during which they feed on digested keratinized

Table 52.4 Clinical Features: Mites

Transmission	• Direct (person to person) *or* • Indirect (through infested bedding or clothing)
Dust and Bedmite	• Survive best in warm humid locations • Feed on skin flakes, mold, fungus, and detritus • Allergic and dermatologic problems when they become airborne from cleaning and vacuuming • Do not bite or sting, nor do they transmit any disease-causing pathogens
Harvest Mite	• Feed on digested keratinized skin during the larval stage only • Attach where clothing fits tightly (waistline, socks, and armpits) • Inject saliva that digests skin, particularly near hair follicles, which causes pruritic welts to develop after 3–6 hours
Bird Mite	• Often called "bird lice" • Cannot infest humans but will bite when no birds are available • Rash, irritation, pruritis, and secondary bacterial infection are common for up to 2 weeks after the birds leave
Chiggers	• Feed on keratinized skin during the larval stage only • Bites around tight-fitting clothes with similar host response to harvest mites
Diagnosis	• Clinical diagnosis *or* • Direct visualization under a microscope of skin scraping or biopsy
Treatment	• Antibiotics for superinfected skin excoriations • Thorough cleaning and vacuuming with a HEPA filter • Wash clothes and linens at 125°F • Symptomatic treatment of pruritis with steroids and antihistamines as needed

Dog, cat, rabbit, fowl, rat, clover and bat mites, straw itch mites, and grain mites can all cause similar medical problems to the species above. HEPA filter, **h**igh-**e**fficiency **p**articulate **a**ir filter.

skin. They tend to attach where clothing fits tightly (waistline, socks and armpits) and do not suck blood but inject saliva, which digests skin, particularly near hair follicles. Severely pruritic welts develop 3–6 hours after exposure and persist up to 2 weeks. Firm red nodules may result from the host immune response. The mites drop off after feeding for 3–4 days.
- **Bird mite:** *Ornithonyssus* species, often called "bird lice," populate bird nests and are parasites of common birds. When birds leave the nest, these hematophagous mites are dispersed and may enter human dwellings and bite humans. They cannot infest humans but will bite when no birds are available. Rash, irritation, pruritis, and secondary bacterial infection are common for up to 2 weeks after bites. Control is best achieved by bird nest control.
- **Chiggers:** *Eutrombicula alfreddugesi* and other species, like the harvest mite, feed only in the larval stage. Common throughout the southeastern United States, they bite around tight-fitting clothes and cause a rash similar to that caused by harvest mites.

- **Dog, cat, rabbit, fowl, rat, clover and bat mites, straw itch mites, and grain mites**: All can cause similar medical problems to the species above. *Cheyletiella* species (including dog, cat, and rabbit mite) infestations tend to appear in very specific patterns on human skin. For example, the pruritis can appear on the arms and across chest after holding a pet animal. This is the most common diagnostic clue.

Differential Diagnosis

The differential diagnosis would include:

- drug eruptions
- furunculosis
- folliculitis
- other contact dermatitis
- other pruritic papular or nodular processes

Laboratory Findings

Mites are usually diagnosed clinically but occasionally require skin scrapings or skin biopsy examined with magnification. Sometimes the larvae can be felt crawling on the skin and can be seen with direct inspection. No laboratory tests exist except allergen testing.

Treatment and Prophylaxis

When superinfected excoriations are found, antimicrobial therapy directed toward *Streptococcus* and *Staphylococcus* (including methicillin-resistant *Staphylococcus aureus* [MRSA]) infection may be warranted. Most ectoparasitic infestations due to mites are self-limited and source control should be the primary target. For bed and dust mites, thorough cleaning and vacuuming with a high-efficiency particulate air (HEPA) filter can provide relief. All bed linens and clothing should be washed at 125°F (52°C), which kills mites. Raising the bed off the floor and air conditioner filter changes may decrease exposures. Allergy treatment with immunotherapy mite extract injections may help decrease allergic symptoms. Pesticide "bombing" will often be ineffective if the sources (bird nests, rodents, domestic animals) are not removed. Household pets can be treated topically (pyrethrin, lime sulfur, etc.) or with ivermectin as advised by a veterinarian.

Treatment of clothing with permethrin and skin with *N,N*-diethyl-*m*-toluamide (DEET)-containing pesticides may provide protection during specific exposures (e.g., field work). Pruritis can be treated with topical or oral steroids and antihistamines.

LICE

Three types of infestation with lice are seen in humans – head lice (*Pediculus humanus capitis*), body lice (*Pediculus humanus corporis*; see Figure 52.1), and pubic lice (*Phthirus pubis*; see Figure 52.2). The head louse infests only the human head, but the pubic louse may be found on any short hair (pubic hair, areolar hair, beard, eyebrow or lash, axillary hairs). The Centers for Disease Control and Prevention (CDC) considers infestation with pubic lice a sexually transmitted disease (STD), and co-infection with other STDs is common.

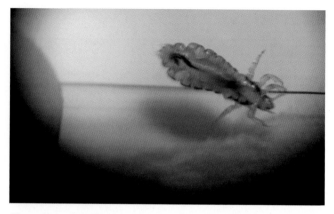

Figure 52.1 *Pediculus corporis* (10×). Courtesy of Dr. Matthew Lewin.

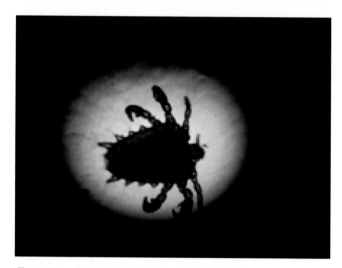

Figure 52.2 *Phthirus pubis* (10×). Courtesy of Dr. Toby Salz.

Life Cycle and Transmission

The adult female head louse lays 1–6 eggs per day for up to 30 days after mating. The eggs are translucent and are attached to a hair shaft close to the scalp. They hatch in 7 days and the 1-mm-long empty egg casings (nits) then become white and are visible. After 9–12 days, the grayish-colored louse becomes an adult about the size of a sesame seed (3–4 mm). Nits (empty egg casings) stay on the hair shaft, and they move away from the scalp as the hair grows. Lice feed on blood and reside close to the scalp.

Head lice are usually transmitted through head-to-head contact but can also be transmitted by fomites (hats, scarves, brushes, etc.). Lice cannot jump or fly. Pubic lice are spread through sexual activity. If pubic lice are discovered in children, sexual abuse should be suspected. Lice or nits found on an eyelash, for example, are almost invariably pubic lice, not head lice.

Clinical Features

The most common symptom of infestation is pruritis (Figure 52.3). It is possible, however, to have an infestation of head lice without itching. A tickling sensation of something moving in the hair may be noticed. Head lice and their nits are most commonly found behind the ears and on the hairs of the

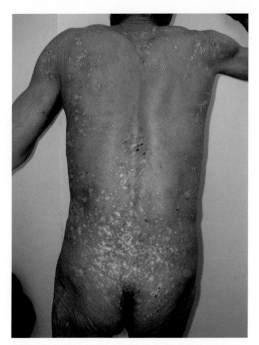

Figure 52.3 Typical distribution of body lice infestation. Courtesy of Dr. Bradley Frazee.

Table 52.5 Clinical Features: Lice

Incubation Period	3–7 days
Head Lice (*Pediculus humanus capitis*)	• Infests only human head • Rare in African Americans • Commonly found behind ears, neck and occiput hair
Body Lice (*Pediculus humanus corporis*)	• Lives in clothing seams • Does not affect hair
Pubic Lice (*Phthiruspubis*)	• Infects any short hair (pubic, areolar, beard, axillary, and eyebrows or lashes) • Lice or nits found on an eyelash are always pubic lice and not head lice • Should suspect sexual abuse if discovered in children
Transmission	• Direct (person to person) *or* • Indirect (through infested bedding or clothing) • Lice cannot jump or fly
Signs and Symptoms	• Pruritis • Visible insects, eggs, feeling of movement on hair or skin
Diagnosis	• Clinical diagnosis *or* • Direct visualization under a light microscope • Skin biopsy

neck and occiput (Table 52.5). Body lice are found on clothing seams (Figure 52.4). Pubic lice will be found attached to the base of the pubic hair and the infestation generally results in severe itching. Often times patients susceptible to lice will have delusional parasitosis. However, they may also have lice or both disorders. Patients with psychiatric disorders are particularly prone to the diagnosis of one or the other, if not both. The presence of delusional parasitosis even in the presence of lice should prompt a psychiatric or toxicological evaluation followed by appropriate counseling.

Laboratory Findings

Infestation with head lice is best diagnosed by isolating parasites with a fine-tooth comb. This is more efficient than direct visualization on the hairs and scalp. The comb should be placed in the hair right at the scalp and then drawn down firmly. The entire head of hair should be combed twice and the comb examined after each stroke. It often takes at least a full minute of combing to find the first louse. Finding nits does not necessarily imply active infestation because nits can persist after treatment. Some sources say that the diagnosis can only be made if a living, moving louse is found.

Treatment and Prophylaxis

Treatment of head lice is somewhat controversial and varies from region to region. Some of these differences lie in different resistance patterns. In the United States, chemical pediculicides are the mainstay of therapy. Treatment should be repeated 10 days after initial application because eggs are less effectively killed than adults and it takes 5–11 days for eggs to hatch. All close contacts should be treated. Permethrin 5% cream or lotion is first-line therapy (Table 52.6). Malathion is also recommended as second-line therapy, though it has a strong odor and cannot be used in young children or in people with asthma or severe eczema. Permethrin is an arthropod specific neurotoxin, but malathion is an acetyl-

cholinesterase inhibitor and can cause severe autonomic dysfunction in humans. Using a nit comb as an adjunct to chemical treatments decreases reinfection rates.

For children younger than 2 years of age, or in cases where parents do not want to use an insecticide, wet combing alone is an alternative. It is not as effective as chemical methods. Brushes, combs, hats, and other possible fomites such as bed sheets and other linens should be cleaned in hot water, but further environmental decontamination is not necessary. Oral ivermectin may also be used and is the preferred treatment in patients unable to comply with topical therapy or who may also have co-infestations (such as scabies). In resistant cases, ivermectin or a combination of topical therapy and oral trimethoprim-sulfamethoxazole may be used. Body lice do

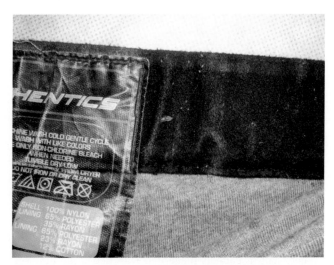

Figure 52.4 Body lice in the seams of clothing. Courtesy of Dr. Bradley Frazee.

Table 52.6 Treatment of Head and Pubic Lice

Drug Name	Dose	Side Effects	Comments
Permethrin (Elimite, Nix)	5% (Elimite) or 1% (Nix) lotion. Nix is OTC and should be applied to hair for 10 minutes and rinse. Elimite is for skin.	Itching, burning, redness may occur.	May comb out lice/nits after treatment. Elimite used for resistant cases.
Pyrethrin/ Piperonyl butoxide (RID, A-200)	Varies (all are OTC). Apply to hair for 10 minutes.	Not common.	Usually requires two treatments. Less effective than permethrin.
Lindane (Kwell)	1% shampoo. Apply to hair, allow to set for 4 minutes, lather for 4 minutes and rinse	Seizures, muscle spasm, aplastic anemia. Not to be used in infants or lactation.	Second or third line therapy
Malathion (Ovide)	0.5% and 1% aqueous-based lotions. Leave on 8–12 hours and rinse.	Flammable, avoid contact with eyes, mucous membranes. Strong odor. Not recommended for children younger than 6 years old.	Second or third line therapy. Is an organophosphate-based poison. Its oxidation product is malaoxon, which is equally toxic.
Ivermectin (Mectizan, Stromectol)	200 μg/kg orally single dose and second dose 10 days later recommended	Rare. Not for children younger than 5 years old.	Usually used in resistant cases.

not require chemical therapy because they live in the clothing, not on the skin (unless severely infested). In most cases, hot-water laundering of all clothing and bedding is sufficient. If lice infest the eyelashes, petroleum jelly can be used to suffocate the parasites.

TICKS

In North America, ticks are widely dispersed in rural and suburban areas. Ticks are arachnids closely related to mites and are hematophagous, taking blood meals from humans and animals. Adult ticks are larger than mites and are visible without magnification. However, smaller, immature forms are also hematophagous and may be overlooked. Both immature and adult forms can be disease vectors. Tick-borne diseases have a wide variety of infectious agents, including viruses, spirochetes, and intracellular bacterial pathogens (*Rickettsia* and Ehrlichiae), gram-negative bacteria (*Francisella tularensis*), and protozoa (*Babesia microti*).

Wherever humans come into contact with ticks, bites and diseases follow. Children are more commonly exposed to ticks, for example, and the peak incidence for Rocky Mountain spotted fever (RMSF) is between ages 5 and 9. Only approximately half of patients diagnosed with tick-borne illnesses will recall having had a tick bite. Lyme disease is now the

most common tick-borne disease in the United States and is a reportable disease. In 2002, 23,763 cases were reported to the CDC (by all states except Hawaii, Montana, and Oklahoma). The national incidence was 8.2 cases per 100,000 population. RMSF is found in all states except Maine, Hawaii, and Alaska and is much more common along the eastern seaboard than the Rocky Mountains. Table 52.7 summarizes the major tick-borne illnesses, the vectors, and their geographic distribution. In some cases, a single bite may transmit multiple diseases (e.g., human granulocytic ehrlichiosis and Lyme disease). If a high proportion of ticks in a given area are infected, a "treat all" prophylactic strategy is warranted for a potentially disabling disease such as Lyme disease. However, this strategy is not appropriate in most cases, and many people receive unnecessary antibiotics and testing.

See also Chapter 4, Systemic Diseases Causing Fever and Rash.

Treatment and Prophylaxis

TICK REMOVAL

Removal of the tick will cure toxin-mediated ascending tick paralysis and may prevent transmission of Lyme disease, which requires that a tick be attached to its host long enough for the infecting pathogen to move from the gut to the salivary tract of the tick – a process that may take hours to days. Thus, the duration of tick attachment is important for disease transmission. Additionally, the longer the ticks are attached, the more difficult they are to remove.

Traction on the tick using a forceps will allow complete removal of some recently attached ticks (Figure 52.5). Later on, the biting apparatus of the tick is cemented in place by its secretions, and pulling on the body will often snap it off, leaving the head behind. A scalpel can be used to core out the head to prevent a foreign-body reaction or superinfection.

MYIASIS

Myiasis is the infestation of skin (and subcutaneous tissues) with fly larvae and is divided into three subtypes: facultative, obligatory, and accidental (Table 52.8). The usual precondition for facultative myiasis is the exposure of a wound to the ubiquitous house fly. Once a fly deposits eggs within a wound, maggots develop and clean the wound. For emergency physicians, the main elements of the epidemiology are homelessness and substance use, which produces an altered sensorium during which flies can access the wound to lay eggs. Obligatory infestations include *Dermatobia hominis* (botfly), *Cordylobia anthropophaga* (tumbu fly), and screw worm infestations. These organisms have larval stages that require the living tissue of an animal host and may cause significant tissue destruction. Accidental myiasis occurs when egg-stage flies are ingested on contaminated food or come into contact with the genitourinary tract.

Clinical Features

Because larvae are visible to the naked eye, the diagnosis of wound-related myiasis is made by careful examination. The most common presentation is a patient with a chronic wound that has obvious maggot infestation when the wound is undressed (Table 52.9).

Table 52.7 Common Tick-Transmitted Diseases

Disease	Causative Agent	Vector	Geography	Signs and Symptoms	Diagnosis and Findings	Selected Treatments	Comments
Lyme Disease	*Borrelia burgdorferi*	Deer tick (black legged) – main reservoir is white-footed mouse	Most in NE or Great Lakes. No cases in Montana.	Erythema migrans, lymphadenopathy, fever, arthritis, CNS late (3 stages)	Clinical. Joint fluid PCR, serology	amoxicillin 250–500 mg tid *or* doxycycline 100 mg bid 10–21 days Doxycycline prophylaxis: 200 mg × 1 dose	Bell's-like palsy should provoke tick bite questions. New vaccine "LymeRix"
Rocky Mountain Spotted Fever (RMSF)	*Rickettsia rickettsii*	Wood tick, dog tick	All states except Maine, Hawaii, and Alaska	Fever, headache, rash involving palms and soles	Thrombocytopenia, hyponatremia, rash biopsy, immunofluorescence	doxycycline 100 mg bid × 7 days	Not in the Rockies primarily and may not be "spotted"
Ehrlichiosis (HME)	*Ehrlichia chaffeensis*	Lone star tick (south central U.S.), dog tick (SE U.S.)	See vector box	Flulike syndrome and a rash	Leukopenia, thrombocytopenia, transaminitis, serology	doxycycline 100 mg bid × 7 days	Treat while diagnostics are pending (RMSF mimic)
Ehrlichiosis (HGE)	*Anaplasma phagocytophilum*	Deer tick	Midwest and NE US	Flulike syndrome and a rash	Leukopenia, thrombocytopenia, transaminitis, serology	doxycycline 100 mg BID × 7 days	Treat while diagnostics are pending (RMSF mimic)
Tularemia	*Francisella tularensis*	Lone star tick, wood tick, dog tick – also deer and horse flies	All states except Hawaii	Fever, headache, sore throat, cough, ARDS, chest pain (pericarditis)	Serology, rabbit exposure, CXR (triad of effusion, adenopathy, ovoid opacities)	aminoglycoside of choice IV 7–14 days *plus* chloramphenicol for meningitis	"Rabbit fever," possible bioweapon
Babesiosis	*Babesia microti, Babesia divergens*	Deer tick (black legged)	NE U.S.	Flulike syndrome, jaundice, renal failure	Hemolytic anemia, "Maltese cross" (on smear), serology, PCR	clindamycin 600 mg PO tid *plus* quinine 650 mg PO tid × 7 days each	Malaria-like
Colorado Tick Fever	RNA orbivirus	Wood tick	Rocky Mountains	Flulike syndrome, "saddleback fever"	Serology, immunofluorescence	Supportive care	Treat while diagnostics are pending
Tick Paralysis	Noninfectious (neurotoxin)	*Dermacentor andersoni, D. variabilis,* and others	Rocky Mountains – NW U.S./Canada	Ascending paralysis	Find feeding tick (usually on a child)	Remove tick	Look for a tick in the scalp region
Relapsing Fever	Borrelial spirochete	*Ornithodoros* genus (main reservoir rabbits and rodents)	West of the Mississippi	Flulike syndrome, epistaxis, myocarditis, iridocyclitis	Splenomegaly, bone marrow aspiration, leukocytosis	doxycycline 100 mg bid until 48 hours no symptoms	Jarish-Herxheimer reaction
North Asian Tick Typhus and African Tick Typhus	*Rickettsia sibirica* and *Rickettsia conorii*	*Ixodes* ticks of Northeast and Central Asia (*R. sibirica*) and subequatorial Africa (*R. conorii*)	Northeast and Central Asia (*R. sibirica*) and subequatorial Africa (*R. conorii*)	Cardinal symptoms of rickettsiosis but not usually fatal or with high morbidity as with RMSF	Fever, headache, rash, eschar, lymphadenopathy are typical	doxycycline 100 mg PO bid for 7 to 10 days	

ARDS, acute respiratory distress syndrome; CNS, central nervous system; CXR, chest x-ray; PCR, polymerase chain reaction.

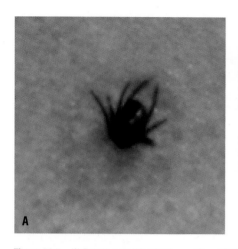
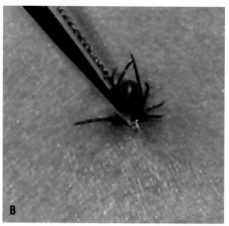
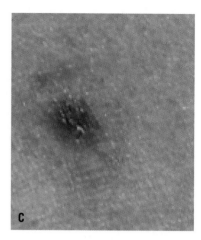

Figure 52.5 (A) Deeply embedded *Ixodes pacificus*. (B) Forceps removal with forceps as close to the head as possible and slow, but firm traction. (C) Successful removal of the tick and its head. The patient had been camping in a Lyme endemic county and was treated with doxycycline for prophylaxis. Courtesy Dr. Matthew Lewin.

Table 52.8 Subtypes of Myiasis Infestation

Facultative (Semi-Specific) Agents	Wounds and ulcers become colonized by maggots but there is limited live tissue damage. *Fannia canicularis* (lesser house fly) and *Musca domestica* (house fly) are commonly involved. Other species such as the green blowfly and humpback flies can also result in facultative myiasis.
Obligatory (or Specific) Agents	Have a larval stage that can grow only in the living tissue of an animal host. Tissue destruction and more rarely, superinfection follow. *Dermatobia hominis* (botfly) and *Cordylobia anthropophaga* (tumbu fly) are the most common agents. Old and New World screw worms are very invasive obligatory agents that can be quite disfiguring and can even invade bone.
Accidental (Nonspecific) Agents	Egg-stage flies are ingested on contaminated food or come into contact with the genitourinary tract.

Furuncular cutaneous myiasis presents as a pruritic papule 2–3 mm across that gradually increases in size with a diameter of 1–3 cm. The respiratory sinuses of the maggot may be seen at the center of this furuncle, and it is through this punctuate opening that the larva breathes. The oft-quoted cure, using a strip of bacon, works because the grease occludes the opening and suffocates the larvae. Because botfly larvae develop for a long period (5–12 weeks) in their host tissues, a chronic furunculosis with persistent pruritic papules not responsive to antibiotics is a common historical feature. In the United States, botfly (*D. hominis*) is more commonly found in a traveler who has returned from Central or South America or in military personnel returning overseas from central Asian republics such as Afghanistan. Infestation often does not become apparent until long after the return from the trip, and patients may not associate the travel history with the lesion.

Differential Diagnosis

Important questions to ask include:

- Any travel history within the last 6 weeks?
- History of exposure to biting flies?
- History of furuncular disease?

Key features that distinguish myiasis from infestation by smaller arthropods such as mites, lice, bedbugs and fleas (Table 52.10) are:

- the size of lesions and degree of inflammation
- the relatively small number of furuncles in the typical traveler (though massive infestations can occur in the intoxicated who fail to notice the biting).

Table 52.9 Clinical Features: Myiasis

Course	Symptoms develop over weeks to months
Transmission	Fly deposits eggs within a wound
Obligatory (i.e., Requires Host to Complete Life Cycle)	• Furuncular myiasis occurs because the larval stage can only grow in living tissue of host • Tissue destruction and rarely superinfection occurs • *Dermatobia hominis* (botfly) and *Cordylobia anthropophaga* (tumbu fly) are most common • Old and New World screw worms are very invasive agents that can be disfiguring and invade bone
Facultative (Semispecific) Agents	• Wounds and ulcers become colonized by maggots • Limited tissue damage • *Fannia canicularis* (lesser house fly), *Musca domestica* (house fly) are commonly involved • Green blowfly and humpback flies are also facultative agents
Accidental (Nonspecific) Agents	Occurs when egg-stage flies are ingested on contaminated food leading to infestation of the GI or GU tract and deposition of larvae into feces. May or may not be symptomatic.
Signs and Symptoms	• Obvious visualization of larvae (maggots) • Pruritic papules ~ 2–3 mm in furuncular cutaneous myiasis
Diagnosis	Direct visualization
Treatment	• Good wound care • Furuncular myiasis – surgical or suffocation removal methods

GI, gastrointestinal; GU, genitourinary.

Table 52.10 Differential Diagnosis of the Persistent Pruritic Papule

Infestation	Physical Characteristics	Location and Historical Features
Scabies	Excoriated papules with burrows	Intertriginous areas with moist, warm skin
Leishmaniasis	Indurated, ulcerated papules and plaques with rolled or raised borders (cheese pizza lesion)	Travel to an area with sandflies (e.g., military returning from Iraq)
Cutaneous myiasis	Tender, ulcerated papules with central punctum. Nodules may move!	Travel to area with botfly or tumbu fly
Furunculosis	Erythematous perifollicular nodules	Current MRSA epidemic in U.S.

- there is commonly a readily identifiable punctate opening at the crown of the pruritic papule and a magnifying glass will allow visualization of the parasite's breathing apparatus

Other conditions to consider are:

- bedbug infestation
- excoriated allergic dermatitis
- primary soft-tissue infection
- skin picking or delusional parasitosis

Laboratory and Radiographic Findings

Exact diagnosis is made by allowing the extracted larvae to pupate and complete its growth to the adult fly, which can then be speciated, though many entomologists can identify species from the larval stages. This is rarely done in practice, however, and diagnosis is usually made based on the history and examination.

Ultrasound may aid in diagnosis and surgical debridement of myiasis. Using a 10-MHz ultrasound probe, a mobile element of a furuncle confirms the presence of the larvae below the skin and may guide surgical removal.

Treatment and Prophylaxis

Myiasis associated with wounds (due to semispecific agents) is usually a self-limited problem easily managed by good wound care. The maggots seen in the wound can usually be irrigated away (along with any other eggs). Good wound care and dressings will prevent reinfestation. The psychological aspects of myiasis may be more difficult to manage and may require referral.

Furuncular myiasis due to obligatory agents is more difficult to manage. Surgical incision and extraction of larvae should be performed under local anesthesia. Injecting the area beneath the larvae with lidocaine may force them to surface and allow tweezer extraction. Suffocation techniques with bacon, petroleum jelly, or mineral oil may also allow removal. These approaches are particularly useful in endemic areas with few resources. Care must be taken to avoid partial removal. Retention of dead larvae can result in local infection and granuloma formation.

COMPLICATIONS AND ADMISSION CRITERIA

It would be unusual to have to admit a patient for primary arthropod infestations such as lice and scabies. However, these patients frequently have concomitant psychiatric or immune-compromised states that place them at risk for complications from compromised dermis. Infections resulting from bites or the transmission of bacterial and/or viral pathogens by arthropods may cause debilitating or life-threatening disease. Some diseases transmitted by ticks such as *Rickettsia sibirica* can present as fever and fixed lymphadenopathy months after exposure and be mistaken for lymphoma with constitutional symptoms. Others, such as RMSF, can be fatal and require a high degree of clinical suspicion and rapid treatment in order to avert disaster. All patients strongly suspected to have RMSF should be admitted.

INFESTATION AND INFECTION CONTROL

Prevention is the cornerstone of infestation and infection control. Fastidious attention to risk factors for exposure and to contact identification can prevent major outbreaks of infestation and disease. For common urban infestations such as lice, personal and public hygiene are paramount. Hospitals, psychiatric facilities, jails and emergency departments are particularly susceptible to minor or major outbreaks of scabies and lice if infested individuals are not treated appropriately, including decontamination of skin, hair, clothes, and bed sheets. Health care workers treating patients suspected to have scabies should use universal precautions. Diseases such as RMSF and Lyme disease are not transmitted by human-to-human contact.

PEARLS AND PITFALLS

1. Treatment failures with scabies and lice are becoming more common because of resistance. Ivermectin has emerged as a simple, effective, albeit more expensive oral treatment option.
2. Mites are ubiquitous ectoparasites that affect humans via their feeding or via their allergenicity, potentially causing asthma, eczema, and dermatitis.
3. Most mites feed in the larval stage, typically resulting in a very pruritic papular or nodular lesion.
4. Ticks are major vectors for a wide array of diseases, and Lyme disease is the most common tick-borne disease in the United States.
5. Most myiasis in the United States is due to facultative organisms that usually cause little or no live tissue damage – these maggots generally debride the wounds they infest.
6. In the United States, obligatory or specific myiasis is primarily a disease of travelers.
7. Delusional parasitosis (Figure 52.6) is common in psychiatric disorders and, in particular, in abusers of sympathomimetic drugs, such as methamphetamine. Patients may present with samples of lint, scabs, or labeled photographs as "evidence."

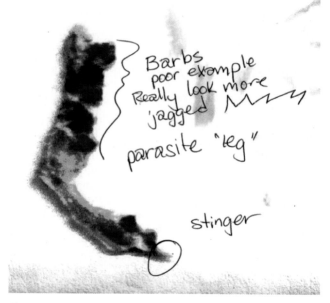

Figure 52.6 Delusional parasitosis. The patient presented with bags and labeled photos of scabs as evidence of infestation. Photograph and copy courtesy of Dr. Matthew Lewin.

REFERENCES

Bratton RL, Corey R. Tick-borne disease. Am Fam Physician 2005 Jun 15;71(12):2323–30.

Caumes E. Skin diseases. In: Travel medicine, 1st ed. New York: Mosby, 2004.

Centers for Disease Control and Prevention (CDC). Epidemiologic notes and reports scabies in health care facilities – Iowa. MMWR 1988;37(11):178–9.

Chin RL. Cellulitis due to bot fly larvae. N Engl J Med 1997;337:429–30.

Chosidow O. Clinical practice. Scabies. N Engl J Med 2006 Apr 20;354(16):1718–27.

Edlow JA. Lyme disease and related tick-borne illnesses. Ann Emerg Med 1999 Jun;33(6):680–93.

Johnston G, Sladden M. Scabies: diagnosis and treatment. BMJ 2005 Sept 17;331(7517):619–22.

Roberts RJ. Clinical practice. Head lice. N Engl J Med 2002 May 23;346(21):1645–50.

ADDITIONAL READINGS

Auerbach PS. Wilderness medicine, 5th ed. New York: Mosby, 2007.

Heukelbach J, Feldmeier H. Ectoparasites – the underestimated realm. Lancet 2004 Mar 13;363(9412):889–91.

Szepietowski JC, et al. Delusional parasitosis in dermatological practice. J Eur Acad Dermatol Venereol 2007;21(4):462–5.

53. Fever in Pregnancy

Shani Delaney, Deborah Cohan, and Patricia A. Robertson

INTRODUCTION

The work-up of fever in pregnancy requires special consideration of the effect of fever itself on the fetus, the impact of the pregnant state on the etiologic illness, the impact of the illness on the pregnancy, and the limitations that concerns for fetal well-being may place on diagnostic and therapeutic modalities.

The definition of fever in pregnancy is 100.4°F or 38.0°C. The normal fetal heart rate is between 110 and 160 beats per minute. Maternal fever often causes a fetal tachycardia, sometimes up to 180–200 beats per minute. It is important to treat maternal fever with antipyretics, especially in the first trimester, to decrease the risk of birth defects. The consequences of an episode of hyperthermia depend on the extent of the temperature elevation, its duration, and the stage of fetal development. Mild exposures during the preimplantation period and more severe exposures during embryonic and fetal development can result in miscarriage. Hyperthermia (usually at a level of 2.0°C elevation over normal) can cause a wide range of structural and functional defects in the fetus, ranging from central nervous system defects to growth issues. Pregnant women are also advised to be cautious about hot tubs or spa use in early pregnancy, based on their possibility of raising core maternal temperature. Although it is important to recognize that most pregnancies exposed to maternal fever will result in a normal neonate, all fever in pregnant women should be aggressively controlled. The most commonly used antipyretic is acetaminophen in standard doses. Avoid nonsteroidal anti-inflammatory agents, such as ibuprofen, because they have been associated with spontaneous abortions, and at high doses later in pregnancy can affect the fetal kidneys and cause premature closure of the ductus arteriosus.

With the exception of chorioamnionitis as a possible etiology, the differential diagnosis for fever in a pregnant woman is similar to that in a nonpregnant woman. Because of the general suppression of the immune system, however, women are more susceptible to infections while pregnant. There are also additional considerations depending on the risk a particular infection may pose to the fetus.

Laboratory Considerations

When diagnosing a fever in pregnancy, interpretation of laboratory values also differs slightly: a mild leukocytosis in pregnancy is normal and will continue approximately 1 week into the postpartum period. There is often a mild anemia and decrease in serum osmolality due to hemodilution. Alkaline phosphatase is produced by the placenta and is usually elevated in pregnancy. Elevation in fibrinogen is also normal in pregnancy, and a fibrinogen level in the low or normal range during pregnancy should raise concern for disseminated intravascular coagulopathy if there is clinical suspicion. Arterial blood gas (ABG) has different ranges of normal because of changes in maternal physiology: increases in minute ventilation elevate PaO_2 levels and cause a mild hyperventilation, resulting in a chronic respiratory alkalosis with metabolic compensation. Normal ABG values in pregnancy are: pH 7.4–7.45, $PaCO_2$ 27–32 mm Hg, serum bicarbonate 18–21 mEq/L. Creatinine and blood urea nitrogen (BUN) should decrease mildly in pregnancy because of an increased glomerular filtration rate. Low thyroid-stimulating hormone (TSH) values are normal in the early first trimester because of cross reactivity of the alpha subunit of human chorionic gonadotropin (HCG) with the TSH receptor, with values returning to normal by the end of the first trimester.

Other findings specific to pregnancy include a holosystolic murmur at the left upper sternal border (due to a 30–50% increase in cardiac output) and a mild maternal tachycardia.

Maternal blood pressure decreases early in pregnancy, with the nadir at 16–20 weeks' gestation, and then slowly rises to prepregnancy levels near term.

Radiologic Considerations

The need for diagnostic imaging to support a diagnosis in pregnancy must be weighed against concerns about radiation exposure to the fetus (Table 53.1). Risks to the fetus depend greatly on the amount of radiation exposure and the gestational age at time of exposure. Small amounts of radiation (equivalent to fewer than 500 chest x-rays) in utero do not cause an increased risk of birth defects. The risk of childhood leukemias may rise from approximately 1 in 3000 to 1 in 2000 after intrauterine exposure to radiation at diagnostic levels.

In early first trimester (up to 2 weeks) the concern for radiation exposure is primarily due to the risk of spontaneous abortion – risks can be described to the patient as an "all or nothing" risk. During organogenesis, between 2 and approximately 15 weeks, concern arises primarily over brain development, malformations, and possible effects on lifetime IQ. However, severe mental retardation has only been seen in very high radiation exposures, such as after the World War II atomic bombs in Hiroshima and Nagasaki. Teratogenic effects on lifetime cancer risk, brain development, adult height, and other malformations still occur during weeks 15–26 of gestation, though the amount of radiation needed to cause these effects is much higher than at earlier gestational ages. From 26 weeks' gestation to delivery, the risk of radiation to the fetus is felt to be equivalent to that of the newborn. Increased risk for major anomalies from diagnostic levels of radiation after 26 weeks' gestation has not been documented. However, the risk for increased incidence of cancer later in life still exists. *The maximum amount of ionizing radiation that a fetus should be exposed to in utero is a cumulative dose of 5 rad.*

Ultrasound and magnetic resonance imaging (MRI) are felt to be safe in pregnancy with no known teratogenic effects.

Medication Prescribing

Medications are classified for use in pregnancy as A, B, C, D, or X. In general, medications classified as A and B are considered safe in pregnancy, and C medications are acceptable to use if the benefit of the treatment outweighs the risk. Medications classified as D and X are contraindicated. However, this classification system is imperfect, because some of the data are based on animal studies rather than human studies, and updates are not always timely.

Surgical Considerations

If surgery is indicated for the treatment of an infection, early intervention is important. This is especially true in the case of appendicitis, because perforation can cause early delivery and fetal sepsis. Anesthesia is safe during pregnancy, as long as medications and doses are appropriately adjusted.

PYELONEPHRITIS

Epidemiology

Urinary tract infection (UTI) is the most common medical complication of pregnancy and, if untreated, places patients

Table 53.1 Estimated Fetal Exposure for Various Diagnostic Imaging Methods

Examination Type	Estimated Fetal Dose per Examination (rad)	Number of Examinations Required for a Cumulative 5-rad Dose
Plain Films		
Skull	0.004	1250
Dental	0.0001	50,000
Cervical spine	0.002	2500
Upper or lower extremity	0.001	5000
Chest (two views)	0.00007	71,429
Mammogram	0.020	250
Abdominal (multiple views)	0.245	20
Thoracic spine	0.009	555
Lumbosacral spine	0.359	13
Intravenous pyelogram	1.398	3
Pelvis	0.040	125
Hip (single view)	0.213	23
CT Scans (Slice Thickness: 10 mm)		
Head (10 slices)	<0.050	>100
Chest (10 slices)	<0.1	>50
Abdomen (10 slices)	2.6	1
Lumbar (5 slices)	3.5	1
Pelvimetry (1 slice with scout film)	0.250	20
Fluoroscopic Studies		
Upper GI series	0.056	89
Barium swallow	0.006	833
Barium enema	3.986	1
Nuclear Medicine Studies		
Most studies using technetium (^{99m}Tc)	<0.5	>10
Hepatobiliary technetium HIDA scan	0.150	33
Ventilation-perfusion scan (total)	0.215	23
Perfusion portion: Technetium	0.175	28
Ventilation portion: xenon (^{133}Xe)	0.040	125
Iodine (^{131}I) at fetal thyroid tissue	590	Contraindicated in pregnancy
Environmental Sources (for Comparison)		
Background radiation (cumulative over 9 months)	0.1	N/A

CT, computed tomographic; GI, gastrointestinal; HIDA, hepatobiliary iminodiacetic acid.
Adapted from Toppenberg, Hill, and Miller, 1999.

at risk of pyelonephritis. A urinary tract infection is always considered a complicated UTI in a pregnant patient.

- *Escherichia coli* is the causative organism in 80–90% of acute infections.
- *Staphylococcus saprophyticus* is the second most common causative organism for UTIs in sexually active women.
- Other common gram-negative organisms are *Klebsiella*, *Enterobacter*, *Proteus*, and *Pseudomonas*.
- Group B *Streptococcus* (GBS) is not typically considered pathogenic outside of pregnancy, but untreated GBS UTI is associated with preterm delivery.

Table 53.2 Urinary Tract Infections in Pregnancy

Organisms	• *Escherichia coli* is responsible for 85–90% of infections. • The remaining 10–15% typically are caused by: ○ *Enterococcus* ○ group B *Streptococcus* ○ *Staphylococcus* ○ *Proteus* ○ *Pseudomonas* ○ *Citrobacter* ○ *Enterobacter*
Cystitis Signs and Symptoms	• Frequency, urgency, dysuria, hematuria • Suprapubic tenderness • Low back pain • Often abrupt onset • *Absence* of fever or chills
Pyelonephritis Signs and Symptoms	• Frequency, urgency, dysuria, hematuria • Back or flank pain* • Fever* and chills • Nausea and vomiting • Costovertebral angle tenderness

*85% of women will present with fever and back pain.

Table 53.3 Laboratory Diagnosis of Pyelonephritis versus Cystitis

	Cystitis	Pyelonephritis
Pyuria	+	+
Bacteriuria	+	+
Hematuria	+/−	+/−
Positive urine culture (>100K colonies of a single organism)	+	+
WBC casts on urinalysis	−	+
Leukocytosis	−	+
Positive blood cultures*	−	+/−

*Debatable utility as only 10–15% positive, and the organism will almost exclusively be the same as that which is isolated from urine, and the duration of treatment is not changed by positive blood cultures.

The incidence of acute pyelonephritis in pregnancy is 1–2.5%. In 10–18% of affected patients, it will recur within the same pregnancy. Asymptomatic bacteriuria (ASB), defined as 10^5 colony-forming units (CFU)/mL *of a single organism* on two successive urine cultures by clean catch or 10^2 CFU *of a single organism* on straight catherization, leads to pyelonephritis in 20–30% of cases, and widespread prenatal screening to detect and treat ASB has greatly reduced the incidence of acute pyelonephritis in pregnancy. Risk factors for pyelonephritis include a prior episode of pyelonephritis, ASB, urinary tract obstructive abnormalities, or calculi.

Clinical Features

Table 53.2 summarizes the most important clinical features of urinary tract infections in pregnancy.

Differential Diagnosis

Key features that distinguish pyelonephritis from cystitis are:

- fever and back pain
- white blood cell (WBC) casts on urinalysis
- leukocytosis
- nausea and vomiting (due to peritoneal irritation)

Other conditions to consider include:

- musculoskeletal pain
- appendicitis
- nephrolithiasis
- preterm premature rupture of membranes (PPROM) with amnionitis
- preterm labor

Laboratory Diagnosis

Table 53.3 summarizes the laboratory diagnosis of cystitis versus pyelonephritis.

Treatment and Prophylaxis

Regional antibiotic resistance rates for common organisms causing urinary tract infections should be considered when choosing an antibiotic regimen.

- In general, cephalosporins and penicillins are considered safe in pregnancy.
- Some sources suggest avoiding sulfonamides near term due to the risk of hyperbilirubinemia in the newborn, though there are no human reports of hyperbilirubinemia in the newborn exposed to third-trimester sulfas. They are considered safe to use throughout pregnancy (though they require folate supplementation for chronic use in first trimester).
- Nitrofurantoin is commonly used to treat lower UTIs in pregnancy; however, it is not effective for treating pyelonephritis and should be reserved for daily bacteriuria suppression following complete treatment of pyelonephritis.
- Tetracyclines are contraindicated in pregnancy because of discoloration of fetal teeth and inhibition of bone growth.
- Aminoglycosides should be avoided in pregnancy because of fetal ototoxicity and risk of congenital deafness. However, in patients with anaphylaxis to penicillins and cephalosporins, aminoglycosides may be the next antibiotic of choice.
- Quinolones should be used with special consideration because of potential bone and cartilage abnormalities in the fetus. However, recent safety data show that these risks are very low and quinolones can be used in pregnancy for UTIs and pyelonephritis, particularly if there are no other options because of bacterial resistance to other antibiotic classes.

Initial treatment of pyelonephritis in pregnancy is usually a broad-spectrum cephalosporin administered intravenously until 24–48 hours after the patient becomes afebrile (Table 53.4). Continuation of treatment with oral antibiotics (determined by final urine culture results) is recommended to complete a 14-day course of therapy. There is some evidence for safe outpatient therapy for pyelonephritis in pregnancy, in select populations. Outpatient regimens include two

Table 53.4 Treatment of UTIs in Pregnancy

Cystitis	cephalexin 500 mg PO qid × 7 days *or* nitrofurantoin 100 mg PO bid × 7 days *or* ampicillin 500 mg PO bid × 7 days (*not* for empiric prescription; use only for known sensitive organisms) *or* amoxicillin 500 mg PO tid × 7 days (*not* for empiric prescription; use only for known sensitive organisms) trimethoprim-sulfamethoxazole if sensitive
Pyelonephritis	**First-line agents**: ceftriaxone 1 g IV or IM q24h until afebrile × 48 hours, then change to PO to complete 14 days *or* cefazolin 1 g IV q8h until afebrile × 48 hours, then change to PO to complete 14 days **Second-line agents**: piperacillin 4 g IV q8h until afebrile 48 hours, then change to PO to complete 14 days *or* ampicillin 2g IV q6h plus gentamicin 3–5 mg/kg/day IV in three divided doses until afebrile × 48 hours, then change to PO to complete 14 days (*Caution*: With gentamicin in pregnancy, use only if no other acceptable coverage based on sensitivities; do not start as empiric therapy) **Followed by**: nitrofurantoin 100 mg PO qd for prophylaxis until delivery *Never* start with an oral agent; always use IV antibiotics for initial treatment for 24–48 hours, or until afebrile

Table 53.5 Prophylaxis for UTIs in Pregnancy

Cystitis	All patients need a repeat urine culture for test of cure after completing treatment – usually a week after completion of antibiotics. If a pregnant patient has two episodes of cystitis within a single pregnancy, she should be placed on antibiotic suppression for the remainder of the pregnancy. Nitrofurantoin 100 mg PO daily is an acceptable regimen.
Pyelonephritis	After completion of a 14-day course of antibiotics determined by the final urine culture, prophylaxis should continue until delivery. Nitrofurantoin 100 mg PO daily is an acceptable regimen.

doses of ceftriaxone 1 g intravenously (IV) or intramuscularly (IM), 24 hours apart, followed by oral antibiotics determined by the final urine culture results to complete a 14-day course (Table 53.5).

Complications and Admission Criteria

Major maternal complications of pyelonephritis in pregnancy include:

- respiratory insufficiency or acute respiratory distress syndrome (ARDS)
- anemia
- renal dysfunction

- bacteremia occurs in 10–15% of pregnant women with acute pyelonephritis; however, it is rare to see overt sepsis

Major fetal complications include:

- preterm labor
- preterm birth
- low birth weight
- fetal demise

Any pregnant patient with pyelonephritis should be evaluated for admission, and threshold for admission beyond 24 weeks gestation should be very low. There is some evidence for safe outpatient management of pyelonephritis in pregnancies at less than 24 weeks gestation with strict criteria. The criteria that *exclude* outpatient management and should always prompt admission for pyelonephritis at less than 24 weeks gestation are:

- diabetes, HIV, or any other form of immunosupression
- clinical signs of sepsis
- respiratory insufficiency
- initial temperature greater than 39.8°C
- blood pressure less than 90/50 mm Hg
- sustained pulse greater than 140 bpm
- creatinine greater than 1.4 mg/dL
- WBC greater than 20×10^9/L
- a known allergy to cephalosporins
- inability to tolerate oral intake
- inability to follow instructions
- inability to reliably follow up
- any serious underlying medical illness, including a known renal or urologic problem

Pearls and Pitfalls

1. Acute pyelonephritis is one of most common serious medical complications of pregnancy, seen in 1–2% of pregnant women, with the majority in second and third trimester.
2. Contraindicated antibiotics in treating UTI during pregnancy include tetracyclines and fluoroquinolones.
3. Treatment of asymptomatic bacteriuria in pregnancy is essential, as it has been associated with pyelonephritis, preterm labor, hypertension in pregnancy, and early pregnancy loss.
4. Avoid urinary catheterization if possible during pregnancy because it may increase the risk of subsequent infection.
5. Hydroureter and mild hydronephrosis of pregnancy is a physiological change of pregnancy. Dilatation begins by the 7th week of pregnancy and progresses until term. Both mechanical and hormonal changes contribute. The right ureter and kidney are more affected than the left because of rotation of the uterus. Postpartum ureters return to normal in most patients by 2 months.
6. There is an increase risk of respiratory distress syndrome in pregnant women with pyelonephritis. The mechanism is not well understood.

RESPIRATORY INFECTIONS
Epidemiology

Viral upper respiratory infection (URI) is common in pregnant women, and only symptomatic treatment is indicated.

Table 53.6 Clinical Features: Respiratory Infections

Viral URI	• Fever, chills, rhinorrhea, myalgias, cough **Treatment:** Supportive. Acetaminophen for fever and guaifenesin for cough
Acute Bronchitis	• Often low-grade fever and cough **Treatment:** Supportive. Acetaminophen for fever and guaifenesin for cough
Influenza	• CBC may show marked leukocytosis • Blood cultures are typically negative • Chest x-ray is usually normal. Anteroposterior neck radiograph may show "steeple sign" or irregularity of the proximal mucosa • Culture secretions/DFA are positive **Treatment:** Supportive
Pneumonia	• See Chapter 32, Community-Acquired Pneumonia, for more details • Chest x-ray with proper shielding has minimal effects on the fetus – do not hesitate to use this modality if needed **Treatment:** Antibiotics as indicated. Cephalosporins and macrolides are safe to use in pregnancy. Hospitalize for suspected varicella pneumonia because maternal morbidity is high.

CBC, complete blood count; DFA, direct fluorescent antibody.

The incidence of lower respiratory tract infections in women of childbearing age is about 64 per 1000, ranging from acute bronchitis, to influenza, to exacerbations of underlying lung disease such as asthma, to pneumonia. The diagnosis of pneumonia represents less than 1.5% of lower respiratory tract infections in pregnant women. Pertussis should always be considered in a pregnant woman when cough is a prominent symptom.

Clinical Features

Acute bronchitis is generally mild and self-limiting (Table 53.6). Chronic bronchitis has been associated with placental abruption and should be treated with inhalers and antibiotics (if bacterial origin is suspected) because it may progress to a parenchymal infection. The development of frank fever after several days of low-grade temperature elevation and cough may represent the development of pneumonia.

Differential Diagnosis

Pneumonia must be considered in any pregnant woman with respiratory symptoms and a fever. Oxygen saturation measurements and chest auscultation are always indicated, and chest radiograph with shielding of the fetus may be indicated. The WBC count may or may not be elevated. If there is a diagnosis of varicella with respiratory distress, it is critical to rule out varicella pneumonia, because significant maternal mortality is associated. Risk factors for the development of varicella pneumonia in pregnant women include smoking and more than 100 cutaneous lesions. Often these patients are admitted to an intensive care unit (ICU) setting and treated with intravenous (IV) acyclovir. All patients suspected of having varicella infection should be isolated from other pregnant women and newborns.

Infants born to pregnant patients with a current or recent pneumonia are born earlier and weigh less. Paroxysmal coughing spasms have been associated with preterm premature rupture of the membranes (PPROM), as well as occasional rib fractures, so medical control of coughing is important. Although the placenta usually acts as an excellent filter to prevent infection of the fetus, occasionally transplacental infection will occur, especially in human immunodeficiency virus (HIV)-infected patients.

Key features that require different management of respiratory distress and fever in pregnancy are:

- Any pregnant woman with respiratory symptoms and fever must be evaluated for pneumonia. Once diagnosed, she should be treated because of the associated risk of prematurity and low birth weight.
- Varicella pneumonia is associated with high maternal mortality, and patients should be admitted to an ICU setting in isolation.
- Paroxysmal coughing has been associated with PPROM and should be treated symptomatically.

Laboratory Diagnosis

Routine laboratory tests are not indicated, although a complete blood count may show marked leukocytosis. Blood cultures are typically negative. A chest radiograph can help in the diagnosis of pneumonia; the radiation exposure is minimal with proper fetal shielding.

Baseline respiratory rate and minute ventilation are increased during pregnancy, because of physiologic changes of pregnancy as well as the pressure of the abdominal contents against the diaphragm. A "normal" adult pCO_2 level should raise alarms in a pregnant woman, because a respiratory alkalosis is expected in pregnancy.

Treatment

For viral URIs, hydration, acetaminophen, and guaifenesin are acceptable treatments. Pseudoephedrine should not be used in the first trimester because of reported increased incidence of limb defects of the fetus, or in the third trimester if there is any maternal hypertension present, because the drug may constrict already compromised placental blood vessels.

Influenza causes significant maternal morbidity and mortality in pregnant women. Safety of the neuraminidase inhibitors for the treatment of influenza has not been established in pregnancy, and they are not routinely recommended. For prevention of influenza during pregnancy, the flu vaccine (killed vaccine) without thimerosal is recommended in all trimesters. Currently, the nasal-spray influenza vaccine (FluMist), which is made with live attenuated influenza viruses, is contraindicated for use in pregnancy.

As always, consider the teratogenicity of antibiotics before choosing a regimen. Cephalosporins and macrolides are safe treatment options for common community-acquired pneumonia in pregnancy. See Chapter 32, Community-Acquired Pneumonia.

Complications and Admission Criteria

Many respiratory complications are similar in the pregnant and nonpregnant patient; however, clinicians should have a lower threshold for admitting pregnant patients with pneumonia, because of potential complications of low birth weight and prematurity. PPROM is a complication associated with paroxysmal coughing.

Infection Control

Respiratory precautions for the pregnant population are similar to those for nonpregnant populations. Any patient with suspected varicella pneumonia should be isolated from other pregnant patients. According to 2006 recommendations from the CDC Advisory Committee on Immunization Practices (ACIP), all pregnant women should receive a Tdap vaccine (tetanus, diphtheria, pertussis) in the second or third trimester or postpartum period as a pertussis prevention campaign. Offer influenza immunization to all pregnant women.

Pearls and Pitfalls

1. Varicella pneumonia carries significant morbidity and mortality for a pregnant woman. Do not hesitate to hospitalize anyone with concern for varicella pneumonia. See later section on TORCH infections for more details.
2. Remember the physiologic changes in ABG findings during pregnancy when interpreting a blood gas. A "normal" CO_2 level on ABG in a pregnant woman should raise alarms, because you should expect a low CO_2 value consistent with a respiratory alkalosis in pregnancy.
3. The risk to the fetus of a chest x-ray is minimal with proper shielding – never withhold diagnostic imaging of the chest in a pregnant woman if it will assist in the diagnosis.

APPENDICITIS

Epidemiology

Appendicitis is the most common nonobstetric condition requiring surgery during pregnancy. Because of changes in physiology and anatomy during pregnancy, diagnosis can be delayed, thereby increasing risk of perforation, preterm labor, preterm delivery, and fetal sepsis and loss. The prevalence of appendicitis in the pregnant population ranges from 0.05% to 0.13%. This is approximately the same rate as in the general population, but the rate of perforation is higher in pregnant women.

Rates of preterm contractions associated with appendicitis are as high as 83% in the third trimester. Preterm labor occurs in up to 13% of pregnant patients with appendicitis in the third trimester. Fetal loss rates in uncomplicated appendicitis are low, ranging from 0% to 1.5%. However, this risk rises significantly in ruptured cases, ranging from 20% to 35%.

Clinical Presentation

Appendicitis commonly presents in pregnancy with signs and symptoms similar to those in nonpregnant women: fever, anorexia, nausea, vomiting, abdominal pain starting in the periumbilical region and migrating to the right lower quadrant, leukocytosis, tachycardia, and rebound and guarding on abdominal examination (Table 53.7). However, normal pregnancy symptoms such as nausea, vomiting, and anorexia can lower clinical suspicion for appendicitis. Several anatomic changes can decrease the incidence of classic physical exam

Table 53.7 Clinical Features: Appendicitis

Signs and Symptoms	**Classic symptoms:** • Fever, anorexia, nausea, vomiting, abdominal pain starting in the periumbilical region and migrating to the right lower quadrant, leukocytosis, tachycardia, rebound and guarding on abdominal examination **Nonclassic symptoms:** • Displacement of the appendix by the gravid uterus can cause abdominal pain in any quadrant • Separation of the visceral and parietal peritoneum in pregnancy further decreases the ability to localize abdominal pain • Laxity of the abdominal muscles in late pregnancy can reduce rebound tenderness and guarding
Laboratory and Radiographic Findings	• Leukocytosis • Abdominal ultrasound, CT scan, or MRI with findings consistent with appendicitis

Treatment	• Appendectomy
	• Antibiotics:
	  Cephalosporins are safe in pregnancy, acceptable regimens include:
	  cefoxitin 1–2 g IV q6 *or*
	  cefotetan 1–2 g IV q12h *or*
	  ticarcillin-clavulanate 3.1 g IV q6h *or*
	  ampicillin-sulbactam 3 g IV q6h *or*
	  piperacillin-tazobactam 3.375 g IV q6h or 4.5 g IV q8h
	  For combination therapy to increase anaerobic coverage, metronidazole is safe in pregnancy: 500 mg IV q6–8h

CT, computed tomographic.

findings: displacement of the appendix by the gravid uterus can cause the abdominal pain of appendicitis to localize to any quadrant, separation of the visceral and parietal peritoneum in pregnancy further decreases the ability to localize abdominal pain, and laxity of the abdominal muscles in late pregnancy can reduce the rebound tenderness and guarding of peritoneal inflammation.

Differential Diagnosis

Any intra-abdominal process can occur in pregnancy and should always be considered, similar to the nonpregnant state. Nonetheless, some of the symptoms of appendicitis can be considered normal for pregnancy.

Key features that may help distinguish appendicitis from other conditions include:

- Hyperemesis gravidarum (refractory anorexia, nausea, and vomiting) is not associated with fever and leukocytosis.
- Septic abortion in its early presentation may include fever and abdominal pain – but it is usually associated with vaginal bleeding.
- Pyelonephritis will almost universally include back pain as a symptom, and the clean catch urinalysis will suggest infection (leukocyte esterase, nitrite, protein, blood).
- Round ligament pain typically occurs in the second trimester as the uterus continues to grow out of the pelvis. Round ligament pain is classically described by the patient as rapid, sharp, often radiating to the groin and

inguinal areas. It is never associated with fever, nausea, vomiting, or any laboratory abnormalities. It will resolve spontaneously, does not require any treatment, except acetaminophen as needed for pain control.

- Acute cholecystitis and hepatitis may present with right upper quadrant pain, fever, and elevated WBC. However, liver function tests should differentiate these diagnoses from appendicitis in pregnancy.
- Pelvic inflammatory disease (PID) and tubo-ovarian abscess (TOA). Although these infectious etiologies may present with abdominal pain, fever, elevated WBC and peritoneal signs, PID and TOA are extremely rare in pregnancy because of the decreased ability of organisms to ascend the genital tract during pregnancy.

Laboratory and Radiologic Diagnosis

Routine leukocytosis or elevated WBC is almost universally present in appendicitis in the general population. In pregnancy, mild elevations in WBC can be present and normal, adding to the difficulty of diagnosis. However, an elevated neutrophil count is never considered normal in pregnancy. Ultrasound is the imaging study of choice to evaluate the appendix in pregnancy. However, if confirmation of diagnosis cannot be made clinically or with ultrasound, a computed tomographic (CT) scan of the abdomen can be considered to increase sensitivity of detection. At institutions where MRI is readily available, as well as a radiologist experienced in interpreting the appearance of appendicitis in this modality, MRI can also be used.

Treatment

Ultimately, appendectomy is the treatment of choice for the pregnant woman, as for the general population. The laparoscopic technique has all the same benefits in pregnancy as in the general population (reduced narcotic use – of particular importance in pregnancy, less postoperative pain, early return of bowel function, early ambulation, and less hospitalization time) without any evidence of adverse effects as compared to open appendectomy. However, once a pregnancy is past 26 weeks, risk of perforation to the pregnant uterus increases with laparoscopy, so a laparotomy may be the preferred option. Antibiotic coverage for common gastrointestinal organisms can be used safely in pregnancy. In general, all cephalosporins are felt to be safe in pregnancy. For additional anaerobic coverage, metronidazole may also be considered.

Complications and Admission Criteria

Complications of appendicitis in pregnancy include perforation, preterm labor, preterm delivery, and fetal loss. Any pregnant woman with a confirmed diagnosis or suspicion for appendicitis should be admitted at any gestational age.

Pearls and Pitfalls

1. Do not delay diagnostic tests and imaging when appendicitis is suspected in a pregnant woman.
2. Appendicitis can be the great masquerader in pregnancy because of physiologic and anatomic differences in the

gravid state – it should always be in your differential diagnosis for abdominal pain and fever in pregnancy.
3. There are higher rates of perforation in pregnancy, likely because of delay in diagnosis of atypical presentations.

CHORIOAMNIONITIS
Epidemiology

Chorioamnionitis is an infection of the two membranes of the placenta (the chorion and the amnion) and the amniotic fluid that surrounds the baby. Chorioamnionitis can cause bacteremia and sepsis in the mother and may lead to preterm birth and serious infection in the newborn baby. Other terms for chorioamnionitis include intra-amniotic infection and amnionitis.

Chorioamnionitis occurs in about 2% of all pregnancies and is usually caused by bacteria that reach the uterus through the vagina. It usually occurs in the setting of ruptured membranes. Rarely intra-amniotic infection can occur with intact membranes, likely through transplacental hematogenous transmission of the infectious agent. For some organisms, such as *Listeria*, this is the most common route of infection. Risk of neonatal infection increases as the duration of ruptured membranes lengthens. Chorioamnionitis may initiate uteroplacental bleeding or a placental abruption. Labor and delivery may be rapid in the presence of chorioamnionitis.

Premature rupture of the membranes (PROM) happens in 5–10% of term pregnancies, and PPROM is the initiating event in 30% preterm births ("premature" refers to prior to the start of labor; "preterm" refers to before 37 weeks gestation). Bacteria causing chorioamnionitis reflect the bacteria inhabiting the vaginal environment: group B *Streptococcus* (GBS; about 30% of women carry this bacterium in their vaginas), *E. coli*, enterococci, *Gardnerella vaginalis*, peptostreptococci, and so forth. The vast majority of chorioamnionitis etiologies are multiorganism infections.

Clinical Features

Any pregnant patient who presents with a fever in the third trimester must be evaluated for uterine tenderness and ruptured membranes (Table 53.8). A dry, thin layer of vaginal fluid should be evaluated by microscopy for the presence of ferning, which suggests the presence of amniotic fluid and thus rupture of membranes. Sterile indicator paper or swabs can be used to check the pH of the vaginal fluid: A blue indicator of basic pH suggests the presence of amniotic fluid and raises concern for rupture of the membranes (although sperm and blood can also increase the pH of vaginal secretions). *Digital exam of the cervix is contraindicated when ruptured membranes are suspected.*

Examination may also reveal uterine irritability or frank contractions. Vaginal bleeding may also be a sign of impending labor or placental abruption in the setting of intrauterine infection.

Differential Diagnosis

Key features that may help distinguish chorioamnionitis from other conditions include:

Table 53.8 Clinical Features: Chorioamnionitis

Organisms (Prevalence %) (often multiorganism)	• Group B *Streptococcus* (GBS) (14.6) • *Escherichia coli* (8.2) • *Enterococcus* (5.4) • *Gardnerella vaginalis* (24.5) • *Peptostreptococcus* (9.4) • *Bacteroides bivius* (29.4) • *Bacteroides fragilis* (3.4) • *Fusobacterium* spp. (5.4) • *Mycoplasma hominis* (30.4) • *Ureaplasma urealyticum* (47.0) • *Listeria* is a rare cause of chorioamnionitis but has serious consequences for the fetus. See later section for more details.

Signs and Symptoms	• Fever
	• Significant maternal tachycardia (>120 bpm)
	• Fetal tachycardia (>160 bpm)
	• Tender or painful uterus
	• Malodorous amniotic fluid
	• Maternal leukocytosis
	• Possible uterine contractions or labor
	• If rupture of membranes:
	  ○ leakage of fluid from vagina
	  ○ pooling of vaginal fluid; vaginal pool fluid is nitrazine positive (blue) on pH paper
	  ○ ferning of dried amniotic fluid from vagina on microscope examination

Treatment	• Antibiotic regimen for chorioamnionitis:
	  ○ second- or third-generation cephalosporin such as cefotetan 2 g IV q12h or cefoxitin 2 g IV q8h
	  ○ ampicillin 2 g q6h *plus* gentamicin 5 mg/kg/24h IV dosed daily or divided q8h
	  ○ consider adding clindamycin 900 mg IV q8h
	• Never tocolyze (stop uterine contractions) in the setting of chorioamnionitis, because delivery is always indicated
	• Refrain from digital vaginal exams to reduce further ascending infections from the vagina
	• Delivery

Table 53.9 Laboratory Results of Chorioamnionitis

Study	Anticipated Results in Amnionitis
CBC with Differential	Leukocytosis – occurs commonly in normal labor, and in normal pregnancy. However, a significant left shift/neutrophil predominance should raise your suspicion for an acute infectious event.
Blood Cultures	Positive in only 10% of cases. Should only be drawn if there is concern for septic physiology.
Urinalysis and Culture	All patients should have a urine culture when amnionitis is suspected to rule out UTIs as an etiology for fever.
Amniocentesis	Should always be performed by an experienced clinician with ultrasound guidance to avoid fetal injury and placental bleeding. May be useful in cases of equivocal clinical diagnosis for chorioamnionitis. Basic amniotic fluid studies should include Gram stain, cell count, culture, glucose, and protein levels.

CBC, complete blood count.

Laboratory Diagnosis

The laboratory diagnosis of chorioamnionitis is limited as it is principally a clinical diagnosis. However, several tests may be useful (Table 53.9).

If not completed in the course of prenatal care, testing for *Chlamydia*, gonorrhea, and GBS should be done (*Chlamydia* and gonorrhea on cervical swabs or urine, and GBS on a swab from the outer third of the vagina and over the rectum).

Treatment

If rupture of membranes is confirmed (usually all three tests are positive: positive pooling of fluid in the vagina, positive indicator test, and positive ferning under the microscope of dried vaginal pool fluid) in the presence of a maternal fever, fetal tachycardia, and uterine tenderness, then the diagnosis is usually chorioamnionitis and the treatment is delivery, no matter what the gestational age.

Antibiotics should be started immediately. A second- or third-generation cephalosporin is an acceptable regimen. Additional regimens include ampicillin and gentamicin with or without clindamycin. If the pregnancy is viable (usually after 24 weeks), the fetus should be placed on a fetal heart monitor as part of the surveillance.

Occasionally a prolapsed umbilical cord can occur with rupture of the membranes and will often cause fetal bradycardia. Emergent delivery in the operating room is indicated.

If the pregnancy is preterm, consider giving steroids, such as betamethasone or dexamethasone, to decrease the risk of respiratory distress syndrome and other complications in the newborn. Never delay delivery in the setting of chorioamnionitis to wait for the effects of steroids.

Complications and Admission Criteria

Complications of chorioamnionitis include PPROM, preterm labor, preterm delivery, maternal sepsis (rare), neonatal sepsis, and fetal loss. Any pregnant woman with a confirmed

- **Appendicitis** – The abdominal exam may reveal significant rebound and abdominal tenderness distant from the uterus. History reveals persistent nausea and vomiting, and radiological imaging is consistent with appendicitis.
- **Pyelonephritis** – Physical exam often reveals unilateral costovertebral angle tenderness. Urine analysis is suspicious for infection and urine culture confirms the diagnosis of UTI.
- **Musculoskeletal pain** – Should not cause a febrile presentation. Pain is not localized only over the uterus. The pain may be exacerbated and/or relieved by positional changes.
- **Labor** – Normal labor may cause abdominal and uterine pain – it should never cause fever. Severe, continuous, unrelenting uterine pain and tenderness may indicate a uterine rupture. Suspicion is higher in the setting of any previous uterine scar.
- **Abruption** – May present with significant bright red vaginal bleeding with associated uterine tenderness. Fever should not be present, though uterine irritability and contractions are common. There may also be a concealed abruption behind the placenta, which will not present with vaginal bleeding. The risk for a maternal consumptive coagulopathy is significant – send serial coagulation studies frequently if this is part of your differential diagnosis.

diagnosis or suspicion for chorioamnionitis should be admitted at any gestational age.

Infection Control

Follow universal precautions. There is no concern for chorioamnionitis transmission to other individuals.

Pearls and Pitfalls

1. Digital vaginal exam is contraindicated in suspected rupture of membranes.
2. Premature rupture of membranes affects 5–10% of pregnancies, whereas chorioamnionitis affects 2% of pregnancies.
3. Group B *Streptococcus* is an important infectious agent for neonatal infection, causing pneumonia, meningitis, enteritis, and sepsis in the newborn – always test for GBS in the mother.
4. Uterine tenderness is never normal – it should raise immediate suspicion for chorioamnionitis.
5. Maternal sepsis is rare in cases of chorioamnionitis, but immediate resuscitation is crucial to both mother and fetus.

Special Consideration for Chorioamnionitis: *Listeria*

Listeria infection is a foodborne illness that usually causes mild febrile gastrointestinal illness in immunocompetent persons, but in pregnant women it may cause more severe infection. In pregnancy, *Listeria* often crosses the placenta to infect the fetus, which frequently results in miscarriage, fetal death, or neonatal morbidity. Because *Listeria* infects the amniotic fluid through transplacental and hematogenous means, *Listeria* chorioamnionitis often occurs in the setting of intact membranes. If a pregnant patient presents with a fever and symptoms of gastroenteritis, it is important to take a careful food history. Foods that have caused *Listeria* outbreaks have included unpasteurized dairy products (e.g., soft cheeses, ice cream), deli meats, and other ready-to-eat foods. If a diagnosis of listeriosis is made in a pregnant woman, it is crucial to begin antibiotics to minimize fetal disease. If an amniocentesis is done to rule out chorioamnionitis, the color of the amniotic fluid associated with a *Listeria* source has been described as "bright green" and *Listeria* should be the presumed diagnosis if gram-positive rods are found in an amniotic fluid sample. First-line therapy for listeriosis is ampicillin.

TORCH INFECTIONS

Epidemiology

The "TORCH" mnemonic describes a group of infections that have teratogenic effects:

- Toxoplasmosis
- Other infections, such as varicella
- Rubella
- Cytomegalovirus
- Herpes simplex virus

TOXOPLASMOSIS

Caused by the intracellular parasite *Toxoplasma gondii*, this infection is uncommon in the United States, and congenital infection rate is low (0.01–0.1%). There is a direct relationship between the likelihood of fetal infection and gestational age: That is, the chance of fetal infection is higher with advancing gestational age at time of maternal infection. The severity of teratogenic effects is inversely related to gestational age, with more severe effects seen in infections that occur at earlier gestational ages. Infectious sources include raw or undercooked meat, unwashed fruits and vegetables, exposure to soil during gardening or farming, and fresh cat feces. Women of lower socioeconomic status, who are over age 30, reside in rural locations, and are of foreign birth have higher risk for acquiring toxoplasmosis. Subclinical infection is common and symptoms are often misdiagnosed as mononucleosis.

VARICELLA (CHICKENPOX)

Varicella is a highly contagious virus spread by respiratory droplets and close contact. The incubation period ranges from 10 to 20 days, and individuals are contagious from 2 days *prior* to appearance of the rash until all skin lesions have crusted over. Since the introduction of the varicella vaccination in 1995, the rate of infection has dropped dramatically in the United States. More than 90% of the general population is immune prior to reproductive age because of previous infection or vaccination. However, maternal varicella infection during pregnancy causes significant risks to the mother, as well as teratogenic risks to the fetus. Adult varicella infections tend to be more severe than childhood infections, with the most severe complication being varicella pneumonia, which carries a mortality risk of approximately 28% in pregnant women in one study. Because varicella zoster is a reactivation illness in previously exposed persons, there is no risk of infection to the fetus during pregnancy, but cutaneous lesions are infectious, so skin-skin contact with the newborn should be avoided if a woman has lesions postpartum.

RUBELLA (GERMAN MEASLES)

Since rubella vaccination became available in 1969, the incidence of rubella infections has dropped dramatically. Since 2001, there have been fewer than 25 cases of rubella per year in the United States. The risk of a congenital defect is as high as 85% if an intrauterine infection occurs at less than 8 weeks gestation, and 50% if an intrauterine infection occurs during the 9th to 12th week of gestation. The risk of congenital rubella syndrome significantly decreases if infection occurs after 20 weeks. Any pregnant woman with a rash and a fever should have serologic testing for rubella, unless she has recent testing demonstrating antibodies for rubella.

CYTOMEGALOVIRUS (CMV)

Approximately 40% of women of reproductive age are susceptible to CMV, with infection and seroconversion more likely to occur among women of lower socioeconomic status. Most infections are subclinical (90%), and many infections in pregnancy are missed or often misdiagnosed as mononucleosis. More severe neonatal disease occurs in cases of primary maternal infection as opposed to a recurrent infection during pregnancy. Approximately 0.5–2.5% of births in the United States are associated with congenital CMV infection, causing approximately 1000 neonatal deaths per year, making it the most common intrauterine infection. Surviving infants have a significantly higher disability rate than the unaffected population.

HERPES SIMPLEX VIRUS (HSV)

As a sexually transmitted infection, genital HSV outbreaks are most commonly caused by HSV-2; however about 15% of outbreaks in the genital area can also be caused by HSV-1. Risk of transmission of HSV infection to the neonate is highest during labor, through direct contact. It is very important to ascertain the type of maternal infection during pregnancy, because this has implications for risk to the fetus and neonate: (1) *Primary infection* is an initial infection of either HSV type, in a patient without existing antibodies from prior exposure to either type. (2) *Nonprimary first episode* is an initial outbreak with one HSV type, where the patient has existing antibodies to the other virus type. (3) *Recurrent infection* is reactivation of latent virus from a previous outbreak and not a new infection. A new primary infection carries the highest risk for the fetus or neonate, with transmission rates possibly as high as 40%. Neonatal infection is very rare, less than 1%, in the setting of recurrent maternal infection.

Clinical Features

Table 53.10 summarizes the clinical features of TORCH Infections.

Differential Diagnosis

Whenever one TORCH infection is suspected, clinicians should be sure to rule out other diagnoses. Syphilis is an important TORCH infection in the "Other" category that does not usually cause fever. Congenital syphilis is extremely detrimental to the fetus, with complications including intrauterine growth restriction (IUGR), bone abnormalities, ocular abnormalities, nonimmune hydrops fetalis, reticuloendothelial abnormalities, significant central nervous system (CNS) anomalies and stillbirth.

Potentially febrile viral exanthems concerning during pregnancy are coxsackieviruses and parvovirus B19, also known as "fifth disease" or "slapped-cheek" rash. (See Chapter 44, Fever and Rash in the Pediatric Population.)

Key features that distinguish TORCH infections from coxsackie- and parvoviruses:

- *Coxsackieviruses* are divided into A and B subtypes – A types rarely have effects on the fetus, whereas B types have both maternal and fetal effects. Maternal coxsackievirus infection begins as a fever followed by a wide range of possible presentations: myocarditis, meningoencephalitis, pleurodynia, pneumonia, hemolytic uremic syndrome, and hepatitis. Typically there is not an associated rash. Fetal coxsackievirus type B infections, even in the absence of maternal symptoms, are potentially teratogenic, causing urogenital malformations, cardiac defects and congenital heart disease, digestive tract abnormalities, myocarditis, and neonatal CNS infections. If suspected, the diagnosis can be confirmed with virus isolation from rectal or throat swabs, or from rising maternal antibody titers.
- *Parvovirus B19* is highly infectious and commonly occurs in outbreaks among day care and school settings. Maternal infection manifests as low-grade prodromal fever and may

Table 53.10 Clinical Features: TORCH Infections

TORCH Infection	Clinical Signs and Symptoms
Toxoplasmosis	• Fever, fatigue, sore throat • Maculopapular rash • Cervical lymphadenopathy • Hepatosplenomegaly • Ocular symptoms (blurriness, photophobia, pain) – chorioretinitis in immunocompromised patients • Pulmonary or CNS symptoms in immunocompromised patients
Varicella	• Fever, malaise (precede rash by several days in the adult, are simultaneous in children) • Rash – successive crops beginning as macules, to papules, to vesicles, to pustules that eventually form crusts and scabs. Typically starts on face and scalp, spreading to trunk; extremities minimally involved • Intense pruritis • Respiratory symptoms (2nd to 6th day after the rash), can rapidly progress to fatal acute respiratory distress syndrome (ARDS) • Chest x-ray: diffuse perihilar nodular or miliary pattern in cases of pneumonia • Symptoms of CNS infection, myocarditis, glomerulonephritis, arthritis
Rubella (Defined by CDC, 1996)	• Temperature >37.2°C, or 99.0°F • Acute onset of generalized maculopapular rash (usually starts on face) – about 16–18 days postexposure • Arthralgias or arthritis • Lymphadenopathy • Conjunctivitis
Cytomegalovirus	• Fever • Leukocytosis (heterophile negative, with lymphocytosis) • Abnormal liver function tests • Malaise, myalgias, chills • Mild pharyngitis • Minimal lymphadenopathy • Absence of hepatosplenomegaly and jaundice
Herpes Simplex Virus	• Fever, malaise, myalgias, adenopathy, headaches, nausea (systemic symptoms only in primary infections) • Local painful vesicles that progress to ulcerations • Prodromal local symptoms of pain, paresthesias, or pruritus (approximately 2–3 days) • Primary infections average 3 weeks' duration • Recurrent infections average 2–7 days

CNS, central nervous system.

be followed by the classical erythematous, warm facial "slapped cheek" rash. Rash is less common in adults as opposed to children. Adults are more likely to be asymptomatic (50%) and to develop arthropathy and swollen joints, and they may have a generalized reticular rash on the trunk – thus, if there is any suspicion for a maternal parvovirus B19 infection, even without the textbook "slapped cheek" appearance, a diagnosis should be pursued. Infection in the fetus causes erythroid hypoplasia, shortened red blood cell life span, and hemolysis leading to severe anemia in the fetus, sometimes requiring intrauterine transfusion. Over weeks, the fetus can develop high output cardiac failure leading to hydrops fetalis and potentially causing intrauterine fetal demise (IUFD). If clinically

Table 53.11 Laboratory Findings of TORCH Infections

Infection	Laboratory Diagnosis
Toxoplasmosis	• Maternal serum IgM positive (1 week to several months postinfection; however, can persist for years) or IgG positive (1–2 months postinfection for years) • Avidity assays through a specific toxoplasmosis reference lab • Complement fixation, Sabin-Feldman dye tests • Toxoplasma antigen detection by immunofluorescence • Histologic diagnosis from lymph node biopsy
Varicella	• IgM or IgG antibodies positive from maternal serum • Isolation of varicella virus from unroofed skin lesion swab or bronchoalveolar lavage • Antigen test from unroofed skin lesion swab or CSF • PCR of CSF sample
Rubella	• Isolation of rubella virus – can be isolated from blood and throat 7–10 days postinfection, shedding continues in throat for approximately 1 week • Significant rise in IgG antibody titers (instruct lab to not report simply "positive" or "negative"; "equivocal" should be considered as susceptible to the virus) • Positive IgM antibody (lasts for 4–5 weeks)
Cytomegalovirus	• Virus isolation by urine or cervical culture (does not distinguish between primary and recurrent infection) • IgM antibody tests (positive if infection occurs in last 4–8 months, may remain positive in up to 10% of women with recurrent CMV) • IgG antibody tests • Direct PCR tests • "Owl's eye" appearance of intranuclear inclusion bodies is pathognomonic for CMV but rare
Herpes Simplex Virus	• Viral culture • Serum antibodies (IgG or IgM) • Direct PCR tests

CSF, cerebrospinal fluid; PCR, polymerase chain reaction.

Table 53.12 Treatment and Prophylaxis of TORCH Infections

Infection	Treatment and Prophylaxis
Toxoplasmosis	• Counseling about risks and clinical features of congenital toxoplasmosis, termination options • Spiramycin for maternal infection (available through the FDA in the United States) • Pyrimethamine and sulfadiazine for fetal treatment, with folic acid • Avoid cat litter boxes, do not eat undercooked or raw meat, hand wash after touching cats, keep household cats indoors and prevent cats' consumption of mice and raw meat, use gloves with gardening, wash all fruits and vegetables
Varicella	• Varicella-zoster immune globulin (VZIG) if exposure is within 96 hours. (If evidence of maternal rash exists, viremia has already occurred and VZIG is not indicated.) • Counseling about risks and clinical features of congenital varicella, termination options • Acyclovir 10–15 mg/kg IV tid for 7 days or 800 mg PO daily if evidence of systemic severe maternal illness or any respiratory symptoms • Supportive care for severe pulmonary disease • As a live-attenuated vaccine, varicella vaccination should *not* be given in pregnancy, and conception should be avoided for 3 months postvaccine (although there is currently no evidence of harm if conception occurs sooner). A pregnant woman in the household is *not* a contraindication to giving varicella vaccine to another individual, because the vaccine virus is not transmissible.
Rubella	• Counseling about risks and clinical features of congenital rubella, termination options • Do not culture amniotic fluid as not indicative of fetal infection • CDC does not recommend routine postexposure immunoglobulin because it does not prevent viremia. However, CDC suggests that immunoglobulin may be useful in exposed nonimmune women for whom pregnancy termination is not an option. • As a live-attenuated vaccine, rubella vaccination should *not* be given in pregnancy, and conception should be avoided for 3 months postvaccine. • All rubella nonimmune women should receive the MMR vaccine postpartum (safe with breastfeeding).
Cytomegalovirus	• Counseling about risks and clinical features of congenital CMV, termination options • No treatment or prophylaxis recommended (ganciclovir is Category D). A live-attenuated vaccine is in testing stages.
Herpes Simplex Virus	• Counseling about risks and clinical features of congenital HSV, termination options • The agent most studied to treat and prevent HSV in pregnancy is acyclovir: *For primary infections*: 400 mg PO tid or 200 mg PO 5 times/day for 7–10 days *For recurrent infections*: 400 mg PO tid, 800 mg PO bid, or 200 mg PO 5 times/day for 5 days *For prevention near term*: 400 mg PO tid until delivery • Intravenous administration of acyclovir can be used in pregnancy for severe systemic infections • There is currently no available vaccine

FDA, Food and Drug Administration; MMR, measles, mumps, rubella.

suspected, parvovirus can be detected by IgM- and IgG-specific enzyme-linked immunosorbent assay (ELISA) antibody tests. Keep in mind that false-positive IgM results are relatively common; results should be interpreted with caution and further testing discussed with the laboratory.

Laboratory Findings

Table 53.11 summarizes the laboratory findings of TORCH infections.

Treatment and Prophylaxis

Table 53.12 summarizes the treatment and prophylaxis of TORCH infections.

Complications and Admission Criteria

TOXOPLASMOSIS

Teratogenic effects include chorioretinitis, intracranial calcifications, IUGR, hydrocephaly, microcephaly, hepatosplenomegaly, and low birth weight in the neonate.

Toxoplasmosis has also been associated with abortion and prematurity.

VARICELLA

Congenital varicella can produce spontaneous abortion, stillbirth, limb hypoplasia, cutaneous scars, mental retardation, ocular abnormalities, growth retardation, and rudimentary digits. Risk of congenital varicella is low, approximately 1%, if primary maternal infection occurs during pregnancy; however, the possible teratogenic infections can be severe.

RUBELLA

Although there are very few cases each year in the United States, rubella is a known teratogenic infection, primarily causing cataracts or glaucoma, patent ductus arteriosus, mental retardation, and deafness in the spectrum of congenital rubella syndrome (CRS).

CYTOMEGALOVIRUS

The teratogenic potential of CMV varies, and the clinical impact on the neonate is often less than with other TORCH infections, such as rubella. However, neonatal disease is more severe when in utero infection occurs prior to 22 weeks' gestation.

HERPES SIMPLEX VIRUS

Although rare, congenital in utero infection can occur, resulting in spontaneous abortion, IUGR, premature birth, skin lesions, and severe CNS malformations such as microcephaly, hydranencephaly, and microphthalmos. Neonatal infection acquired during labor and delivery can cause ocular infections, skin lesions, CNS infections, seizures, respiratory difficulties, liver dysfunction, sepsis, and disseminated intravascular coagulopathy (DIC).

ADMISSION CRITERIA FOR TORCH INFECTIONS

Serious maternal compromise with a TORCH infection is rare in an immunocompetent host, and admission is rarely required. The most important exception is when there is any concern for varicella pneumonia; in these cases hospital admission is required at any gestational age for close maternal monitoring.

Infection Control

TOXOPLASMOSIS

Educate pregnant women to avoid sources of toxoplasmosis such as raw or undercooked meat, unwashed fruits and vegetables, exposure to soil during gardening or farming, and fresh cat feces.

VARICELLA

Ask all pregnant women if they have had a personal history of varicella. If not, or if prior infection is uncertain, send a varicella antibody test with prenatal labs. If the antibody is negative, vaccinate the mother *postpartum.*

RUBELLA

Send rubella titers with all standard prenatal labs. Vaccinate all nonimmune mothers *postpartum.*

CYTOMEGALOVIRUS

There are no special prophylaxis or prevention strategies for CMV in pregnancy.

HERPES SIMPLEX VIRUS

Ask all pregnant woman about a personal or partner's history of genital HSV. If the pregnant patient's partner has a history of genital herpes and the patient does not, test for the presence of antibodies of the patient. If the antibodies of the patient are negative for herpes, counsel the couple to use condoms throughout the pregnancy to avoid a primary infection from asymptomatic shedding. If either the patient or her partner has had a prior HSV outbreak, start prophylaxis at 36 weeks' gestation with acyclovir 400 mg by mouth (PO) tid until delivery.

Pearls and Pitfalls

1. Although TORCH infections are relatively rare, never hesitate to send diagnostic tests if there is even a remote suspicion for a TORCH infection, because the consequences can be devastating for the fetus.
2. *Never* give live vaccines in pregnancy (e.g., rubella and varicella). It is not contraindicated to give these vaccines to other individuals when there is a pregnant woman in the house, because the vaccine form is not transmissible. If accidental vaccination occurs during pregnancy, providers should counsel patients on the rare, but important, risks of congenital infection.

HEPATITIS

Epidemiology

Hepatitis A virus (HAV) occurs in approximately 1 in 1000 pregnancies and is transmitted predominantly through a fecal-oral route. The clinical presentation and course are similar to those in nonpregnant women, and there are only case reports of transmission to the fetus. There are no known teratogenic effects.

Acute hepatitis B virus (HBV) occurs in 1–2 in 1000 pregnancies; approximately 1% of pregnant women in the Unites States are chronic carriers of HBV. Acquisition is by perinatal and sexual routes, with vertical transmission from mother to fetus being the primary concern during pregnancy. Mothers who are co-infected with HIV and/or hepatitis B have higher rates of vertical transmission. New active infections of HBV in pregnancy have a similar presentation to that in nonpregnant women, and there are no known teratogenic effects. According to the American Academy of Pediatrics, breastfeeding is not contraindicated in the setting of hepatitis B infection.

Overall seroprevalence of hepatitis C virus (HCV) in pregnant women in the United States ranges between 2% and 5%, with rates being much higher in women co-infected with HIV. Clinical course is usually not affected by pregnancy; however, there is some evidence of postpartum flares. Chronic active HCV can infrequently increase rates of preterm delivery and intrauterine growth. The CDC reports rates of perinatal vertical transmission around 5% in HIV-negative women, and as high as 17% in HIV co-infected women. There are no known teratogenic effects. There is rare evidence of hepatitis C transmission through breastfeeding, though according

Table 53.13 Clinical Features: Hepatitis

Organisms	Hepatitis A, B, and C
Signs and Symptoms	• Weakness and malaise • Nausea, vomiting, anorexia, and right upper quadrant pain • In a small subset of patients, a syndrome similar to serum sickness can occur: fever, an urticarial, rash, and migratory polyarticular arthritis

Table 53.14 Hepatitis Treatment and Prophylaxis

Hepatitis A, B and C	• Supportive care • HAV and HBV vaccination if nonimmune • HBIG and HBV vaccine to neonate within 12 hours of birth

to the American Academy of Pediatrics, breastfeeding is not contraindicated in hepatitis C infections.

Clinical Features

Clinical presentation for acute viral hepatitis in pregnancy is similar across all types and is not affected by pregnancy. Systemic symptoms such as weakness and malaise are common, as well as nausea, vomiting, anorexia, and right upper quadrant pain (Table 53.13). In a small subset of patients, a syndrome similar to serum sickness can occur, which includes fever, an urticarial rash, and migratory polyarticular arthritis. Immune complex mediated diseases can also occur in the setting of acute viral hepatitis. Icterus occurs in 20–50% of acute viral hepatitis infections, usually following onset of systemic symptoms. Mild liver enlargement, right upper quadrant tenderness, rash, warm and tender joints, and spider angiomata can be found on exam. Most concerning is the rare presentation of fulminant viral hepatitis, which can progress to hepatic encephalopathy and coma.

Differential Diagnosis

The differential diagnosis for hepatitis in pregnancy is similar to that in the nonpregnant state. However, there are some special additions and considerations in pregnancy to add to the differential diagnosis.

Key features that help distinguish viral hepatitis from other conditions:

- **Appendicitis** – Keep in mind that appendicitis in pregnancy can present in atypical locations in pregnancy, such as the right upper quadrant. However, liver function tests are normal in appendicitis.
- **Hyperemesis gravidarum** does not cause fever; however, it can have other symptoms similar to those of acute viral hepatitis, excluding a serum sickness-like presentation.
- At later gestations in pregnancy, diffuse symptoms such as nausea, vomiting, and right upper quadrant pain can be a presentation of **preeclampsia**. Preeclampsia can reveal abnormal liver function tests, similar to viral hepatitis. However, preeclampsia is additionally defined by elevated blood pressures of 140/90 or higher, and significant proteinuria on urinalysis. The more severe form of preeclampsia, **HELLP syndrome** (hemolysis, elevated liver enzymes, and low platelets), can also demonstrate anemia, elevated D-dimers, low fibrinogen, coagulopathy and low platelets and sometimes is not accompanied by hypertension.
- **Fatty liver of pregnancy** is associated with stillbirth, elevated ammonia, and hypoglycemia. Liver function tests

are elevated, and mental status changes can occur in severe cases.

Laboratory Diagnosis

There are no differences in the laboratory diagnosis of viral hepatitis in the pregnant state. See Chapter 13 on viral hepatitis for further details of laboratory diagnosis. Keep in mind that alkaline phosphatase (ALP) is produced by the placenta, and normally is elevated in pregnancy, however, aspartate aminotransferase (AST) and alanine aminotransferase (ALT) are unaffected by normal pregnancy. Pregnant women who are HBV or HCV antibody positive should have a hepatic work-up as for any infected, nonpregnant adult and should not be delayed because of pregnancy.

Treatment and Prophylaxis

Supportive care is the primary treatment for acute viral hepatitis in pregnancy (Table 53.14). Vaccines against HAV and HBV are safe to administer during pregnancy. It is essential to inform both the patient and the pediatric team if you have diagnosed hepatitis in pregnancy, both to prevent neonatal infection during birth as well as to discuss the risks and benefits of breastfeeding. In the case of HBV, hepatitis B immune globulin (HBIG) and HBV vaccine administration to the neonate are effective in preventing vertical transmission of HBV in 85–95% of cases if given within 12 hours of birth. The World Health Organization (WHO) supports breastfeeding among neonates who have received HBIG and HBV vaccine, because these treatments substantially reduce the risk of HBV perinatal transmission through breast milk. Lamivudine is considered safe in pregnancy. Neither the CDC nor the American Academy of Pediatrics recommends against breastfeeding in HCV-positive mothers as prevention of transmission.

Complications and Admission Criteria

Maternal complications of hepatitis infection are similar in both the pregnant and nonpregnant populations, although there is some evidence of increased risk of hepatitis flares in the postpartum period for chronic carriers of HBV and HCV. Worsening hepatic function and concern for fulminant hepatic failure are criteria for admission in pregnant patients of any gestational age.

Infection Control

One of the most important infection control measures for hepatitis in pregnancy is to identify mothers who are chronic carriers of hepatitis B, because vertical transmission can be prevented in 85–95% of births by neonatal administration of HBIG and HBV vaccine within 12 hours of birth. Hepatitis B vaccinations should be offered to all household contacts of infected mothers. All individuals should use gloves when handling babies delivered by Hepatitis B positive mothers until the infant's first bath. It is also important to identify mothers who are at risk for HCV infection and to test for the presence of HCV antibody in order to take appropriate measures to reduce the risk of vertical transmission in labor and delivery.

SPECIAL CONSIDERATIONS: COMMON IMMIGRANT AND TRAVEL ILLNESSES

Malaria

Malaria is an important infectious cause of fever in pregnancy that has a significant effect on both maternal and fetal health (see Chapter 54, Fever in the Returning Traveler). Febrile travelers or immigrants from malaria-endemic areas should be tested, since the complications of maternal infection include preterm birth, low birth weight, spontaneous abortion, stillbirth, IUGR, congenital malaria, and significant maternal anemia. *Plasmodium* species can be found in the following areas:

- *Plasmodium falciparum* – sub-Saharan Africa, the Dominican Republic, Haiti, New Guinea, South America, Southeast Asia, and Oceania
- *Plasmodium ovale* – sub-Saharan Africa
- *Plasmodium vivax* – South America, Southeast Asia, and Oceania
- *Plasmodium malariae* – worldwide

EPIDEMIOLOGY

In the Unites States, approximately 1300 cases of malaria are seen per year. Approximately half of these cases are in U.S. citizens who have recently traveled to malaria-endemic areas, and the other half are seen in non-U.S. citizens. The largest areas of malaria diagnoses in the United States are in New York, California, and Maryland. Acquired immunity to malaria can be lost or impaired in pregnancy. Because of decreased immune responses in pregnancy, pregnant women are three times more likely to develop severe malarial infections than nonpregnant women with infections from the same region.

CLINICAL FEATURES

There is a spectrum of disease presentation in pregnant women (Table 53.15). Reactivated latent disease will have a milder illness with decreased likelihood of fetal infection, whereas new infection in a non-immune woman can be life

Table 53.15 Clinical Features: Malaria

Signs and Symptoms	• Cyclic fevers every 48–72 hours (late stages) • "Cold stage," followed by "hot stage," followed by "sweating stage" • Tachycardia and tachypnea • Abdominal pain, back pain • Nausea and vomiting • Delirium • Orthostatic hypotension • Jaundice

Table 53.16 Laboratory Findings of Malaria Infections

Laboratory Test	Possible Findings
CBC	Anemia – may be severe
Electrolyte Panel	Elevated BUN and creatinine Hypoglycemia*
Liver Function Tests†	Elevated total bilirubin – indicative of hemolysis
Blood Smear	Thick – used to identify the presence of parasites Thin – used to make specific diagnosis
ABG	Metabolic acidosis (lactic acidosis)
Chest X-ray	Pulmonary edema
Obstetric Ultrasound	Hydrops fetalis in the case of severe fetal anemia due to congenital infection, IUGR

*May be severe with *Plasmodium falciparum*.
†Alkaline phosphatase elevation is normal in pregnancy because of production by the placenta.
CBC, complete blood count.

threatening, with a high risk for stillbirth and spontaneous abortion. Fetal infection is *extremely* rare.

DIFFERENTIAL DIAGNOSIS

In the setting of pregnancy, fever, and recent travel or immigration, there is a vast differential for any infectious etiology that is endemic to the region of origin. See Chapter 54, Fever in the Returning Traveler.

LABORATORY FINDINGS

Table 53.16 summarizes the laboratory findings of malaria infections.

TREATMENT AND PROPHYLAXIS

Ultimately, prophylaxis and treatment are recommended for pregnant women, as for nonpregnant individuals, with some special considerations of teratogenicity and side effects as outlined in Table 53.17. Check for updated prophylaxis regimens based on region of travel and specifics of dosing from the Centers for Disease Control and Prevention website: http://www.cdc.gov.

Table 53.17 Malaria Treatment and Prophylaxis Drugs in Pregnancy

Safe in Pregnancy*	Chloroquine, pyrimethamine-sulfadoxine, quinine, quinidine, clindamycin
Use with Caution in Pregnancy	Mefloquine,† artemisinin derivatives‡
Contraindicated in Pregnancy	Primaquine, tetracycline, doxycycline, halofantrine

*Considered safe at therapeutic doses. Some association between chloroquine and retinal or cochleovestibular damage; quinine and ototoxicity; primaquine and hemolysis in glucose-6-phosphate dehydrogenase (G6PD)-deficient patients.
†Single report showing association with increase in stillbirths.
‡Not well studied in pregnancy.

Special Populations

COMPLICATIONS AND ADMISSION CRITERIA

Complications of malarial infections include preterm birth, low birth weight, spontaneous abortion, stillbirth, IUGR, congenital malaria, and maternal anemia. All pregnant women with malaria should be admitted.

INFECTION CONTROL

Before traveling to endemic areas, pregnant women should be advised to take appropriate malaria prophylaxis as recommended by the CDC based on their region of travel. There are no restrictions or transmission precautions for patients with malaria.

PEARLS AND PITFALLS

1. Send both a thick and thin smear to aid in diagnosis of type of malaria.
2. Take a good travel history and always check for updated information for treatment resistance patterns depending on the area of travel or origin.
3. Pregnant women may have a more severe presentation and course than nonpregnant women because of a mild immunosuppressed state.

Tuberculosis

There has been a dramatic rise on the rate of tuberculosis (TB) in the United States since the mid-1990s, largely due to the HIV epidemic. The overall increased prevalence has increased the risk of transmission in all populations, and clinicians should always be vigilant about diagnosing both latent and active TB in pregnant women (see Chapter 33, Tuberculosis). Although maternal morbidity is not significantly different in the pregnant state and the risk of congenital TB is low, the mortality from congenital TB is very high: approximately 38% from CDC data.

CLINICAL PRESENTATION

Symptoms in pregnancy are the same as in the general population: fever, weight loss, night sweats, cough, hemoptysis, shortness of breath, fatigue, and general malaise. Chest radiograph findings may include cavitary lesions, infiltrates or consolidations, and/or cavities, especially in the upper lobes. Mediastinal or hilar lymphadenopathy may be present. However, lesions may appear anywhere in the lungs. In HIV-infected and other immunosuppressed persons, any radiographic abnormality may indicate TB, or the chest radiograph may appear normal. Old healed tuberculosis usually manifests as pulmonary nodules in the hilar area or upper lobes. Bronchiectasis, fibrotic scars, volume loss, and pleural scarring may be present.

DIFFERENTIAL DIAGNOSIS

TB may present similarly to a wide variety of other pulmonary, cardiac, and other infectious etiologies. All pregnant women should be screened for TB to avoid the risk of congenital and neonatal infection.

LABORATORY FINDINGS

Ultimately, positive culture or PCR for *Mycobacterium tuberculosis* is needed for confirmation of infection. Presence or absence of acid-fast bacilli on AFB smear is not definitive for diagnosis, and culture must always be performed.

Table 53.18 TB Treatment Regimens in Pregnancy*

Latent Tuberculosis	Isoniazid† daily for 6–9 months (Rifampin is likely safe in pregnancy, although there is minimal evidence on its use compared to the preferred latency treatment of isoniazid in pregnancy. Pyrazinamide should be avoided in the first trimester as teratogenicity is unknown.)
Active Tuberculosis	Isoniazid† 300 mg daily, rifampin 600 mg daily Add ethambutol 2.5 g daily if resistance to isoniazid potentially exists Treatment duration is 9 months for all drugs (Streptomycin is associated with congenital deafness)

*Always consider HIV status and geographic region when choosing a treatment regimen to cover possible immunocompromised states and geographic resistance patterns.
†Always supplement isoniazid with pyridoxine 50 mg daily.

TREATMENT AND PROPHYLAXIS

Tuberculin skin test has no known detrimental effects in pregnancy and should be not withheld. Treatment of latent TB infection is safe during pregnancy and should not be delayed (Table 53.18). Breastfeeding is *not* contraindicated and should *not* be discouraged during the treatment of latent or active TB infection. Treatment of active TB infection should always be carried out, regardless of pregnancy status, with consideration of the teratogenicity of treatment regimens.

COMPLICATIONS AND ADMISSION CRITERIA

Maternal or antepartum complications from active TB are not significantly different from those in the nonpregnant population. Congenital TB in the newborn is rare; however, morbidity and mortality is high.

INFECTION CONTROL

Transmission precautions are the same for nonpregnant and pregnant populations: All patients with suspicion for active TB should be placed in respiratory isolation until sputum AFB smears rule out active infection. All medical providers for these patients should take respiratory precautions when evaluating such patients. Providers should not withhold treatment of TB because of pregnancy or breastfeeding. Most TB treatment regimens are safe during pregnancy and breastfeeding.

PEARLS AND PITFALLS

1. Every pregnant woman should have a purified protein derivative (PPD) placed during each pregnancy. Exceptions include those with known previous PPD positive status that is not related to bacille Calmette-Guérin (BCG) vaccine. Only 15% of patients who have received a BCG vaccine have a persistently positive PPD, so this is not a contraindication to placing a PPD. Women with a positive PPD and a prior BCG vaccination should still be considered as exposed to TB and need a chest radiograph.
2. Every pregnant woman with a positive PPD needs a chest radiograph to rule out evidence of active disease – this can be done in any trimester with the fetus shielded. Exceptions include a patient with a documented negative chest radiograph in the past 2 years and no symptoms of active TB.

3. Do not delay treatment until breastfeeding is completed, because neonatal TB can be severe.

REFERENCES

Centers for Disease Control and Prevention (CDC). Appendix D – vaccine administration, http://www.cdc.gov/vaccines/pubs/pinkbook/downloads/appendices/appdx-full-d.pdf. Retrieved October 31, 2007.

Centers for Disease Control and Prevention (CDC). Measles, mumps, and rubella – vaccine use and strategies for elimination of measles, rubella and congenital rubella syndrome and control of mumps: recommendations of the Advisory Committee on Immunization Practices (ACIP). MMWR 1984;33:301.

Centers for Disease Control and Prevention (CDC). Guideline for vaccinating pregnant women from recommendations of the Advisory Committee on Immunization Practices (ACIP), http://www.cdc.gov/vaccines/pubs/downloads/b_preg_guide.pdf. Retrieved December 28, 2007.

Centers for Disease Control and Prevention (CDC). Radiation emergencies fact sheet, http://www.bt.cdc.gov/radiation/pdf/prenatalphysician.pdf. Retrieved December 28, 2007. Centers for Disease Control and Prevention (CDC). Treatment of malaria guidelines for clinicians, http://www.cdc.gov/malaria/pdf/clinicalguidance.pdf. Retrieved December 28, 2007.

Gershan AA. Chicken pox, measles and mumps. In: Remington JS, Klein JO, eds, Infectious diseases of the fetus and newborn. Philadelphia: WB Saunders, 2001:683–732.

Guttman R, Goldman R, Koren G. Appendicitis during pregnancy. Can Fam Physician 2004;50:355–7.

Johns Hopkins. Antibiotic guide. Available at: http://www.hopkins-abxguide.org.

Smoak B, Writer JV, Keep LW. The effects of inadvertent exposure of mefloquine chemoprophylaxis on pregnancy outcomes and infants of U.S. Army servicewomen. J Infect Dis 1997;176:831–3.

Sperling RS, Newton E, Gibbs RS. Intraamniotic infection in low birth weight infants. J Infect Dis 1988;157:113.

Sweet R, Gibbs R. Perinatal infections. In: Sweet R, Gibbs R, eds. Infectious diseases of the female genital tract. Philadelphia: Lippincott Williams & Wilkins, 2002:449–500.

Sweet R, Gibbs R. Urinary tract infection. In: Sweet R, Gibbs R, eds. Infectious diseases of the female genital tract. Philadelphia: Lippincott Williams & Wilkins, 2002:413–48.

Toppenberg K, Hill A, Miller D. Safety of radiographic imaging during pregnancy. Am Fam Physician 1999;59(7):1813–22.

Tracey M, Fletcher HS. Appendicitis in pregnancy. Am Surg 2000;66:555–9.

Wing DA, Hendershott CM, Debuque L, Millar LK. Outpatient treatment of acute pyelonephritis in pregnancy after 24 weeks. Obstet Gynecol 1999;94:683–8.

ADDITIONAL READINGS

Edwards, MJ. Review: Hyperthermia and fever during pregnancy. Birth Defects Res A Clin Mol Teratol 2006 July;76(7):507–16.

Gabbe SG, Niebyl JR, Simpson JL, eds. Obstetrics: normal and problem pregnancies, 4th ed. New York: Churchill Livingstone, 2002.

Harper JT, Ernest JM, Thurnau GR, et al. Risk factors and outcomes of varicella-zoster virus pneumonia in pregnant women. J Infect Dis 2002 Feb;185(4):422–7.

Lim WS, Macfarlane JT, Colthorpe CL. Treatment of community-acquired lower respiratory tract infections during pregnancy. Am J Respir Med 2003;2(3):221.

54. Fever in the Returning Traveler

Derek Ward, Alex Blau, and Matthew Lewin

INTRODUCTION

Each year millions of people travel internationally from, and visit or immigrate to, the United States. As a group, travelers are exposed to numerous infectious agents, and eliciting a travel history is crucial in any recent traveler with presenting complaints suspicious for infectious disease, because appropriate clinical management may be highly specific to the locality of exposure.

The five most commonly identified causes of systemic febrile illness in returning travelers, in order of prevalence, are malaria, dengue fever, mononucleosis (Epstein-Barr or cytomegalovirus), rickettsial infections, and enteric fever caused by *Salmonella typhi* or *Salmonella paratyphi*. Tuberculosis and leptospirosis are also common, treatable diagnoses.

EPIDEMIOLOGY

A thorough travel history begins with identification of the region of travel and includes stops made during transit, as well as other factors that may affect the risk of contracting disease:

- type of travel (urban, rural, wilderness)
- food and beverage consumed (unfiltered water and ice cubes, uncooked or undercooked foods, and unpeeled fruits and vegetables)
- activities (camping, hiking, fishing, swimming, etc.)
- hygiene practices and availability of soap and toilet facilities
- exposure to animals and insects
- timing of exposure
- sexual contact with local population (primarily or secondarily)
- prophylactic medications taken during travel
- vaccination history (including childhood immunizations)

The following list of disease entities is intended to help identify exposure risk in the returning traveler. This listing is not comprehensive, and information changes frequently. Practitioners should refer to the Centers for Disease Control and Prevention (CDC) for complete and up-to-date information (http://www.cdc.gov, 1–877–394–8747).

Africa, Central

Diseases – Malaria, yellow fever, traveler's diarrhea (*Escherichia coli* infection, salmonellosis, cholera, parasitic infection), typhoid fever, toxoplasmosis, hepatitis A and B, dengue fever, filariasis, leishmaniasis, onchocerciasis, dracunculiasis, trypanosomiasis, rickettsial infections, schistosomiasis, tuberculosis, human immunodeficiency virus (HIV), rabies, plague, cryptosporidiosis.

Africa, East

Diseases – Malaria, yellow fever, traveler's diarrhea (*E. coli* infection, salmonellosis, cholera, parasitic infection), typhoid fever, toxoplasmosis, hepatitis A and B, dengue fever, filariasis, leishmaniasis, onchocerciasis, dracunculiasis, Rift Valley fever, trypanosomiasis, rickettsial infections, schistosomiasis, polio (Ethiopia only), tuberculosis, HIV, cryptosporidiosis.

Africa, North

Diseases – Malaria, traveler's diarrhea (*E. coli* infection, salmonellosis, cholera, parasitic infection), typhoid fever, hepatitis A, B, and C, dengue fever, filariasis, leishmaniasis, onchocerciasis, schistosomiasis, tuberculosis, polio (Egypt only).

Africa, South

Diseases – Malaria, traveler's diarrhea (*E. coli* infection, salmonellosis, cholera, parasitic infection), typhoid fever, toxoplasmosis, hepatitis A and B, HIV, dengue fever, filariasis, leishmaniasis, onchocerciasis, dracunculiasis, trypanosomiasis, rickettsial infections, schistosomiasis, cryptosporidiosis.

Africa, West

Diseases – Malaria, yellow fever, traveler's diarrhea (*E. coli* infection, salmonellosis, cholera, parasitic infection), typhoid fever, toxoplasmosis, hepatitis A and B, dengue fever, filariasis, leishmaniasis, onchocerciasis, dracunculiasis, trypanosomiasis, rickettsial infections, schistosomiasis, plague, tuberculosis, HIV, cryptosporidiosis.

Asia, East/North

Diseases – Malaria, traveler's diarrhea (*E. coli* infection, salmonellosis, cholera, parasitic infection), typhoid Fever, toxoplasmosis, hepatitis A and B, dengue fever, filariasis, Japanese encephalitis, leishmaniasis, plague, avian influenza (H5N1), SARS, cryptosporidiosis, clonorchiasis, Lyme disease.

Asia, South

Diseases – Malaria, traveler's diarrhea (*E. coli* infection, salmonellosis, cholera, parasitic infection), typhoid fever, toxoplasmosis, hepatitis A and B, filariasis, leishmaniasis, dengue fever, Japanese encephalitis, polio, rabies, leptospirosis, cryptosporidiosis, clonorchiasis, onchocerciasis.

Asia, Southeast

Diseases – Malaria, traveler's diarrhea (*E. coli* infection, salmonellosis, cholera, parasitic infection), typhoid fever, toxoplasmosis, hepatitis A and B, filariasis, dengue fever, Japanese encephalitis, polio, rabies, leptospirosis, schistosomiasis, cryptosporidiosis, onchocerciasis, leishmaniasis.

Australia and Southeast Asia

Diseases – Malaria (found only in Papua New Guinea, the Solomon Islands, and Vanuatu), traveler's diarrhea (*E. coli* infection, salmonellosis, cholera, parasitic infection), typhoid fever, toxoplasmosis, hepatitis A and B, dengue fever, filariasis, Ross River virus, Murray Valley encephalitis, scrub typhus and other rickettsial infections, Japanese encephalitis, ciguatera poisoning, cryptosporidiosis, onchocerciasis, leishmaniasis.

Caribbean

Diseases – Malaria (Haiti and Dominican Republic only), traveler's diarrhea (*E. coli* infection, salmonellosis, cholera, parasitic infection), typhoid fever, toxoplasmosis, hepatitis A and B, dengue fever, cutaneous larva migrans, leptospirosis, eosinophilic meningitis caused by *Angiostrongylus cantonensis*, anthrax (Haiti), lymphatic filariasis (Dominican Republic and Haiti), cutaneous leishmaniasis (Dominican Republic), tuberculosis (Haiti), HIV (Haiti), hepatitis B (Haiti and the Dominican Republic), dengue fever, filariasis, leishmaniasis, onchocerciasis, cryptosporidiosis.

Mexico and Central America

Diseases – Malaria, yellow fever (Panama), traveler's diarrhea (*E. coli* infection, salmonellosis, cholera, parasitic infection), typhoid fever, toxoplasmosis, hepatitis A and B, gnathostomiasis, dengue fever, filariasis, leishmaniasis, onchocerciasis, American trypanosomiasis (Chagas disease), myiasis, cryptosporidiosis.

Eastern Europe and Northern Asia

Diseases – Malaria (Armenia, Azerbaijan, Georgia, Kyrgyzstan, Tajikistan, Turkmenistan, Uzbekistan), traveler's diarrhea (*E. coli* infection, salmonellosis, cholera, parasitic infection), typhoid fever, toxoplasmosis, hepatitis A, B, and C, tick-borne encephalitis, rickettsial infections, tuberculosis, leishmaniasis (cutaneous and visceral), diphtheria, cryptosporidiosis, Lyme disease.

Western Europe

Diseases – Mumps (UK), tick-borne encephalitis, Lyme disease, leishmaniasis (cutaneous and visceral), *Legionella* infection, traveler's diarrhea (*E. coli* infection, salmonellosis, cholera, parasitic infection), variant Creutzfeldt-Jakob disease, trichinosis, Lyme disease.

Middle East

Diseases – Malaria (Iran, Iraq, Oman, Saudi Arabia, the Syrian Arab Republic, Turkey, and Yemen), traveler's diarrhea (*E. coli* infection, salmonellosis, cholera, parasitic infection), typhoid fever, toxoplasmosis, hepatitis A and B, leishmaniasis (cutaneous and visceral), West Nile fever, dengue fever, tuberculosis (Yemen), lymphatic filariasis (Yemen), schistosomiasis (Saudi Arabia, Yemen, Iraq, and Syria), polio (Yemen), meningococcal infection (serotypes A and W-135), filariasis, onchocerciasis, cryptosporidiosis.

North America and Hawaii

Diseases – Plague, rabies, Rocky Mountain spotted fever, tularemia, arthropod-borne encephalitis, seasonal influenza, coccidioidomycosis, histoplasmosis, rodent-borne hantavirus pulmonary syndrome, Lyme disease, West Nile fever, enterohemorrhagic *E. coli* infection (*E. coli* O157:H7), salmonellosis, hepatitis A, leptospirosis (especially in Hawaii).

Temperate South America

Diseases – Malaria (Argentina), yellow fever (Argentina), traveler's diarrhea, (*E. coli* infection, salmonellosis, cholera, parasitic infection), typhoid fever, toxoplasmosis, hepatitis A and B, dengue fever, American trypanosomiasis (Chagas disease), leishmaniasis, rodent-borne hantavirus pulmonary syndrome, dengue fever, filariasis, onchocerciasis, cryptosporidiosis.

Tropical South America

Diseases – Malaria, yellow fever, traveler's diarrhea (*E. coli* infection, salmonellosis, cholera, parasitic infection), typhoid fever, toxoplasmosis, hepatitis A and B, brucellosis, dengue, filariasis, leishmaniasis, onchocerciasis (in Venezuela, Brazil, Ecuador, and Colombia), American trypanosomiasis (Chagas disease), bartonellosis, epidemic typhus (louse-borne), schistosomiasis, onchocerciasis, cryptosporidiosis.

CLINICAL FEATURES

Although some patients with travel-related febrile illness present with highly specific signs and symptoms, nonspecific symptoms – cough, shortness of breath, diarrhea, constipation, nausea, vomiting, rash – are common. Physical exam is often unremarkable or nonspecific, but dermatologic findings and other specific signs may aid in narrowing the differential diagnosis.

Physical exam pearls:

1. *Vital signs* – Pulse-temperature dissociation (slow heart rate in spite of high fever) may suggest typhoid fever or a rickettsial disease. Periodic fevers are typical of several travel-related infections, including malaria.
2. *Dermatologic* –

   - Maculopapular rash may be present in dengue fever, leptospirosis, typhus, acute HIV infection, acute hepatitis B, and many drug reactions.
   - Rose spots (small pink macules on the chest or abdomen) suggest typhoid fever.
   - An eschar (black necrotic ulcer with erythematous margins) suggests a number of rickettsial infections. Hemorrhage may occur in dengue fever, meningococcemia, and viral hemorrhagic fevers.
   - Fine serpiginous subcutaneous tracks are characteristic of cutaneous larva migrans.

3. *Ocular* – Conjunctivitis is seen in leptospirosis; conjunctival injection may indicate dengue fever; itching, photophobia, and ocular lesions may be seen in roundworm invasion of the eye (onchocerciasis, loiasis).
4. *Sinus and auditory* – Sinuses, ears, and teeth are common sites of occult infection (sinusitis, otitis media, abscess).
5. *Chest* – New murmurs may appear in bacterial endocarditis.
6. *Abdominal* – Splenomegaly is associated with mononucleosis, malaria, visceral leishmaniasis, typhoid fever, and brucellosis.
7. *Lymphatic* – Bilateral cervical lymphadenopathy may appear in classic Epstein-Barr mononucleosis.
8. *Neurologic* – Fever with altered mental status in the returning traveler is a medical emergency. It may indicate infection by a number of potentially life-threatening species, including *Plasmodium falciparum*.

CLINICAL PRESENTATION OF SPECIFIC DISEASES

Dengue Fever

Clinical presentation of dengue fever ranges from asymptomatic, to the self-limited dengue fever (DF), to the life-threatening dengue hemorrhagic fever (DHF) with shock syndrome (Table 54.1). The risk of severe disease is much higher in recurrent bouts (immunity after the primary infection does not protect against other serotypes).

Symptoms typically develop between 4 and 7 days after exposure. Classic DF presents with an acute fever accompanied by headache, retro-orbital pain, extreme fatigue, and marked muscle and joint pains. The severity of musculoskeletal symptoms accounts for its historical name: "break-bone fever." Fever typically lasts for 5 to 7 days and may be biphasic ("saddleback fever"). Other symptoms may include maculopapular rash, nausea, vomiting, diarrhea, cough, sore throat, and sinus congestion. Physical exam may reveal conjunctival injection, pharyngeal erythema, lymphadenopathy, and hepatomegaly. Neurological manifestations of dengue virus infection occur more rarely and include encephalopathy, seizures, and acute motor weakness. Abdominal pain has been described as the predominant clinical feature in a small subset of patients with DF, mimicking an

Table 54.1 Clinical Features: Dengue

Organism	Any one of four serotypes of dengue virus (DV1–4)
Incubation Period	4–7 days
Signs and Symptoms	**Classic dengue fever (DF):** • Fever with headache • Retro-orbital pain • Extreme fatigue • Marked muscle and joint pain • Maculopapular rash • Nausea, vomiting, diarrhea • Cough, sore throat, sinus congestion • Conjunctival injection, pharyngeal erythema • Lymphadenopathy, hepatomegaly • Encephalopathy, seizures or acute motor weakness **Dengue hemorrhagic fever (DHF):** • Fever lasting 2 to 7 days • Manifestations of increased vascular permeability • Pleural effusion or ascites • Thrombocytopenia • Spontaneous bleeding or a hemorrhagic tendency (positive tourniquet test)
Laboratory Findings	• Cell culture virus isolation • Serology with presence of IgM antibodies • 4-fold rise in antibody titer • Leukopenia is common • Hyponatremia is also common • Thrombocytopenia • Moderate elevation (2- to 8-fold rise) of serum aspartate transaminase (AST)
Prevention	There is no vaccine currently available, so prevention lies in risk reduction. The *Aedes aegypti* mosquito is most active during the day, so although bed-netting is always a good idea, protective clothing and insect repellent are the most important preventative measures.
Treatment	• There is no specific treatment for dengue virus infection • The primary goals of therapy are fever reduction, rehydration, volume replacement, and prevention and treatment of hemorrhage and shock • Because plasma leakage syndrome is the most dangerous complication of DHF, plasma volume replacement is crucial • Shock should be recognized as early as possible

acute abdomen, so clinical suspicion is crucial. It is important to note that spontaneous bleeding can occur even in DF and must be distinguished from DHF.

Dengue hemorrhagic fever is the most serious manifestation of dengue virus infection and may lead to shock. The five features of DHF, as defined by the World Health Organization (WHO), include increased vascular permeability (plasma leakage syndrome, evidenced by 20% or greater rise in hematocrit above baseline value), pleural effusion or ascites, marked thrombocytopenia, fever lasting 2 to 7 days, and hemorrhagic diathesis (positive tourniquet test). (This involves inflating a blood pressure cuff around the arm at a pressure midway between systolic and diastolic for

5 minutes. More than 20 petechiae/square inch is positive. See http://www.who.int/csr/resources/publications/dengue/Denguepublication/en/index.html.) Of these features, plasma leakage syndrome poses the greatest mortality risk to the DHF patient. It coincides with elevation of aminotransferases and severe abdominal pain. Bleeding may manifest as petechiae, ecchymoses, hematemesis, metrorrhagia, melena, or epistaxis.

Clinicians should note the presence of intense abdominal pain, persistent vomiting, a sudden change from fever to hypothermia, and marked restlessness or lethargy, because any of these may signal onset of dengue shock syndrome (DHF with shock).

Malaria

Malaria is an acute, febrile, mosquito-borne illness with an incubation period of 7 days or longer (a fever presenting less than a week after exposure is not malaria). The disease is caused by one of four species of the protozoan genus *Plasmodium*: *P. falciparum*, *P. vivax*, *P. ovale*, or *P. malariae*. The most severe form is caused by *P. falciparum*, the dominant species in tropical Africa, Southeast Asia, Oceania, Haiti, the Amazon basin of South America, and the Dominican Republic.

Symptoms of *P. falciparum* malaria include fever, chills, headache, muscle aches and weakness, vomiting, cough, diarrhea, abdominal pain, and hepatosplenomegaly (Table 54.2). If the infection is active for several days post-incubation, a particular pattern of fever may occur (i.e., patients may notice that the fever peaks at specific times of day). Altered mental status suggests cerebral malaria, a serious complication that is universally fatal without treatment. In advanced infection, signs and symptoms of organ failure may dominate the clinical presentation. Disease progression may include acute renal failure, generalized convulsions, and cardiovascular compromise, followed by coma and death. In endemic areas it is estimated that about 1% of patients with *P. falciparum* infection die. Mortality in nonimmune travelers is significantly higher, especially if treatment is delayed (even for as little as 24 hours). Thus, malaria should be considered with any unexplained fever in a returning traveler, even up to 3 months after the last possible exposure. Importantly, malaria in pregnant travelers increases the risk of maternal death, miscarriage, stillbirth, and neonatal death.

A history of antimalarial chemoprophylaxis is insufficient to exclude a diagnosis of *P. falciparum* malaria, because the prevalence of resistant strains is rising. Numerous strains have acquired resistance to chloroquine, and there are now several regions where intense multidrug resistance has emerged. In border areas between Cambodia, Myanmar, and Thailand, *P. falciparum* infections do not respond to treatment with either chloroquine or sulfadoxine-pyrimethamine, have up to a 50% failure rate with mefloquine, and show a reduced sensitivity to quinine. In these areas, doxycycline or atovaquone-proguanil should be used. Multidrug-resistant malaria has also been reported in Vietnam, Brazil, French Guiana, and Suriname.

Of note, an exoerythrocytic hypnozoite stage of *P. vivax* and *P. ovale* can remain quiescent in the liver following initial infection. Patients may present with relapses caused by activation of these persistent liver forms for months to years after exposure. These dormant organisms require long-term treatment.

PROPHYLAXIS

There are a number of available drugs for malaria prevention. Choice of prophylactic agent should take into account the patient's travel itinerary, psychiatric diagnoses, documented glucose-6-phosphate dehydrogenase (G6PD) deficiency, and other relevant patient information.

The accompanying table of prophylactic antimalarial regimens (Table 54.3) is drawn from CDC guidelines at the time of publication. Clinicians are advised to check the CDC website (http://www.cdc.gov) for the most up-to-date recommendations, because these may change frequently.

TREATMENT

The following treatment information is drawn from the CDC guidelines. Clinicians should refer to the CDC recommendations (http://www.cdc.gov) for the most current and complete information when making patient management decisions (Table 54.4).

Treatment design is dependent on the infecting species, the clinical status of the patient, and likely resistance patterns, based on the geographic regions visited. Identification of the infecting species is critical for several reasons: (1) *P. falciparum* infections require extremely aggressive treatment because of the potential for development of severe clinical malaria; (2) *P. ovale* and *P. vivax* infections generate dormant liver forms (hypnozoites) that may cause recurrent episodes unless treated with primaquine; and (3) geographic drug resistance patterns differ among species.

Table 54.2 Clinical Features: Malaria

Organisms	• *Plasmodium falciparum* • *P. vivax* • *P. ovale* • *P. malariae*
Incubation Period	7 days or longer
Signs and Symptoms	**Generalized illness:** • Fever, chills (a cyclic pattern of febrile episodes may emerge with persistent fevers, commonly repeating every 2–3 days) • Headache • Myalgias, weakness • Cough, vomiting, diarrhea • Abdominal pain • Hepatosplenomegaly • Altered mental status (cerebral infection, universally fatal if untreated) **Advanced disease:** • Acute renal failure • Generalized convulsions • Cardiovascular compromise • Coma
Laboratory Findings	• A thick and thin blood smear should be examined for malarial parasites; if the first sample is negative, serial blood samples should be drawn over several 6-hour intervals, preferably during a febrile episode • Hyperbilirubinemia • Elevated lactate dehydrogenase • Rapid diagnostic tests are available, but are prone to false negative results

Table 54.3 Prophylactic Antimalarial Regimens

Drug	Use	Adult Dose	Pediatric Dose
Atovaquone-proguanil (Malarone)	Prophylaxis in areas with chloroquine- or mefloquine-resistant *Plasmodium falciparum*	One tablet, PO, daily. Adult tablets contain 250 mg atovaquone and 100 mg proguanil hydrochloride.	Pediatric tablets contain 62.5 mg atovaquone and 25 mg proguanil hydrochloride. Dosing is weight-based: • 11–20 kg: one tablet • 21–30 kg: two tablets • 31–40 kg: three tablets • 41 kg or more: one adult tablet daily
	Timeline Begin 1–2 days before travel. Take daily at the same time each day during travel and for 7 days after returning.	**Contraindications** Severe renal impairment (creatinine clearance <30 mL/min)	**Notes** Not recommended for prophylaxis of children <11 kg, pregnant women, or women breastfeeding infants <11 kg. Atovaquone-proguanil should be taken with food or a milky drink.
Chloroquine phosphate (Aralen and generic)	Prophylaxis in areas with chloroquine-sensitive *Plasmodium falciparum*	5 mg/kg base (8.3 mg/kg salt), up to maximum adult dose of 300 mg base, PO, once per week	
	Timeline Begin 1–2 weeks before travel. Take weekly on the same day of the week, during travel and for 4 weeks after returning.	**Contraindications**	**Notes** May exacerbate psoriasis.
Doxycycline	Prophylaxis in areas with chloroquine- or mefloquine-resistant *Plasmodium falciparum*	100 mg, PO, daily	For children 8 years old and over, use 2 mg/kg up to adult dose of 100 mg/day
	Timeline Begin 1–2 days before travel. Take daily at the same time each day while traveling and for 4 weeks after returning.	**Contraindications** Contraindicated in pregnant women and children <8 years of age	**Notes** Patients should be warned about photosensitivity reactions
Hydroxychloroquine sulfate (Plaquenil and generic)	An alternative to chloroquine for prophylaxis in areas with chloroquine-sensitive *Plasmodium falciparum*	5 mg/kg base (6.5 mg/kg salt), PO, once per week, up to maximum dose of 310 mg base	
	Timeline Begin 1–2 weeks before travel. Take weekly on the same day of the week while traveling and for 4 weeks after returning.	**Contraindications**	**Notes**
Mefloquine (Lariam and generic)	Prophylaxis in areas with chloroquine-resistant *Plasmodium falciparum*	228 mg base (250 mg salt), PO, once per week	Pediatric dosing is weight-based: • <10 kg: 4.6 mg/kg base (5 mg/kg salt), once/week. • 10–19 kg: 1/4 adult tablet, once/week • 20–30 kg: 1/2 adult tablet, once/week • 31–45 kg: 3/4 adult tablet, once/week • >45 kg: 1 adult tablet, once/week
	Timeline Begin 1–2 weeks before travel. Take weekly on the same day of the week while traveling and for 4 weeks after returning.	**Contraindications** Contraindicated in persons allergic to mefloquine or related compounds (e.g., quinine and quinidine). Contraindicated in persons with active or recent history of depression, generalized anxiety disorder, psychosis, schizophrenia, other major psychiatric disorders, or seizures.	**Notes** Not recommended for persons with cardiac conduction abnormalities. May reduce serum levels of common seizure medications.
Primaquine	Used for presumptive antirelapse therapy (terminal prophylaxis) to decrease the risk of recurrent illness in *Plasmodium vivax* and *P. ovale* infection. Call malaria hotline (770–488–7788) for additional information.	0.6 mg/kg base (1.0 mg/kg salt), up to maximum dose of 30 mg base (52.6 mg salt), PO, daily	
	Timeline Begin 1–2 days before travel. Take daily at the same time each day while traveling and for 7 days after returning.	**Contraindications** May cause hemolytic episode in patients with G6PD deficiency. Contraindicated during pregnancy and lactation, unless the infant being breastfed has a documented normal G6PD level. Use in consultation with malaria experts.	**Notes**

Special Populations

Table 54.4 Treatment of Malaria

Species	Drug Sensitivity	Adult Treatment*	Pediatric Treatment* (Never to Exceed Adult Dose)
Plasmodium falciparum	Chloroquine-sensitive (Central America west of Panama Canal; Haiti; the Dominican Republic; most of the Middle East)	Chloroquine phosphate (Aralen): • 600 mg base PO immediately • 300 mg base PO at 6, 24, 48 hours Second-line alternative: Hydroxychloroquine (Plaquenil): • 620 mg base PO immediately • 310 mg base PO at 6, 24, 48 hours	Chloroquine phosphate (Aralen): • 10 mg base/kg PO immediately • 5 mg base/kg PO at 6, 24, 48 hours Second-line alternative: Hydroxychloroquine (Plaquenil): • 10 mg base/kg PO immediately • 5 mg base/kg PO at 6, 24, 48 hours
	Chloroquine-resistant (all malarious regions except those listed above)	Any of the following three treatment regimens is considered first line: 1. Quinine sulfate plus one of the following: doxycycline, tetracycline, clindamycin: ○ quinine sulfate: 542 mg base PO tid × 3–7 days ○ doxycycline: 100 mg PO bid × 7 days ○ tetracycline: 250 mg PO qid × 7 days ○ clindamycin: 20 mg base/kg/day PO divided tid × 7 days 2. Atovaquone-proguanil (Malarone): ○ 4 adult tabs PO qd × 3 days 3. Mefloquine (Lariam): ○ 684 mg base PO immediately ○ 456 mg base PO 6–12 hours later	Any of the following three treatment regimens is considered first line: 1. Quinine sulfate plus one of the following: doxycycline, tetracycline, clindamycin ○ quinine sulfate: 8.3 mg base/kg PO tid × 3–7 days ○ doxycycline: 2.2 mg/kg PO bid × 7 days ○ tetracycline: 25 mg/kg/day PO divided qid × 7 days ○ clindamycin: 20 mg base/kg/day PO divided tid × 7 days 2. Atovaquone-proguanil (Malarone): ○ 5–8 kg: 2 peds tabs PO qd × 3 days ○ 9–10 kg: 3 peds tabs PO qd × 3 days ○ 11–20 kg: 1 adult tab PO qd × 3 days ○ 21–30 kg: 2 adult tabs PO qd × 3 days ○ 31–40 kg: 3 adult tabs PO qd × 3 days ○ >40 kg: 4 adult tabs PO qd × 3 days 3. Mefloquine (Lariam): ○ 13.7 mg base/kg PO immediately ○ 9.1 mg base/kg PO 6–12 hours later
Plasmodium malariae	Chloroquine-sensitive[†]	Chloroquine phosphate (as above) Second-line alternative: hydroxychloroquine (as above)	Chloroquine phosphate (as above) Second-line alternative: hydroxychloroquine (as above)
Plasmodium vivax, *Plasmodium ovale*	Chloroquine-sensitive	Chloroquine phosphate *plus* primaquine phosphate: • chloroquine phosphate (as above) • primaquine phosphate: 30 mg base PO qd × 14 days Second-line alternative: Hydroxychloroquine *plus* primaquine phosphate: • hydroxychloroquine (as above) • primaquine phosphate (as above)	Chloroquine phosphate *plus* primaquine phosphate • chloroquine phosphate (as above) • primaquine phosphate: 0.5 mg base/kg PO qd × 14 days Second-line alternative: Hydroxychloroquine *plus* primaquine phosphate: • hydroxychloroquine (as above) • primaquine phosphate (as above)
Plasmodium vivax	Chloroquine-resistant (Papua New Guinea and Indonesia)	Either of the following two treatment regimens are considered first line:	Either of the following two treatment regimens are considered first line:
Severe Infection[‡]		**Adult Treatment**	**Pediatric Treatment**
		Quinidine gluconate plus one of the following: doxycycline, tetracycline, *or* clindamycin • quinidine gluconate: 6.25 mg base/kg loading dose IV over 1–2 hours, 0.0125 mg base/kg/min continuous infusion × at least 24 hours • doxycycline (as above) • tetracycline (as above) • clindamycin (as above)	Quinidine gluconate plus one of the following: doxycycline, tetracycline, *or* clindamycin • quinidine gluconate: same as adult • doxycycline (as above) • tetracycline (as above) • clindamycin (as above)

*Where applicable, medication dosages have been reported in base form. Conversions to appropriate doses of the corresponding salt can be made using updated CDC treatment guidelines as a reference. Care should taken in making these calculations as they are a common source of error.

[†] There have been no reports to date of chloroquine resistance in any strains of *P. malariae*.

[‡] Severe malaria is almost universally caused by strains of *P. falciparum*. Severe infection is distinguished by the presence of one or more of the following: impaired consciousness or coma, severe normocytic anemia, renal failure, pulmonary edema, acute respiratory distress syndrome, circulatory shock, disseminated intravascular coagulation, spontaneous bleeding, acidosis, hemoglobinuria, jaundice, repeated generalized convulsions, and/or parasitemia of >5%.

For the management of malaria in pregnant women, refer to the latest CDC guidelines or consult with a specialist via the CDC Malaria Hotline: (770) 488–7788. Clinicians should also be aware that malaria is a reportable illness nationally and should be promptly reported to the relevant health department.

Rickettsial Infections

Early symptoms, including fever, headache, and malaise, are generally nonspecific. Clinical presentation of rickettsial infections differs among organisms, and laboratory diagnosis is necessary for identification of a particular agent. Hallmark dermatologic signs include rash and an eschar at the site of the tick bite, which may appear in scrub typhus and several of the spotted fevers.

Rickettsial infections can be life threatening. For instance, *Rickettsia rickettsii* invades endothelial cells and causes vasculitis, resulting in the characteristic rash and potentially damaging the brain, lungs, and other organs.

Accurate diagnosis hinges on assessment of exposure risk, because rickettsial infections are specific to geography and vector. Relevant information on the various rickettsioses and their respective vectors, reservoirs, geographic distributions, and major signs and symptoms are elaborated in Tables 54.5 and 54.6.

Infectious Mononucleosis

Infectious mononucleosis (IM) in the returning traveler is caused primarily (90%) by EBV, with a significant subset due to CMV infection. Initial symptoms of classic IM include malaise, headache, and low-grade fever (Table 54.7). Tonsillitis, pharyngitis, cervical lymphadenopathy (usually symmetrical, involving the posterior chain), and moderate to high fevers develop subsequently. Severe fatigue is a prominent and characteristic complaint. Tonsillar exudates (white, gray, green, or necrotic in appearance) are a frequent component of the pharyngitis and can be a source of significant discomfort. Nausea, vomiting, anorexia, and splenomegaly are common.

Other, less common findings include palatal petechiae, periorbital or palpebral edema, and maculopapular or morbilliform rashes (rashes commonly appear after treatment with ampicillin). Neurologic complications can include Guillain-Barré syndrome, facial nerve palsy, meningoencephalitis, aseptic meningitis, transverse myelitis, peripheral neuritis, and optic neuritis. Potential hematologic abnormalities include hemolytic anemia, thrombocytopenia, aplastic anemia, thrombotic thrombocytopenic purpura, and disseminated intravascular coagulation.

Splenic rupture is a rare but potentially fatal complication of IM. Management is similar to other forms of splenic injury. Nonoperative treatment with intensive supportive care and splenic preservation has been successfully carried out in select cases, whereas others have required splenectomy.

Upper airway obstruction due to massive lymphoid hyperplasia and mucosal edema is another uncommon but serious complication. Corticosteroids may be useful in patients who develop or are at significant risk of obstruction. Principles of emergency airway management should be observed.

The vast majority of individuals with IM recover uneventfully. Acute symptoms resolve in 1 to 2 weeks, whereas fatigue often persists for months.

Table 54.5 Clinical Features: Rickettsial Infections

Incubation Period	Generally shorter than 4 weeks
Signs and Symptoms	• Fever, headache, and malaise • Rashes are seen with a number of rickettsioses • An eschar may be seen in scrub typhus and several of the spotted fevers
Laboratory Findings	• Rickettsia do not stain with most conventional methods • Positive DFA, positive ELISA, or a rise in antibody titer are diagnostic • WBC count is generally normal in patients with *R. rickettsii* infection, but the differential is often remarkable for bandemia • Thrombocytopenia • Mild elevations in hepatic transaminases • Hyponatremia • CSF pleocytosis (with polymorphonuclear or lymphocytic predominance)*
Prevention	Prevention of rickettsial infection is limited to avoidance of the infectious vector. Travelers in endemic regions are advised to use repellents and wear protective clothing. If a tick is detected, rapid and appropriate removal should ensue.
Treatment	Treatment of all rickettsial illness is with a tetracycline (doxycycline 100 mg twice daily, PO or IV). In pregnant women, chloramphenicol (50 mg/kg in four divided doses, up to a maximum of 2.0 g) should be used in cases where the clinical course is not expected to be self-limited.

*Laboratory diagnosis of CNS rickettsial infections is difficult and empiric treatment for other causes (e.g., meningococcemia) should be administered until the causative organism is isolated.
CNS, central nervous system; CSF, cerebrospinal fluid; DFA, direct fluorescent antibody; ELISA, enzyme-linked immunosorbent assay; WBC, white blood cell.

A positive heterophile antibody assay (monospot test) supports the clinical diagnosis of EBV-induced IM (though CMV disease is heterophile negative). Although monospot testing is highly specific, false negatives are common, especially early in the clinical course. A negative test in the setting of high clinical suspicion warrants either repeat testing or an assay of EBV-specific IgG and IgM (97% sensitivity). Heterophile-negative IM is seen with CMV, toxoplasmosis, acute HIV infection, hepatitis B, and human herpesvirus (HHV)-6 infection.

As with EBV, CMV-induced IM can be accompanied by numerous dermatologic manifestations, including maculopapular, rubelliform, morbilliform, and scarlatiniform eruptions (some of these appear with ampicillin use). CMV infection has additionally been associated with neurologic sequelae such as encephalitis, Guillain-Barré syndrome and various focal deficits (i.e., Horner's syndrome and peripheral neuropathy).

Enteric Fever

Enteric fever, commonly called typhoid fever, is caused by a group of *Salmonella* species, including *S. typhi* and *S. paratyphi*. Infection manifests as a sustained febrile illness with

Table 54.6 Specific Rickettsial Infections Disease

	Organism	Vector	Reservoir	Geographic Distribution	Signs and Symptoms
Typhus Fevers					
Epidemic typhus, sylvatic typhus	*Rickettsia prowazekii*	Human body louse, squirrel flea, squirrel louse	Humans, flying squirrels	Mountainous regions of Africa, Asia, and Central and South America	Headache, chills, fever, weakness, confusion, photophobia, vomiting, rash (generally starting on trunk)
Murine typhus	*Rickettsia typhi*	Rat flea	Rats, mice	Worldwide	Headache, chills, fever, weakness, confusion, photophobia, vomiting, rash (generally appearing first on the trunk), generally less severe than epidemic typhus
Spotted Fevers					
Rocky Mountain spotted fever	*Rickettsia rickettsii*	Tick	Rodents	United States (particularly in the southeastern and south central states), Canada, Mexico, Central and South America	Headache, fever, abdominal pain, rash (generally appearing first on the extremities)
Mediterranean spotted fever	*Rickettsia conorii*	Tick	Rodents	Africa, India, Europe, Middle East, Mediterranean	Fever, eschar, regional adenopathy, rash on extremities
African tick-bite fever	*Rickettsia africae*	Tick	Rodents	Sub-Saharan Africa	Fever, eschar, regional adenopathy, rash (subtle or absent)
North Asian tick typhus	*Rickettsia sibirica*	Tick	Rodents	Russia, China, Mongolia	Fever, eschar, regional adenopathy, rash (subtle or absent)
Oriental spotted fever	*Rickettsia japonica*	Tick	Rodents	Japan	Fever, eschar, regional adenopathy, rash subtle or absent
Rickettsial pox	*Rickettsia akari*	Mite	House mice	Russia, South Africa, Korea	Fever, eschar, adenopathy, disseminated vesicular rash
Tick-borne disease	*Rickettsia slovaca*	Tick	Lagomorphs (rabbits, pikas), rodents	Europe	Necrosis, erythema, lymphadenopathy
Aneruptive fever	*Rickettsia helvetica*	Tick	Rodents	Europe, Asia, and Africa	Fever, headache, myalgia
Cat flea rickettsiosis	*Rickettsia felis*	Cat and dog flea	Domestic cats, opossums	Europe, South America	Headache, chills, fever, weakness, confusion, photophobia, vomiting, rash (generally starting on trunk) generally less severe than epidemic typhus
Queensland tick typhus	*Rickettsia australis*	Tick	Rodents	Australia, Tasmania	Fever, eschar, regional adenopathy, rash on extremities
Flinders Island spotted fever, Thai tick typhus	*Rickettsia honei*	Tick	Not defined	Australia, Thailand	Fever, rash on extremities, eschar and adenopathy are rare
Orientia					
Scrub typhus	*Orientia tsutsugamushi*	Mite	Rodents	Indian subcontinent, Central, Eastern, and Southeast Asia and Australia	Fever, headache, sweating, conjunctival injection, adenopathy, eschar, rash (nascent on trunk), respiratory distress
Coxiella					
Q fever	*Coxiella burnetii*	Most human infections are acquired via inhalation of contaminated aerosols	Goats, sheep, cattle, domestic cats, other	Worldwide	Fever, headache, chills, sweating, pneumonia, hepatitis, endocarditis

Special Populations

Table 54.7 Clinical Features: Infectious Mononucleosis

Organisms	EBV, CMV, and more rarely HIV (seen in acute infection), *Toxoplasma gondii*, hepatitis B virus, and HHV-6
Incubation Period	Generally shorter than 4 weeks, but variable
Signs and Symptoms	**Common**: • Malaise, headache, fever • Tonsillitis, pharyngitis (with white, gray, green, or necrotic exudate) • Symmetrical, posterior chain cervical lymphadenopathy • Severe fatigue • Nausea, vomiting, anorexia • Splenomegaly **Less common**: • Palatal petechiae • Periorbital or palpebral edema • Maculopapular or morbilliform rashes • Guillain-Barré syndrome, facial nerve palsy, meningoencephalitis, aseptic meningitis, transverse myelitis, peripheral neuritis, optic neuritis • Hemolytic anemia, thrombocytopenia, aplastic anemia, thrombotic thrombocytopenic purpura • Disseminated intravascular coagulation
Laboratory Findings	**Virus-specific findings**: • EBV – heterophile antibody positive, IgG and IgM serologies • CMV – heterophile antibody negative, IgG and IgM serologies, early antigen detection can be accomplished via shell vial cultures **Both**: • Absolute lymphocytosis with >50% mononuclear cells and >10% atypical lymphocytes • Reduced haptoglobin levels • Cold agglutinins • Elevated rheumatoid factor • Positive ANA
Prevention	There is no known prophylaxis. Precautions should be taken to avoid contact with body fluids of infected patients.
Treatment	**EBV**: • Generally limited to supportive, symptomatic therapy. Use of corticosteroids and acyclovir is controversial but may be helpful in reducing discomfort from lymphoid and mucosal swelling. Because of the risk of traumatic splenic rupture, patients should be advised not to participate in physical activities that put them at risk for injury. **CMV**: • No specific treatment is indicated unless the patient is immunocompromised. In such patients, ganciclovir, valganciclovir, foscarnet, and cidofovir can be used.

ANA, antinuclear antibodies.

Table 54.8 Clinical Features: Enteric Fever

Organisms	• *Salmonella typhi* • *S. paratyphi*
Incubation	5 to 21 days
Signs and Symptoms	• Week 1 – rising ("stepwise") fever • Week 2 – abdominal pain, rose spots • Week 3 – hepatosplenomegaly, intestinal bleeding, bowel perforation • Constipation followed by diarrhea • Relative bradycardia, pulse-temperature dissociation • Other features include septic shock, altered level of consciousness, acute psychosis, myelitis, rigidity
Laboratory Findings	• Blood culture isolation of the causative microorganism (*S. typhi, S. paratyphi*) • Culturing stool, urine, and rose spots may also yield organisms. If clinical suspicion is high, but cultures are negative, bone marrow aspiration is recommended. • Leukopenia • Leukocytosis • Abnormal liver function tests
Prevention	Two typhoid vaccines (oral and intramuscular) are available. Neither provides protection against paratyphoid infection and neither is completely effective against *S. typhi*.
Treatment	Many *Salmonella* strains are resistant to ampicillin, trimethoprim-sulfamethoxazole, and chloramphenicol. More recently, resistance to fluoroquinolones has begun to emerge. In planning treatment, antibiotic susceptibility testing should be performed. Appropriate first-line therapies include: • ciprofloxacin (500 mg twice/day) or ofloxacin (400 mg twice/day) either PO or parenterally × 7–10 days • ceftriaxone (2–3 g once/day parenterally × 7–14 days) Second-line treatment options: • cefixime (20–30 mg/kg per day PO, bid, × 7–14 days) • azithromycin (1 g PO, single dose, followed by 500 mg once/day × 7–14 days or 1 g PO qd × 5 days) • chloramphenicol (2–3 g per day PO, qid, × 14 days) For U.S. pediatric patients, the following agents are considered first-line: • ceftriaxone (100 mg/kg per day IV, maximum 4 g per day × 10–14 days) • cefotaxime (150–200 mg/kg per day IV, maximum 12 g per day × 10–14 days) • cefixime (20 mg/kg per day PO, bid, maximum 400 mg per day × 10–14 days) • ciprofloxacin (30 mg/kg daily, PO or parenterally, maximum 1000 mg per day × 7–10 days) • ofloxacin (30 mg/kg daily, PO or parenterally, maximum 800 mg per day × 7–10 days) For severe typhoid fever (disease with associated mental status changes) in both children and adults corticosteroid therapy is indicated: • dexamethasone (loading dose of 3 mg/kg followed by 1 mg/kg IV q6h × a total of 48 hours)

abdominal symptoms 5 to 21 days after ingestion of the causative microorganism (Table 54.8).

The classic presentation in untreated individuals follows a timed progression: week 1 — rising ("stepwise") fever; week 2 — abdominal pain and rose spots; week 3 — organomegaly, intestinal bleeding, and bowel perforation (related to

Special Populations

ileocecal lymphatic hyperplasia), which may result in secondary bacteremia and peritonitis. Although most infections eventually cause diarrhea, a large number manifest initially with constipation. Relative bradycardia and pulse-temperature dissociation, although not diagnostic, are classically associated with enteric fever.

Less common complications include septic shock, altered level of consciousness, acute psychosis, myelitis, and rigidity. As a result of bacteremia, focal extraintestinal complications may occur, extending potentially to all organ systems.

DIFFERENTIAL DIAGNOSIS

The differential diagnosis of fever in the returning traveler is based largely on likely exposure. Clinical symptoms increase suspicion and laboratory diagnosis is confirmatory for many diseases. The following tables may be helpful in beginning a differential.

Table 54.9 divides a number of travel-related diseases by length of time from exposure to onset of symptoms. Table 54.10 links exposure risk to type of contact.

LABORATORY DIAGNOSIS

Fever in the returning traveler is often treated empirically, though a number of laboratory tests may be obtained to narrow the differential and aid in choice of therapy:

- complete blood count with differential and/or thick and thin smears to inspect for intracellular parasites
- chemistry panel (electrolytes, blood urea nitrogen, creatinine)
- serum glucose
- liver panel (alanine aminotransferase, aspartate aminotransferase, total bilirubin, alkaline phosphatase)
- urinalysis
- chest x-ray
- blood culture

Table 54.9 Typical Incubation Times for Travel-Related Infections

Incubation Period	Diseases
Short (<4 Weeks)	Insect-borne virus infection (e.g., dengue fever), bacterial dysentery, brucellosis, EBV infection, hepatitis A, influenza, leptospirosis, plague, Q fever, relapsing fever, rickettsial spotted fevers, rubella, rubeola, tularemia, typhoid fever, typhus, yellow fever
Long (>4 Weeks)	Trypanosomiasis (African and American), amebiasis, brucellosis, filariasis, hepatitis B and C, leishmaniasis, melioidosis, paragonimiasis, rabies, strongyloidiasis, tuberculosis
Variable	Malaria (generally short without chemoprophylaxis), schistosomiasis, some sexually transmitted diseases (e.g., syphilis)

Adapted from the CDC Traveler's Health Yellow Book: Health Information for International Travel, 2005–2006. Available at: http://www2.ncid.cdc.gov/travel/yb/utils/ybGet.asp?section = dis&obj = rickettsial.htm&cssNav = browseoyb. Retrieved December 11, 2006.

Table 54.10 Travel-Related Disease: Exposure Risk by Type of Contact

Sexual Contact	Chancroid, gonorrhea, hepatitis B, HIV infection, syphilis
Animal Contact	
Monkeys	B-virus (cercopithecine herpesvirus 1) infection
Deer mice	Hantavirus pulmonary syndrome
Dogs	Rabies (in developing countries), Rocky Mountain spotted fever (*Rickettsia rickettsii*)
Skunks, raccoons, bats	Rabies (in the United States)
Civet cat	SARS, coronavirus infection
Chickens/fowl	Avian influenza
Wild birds	Avian influenza, West Nile fever
Rodents	Rocky Mountain spotted fever (*R. rickettsii*), epidemic typhus (*R. prowazekii*), endemic typhus (*R. typhi*), plague (especially prairie dogs)
Insect Contact	
Mosquitoes	Malaria, dengue fever, yellow fever, Rift Valley fever, arboviral encephalitides (including West Nile fever, Japanese encephalitis, and Venezuelan equine encephalitis)
Ticks	Rocky Mountain spotted fever (*Rickettsia rickettsii*), tularemia
Mites	Rickettsial pox (*R. akari*), scrub typhus (*R. tsutsugamushi*)
Fleas	Endemic typhus (*R. typhi*)
Lice	Epidemic typhus (*R. prowazekii*)
Tsetse flies	African trypanosomiasis
Ingested	
Undercooked food	Cholera, nontyphoidal salmonellosis, trichinosis, typhoid fever (*Salmonella typhi*, *S. paratyphi*)
Untreated water	Cholera, hepatitis A, nontyphoidal salmonellosis, typhoid fever (*S. typhi*, *S. paratyphi*), giardiasis
Unpasteurized dairy	Brucellosis, tuberculosis
Fresh Water Contact	Leptospirosis, schistosomiasis, *Naegleria* or *Acanthamoeba* infection

SARS, severe acute respiratory syndrome.

Less commonly indicated tests that should be ordered based on clinical suspicion include:

- stool ova and parasites should be ordered for patients at risk for parasites
- hepatitis serologies
- coagulation studies
- HIV and sexually transmitted disease tests
- purified protein derivative (PPD)

PEARLS AND PITFALLS

1. History, physical examination, and a knowledge of the geographic distribution of common pathogens are critical to proper diagnosis and treatment of the majority of travel-related febrile illnesses.
2. Travelers should be educated and given appropriate vaccines and medications prior to departure. Travelers should be further advised to bring a thermometer and to keep a diary of signs and symptoms.
3. Not every fever in the returning traveler is related to travel.
4. Remote travel history may be important (e.g., liver flukes or malaria can lie dormant for decades).

5. The CDC and the International Society for Travel Medicine (ISTM) are excellent resources for physicians and patients.

REFERENCES

Birnbaumer DM. Fever in the returning traveler. In: Slaven EM, Stone SC, Lopez FA, eds, Infectious diseases: emergency department diagnosis & management, 1st ed. New York: McGraw-Hill, 2007.

Brandfonbrener A, Epstein A, Wu S, Phair J. Corticosteroid therapy in Epstein-Barr virus infection. Arch Intern Med 1986;146:337.

Chaijaroenkul W, Bangchang KN, Mungthin M, Ward SA. In vitro antimalarial drug susceptibility in Thai border areas from 1998–2003. Malar J 2005 Aug 2;4:37.

Chapman AS, in collaboration with the Tickborne Rickettsial Diseases Working Group. CDC guidelines. Diagnosis and management of tickborne rickettsial diseases: Rocky Mountain spotted fever, ehrlichioses, and anaplasmosis – United States: a practical guide for physicians and other health-care and public health professionals. Available at: http://www.cdc.gov/mmwr/preview/mmwrhtml/rr5504a1.htm. Retrieved March 25, 2008.

Freedman DO, Weld LH, Kozarsky PE, et al. Spectrum of disease and relation to place of exposure among ill returned travelers. N Engl J Med 2006;354:119.

Khan MA, Smego RA Jr, Razi ST, Beg MA. Emerging drug-resistance and guidelines for treatment of malaria [Review]. J Coll Physician Surg Pak 2004 May;14(5):319–24.

Khor BS, Liu JW, Lee IK, Yang KD. Dengue hemorrhagic fever patients with acute abdomen: clinical experience of 14 cases. Am J Trop Med Hyg 2006 May;74(5):901–4.

Lo Re V 3rd, Gluckman SJ. Fever in the returned traveler [Review]. Am Fam Physician 2003 Oct 1;68(7):1343–50.

Tynell E, Aurelius E, Brandell A, et al. Acyclovir and prednisolone treatment of acute infectious mononucleosis: a multicenter, double-blind, placebo-controlled study. J Infect Dis 1996;174:324.

World Health Organization. Guidelines for the diagnosis and treatment of malaria. Available at: http://whqlibdoc.who.int/publications/2005/9241580364_chap7.pdf. Retrieved December 10, 2006.

ADDITIONAL READINGS

Mensah GA, Grant AO, Pepine CJ, et al. ACCF/AHA/CDC conference report on emerging infectious diseases and biological terrorism threats: the clinical and public health implications for the prevention and control of cardiovascular diseases. Circulation 2007 Mar 27;115(12):1656–95.

Saxe SE, Gardner P. The returning traveler with fever [Review]. Infect Dis Clin North Am 1992 Jun;6(2):427–39.

Spicuzza L, Spicuzza A, La Rosa M, et al. New and emerging infectious diseases [Review]. Allergy Asthma Proc. 2007 Jan–Feb;28(1):28–34.

Stone L, Olinky R, Huppert A. Seasonal dynamics of recurrent epidemics. Nature 2007 Mar 29;446(7135):533–6.

Watt G, Parola P. Scrub typhus and tropical rickettsioses [Review]. Curr Opin Infect Dis 2003 Oct;16(5):429–36.

55. Infectious Complications of Injection Drug Use

Ralph Wang and Bradley W. Frazee

INTRODUCTION

It is estimated that 3 million Americans have used heroin in their lifetime, and that there were 400,000 active heroin users in the United States in the year 2000, many of whom inject the drug. There are about half as many cocaine and methamphetamine injection drug users (IDUs). Emergency departments (EDs) serve as a regular source of medical care for this patient population, and at some urban hospitals, as many as 10% of admissions are related to injection drug use (IDU).

The list of infections resulting from IDU spans the entire spectrum of infectious disease – from common viral infections, such as hepatitis C, to rare bacterial infections. This chapter will describe the infectious diseases that are commonly encountered in the acute care setting in patients who are IDUs. These include infectious endocarditis, cutaneous abscess, necrotizing fasciitis, septic arthritis and osteomyelitis, spinal epidural abscess, wound botulism, and tetanus.

Common to many of the infections discussed in this chapter is the difficulty of making a correct diagnosis and the high risk of morbidity. IDU-associated soft-tissue infections include not only simple subcutaneous abscess and cellulitis, but also necrotizing fasciitis, which may be fatal if not rapidly diagnosed and treated. Wound botulism related to IDU is easily misdiagnosed, and failure to initiate specific therapy can lead to respiratory failure. Similarly, a delay in the diagnosis of spinal epidural abscess – a notorious complication of injection drug use that may present simply as back pain – can result in irreversible paralysis.

Roughly 40% of febrile IDUs who present to the acute care setting have no apparent source of fever and seem well enough to be discharged. However, a significant proportion of these patients harbor an occult serious infection, and even a thorough work-up cannot exclude the possibility of bacteremia and endocarditis. The issue of appropriate management and disposition of the IDU with fever that has no apparent source is discussed below.

INJECTION DRUG USE–ASSOCIATED ENDOCARDITIS

Infective endocarditis (IE), defined as a bacterial or fungal infection of the heart valves and perivalvular tissue, is a notorious complication of IDU. Endocarditis due to IDU differs from non-IDU-related disease. In the absence of IDU, endocarditis occurs almost exclusively in the setting of underlying valve pathology or prosthesis, whereas such abnormalities are present in less than 25% of IDU-associated cases (see Chapter 1, Infective Endocarditis). It is speculated that injected material may produce subtle valve damage, particularly of the tricuspid valve, that is not evident in echocardiography studies. The frequent bacteremia caused by IDU, which then leads to IE, usually results from introduction of skin flora, and less often from contaminated drugs or syringes.

Staphylococcus aureus causes 51–82% of cases of IE in IDUs, in contrast to non-IDU cases where *Streptococcus viridans* species are the predominant pathogen. The percentage of IDU-related endocarditis caused by methicillin-resistant *Staphylococcus aureus* (MRSA) continues to rise. MRSA was recently estimated to account for up to 37% of *S. aureus* endocarditis in the United States. *Pseudomonas*, a frequent pathogen in some early case series involving IDU, is found in only 5–10% of cases in recent studies. Other organisms found in IDU-related IE include streptococcal species, *Enterococcus*, enteric gram-negatives, and fungi, particularly *Candida* species. Culture-negative endocarditis, which may be caused by the HACEK organisms or by any organism whose growth in culture is suppressed by prior antibiotic use, accounts for 5–10% of cases in IDUs.

The pattern of valvular involvement in IDU-related endocarditis differs from that in non-IDUs in that vegetations are more commonly located on the tricuspid valve. Right-sided endocarditis has a distinctive pathophysiology and clinical presentation. Left-sided endocarditis usually produces significant mitral or aortic valve regurgitation with an audible murmur and may lead to pump failure. Tricuspid regurgitation is of lesser hemodynamic consequence and may be clinically silent. Similarly, whereas left-sided IE is associated with prominent vascular and immune phenomena, such as splinter hemorrhages, these findings are absent in isolated right-sided disease. Instead, right-sided endocarditis tends to produce pulmonary signs and symptoms such as chest pain and infiltrates on chest x-ray from septic pulmonary emboli.

Another fairly common form of endocarditis in IDUs is *S. aureus* infection of the aortic or mitral valves, which results in so-called acute bacterial endocarditis. In contrast to isolated tricuspid disease, or subacute bacterial endocarditis with *Streptococcus viridans* species, aortic and mitral valve infection by *S. aureus* is associated with a more aggressive course and high morbidity and mortality (see later discussion). *S. aureus* aortic valve endocarditis results in heart failure, valve destruction requiring surgical replacement, or death, in up to 40% of cases. Septic embolization to the brain, coronary arteries, or kidneys can occur. IE presenting with altered mental status or heart failure is considered an ominous sign, indicating likely infection of the aortic valve.

Epidemiology

Infective endocarditis, although a well-recognized complication of injection drug use, is actually fairly uncommon, with an incidence of 1–20 per 10,000 users per year. IE accounts for 5–15% of hospitalizations for IDU-related infections. IDUs who are positive for human immunodeficiency virus (HIV) are at substantial increased risk for IE, and cocaine injection may present a higher risk than heroin.

Clinical Features

Endocarditis typically presents with nonspecific symptoms such as arthralgias, malaise, back pain, and weight loss (Table 55.1). Pulmonary symptoms such as cough, dyspnea, and chest pain are more common in tricuspid disease. Fever is a cardinal sign, found at presentation in more than 94% of patients.

Table 55.1 Clinical Features: IDU Endocarditis

Organisms	• *Staphylococcus aureus* (MSSA and MRSA) • *Streptococcus* species • *Enterococcus* species • Enteric gram-negatives • Fungi
Signs and Symptoms	• Fever • Malaise, weight loss • Cough (tricuspid vegetation) • Dyspnea • Chest pain, back pain • Murmur (30–50% of patients) • Heart failure (left-sided *S. aureus*) • Altered mental status (left-sided *S. aureus*)
Laboratory and Radiologic Findings	• Persistent bacteremia • Echocardiography: oscillating intracardiac mass attached to a valve (definitive), valvular incompetence, reduced ventricular function, perivalvular abscess

MRSA, methicillin-resistant *Staphylococcus aureus*; MSSA, methicillin-sensitive *Staphylococcus aureus*.

A murmur is heard at the time of presentation in only 30–50% of IDU-related cases, and in even fewer of those with isolated right-sided disease. Classic vascular and immune phenomena are often absent in IDU-related disease.

Differential Diagnosis

Rarely is endocarditis obvious at the time of acute care presentation. More often a broad differential for the source of the patient's fever must be considered. Common infections in the IDU population that may present similarly include the following:

- community-acquired pneumonia
- skin and soft-tissue infection
- septic arthritis, osteomyelitis, spinal epidural abscess
- pyelonephritis and pelvic inflammatory disease
- HIV-related opportunistic infections
- transient *S. aureus* bacteremia
- viral syndromes, including hepatitis
- pyrogen reaction to injected material ("cotton fever")

Laboratory and Radiographic Findings

The chest x-ray is an essential diagnostic study in the evaluation of possible endocarditis because the chest radiograph is abnormal in up to 72% of IDUs with IE, possibly due to the high proportion of right-sided disease. Septic pulmonary emboli classically appear as multiple round infiltrates that may show evidence of cavitation. Other findings on chest radiograph include nonspecific infiltrates, pleural effusions and pulmonary edema. Laboratory abnormalities that support the diagnosis of IE include hematuria, proteinuria and anemia. On electrocardiogram (ECG), conduction abnormalities, particularly atrioventricular (AV) block, may be seen because of an associated valve ring abscess that erodes into the conducting system.

Blood cultures are a cornerstone of diagnosis in IE. Endocarditis produces a continuous bacteremia, and blood cultures are positive in 80–95% of cases of infectious endocarditis diagnosed by Duke criteria. Proper blood culture collection prior to administration of antibiotics is essential. At least two separate cultures should be obtained, each containing 10 mL of blood, although the recommendation that they be separated in time by as much as 1 hour may be difficult to adhere to in the ED.

Echocardiography is used both for definitive diagnosis and to assess complications and prognosis. The finding of an oscillating intracardiac mass attached to a valve is considered definitive evidence of endocarditis. Other possible echocardiographic findings include valvular incompetence, reduced ventricular function, and perivalvular abscess. Diagnostic criteria, such as the Duke criteria, that incorporate both clinical and echocardiographic findings assist in making the diagnosis of IE.

Treatment and Prophylaxis

Empiric treatment of suspected IE related to IDU should cover *S. aureus* (usually including MRSA) and streptococcal species. The regimen of choice is nafcillin plus gentamicin, or vancomycin plus gentamicin, depending on the local prevalence

Table 55.2 Initial IV Therapy for IDU Endocarditis

Patient Category	Therapy Recommendation
Adults	nafcillin 2 g IV q4h or vancomycin 1 g IV q12h (if high prevalence of MRSA or PCN allergy) *plus* gentamicin 1–1.7 mg/kg IV q8h
Immunocompromised	Same as for nonimmunocompromised persons

PCN, penicillin.

of MRSA (Table 55.2). The regimen of vancomycin and gentamicin is also used in patients with proven penicillin allergy. Unfortunately, vancomycin has been shown to be less effective than nafcillin in eradicating methicillin-sensitive *S. aureus*, and empirical therapy should be tailored as soon as blood culture results become available. The addition of gentamicin to nafcillin shortens the time to negative blood cultures, and a 2-week course of nafcillin and gentamicin has been shown to effectively treat isolated tricuspid valve IE in IDUs, provided the vegetation is small and there is no evidence of pulmonary emboli. In well-appearing patients, treatment can be delayed until culture results are known; however, empirical treatment should be started immediately for all ill-appearing patients and those with heart failure.

Complications and Admission Criteria

Serious complications of endocarditis are more common with left-sided disease. Intracardiac complications include valvular destruction and resultant heart failure, intracardiac abscess, purulent pericarditis, and septic embolization to the coronary arteries. Septic embolic complications are often seen in left-sided *S. aureus* endocarditis. Septic cerebral emboli may present with delirium or focal neurological findings. Meningitis may occur in association with IE and likely results from microemboli to the meningeal arteries. Spinal epidural abscess is a feared rare complication of IE. Renal sequelae include glomerulonephritis as well as renal infarction. Right-sided IE causes downstream pulmonary complications such as septic pulmonary embolism, pneumonia, empyema, and pyopneumothorax. Mortality from endocarditis in IDUs ranges from 2% to 39%. Isolated right-sided disease has a mortality of less than 10%.

Special Considerations – Disposition of the Injection Drug User with a Fever

The proper evaluation and disposition of the IDU with a fever can be difficult. In many cases there is an underlying infection that requires admission; often, it can be diagnosed after a thorough ED evaluation. Patients should be carefully examined for signs of a soft-tissue infection and a thorough heart and lung exam performed. Any musculoskeletal or neurologic complaint including pain should be viewed as a possible indicator of infection. Findings such as decreased range of motion in a joint, weakness, or numbness may point to an infectious source. The chest radiograph has a high yield in this patient population, because pneumonia and HIV-related diseases such as tuberculosis are common, and because endocarditis frequently produces chest radiograph abnormalities. Occa-

sionally, more complicated diagnostic testing (e.g., magnetic resonance imaging [MRI]) is required to make the correct diagnosis. Despite a thorough work-up, however, in about 40% of IDUs with fever, no apparent source can be found and the patient seems well enough to be discharged. Unfortunately, a significant proportion of these well-appearing patients harbor an occult serious infection, such as bacteremia or endocarditis.

The problem of proper disposition of febrile but well-appearing IDUs with no apparent source of fever has been examined in four prospective studies involving a total of approximately 500 patients. Six to 13% of such patients were eventually diagnosed with IE. Unfortunately, it is often difficult to predict which patients actually have endocarditis. To complicate matters, IDUs may not follow up reliably, if, for example, blood cultures turn positive after discharge. This forms the basis for the recommendation that all febrile IDUs without an obvious source of fever, even if they appear well, should have 2 blood cultures drawn and should be admitted to the hospital until cultures remain negative for 48 hours. This approach remains the standard of practice at urban teaching hospitals that serve large IDU populations.

SUBCUTANEOUS ABSCESS

Abscesses are collections of pus or infected material found within the cutaneous or subcutaneous spaces. (See also Chapter 43, Bacterial Skin and Soft-Tissue Infections.) Despite the fact that antibiotics are rarely necessary because surgical drainage is usually sufficient treatment, the bacteriology of IDU abscesses has been well studied. Skin flora and oral flora account for the majority of pathogens. *Staphylococcus aureus* and *Streptococcus* species are the predominant aerobes. MRSA is now a common pathogen in IDU-related abscesses, even if the patient lacks traditional risk factors, such as recent hospitalization. *Eikenella*, a gram-negative aerobe that is found in "fight bites," is commonly found. *Peptostreptococcus* and *Fusobacterium* are the predominant anaerobes. *Bacteroides fragilis*, an antibiotic-resistant anaerobe, is less commonly found in abscesses above the diaphragm.

Epidemiology

Subcutaneous abscess is the most common bacterial complication of IDU. A recent study reported a 32% prevalence of abscess among active IDUs. The practice of subcutaneous injection, or "skin popping," increases the risk of abscess approximately five fold. Needle licking, another common practice, probably accounts for the high percentage of oral flora found in IDU-related abscesses. Other risk factors for abscesses formation include cocaine injection, lack of skin preparation, and use of dirty needles.

Clinical Features

Most patients complain of a painful mass at a previous injection site (Table 55.3). Large abscesses that typically occur in the upper arm and gluteal regions may produce a low-grade fever. Erythema, fluctuance, and drainage are confirmatory physical findings, present in a majority of cases. However, early abscesses, or deep, often intramuscular, collections may exhibit no fluctuance and are easily misdiagnosed as cellulitis or a septic joint.

Table 55.3 Clinical Features: Subcutaneous Abscesses

Organisms	• *Staphylococcus aureus* (MSSA and MRSA) • *Streptococcus* species • *Eikenella* • *Peptostreptococcus* • *Fusobacterium*
Signs and Symptoms	• Pain at a previous injection site • Fever (low grade, associated with large abscesses) • Erythema • Fluctuance • Drainage • Superficial necrosis
Laboratory and Radiologic Studies	• Blood cultures: positive in approximately 20% of febrile patients • Leukocytosis • Ultrasound: hypoechoic collection • Plain x-ray: foreign body (e.g., needle), gas bubble

MRSA, methicillin-resistant *Staphylococcus aureus*; MSSA, methicillin-sensitive *Staphylococcus aureus*.

Differential Diagnosis

The diagnosis of a subcutaneous abscess is usually straightforward. Complications and coexisting infections can occur, however. These include necrotizing soft-tissue infection, septic arthritis, osteomyelitis, epidural abscess, and endocarditis. Among these, by far the most important is a necrotizing soft-tissue infection, which can appear initially as a simple abscess, yet requires immediate and extensive surgical debridement.

Laboratory and Radiographic Findings

Ultrasound can be indispensable in revealing the correct diagnosis, and, where available, this modality has largely replaced needle aspiration to confirm and localize a pus collection. Abscess cavities are visualized as a hypoechoic mass with posterior acoustic enhancement. Plain radiographs, although unnecessary in routine management, may reveal a subcutaneous needle or soft-tissue gas. A single gas bubble is sometimes seen in an abscess cavity, but gas within the tissues should always raise the possibility of a necrotizing infection.

Abscess cultures from the incision and drainage are indicated if the prevalence of MRSA in a particular community has not been previously established. Although blood cultures are rarely indicated in the management of abscesses, studies have shown that bacteremia is present in up to 20% of patients with large abscesses associated with fever and requiring drainage in the operating room. Bacteremia is almost never present if there is no associated fever.

Treatment and Prophylaxis

Incision and drainage is the primary treatment for IDU-related abscess (Table 55.4). In most cases this can be performed in the acute care setting. Achieving adequate anesthesia is often a challenge. A generous incision should be made and the abscess cavity bluntly dissected and explored. Patients are instructed to return at least once, at 24–48 hours, for wound check, dressing change, and to review wound care procedures.

Table 55.4 Initial Treatment for Abscess Complicated by Cellulitis or Underlying Immunosuppression

Patient Category	Therapy Recommendation

Adults	• Incision and drainage in all patients
	• Oral antibiotics:
	  cephalexin 500 mg PO qid *plus* TMP-SMX DS bid
	  or
	  dicloxacillin 500 mg qid *plus* TMP-SMX DS bid
	  or
	  clindamycin 300–450 mg tid, alone
	• IV antibiotics:
	  clindamycin 600 mg q8h *plus* vancomycin 1 g q12h

DS, double strength.

The need for prophylactic antibiotics prior to incision and drainage, to suppress bacteremia and prevent endocarditis, is controversial. American Heart Association guidelines list abscess incision and drainage among the procedures for which preoperative antibiotics should be considered in patients with high-risk cardiac abnormalities. However, there is very little evidence to suggest that abscess incision and drainage causes persistent bacteremia. Pre-incision and drainage antibiotics can be limited to patients at highest risk for endocarditis: those with prosthetic valves, congenital cardiac abnormalities, or a prior history of endocarditis.

Treatment of uncomplicated abscesses with a course of oral antibiotics, following incision and drainage, is usually not indicated. Antibiotics should be given when there appears to be significant surrounding cellulitis and should be given in patients with diabetes or HIV infection. Adequate staphylococcal (including MRSA) and streptococcal coverage can be achieved with a combination of a first generation cephalosporin or dicloxacillin plus trimethoprim-sulfamethoxazole (TMP-SMX) or with clindamycin alone. Gram-negative and anaerobic coverage, such as with amoxicillin-clavulanate or a quinolone, is usually not necessary. If the abscess is accompanied by fever or if the patient is ill appearing, parenteral antibiotics and admission to a surgical service are indicated.

INJECTION DRUG USE–ASSOCIATED NECROTIZING SOFT-TISSUE INFECTIONS

(See also Chapter 43, Bacterial Skin and Soft-Tissue Infections.) Necrotizing soft-tissue infections (NSTIs) include necrotizing fasciitis, myositis, and necrotizing cellulitis. These are rapidly progressive, life-threatening soft-tissue infections involving deep subcutaneous tissue, fascia, and muscle and are associated with systemic toxicity. Immediate surgical exploration is generally required for diagnosis, and if necrotizing fasciitis is found, aggressive debridement is required for cure. A definitive diagnosis is made intraoperatively when friable, necrotic fascia or muscle, often with associated vascular thrombosis, is found.

Bacteriology studies reveal that 60–85% of NSTIs are polymicrobial. Aerobes include *Staphylococcus aureus* and group A *Streptococcus*; anaerobes include gas-forming *Clostridium* species, *Peptostreptococcus*, and other so-called oral anaerobes. In cases caused by IDU, staphylococcal species and clostridial species are the dominant pathogens isolated.

Special Populations

Table 55.5 Clinical Features: Necrotizing Soft-Tissue Infections

Organisms	• Usually polymicrobial • *Staphylococcus aureus* (including MRSA) • *Streptococcus* species • *Clostridium* species • Oral anaerobes
Signs and Symptoms	• Pain (out of proportion to exam) • Erythema • Edema (circumferential; "woody") • Skin necrosis, bullae • Cutaneous sensory deficit
Laboratory and Radiologic Findings	• WBC >14,000/mm³ • Subcutaneous gas on plain x-ray • Elevated BUN and sodium <135

BUN, blood urea nitrogen; WBC, white blood (cell) count.

Table 55.6 Initial IV Therapy for Necrotizing Fasciitis

Patient Category	Therapy Recommendation
Adults	• Prompt surgical debridement • Aggressive fluid resuscitation • Antibiotics: piperacillin-tazobactam 3.375 g IV q6h or cefepime 1 g IV q8h or imipenem 500 mg IV q6h *plus* clindamycin 900 mg IV q6h *plus* vancomycin 1 g IV q12h
Immunocompromised	Same as for nonimmunocompromised persons

Epidemiology

In community-acquired cases of NSTI (as opposed to hospital-acquired or postoperative cases), the most prevalent risk factor is IDU. Use of black tar heroin, a highly contaminated drug produced in Mexico, and the practice of "skin popping" (intradermal or intramuscular injection) are linked to outbreaks of severe NSTI in which clostridial species are isolated in a high proportion of cases.

Clinical Features

The timely diagnosis of NSTI is critical, yet often difficult. Patients may present with a variety of nonspecific symptoms and signs that lead to initial misdiagnosis. Nonspecific signs and symptoms include pain, warmth, and edema (Table 55.5). Fever is present at presentation in only 30–80%. Findings more specific for NSTI, but often absent, include pain out of proportion to skin findings, skin necrosis, bullae, crepitus from subcutaneous gas, and a cutaneous sensory deficit. Tense circumferential edema of an extremity, often spreading onto the trunk, is highly characteristic of NSTI due to IDU. Signs of shock or organ dysfunction are found at the time of presentation in 0–40% of cases.

Laboratory and Radiographic Findings

Marked leukocytosis is highly characteristic of NSTI, with a white blood cell count (WBC) above 20,000/mm³ found in about 50% of cases. Whereas extreme leukocytosis should raise concern for NSTI, its absence does not exclude the diagnosis. Other objective criteria reported to be useful in differentiating necrotizing from non-necrotizing skin infections include WBC greater than 14,000/mm³, gas on plain soft-tissue x-ray, elevated blood urea nitrogen (BUN), and sodium less than 135 mEq/L.

Imaging can help differentiate NSTI from less severe skin infections. Plain film demonstrates subcutaneous gas in a stippled pattern in 20–60% of cases. Computed tomographic (CT) scan is somewhat more sensitive than plain film in demonstrating gas in the tissue and may reveal unsuspected deep fluid collections or phlegmon. The typical CT finding in NSTI is asymmetric thickening of deep fascia associated with gas.

MRI, although expensive and time consuming, may be useful in differentiating NSTI from non-necrotizing infections.

Although a positive result from an imaging study is useful, indicating the need for immediate operation, a negative result cannot be relied on to exclude the diagnosis. Moreover, delays associated with obtaining a CT scan or MRI should not delay surgical exploration, once NSTI is suspected. The proper approach to diagnosis combines the following: a high index of suspicion on the part of the emergency physician, prompt surgical consultation, and a low threshold for operative exploration.

Treatment and Prophylaxis

Initial management of NSTI includes aggressive fluid resuscitation and early broad-spectrum antibiotics. Prompt surgical debridement is the cornerstone of therapy (Table 55.6). A delay to surgical debridement is the single most important risk for increased morbidity and mortality. Even a 1-day delay may increase mortality fourfold.

Complications and Admission Criteria

Death is the major complication of NSTI, which has an overall mortality rate of around 25%. Comparison of IDU-related NSTI versus non-IDU NSTI at one institution revealed a lower mortality among IDUs (10% vs. 21%), which may be explained by their younger age and lack of comorbidities. Other complications include extremity amputation, extensive debridement, septic shock, and prolonged intensive care unit (ICU) stay.

INJECTION DRUG USE–ASSOCIATED SEPTIC ARTHRITIS AND OSTEOMYELITIS

Both septic arthritis (SA) and osteomyelitis (OM) may result from injection drug use, usually as a result of hematogenous seeding. Bacteremia may occur transiently after drug injection or may be due to endocarditis. Bone and joint infections related to IDU typically affect the axial skeleton. In SA, the sacroiliac, costochondral, hip, and sternoclavicular joints are common sites, followed by the knee and shoulder joint. OM occurs more commonly in the lumbar and cervical spines. The bacteriology is similar for both infections. *Staphylococcus aureus* predominates. Cases of IDU-related OM due to *Pseudomonas aeruginosa*, *Eikenella corrodens*, and *Streptococcus viridans* species also have been reported. (See Chapter 21, Adult Septic Arthritis, and Chapter 23, Osteomyelitis.)

Table 55.7 Clinical Features: IDU-Related Osteomyelitis and Septic Arthritis

Organisms	**Septic arthritis:** • *Staphylococcus aureus* (including MRSA) **Osteomyelitis:** • *Staphylococcus aureus* (including MRSA) • *Pseudomonas* • *Eikenella corrodens*
Signs and Symptoms	**Septic arthritis:** • Joint pain, swelling, tenderness, decreased range of motion, fever **Osteomyelitis:** • Back pain, bone pain, fever
Laboratory and Radiologic Findings	**Septic arthritis:** • Leukocytosis • Positive arthrocentesis **Osteomyelitis:** • Elevated ESR • Positive blood cultures • Abnormal plain films • Abnormal scintigraphy • Abnormal MRI

ESR, erythrocyte sedimentation rate.

Epidemiology

The incidence of SA and OM has not been well established, but in one report they together accounted for 4% of IDU-related hospital admissions. SA appears to be more common, occurring five times as often in one case series.

Clinical Features

Septic arthritis usually presents as an acute infection, with rapid onset of pain, tenderness, and decreased range of motion at a joint (Table 55.7). By contrast, OM is often indolent, with patients presenting as late as 3 months after the onset of infection. Back pain is the most common chief complaint in spinal OM. Fever is common in both infections, but may be absent at the time of presentation.

Differential Diagnosis

Musculoskeletal complaints in IDUs are often due to infection. SA, OM, and spinal epidural abscess (see below) are primary considerations when an IDU complains of back or joint pain. A high degree of suspicion should be maintained even if the presentation does not include fever or leukocytosis. Gonococcal arthritis remains a consideration in monoarticular and oligoarticular arthritis in this population. *Mycobacterium tuberculosis* osteomyelitis has been reported in IDU, albeit rarely. Noninfectious entities include gout, pseudogout, and rheumatoid arthritis.

Laboratory and Radiographic Findings

The work up of both SA and OM includes an erythrocyte sedimentation rate (ESR), blood cultures, and x-rays of the symptomatic area. The ESR, although nonspecific, is elevated above 20 mm/hr in about 90% of cases of SA and OM. Although positive in only 20–30% of cases, blood cultures are particularly important in osteomyelitis because they may establish the etiology and obviate bone biopsy. A positive blood culture

in the setting of SA or OM generally mandates a search for endocarditis.

Plain radiographs are insensitive for acute OM. There is a "lag period" of 10 days to 3 weeks or more before the lytic and demineralizing effects of infection become apparent radiographically. In one study fewer than 5% of plain films were positive on presentation, whereas radiographic signs of OM were present in 90% of cases after 3–4 weeks. Radionuclide scintigraphy, using technetium-, gallium-, or indium-tagged WBCs to visualize areas of infection, has a sensitivity of 50% for chronic infections and as high as 90% in acute infection. Compared with scintigraphy, MRI can better differentiate soft-tissue infection from osteomyelitis and can assess for coexistent spinal epidural abscess and osteomyelitis. The sensitivity and specificity of MRI for osteomyelitis range from 60% to 100% and from 50% to 90%, respectively.

Arthrocentesis remains the main diagnostic test for suspected SA. Synovial fluid WBC above $50,000/mm^3$ (in the absence of crystals) or positive Gram stain generally indicates SA. Synovial fluid culture reveals the etiology in approximately 75% of cases, provided that arthrocentesis is performed prior to antibiotic administration. In the case of a suspected septic hip joint, ultrasound guidance may permit successful arthrocentesis.

Treatment

Initial treatment for suspected OM is usually empirical (Table 55.8). Care should be taken to obtain blood cultures and, if possible, bone cultures, before starting antibiotics. In the case of SA, Gram stain of synovial fluid can be used to guide initial therapy. If the Gram stain is unrevealing, therapy should be directed against *S. aureus*, including MRSA, and gram-negative bacilli including pseudomonal species. Joint drainage is an essential part of therapy for septic arthritis,

Table 55.8 Initial Empirical IV Therapy for Osteomyelitis and Septic Arthritis

Patient Category	Therapy Recommendation
Adults	**Osteomyelitis:** • Antibiotics may be sufficient for acute hematogenous osteomyelitis • Operative drainage and debridement are usually necessary for chronic osteomyelitis • IV antibiotics for 4–6 weeks. Initial antibiotics selection should cover *Staphylococcus aureus*: nafcillin 2 g IV q6h *or* cefazolin 1–2 g IV q8h *or* vancomycin (for MRSA) 10–15 mg/kg IV q12h (trough goal of 15–25 μg/ml) **Septic arthritis:** • Joint drainage with or without irrigation • Empiric IV antibiotics after synovial fluid obtained for culture and Gram stain: piperacillin-tazobactam 3.375 g IV q6h *or* (for MRSA) vancomycin 1 g IV q12h *plus* ceftriaxone 1 g IV q24h *or* (for gonococcal arthritis) ceftriaxone 1 g IV q24h
Immunocompromised	Same as for nonimmunocompromised persons

and options include repeated needle aspiration, arthroscopic drainage, or arthrotomy.

SPINAL EPIDURAL ABSCESS

Spinal epidural abscess (SEA) is a rare but feared complication of IDU. SEA is a diagnostic challenge because it may present simply as back pain, because MRI is generally required for diagnosis, and because diagnostic delay can be associated with sudden and irreversible neurologic damage.

Most SEAs are due to hematogenous seeding of the vertebrae or epidural space. Common sources of bacteremia, besides the frequent transient bacteremia of IDU, include skin and soft-tissue infections, dental infections, urinary tract infections, and endocarditis. *S. aureus* (including MRSA) is the predominant pathogen in SEA, implicated in 50–65% of cases and in an even higher percentage of IDU-related cases. *Pseudomonas* and tuberculosis also have been isolated in IDU-related SEA. Adjacent bone or soft-tissue infections, such as osteomyelitis, diskitis, or psoas abscess, are common.

There are two proposed mechanisms of cord injury in SEA, which may explain the wide variation in the time of onset of neurologic deficits: direct compression and vascular ischemia. Compression due to mass effect may produce a subacute course, whereas thrombosis and vascular injury may result in a rapid paralysis.

Epidemiology

The incidence of SEA in the general population is estimated at 0.2–1.0 per 10,000 hospital admissions. Although IDU is considered a major risk factor for SEA, no study has specifically addressed the incidence in this patient population.

Clinical Features

Although the classic presentation of SEA includes back pain, fever, and neurologic symptoms, the presence of this triad is far from universal (Table 55.9). Back pain is present in greater than 90% of patients, whereas fever is present in 60–76%, and neurologic deficits are found at presentation in 57–70%. Neurologic findings include radicular pain, urinary incontinence, leg weakness and para- or quadriplegia. Patients may occasionally present with sepsis or encephalitis, further confounding and delaying the diagnosis.

Table 55.9 Clinical Features: Spinal Epidural Abscess

Organisms	• *Staphylococcus aureus* (including MRSA) • Gram-negative rods • Streptococci
Signs and Symptoms	• Back pain • Fever • Neurologic findings: radicular pain, weakness, urinary incontinence
Laboratory and Radiologic Findings	• Elevated ESR • Positive blood cultures • MRI showing phlegmon or frank pus in the epidural space
Treatment	Urgent neurosurgical consultation for possible surgical drainage if cord impingement occurring

Differential Diagnosis

The differential diagnosis for spinal epidural abscess includes:

- osteomyelitis and diskitis
- metastatic cancer
- spinal fracture or disk disease
- meningitis
- herpes zoster

Laboratory and Radiographic Findings

Emergent imaging is required to exclude or establish the diagnosis of SEA, and contrast MRI is now the study of choice. With a sensitivity of 90%, it has replaced the equally sensitive but more invasive CT-myelogram. MRI provides images of the abscess and the cord itself and may identify an alternative diagnosis. Plain radiographs cannot be relied on to exclude the diagnosis of SEA, although they may be abnormal if there is associated vertebral osteomyelitis. In such cases, end plate destruction or a narrowed disk space may be evident.

An ESR above 30 mm/hr, although nonspecific, is almost always present in SEA. Some authors advocate ESR as a screening test for SEA in patients who are at risk, such as IDUs, who present with unexplained back pain. No prospective data exist to support this approach. Blood cultures are positive in approximately 60% of cases of SEA and may provide an etiologic diagnosis. It is therefore critical that blood cultures be obtained prior to beginning empiric antibiotics whenever the diagnosis of SEA is being considered.

Treatment and Prophylaxis

Treatment of SEA involves both surgical decompression and appropriate antibiotic therapy (Table 55.10). Although conservative, nonoperative management has been described, surgical drainage remains the treatment of choice in many cases. Indications for surgery include neurologic deficits, negative blood cultures, and failure of conservative therapy. In one series of IDU-related SEAs, permanent neurologic damage occurred in 25% of cases. The only modifiable determinant of neurologic outcome is time from presentation to operative decompression. In one study, all patients who had surgery within 36 hours of the development of neurologic deficit showed some degree of recovery, whereas recovery was

Table 55.10 Initial Therapy for IDU-Related Spinal Epidural Abscess

Patient Category	Therapy Recommendation
Adults	• Surgical drainage and decompression • Antibiotics: vancomycin 1–1.5 g IV q12 *plus* cefepime 2 g IV q12h *or* vancomycin *plus* piperacillin-tazobactam (Zosyn) 3.375 g IV q12h *or* vancomycin *plus* ciprofloxacin 400 mg IV q12 *plus* metronidazole (Flagyl) 500 mg IV q8h *or* vancomycin *plus* meropenem 1 g IV q8h
Immunocompromised	Same as for nonimmunocompromised persons

limited (2 of 11) in those whose surgery was delayed beyond 36 hours.

Antibiotic therapy is optimally guided by the results of operative or blood cultures. The combination of vancomycin and an anti-pseudomonal antibiotic, such as cefepime, is the recommended initial empiric regimen.

BOTULISM

Botulism is an illness of descending paralysis and autonomic dysfunction due to a neurotoxin produced by *Clostridium botulinum*, a gram-positive rod (see Chapter 65, Botulism). Wound botulism is an increasingly frequent complication of IDU. *Clostridium botulinum* requires anaerobic conditions to propagate and elaborate toxin, and abscess cavities and subcutaneous pockets formed by IDU seem to be an ideal environment. Botulinum toxin binds to the presynaptic terminal, irreversibly blocking acetylcholine release at cranial nerves, autonomic nerves, and neuromuscular junctions.

Epidemiology

First reported in 1982, the incidence of wound botulism associated with IDU has risen steadily since 1988, with about 20 cases a year in California alone over the past decade. Subcutaneous injection of black tar heroin appears to be the primary risk factor for development of botulism in IDU. Black tar heroin is contaminated by *Clostridium* spores in the process of "cutting" the drug.

Clinical Features

Patients present with three types of neurologic deficits: cranial nerve dysfunction, autonomic dysfunction, and symmetric motor weakness (Table 55.11). Cranial nerve symptoms include dysphagia (80%), dysarthria/hoarseness (70%), and diplopia (40%). Autonomic dysfunction may manifest as dry mouth and dilated pupils. Eighty percent of patients complain of shortness of breath. Respiratory muscle weakness occurs in up to 75% of patients, most of whom require mechanical ventilation.

Table 55.11 Clinical Features: Wound Botulism

Organism	*Clostridium botulinum*
Signs and Symptoms	• Cranial nerve abnormalities • Dysphagia • Dysarthria and hoarseness • Diplopia • Autonomic dysfunction • Dry mouth • Dilated pupils • Symmetric motor weakness
Laboratory and Radiologic Findings	• CSF normal • Wound culture (specify for *Clostridium tetani*) • Serum mouse bioassay for botulinum toxin
CSF, cerebrospinal fluid.	

Differential Diagnosis

Diagnosis of botulism during the initial stages requires a high index of suspicion because of the lack of readily available rapid confirmatory tests. The differential for descending paralysis with prominent bulbar weakness includes myasthenia gravis or Miller-Fisher variant of Guillain-Barré syndrome. In the IDU patient, wound botulism must be considered while tests that exclude other diagnoses, such as cerebrospinal fluid (CSF) analysis, are undertaken.

Key features that distinguish botulism from other neuromuscular diseases are:

- afebrile illness
- normal mental status
- cranial nerves involved
- descending paralysis
- symmetric bilateral impairment
- absence of paresthesias
- normal CSF studies
- characteristic electromyographic findings

Laboratory and Radiographic Findings

Confirmatory studies include wound cultures for *Clostridium botulinum* and a bioassay for botulinum toxin, performed on patient serum. Wound cultures are positive in 60% of cases, whereas the bioassay has a reported sensitivity of greater than 90%.

Treatment and Prophylaxis

The management of botulism consists of (1) minimizing toxin binding, (2) removing the toxin source, and (3) supportive care (Table 55.12). Botulism antitoxin, the only specific treatment for botulism, is a trivalent horse serum against toxin types A, B, and E. It binds only extraneuronal toxin and therefore is most effective when given early in the course. One vial contains more than 100 times the amount of antitoxin needed to neutralize the largest amount of toxin ever reported to the Centers for Disease Control and Prevention (CDC). To obtain the antitoxin, contact the local department of public health. It can be given intravenously (IV) or intramuscularly (IM). Patients given antitoxin within 24 hours of presentation had a 10% mortality, whereas patients treated beyond 24 hours had 15% mortality, and untreated patients had 46% mortality. In a study of 20 IDU patients with proven botulism, those treated within 12 hours experienced a lower rate of respiratory failure than those treated late. The antitoxin causes anaphylaxis in 2% of cases, prompting some authors to recommend cautious pretesting as well as prophylactic subcutaneous epinephrine.

Table 55.12 Initial IV Therapy for Botulism

Patient Category	Therapy Recommendation
Adults	• Botulism antitoxin • Incision and drainage of cutaneous abscesses • Penicillin IV 24 million units/day divided q6h
Immunocompromised	Same as for nonimmunocompromised persons

To eliminate ongoing toxin production, all suspicious skin lesions should be drained or excised and IV penicillin given.

Complications and Admission Criteria

The most important complication of botulism is ventilatory failure. Respiratory weakness should be assessed by measuring negative inspiratory forces or forced vital capacities. A negative inspiratory force of 20 cm H_2O or less, or a worsening trend, indicates the need for intubation. Ventilatory support is a temporizing measure while synaptic receptors regenerate. Unfortunately, patients may require months of mechanical ventilation before adequate inspiratory strength returns. With the use of mechanical ventilation, mortality due to all forms of botulism has been reduced to approximately 10%. Nonetheless, morbidity remains high because of long-term paralysis and the complications of critical care.

TETANUS

Tetanus is a rare but dreaded complication of IDU and under-immunization. It is a syndrome of uncontrolled muscle spasm and autonomic dysfunction as a result of *Clostridium tetani* infection and toxin elaboration.

The pathophysiology of tetanus begins with the introduction of *Clostridium tetani* spores into a wound – subcutaneous injection of heroin is thought to produce favorable conditions for the bacterial growth. These spores germinate and elaborate the exotoxin tetanospasmin. Tetanospasmin is transported in retrograde fashion to the spinal cord, where the toxin inhibits neurotransmission, ultimately causing muscle spasm and autonomic instability. (See Chapter 63, Tetanus.)

Epidemiology

Although tetanus is now a rare disease in the United States, IDUs remain at significant risk for developing the disease. Of 124 cases reported in the United States between 1995 and 1997, 11% were associated with IDU. IDU-related tetanus occurred exclusively in undervaccinated individuals. The practice of skin popping also appears to be associated with tetanus. Clinicians who regularly see IDUs must ensure that this group of patients is immunized.

Clinical Features

Presenting symptoms are due to muscle spasm, which may be localized – so-called cephalic tetanus – or generalized. Trismus and neck or back pain are the initial symptoms in 85% of cases (Table 55.13). Physical exam reveals palpable muscle rigidity and hyperreflexia. Other findings include opisthotonos (hyperextension and spasm of the neck and back), risus sardonicus (appearance of a sardonic smile from facial muscle spasm), dysphagia, and drooling.

Differential Diagnosis

The diagnosis of tetanus is clinical. Disorders that may present similarly include seizures, meningitis/encephalitis, drug withdrawal, sepsis, and strychnine poisoning. The differential diagnosis of localized tetanus includes peritonsillar abscess, mandibular disorders, and dystonic reactions. A history and physical consistent with tetanus in an IDU, combined with negative results on CT scan and lumbar puncture, is sufficient to establish the diagnosis.

Table 55.13 Clinical Features: Tetanus

Organism	*Clostridium tetani*
Signs and Symptoms	• Neck pain • Back pain • Trismus • Opisthotonos • Risus sardonicus • Dysphagia and drooling • Muscle rigidity • Hyperreflexia
Laboratory and Radiologic Findings	• Initial diagnosis is clinical • CT negative • CSF negative • Tetanus toxoid antibody titers • Wound culture

Laboratory and Radiographic Findings

Wound cultures for *C. tetani* are insensitive. Antibody titers against tetanus toxoid should be ordered, although results will not be available to assist with immediate diagnosis.

Treatment and Prophylaxis

As in wound botulism, the treatment of tetanus primarily involves three strategies (Table 55.14): (1) Elimination of all potential sources of toxin production is accomplished by drainage of skin abscesses and administration of antibiotics active against *Clostridium*. Metronidazole is the usual first-line agent. (2) Clearance of extraneuronal tetanus toxin is achieved by administration of tetanus immunoglobulin (TIG). Intrathecal plus intravenous administration of TIG probably offers an advantage over the intravenous route alone. Active immunization with tetanus toxoid also should be initiated immediately. (3) Aggressive supportive care is critical to prevent morbidity and mortality. Patients with severe, generalized, or rapidly progressing muscle spasm should be intubated, sedated and paralyzed if necessary. Long-term ventilatory support and tracheostomy are often required. Muscle spasm is controlled with benzodiazepines or propofol. Labetalol, a combined beta and alpha adrenergic blocker, can be used to manage autonomic instability.

Table 55.14 Initial IV Therapy for Tetanus

Patient Category	Therapy Recommendation
Adults	• Wound debridement • Metronidazole 500 mg IV q8h • Human tetanus immunoglobulin (neutralize unbound toxin) • Tetanus toxoid (active immunization) • Treatment of muscle spasm • Sedatives (diazepam, propofol) • Neuromuscular blockade (and intubation) • Treatment of autonomic instability • Labetalol • Magnesium
Immunocompromised	Same as for nonimmunocompromised persons

PEARLS AND PITFALLS

1. IDUs presenting with fever have a serious infection warranting admission about 60% of the time; the majority of these infections can be diagnosed with a thorough ED evaluation.

2. Even if the acute evaluation is negative, febrile IDUs generally require hospital admission because occult bacteremia and endocarditis are difficult to exclude.

3. Endocarditis related to IDU often occurs on the tricuspid valve, resulting in pulmonary symptoms and signs and an abnormal chest x-ray.

4. Abscesses may not demonstrate fluctuance; consider the use of bedside ultrasound to identify and localize a pus collection for drainage.

5. Necrotizing soft-tissue infections secondary to IDU are typified by tense edema and extreme leukocytosis.

6. Once the diagnosis of necrotizing fasciitis is entertained, there is no diagnostic test that can reliably exclude the diagnosis except operative exploration.

7. Mortality in necrotizing soft-tissue infections is directly related to the time between presentation and operative debridement.

8. Musculoskeletal complaints in IDUs are frequently due to an infection; a musculoskeletal complaint plus fever mandates a search for an infection including osteomyelitis or septic arthritis.

9. Back pain plus fever in an IDU mandates evaluation for spinal epidural abscess; the diagnosis should be made prior to the onset of neurologic symptoms; MRI is usually required to exclude the diagnosis.

10. Bulbar neurologic symptoms in an IDU indicate wound botulism until proven otherwise.

REFERENCES

Anderson MW, Sharma K, Feeney CM. Wound botulism associated with black tar heroin. Acad Emerg Med 1997;4:805–9.

Binswanger IA, Kral AH, Bluthenthal RN, et al. High prevalence of abscesses and cellulitis among community-recruited injection drug users in San Francisco. Clin Infect Dis 2000 Mar;30(3):579–81.

Callahan TE, Schecter WP, Horn JK. Necrotizing soft tissue infections masquerading as cutaneous abscess following illicit drug injection. Arch Surg 1998;133:812–8.

Chandrasekar PH, Narula AP. Bone and joint infections in intravenous drug abusers. Rev Infect Dis 1986 Nov–Dec;8(6):904–11.

Chen JL, Fullerton KE, Flynn NM. Necrotizing fasciitis associated with injection drug use. Clin Infect Dis 2001;1(33):6–15.

Hecht SR, Berger M. Right-sided endocarditis in intravenous drug users. Ann Intern Med 1992;117:560–6.

Koppel BS, Tuchman AJ, Mangiardi JR, et al. Epidural spinal infection in intravenous drug abusers. Arch Neurol 1988. Dec;45(12):1331–7.

Marantz PR, Linzer M, Feiner CJ, et al. Inability to predict diagnosis in febrile intravenous drug abusers. Ann Intern Med 1987;106(6):823–8.

Mathew J, Addai T, Anand A, et al. Clinical features, site of involvement, bacteriologic findings, and outcome of infective endocarditis in intravenous drug users. Arch Intern Med 1995;155:1641–8.

McGuigan CC, Penrice GM, Gruer L, et al. Lethal outbreak of infection with *Clostridium novyi* type A and other spore-forming organisms in Scottish injecting drug users. J Med Microbiol 2002;51(11):971–7.

Samet JH, Shevitz A, Fowle J, Singer DE. Hospitalization decisions in febrile intravenous drug users. Am J Med 1990;89:53–7.

Weisse AB, Heller DR, Schhimenti RJ, et al. The febrile parenteral drug user: a prospective study in 121 patients. Am J Med 1993;94:274–80.

Werner SB, Passaro D, McGee J, et al. Wound botulism in California, 1951–1998: recent epidemic in heroin injectors. Clin Infect Dis 2000 Oct;31(4):1018–24.

Special Populations

56. Blood or Body Fluid Exposure Management and Postexposure Prophylaxis for Hepatitis B and HIV

Roland C. Merchant and Michelle E. Roland

INTRODUCTION

Because the efficacy of prophylactic therapy may be highly time-dependent, the acute care management of occupational or other blood and body fluid exposures must include rapid determination of the need for prophylaxis, testing, and treatment. Attention to wound care principles and referral for social, medical, or advocacy services remain important in all cases.

EXPOSURE EPIDEMIOLOGY AND TRANSMISSION RISK

There were an estimated 78,123 visits to United States emergency departments (EDs) annually during 1998–2000 for work-related exposures to blood or body fluids. More than 90,000 females of all ages present annually for medical care after sexual assault. The frequency of ED visits for other populations and for other types of blood or body fluid exposures is not well known.

Hepatitis B

The Centers for Disease Control and Prevention (CDC) estimates that 5.6% of 20- to 59-year-olds in the United States have been infected with hepatitis B, though the prevalence and incidence has decreased over the past 20 years (see Chapter 13, Viral Hepatitis). This reduction is likely due to widespread use of the hepatitis B vaccination, universal precautions in health care settings, and educational campaigns to increase condom usage and reduce injection-needle sharing.

Although it is found in other body fluids (e.g., bile, breast milk, cerebrospinal fluid, saliva, semen, and sweat), hepatitis B is primarily transmitted through contact with blood. Hepatitis B can be transmitted through:

- shared injection-drug use equipment
- unprotected sexual intercourse
- perinatal transmission
- percutaneous injuries

- blood or body fluid splashes to mucous membranes or non-intact skin
- improper hemodialysis procedures
- transfusions with infected blood products

Among healthy adults acutely infected with hepatitis B, about 95% resolve their infection. The remainder become chronic carriers and about 20% of these develop cirrhosis.

The risk of hepatitis B infection from a blood or body fluid exposure is directly related to the infectivity of the source (Table 56.1). The risk from a percutaneous injury is greatly increased when the source harbors the hepatitis B e (envelope) antigen, which is a marker of active viral replication.

Hepatitis C

According to estimates from the CDC, 2.4% of 20- to 59-year-olds in the United States have hepatitis C antibodies indicating prior or current infection with the virus. The mechanisms of hepatitis C transmission are less well understood than those of hepatitis B and human immunodeficiency virus (HIV), but are believed to be similar. Hepatitis C can be transmitted through transfusion of blood products; however, since screening of blood products for hepatitis C began in 1990, this has become a rare form of transmission in the United States. According to the CDC, the average incidence of hepatitis C infection through a percutaneous exposure to a known hepatitis C–infected source is 1.8% (0–7%). There are no comparable CDC estimates for other types of exposures to hepatitis C.

Table 56.1 Risk of HBV Infection with Antigen Status of Infected Material

Antigen Status	Clinical Hepatitis Risk	Serologic Hepatitis Risk
HBsAg (−) and HBeAg (+)	22–31%	37–62%
HBsAg (+) and HBeAg (−)	1–6%	23–37%

HIV

The CDC estimates that at the end of 2003, 0.4% of people in the United States were living with an HIV infection and 24–27% of these persons were unaware of their infection. Approximately 40,000 people each year in the United States are newly diagnosed with an HIV infection.

HIV can be transmitted through:

- unprotected sexual intercourse
- shared injection-drug use equipment
- perinatal transmission
- percutaneous injuries
- blood or body fluid splashes to mucous membranes or nonintact skin
- transfusions with HIV-infected blood products

HIV is primarily transmitted through contact with blood, seminal or vaginal fluids, and breast milk. Although HIV can also be recovered from cerebrospinal, synovial, pleural, peritoneal, pericardial, and amniotic fluid, these body fluids are unlikely sources of HIV transmission. Feces, nasal secretions, saliva, sputum, sweat, tears, urine, and vomitus are not considered to be infectious unless they are visibly bloody.

Because blood products in the United States have been screened for HIV since the mid-1980s, the risk of HIV-related transfusion transmission is exceedingly low. The estimated risk of transfusion of an infected unit is 1 infection per 2.3 million transfusion donations.

CDC-estimated risks of an HIV infection after selected exposures are shown in Table 56.2.

There are many factors that could potentially moderate transmission of these viruses. Some factors that might increase transmission risk are listed in Table 56.3.

EXPOSURE WOUND MANAGEMENT

Basic wound care including irrigation with normal saline or clean water should be initiated immediately for patients with percutaneous injuries, and for skin and non-genital mucous membrane exposures. Patients with anal or vaginal sexual exposures should not irrigate the sites of their exposure as this may further disrupt mucosa. Hydrogen peroxide and caustic agents (e.g., bleach) should not be used to clean wounds, and there is no evidence that antiseptic solutions reduce transmission. Wounds should not be bled or "milked" or widened, as this may enhance exposures to infectious agents. Since there is no evidence that the timing of closure of open wounds affects

Table 56.2 Risks of HIV Infection

Exposure Route	Risk per 10,000 Exposures
Screened blood transfusion in the United States	<0.005
Contaminated blood transfusion	9000
Needle-sharing injection drug use	67
Receptive anal intercourse	50
Percutaneous needle stick	30
Receptive penile-vaginal intercourse	10
Insertive anal intercourse	6.5
Insertive penile-vaginal intercourse	10
Receptive oral intercourse	1
Insertive oral intercourse	0.5

Table 56.3 Factors Moderating Risk of HIV and Hepatitis Transmission

Factor	Nonsexual Exposures	Sexual Exposures
Volume and Type of Exposure	For percutaneous exposures: • Large, hollow bore needle • Blood visible on the percutaneous device • Percutaneous device used in artery or vein • Large amount of blood For splash exposures: • Large amount of blood	Exposures involving blood as well as seminal or vaginal fluids Exposures to large amounts of seminal or vaginal fluids
Surface Area of Exposure Site	Deep percutaneous injuries Mucous membrane exposures, particularly eye exposures Nonintact skin	Cervical ectopy Uncircumcised penis Traumatic sexual intercourse (anal and vaginal)
Exposure Source and Exposed Person Factors	Higher viral load in source fluid	Higher viral load in source fluid* Sexually transmitted diseases in source and/or exposed person

*Caution: Viral load in serum may not be reflective of the viral load in genital secretions; patients may have an undetectable serum viral load yet have virus in their genital secretions.

infection rates, usual approaches to wound irrigation and closure are appropriate.

EXPOSURE EVALUATION

Evaluation begins with a complete history of the exposure and examination of the exposure site to determine whether the exposure could result in transmission of hepatitis or HIV. If transmission is possible, the hepatitis B and C and HIV status of the exposed person and the source should be assessed and prophylaxis considered. Prophylaxis for a given agent is not warranted when the exposed person is known to be already infected with that agent.

Assessment of the Hepatitis B, Hepatitis C, and HIV Status of the Source

In most cases, the hepatitis and HIV status of the source will not be known during the patient's ED evaluation. When the source is available, he or she should be asked about hepatitis and HIV risk factors and asked to undergo testing unless recent results are already available. There is no accepted rule for deciding when a patient's prior hepatitis B or C or HIV test is current enough for an assessment of their status. An antibody test can determine infections that occurred several weeks to months before, but cannot assess whether the person tested has been recently infected. Unfortunately, a person infected with HIV is usually highly infectious prior to the appearance of serum antibodies and, hence, before antibody-based detection tests become positive. Although a source with negative serologies within the prior 3 to 6 months and no

Special Populations

high-risk behaviors is probably not infected, given the paucity of data, all sources should be offered retesting at the time of the exposure. If the source cannot be tested, local prevalence rates and source population risk factors may provide guidance. Clinicians should be aware of the limitations of applying these estimates to individual cases and rely on actual test results whenever possible.

Testing

Hepatitis B and C testing involves examining the source's blood for markers of viral infection and for evidence of immunity. Hepatitis B testing assesses for the presence of the hepatitis B surface antibody (which indicates immunity to hepatitis B), surface (s) antigen, and envelope (e) antigen (which indicates active viral replication). The interpretation of hepatitis C testing is more complex, and clinicians should refer to current CDC recommendations. In general, if the source has a negative enzyme immunoassay (EIA) for hepatitis C, then they are likely not infected. Rapid HIV antibody tests of whole blood, plasma, and oral fluid are now available, and the CDC now recommends these tests as a part of occupational exposure evaluations. The tests provide results in approximately 20 minutes and have test performance characteristics that are similar to standard or conventional tests for HIV. A preliminary positive rapid HIV test result should be confirmed using Western blot or EIA.

In the absence of rapid HIV tests, a standard HIV test can be used to determine the source's HIV status. The use of unpooled tests for HIV ribonucleic acid (RNA) instead of HIV antibodies is not recommended for most exposure evaluations because of their relatively high rates of false-positive test results. However, these tests can be helpful when run in real time and without pooling strategies when acute HIV infection is suspected – that is, when there is evidence of an acute "flulike" illness with fever, malaise, myalgias, and/or adenopathy not explained by another etiology, in the presence of recent high-risk behaviors. Expert consultation is advised when using these tests.

POSTEXPOSURE PROPHYLAXIS FOR HEPATITIS B AND HIV

Postexposure prophylaxis (PEP) is currently available only for hepatitis B and HIV. There is no current recommended prophylaxis against hepatitis C. Because the treatment of acute hepatitis C is much more effective than treatment of chronic hepatitis C, exposed patients should be monitored for seroconversion and referred for treatment if an infection is detected.

Timing of PEP Delivery

If PEP for hepatitis B or HIV is indicated for an exposure, then it should be given as soon as possible after the exposure – ideally, within one hour, although this is not possible for many types of exposures. The results of animal and immunologic studies suggest that HIV PEP might not be effective if given more than 72 hours after exposure. The optimal time for administering hepatitis B prophylaxis is not known, but studies of health care workers given hepatitis B immunoglobulin within 1 week of exposure and of infants given hepatitis B immunoglobulin and vaccine at birth indicate 70–75% and

Table 56.4 CDC Hepatitis B Prophylaxis Recommendations

Vaccination Status of Exposed Individual	Prophylaxis
Previously Unvaccinated	
HBsAg(+) source	HBIG × 1 and hepatitis B vaccine series
Unknown HBsAg source	Hepatitis B vaccine series
Previously Vaccinated	
Known responder	No treatment
Known nonresponder	
HBsAg(+) source	HBIG × 1 and revaccination or HBIG × 2
Unknown HBsAg source	If high-risk source, treat as if HBsAg(+)
Unknown responder	
HBsAg(+) source	Test exposed individual for hepatitis B surface antibody • If adequate antibody response, then no treatment • If inadequate antibody response, then HBIG × 1 and vaccine booster
Unknown HBsAg source	Test exposed individual for hepatitis B surface antibody • If adequate antibody response, then no treatment • If inadequate antibody response, then administer hepatitis B vaccine and recheck antibody titer in 1–2 months

85–95% effectiveness, respectively. Hepatitis B PEP may not be effective if given more than 1 week after perinatal and percutaneous exposures or more than 2 weeks after sexual exposures.

Postexposure prophylaxis should be initiated in the ED because the medications are likely more effective when taken soon after exposure. All patients who decline HIV PEP when it is recommended should have follow-up scheduled within 24 hours with a clinician experienced in prescribing HIV PEP, so that they have a second opportunity to take prophylaxis while it might still be effective.

Hepatitis B PEP Regimens

Hepatitis B prophylaxis (Table 56.4) consists of postexposure vaccination alone or vaccination plus hepatitis B immunoglobulin (HBIG). Most patients should receive only the hepatitis B vaccine. The idea underlying this practice is that the immune system can be adequately stimulated by the vaccine to help contain the virus before it can replicate enough to infect the exposed person. HBIG is reserved for exposures in which the perceived infection risk is high (i.e., when the source has detectable hepatitis B virus DNA, hepatitis B e or s antigen) or when the exposed person will likely not respond to the hepatitis B vaccine (i.e., known prior vaccine nonresponders).

Clinicians should advise patients who are vaccinated against hepatitis B in the setting of an exposure that they must receive two additional hepatitis B vaccinations at 1 and 6 months to be fully immunized. All health care workers and others at increased risk of being exposed to blood or body fluids should be vaccinated and have their hepatitis B titers checked 1 month after the final vaccination to verify immunity. Patients who fail to acquire immunity can receive second

Table 56.5 CDC Occupational HIV PEP Guidelines

Exposure Type	Infection Status of Score			
	HIV+ Class 1*	HIV+ Class 2†	Unknown HIV Status of Source	Source Unknown
Percutaneous Exposures				
Less severe	• Basic 2-drug PEP	• Expanded ≥3-drug PEP	• Generally, no PEP • Consider basic 2-drug PEP for sources with HIV risk factors	• Generally, no PEP • Consider basic 2-drug PEP where exposure to HIV-infected persons is likely
More severe	• Expanded 3-drug PEP	• Expanded ≥3-drug PEP	• Generally no PEP • Consider basic 2-drug PEP for sources with HIV risk factors	• Generally, no PEP • Consider basic 2-drug PEP where exposure to HIV-infected persons is likely
Mucous Membrane and Nonintact Skin Exposure				
Small volume	• Consider basic 2-drug PEP	• Basic 2-drug PEP	• Generally, no PEP	• Generally, no PEP
Large volume	• Basic 2-drug PEP	• Expanded ≥3-drug PEP	• Generally, no PEP • Consider basic 2-drug PEP for sources with HIV risk factors	• Generally, no PEP • Consider basic 2-drug PEP where exposure to HIV-infected persons is likely

*HIV-Positive, Class 1: asymptomatic HIV infection or known low viral load (e.g., <1500 RNA copies/mL)
†HIV-Positive, Class 2: symptomatic HIV infection, AIDS, acute seroconversion, or known high viral load

Table 56.6 CDC Occupational HIV PEP Regimens

Preferred Basic Regimen	Alternate Basic Regimens	Preferred Expanded Regimen	Alternate Expanded Regimens
zidovudine (Retrovir; ZDV; AZT) *plus* lamivudine (Epivir; 3TC); available as Combivir: • ZDV: 300 mg twice daily or 200 mg three times daily • 3TC: 300 mg once daily or 150 mg twice daily • Combivir: one tablet twice daily *or* zidovudine (Retrovir; ZDV; AZT) *plus* emtricitabine (Emtriva; FTC): • ZDV: 300 mg twice daily or 200 mg three times daily, with food • FTC: 200 mg (one capsule) once daily *or* tenofovir DF (Viread; TDF) *plus* lamivudine (Epivir; 3TC): • TDF: 300 mg once daily • 3TC: 300 mg once daily or 150 mg twice daily *or* tenofovir DF (Viread; TDF) *plus* emtricitabine (Emtriva; FTC); available as Truvada • TDF: 300 mg once daily • FTC: 200 mg once daily • As Truvada: one tablet daily	lamivudine (Epivir; 3TC) *plus* stavudine (Zerit; d4T): • 3TC: 300 mg once daily or 150 mg twice daily • d4T: 40 mg twice daily • 30 mg twice daily if body weight is <60 kg *or* emtricitabine (Emtriva; FTC) *plus* stavudine (Zerit; d4T): • FTC: 200 mg daily • d4T: 40 mg twice daily • If body weight is <60 kg, 30 mg twice daily *or* lamivudine (Epivir; 3TC) *plus* didanosine (Videx; ddI): • 3TC: 300 mg once daily or 150 mg twice daily • ddI: Videx chewable/dispersible buffered tablets can be administered on an empty stomach. The dose is either 200 mg twice daily or 400 mg once daily for patients weighing >60 kg and 125 mg twice daily or 250 mg once daily for patients weighing >60 kg. *or* emtricitabine (Emtriva; FTC) *plus* didanosine (Videx; ddI): • FTC: 200 mg once daily • ddI: see above	Basic regimen plus: lopinavir/ritonavir (Kaletra; LPV/RTV): • LPV/RTV: 400/100 mg = 3 capsules twice daily with food	Basic regimen plus one of the following: atazanavir (Reyataz; ATV) *plus* ritonavir (Norvir; RTV): • ATV: 400 mg once daily, unless used in combination with TDF, in which case ATV should be boosted with RTV, preferred dosing of ATV 300 mg *plus* RTV: 100 mg once daily *or* fosamprenavir (Lexiva; FOSAPV) *plus* ritonavir (Norvir; RTV): • FOSAPV: 1400 mg twice daily (without RTV) • FOSAPV: 1400 mg once daily *plus* RTV 200 mg once daily • FOSAPV: 700 mg twice daily *plus* RTV 100 mg twice daily *or* indinavir (Crixivan; IDV) *plus* ritonavir (Norvir; RTV): • IDV 800 mg *plus* RTV 100 mg twice daily without regard to food *or* saquinavir (Invirase; SQV) *plus* ritonavir (Norvir; RTV): • SQV: 1000 mg (given as Invirase) *plus* RTV 100 mg, twice daily • SQV: five capsules twice daily *plus* RTV: one capsule twice daily *or* nelfinavir (Viracept; NFV): • NFV: 1250 mg (2 × 625 mg or 5 × 250 mg tablets), twice daily with a meal *or* efavirenz (Sustiva; EFV): • EFV: 600 mg daily, at bedtime

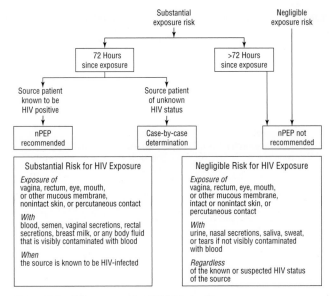

Substantial Risk for HIV Exposure

Exposure of
vagina, rectum, eye, mouth, or other mucous membrane, nonintact skin, or percutaneous contact

With
blood, semen, vaginal secretions, rectal secretions, breast milk, or any body fluid that is visibly contaminated with blood

When
the source is known to be HIV-infected

Negligible Risk for HIV Exposure

Exposure of
vagina, rectum, eye, mouth, or other mucous membrane, intact or nonintact skin, or percutaneous contact

With
urine, nasal secretions, saliva, sweat, or tears if not visibly contaminated with blood

Regardless
of the known or suspected HIV status of the source

Figure 56.1 CDC nonoccupational HIV PEP algorithm.

series of hepatitis B vaccination. If they again fail to acquire immunity, they are deemed vaccine "non-responders" and should be given hepatitis B immunoglobulin after any suspected hepatitis B exposure.

HIV PEP Regimens

Regimens for HIV PEP typically consist of two nucleotide or nucleoside reverse transcriptase inhibitors (NRTIs) for the basic regimen and the addition of a protease inhibitor (PI) or nonnucleoside reverse transcriptase inhibitor (NNRTI) for the expanded regimen (Tables 56.5 and 56.6). Nevirapine should not be used for PEP because it has been associated with severe to fatal hepatic and dermatologic toxicities in HIV-uninfected individuals. The CDC and other groups recommend a 28-day course of therapy, unless severe adverse side effects occur, or the source of the exposure is found to be uninfected. In addition to the CDC guidelines, institutional PEP protocols should take into account national, state, and local guidelines, which may vary based on the risk of infection and differ for occupational and nonoccupational exposures.

CDC Nonoccupational HIV PEP Guidelines

The CDC nonoccupational HIV PEP guidelines specifically address exposures to known HIV-infected persons. Persons who had consensual sex with a known HIV-infected person and a condom failure occurred, or who sustained a needle stick while caring for an HIV-infected person, or an inmate who was sexually assaulted while in prison by another inmate known to be HIV infected are three examples of patients who might present to the ED after an exposure to a known HIV-infected person. The CDC algorithm shown in Figure 56.1 suggests when HIV PEP might be prescribed under these or similar circumstances:

The management of patients with nonoccupational exposures to persons of unknown HIV status is not delineated in these guidelines. Clinicians are advised to make case-by-case evaluations with the assistance of a clinician experienced in HIV PEP.

Table 56.7 CDC Nonoccupational HIV PEP Antiretroviral Regimens

Regimens	Drug Combinations
Preferred	
Nonnucleoside reverse transcriptase inhibitor–based	• efavirenz *plus* (lamivudine or emtricitabine) *plus* (zidovudine or tenofovir)
Protease inhibitor–based	• lopinavir/ritonavir *plus* (lamivudine or emtricitabine) *plus* zidovudine
Alternative	
Nonnucleoside reverse transcriptase inhibitor–based	• efavirenz *plus* (lamivudine or emtricitabine) *plus* abacavir or didanosine or stavudine
Protease inhibitor–based	• atazanavir *plus* (lamivudine or emtricitabine) *plus* (zidovudine or stavudine or abacavir or didanosine) or (tenofovir *plus* ritonavir [100 mg/day])
	• fosamprenavir *plus* (lamivudine or emtricitabine) *plus* (zidovudine or stavudine) *plus* (abacavir or tenofovir or didanosine)
	• fosamprenavir/ritonavir *plus* (lamivudine or emtricitabine) *plus* (zidovudine or stavudine or abacavir or tenofovir or didanosine)
	• indinavir/ritonavir *plus* (lamivudine or emtricitabine) *plus* (zidovudine or stavudine or abacavir or tenofovir or didanosine)
	• lopinavir/ritonavir *plus* (lamivudine or emtricitabine) *plus* (stavudine or abacavir or tenofovir or didanosine)
	• nelfinavir *plus* (lamivudine or emtricitabine) *plus* (zidovudine or stavudine or abacavir or tenofovir or didanosine)
	• saquinavir/ritonavir *plus* (lamivudine or emtricitabine) *plus* (zidovudine or stavudine or abacavir or tenofovir or didanosine)
Triple nucleoside reverse transcriptase inhibitor	• abacavir *plus* lamivudine *plus* zidovudine (only when a nonnucleoside or protease inhibitor-based regimen cannot or should not be used)

The CDC-recommended HIV PEP medications for nonoccupational exposures are similar to those for occupational exposures. Although the preferred regimens vary slightly, they are all believed to be equally effective. The medication regimens are presented in Table 56.7, and the dosings are the same as for occupational HIV PEP.

Discontinuation of HIV PEP

Discontinue HIV PEP:

- if the source of the infection is known or found to be HIV uninfected
- at the completion of 28 days of uninterrupted therapy
- if serious adverse side effects occur

If a source's HIV test at the time of exposure is negative, the CDC recommends that HIV PEP be discontinued. The CDC acknowledges that "although concerns have been expressed regarding HIV-negative sources being in the window period for seroconversion, no case of transmission involving an exposure source during the window period has been reported in the United States." Despite this recommendation, some clinicians and patients may feel uncomfortable deferring or discontinuing HIV PEP when the source is at high risk, even with a negative test at the time of exposure. For these patients, clinicians should attempt to evaluate the source's recent risk factors for HIV (i.e., high-risk sexual and injection-drug behaviors within the prior 3–6 months), and be on the alert for any signs or symptoms of an acute HIV infection in the source. Consultation with an expert in HIV medicine is advised under these circumstances.

Adverse Side Effects of HIV PEP

Tables 56.8 and 56.9, from the CDC's occupational HIV PEP guidelines, list the primary adverse effects and toxicities of

Table 56.8 Primary Side Effects and Toxicities Associated with HIV PEP

Class and Agent	Side Effect and Toxicity
Nucleoside Reverse Transcriptase Inhibitors	
Zidovudine	Anemia, neutropenia, nausea, headache, insomnia, muscle pain, and weakness
Lamivudine	Abdominal pain, nausea, diarrhea, rash, and pancreatitis
Stavudine	Peripheral neuropathy, headache, diarrhea, nausea, insomnia, anorexia, pancreatitis, elevated liver function tests (LFTs), anemia, and neutropenia
Didanosine	Pancreatitis, lactic acidosis, neuropathy, diarrhea, abdominal pain, and nausea
Emtricitabine	Headache, nausea, vomiting, diarrhea, and rash. Skin discoloration (mild hyperpigmentation on palms and soles), primarily among nonwhites
Nucleotide Analogue Reverse Transcriptase Inhibitors	
Tenofovir	Nausea, diarrhea, vomiting, flatulence, and headache
Nonnucleoside Reverse Transcriptase Inhibitors	
Efavirenz	Rash (including cases of Stevens-Johnson syndrome), insomnia, somnolence, dizziness, trouble concentrating, abnormal dreaming, and teratogenicity
Protease Inhibitors	
Indinavir	Nausea, abdominal pain, nephrolithiasis, and indirect hyperbilirubinemia
Nelfinavir	Diarrhea, nausea, abdominal pain, weakness, and rash
Ritonavir	Weakness, diarrhea, nausea, circumoral paresthesia, taste alteration, and elevated cholesterol and triglycerides
Saquinavir	Diarrhea, abdominal pain, nausea, hyperglycemia, and elevated LFTs
Fosamprenavir	Nausea, diarrhea, rash, circumoral paresthesia, taste alteration, and depression
Atazanavir	Nausea, headache, rash, abdominal pain, diarrhea, vomiting, and indirect hyperbilirubinemia
Lopinavir/ritonavir	Diarrhea, fatigue, headache, nausea, and increased cholesterol and triglycerides
Fusion Inhibitor	
Enfuvirtide	Local injection site reactions, bacterial pneumonia, insomnia, depression, peripheral neuropathy, and cough

Table 56.9 Potential Adverse Drug Interactions with Protease Inhibitors

Drug Class	Agent
Antimycobacterials	• rifampin
Benzodiazepines	• midazolam • triazolam
Ergot derivatives	• dihydroergotamine • ergotamine • ergonovine • methylergonovine
Gastrointestinal motility agents	• cisapride
HMG-CoA reductase inhibitors (statins)	• lovastatin • simvastatin
Neuroleptics	• pimozide
Inhaled steroids	• fluticasone
Herbal products	• St. John's wort (*Hypericum perforatum*) • garlic

protease inhibitors, and list medications that should not be taken concomitantly.

The occurrence of adverse effects is a function of the type and number of medications used for HIV PEP. Many patients do not complete HIV PEP because of adverse side effects. Additional symptoms may result from the anxiety and distress associated with the HIV exposure. Some tips to reduce side effects include:

- taking antimotility and/or antiemetic agents
- changing the time of day the dose is taken
- taking the medications with food

Failure of HIV PEP

Patients being prescribed HIV PEP should be aware that there have been documented prophylaxis failures. As of 2005, there were six cases worldwide of health care workers who became HIV infected despite taking two or more antiretroviral medications for HIV PEP. There also have been nonoccupational HIV PEP failures. Possible reasons for failure of HIV PEP include:

- exposure to a strain of HIV resistant to the antiretroviral regimen prescribed
- exposure to a large inoculum of virus
- delay to initiation or shortened duration of HIV PEP
- factors related to the immune system of the exposed person and the viral strain
- incomplete efficacy of PEP

Expert Consultation

The CDC specifically recommends consulting an expert in HIV PEP under the following circumstances:

- delay from time of exposure to time of evaluation is beyond 72 hours

- exposures to unknown sources (e.g., needles from unknown sources found in sharps disposal container or laundry)
- known or suspected pregnancy in the exposed person
- the exposed person is breastfeeding
- the source is or was on antiretroviral medications (i.e., possible resistance of the source virus to antiretroviral agents)
- the initial PEP regimen causes severe adverse reactions

Consultation is also advisable when:

- an acute HIV infection is suspected
- the source of the exposure has a negative HIV test but has a high-risk social or medical history
- the ED clinician is unfamiliar with prescribing HIV PEP

Consultations should not delay the onset of HIV PEP. If HIV PEP appears warranted, it is better to give the first dose of HIV PEP (unless there are obvious contraindications such as a medication allergy) and then wait for expert consultation. EDs should establish relationships with local experts in this field, if available, and design protocols that help facilitate rapid consultations. If local experts are not available, ED clinicians are encouraged to seek advice from the 24-hour National Clinicians' Post-exposure Prophylaxis Hotline (PEPline) at (888) 448–4911.

ADDITIONAL INTERVENTIONS AND PROPHYLAXIS

Patients who sustain blood or body fluid exposures are at risk for infections or preventable occurrences besides hepatitis B or HIV. Some additional interventions and prophylaxis that can be provided include:

- emergency contraception: levonorgestrel-only or ethinyl estradiol/norgestrel or ethinyl estradiol/levonorgestrel regimens (first dose should be given in the ED)
- prophylaxis against other sexually transmitted diseases including gonorrhea, *Chlamydia*, *Trichomonas*, and bacterial vaginosis (see Chapters 17 and 18 on sexually transmitted diseases)
- hepatitis A: hepatitis A vaccination at exposure and 6 months postexposure; can be considered for men who have sex with men and others at higher risk

Many of these medications may cause nausea. If HIV PEP is indicated, it should be administered first, followed by an antiemetic, before emergency contraception and/or other prophylaxis are administered.

ED LABORATORY TESTING

Table 56.10 provides a list of baseline laboratory tests that should be performed for patients exposed to blood or body fluids.

It is not necessary for patients to have an HIV test or a hepatitis panel sample drawn prior to receiving PEP. These tests check for antibodies so they are not affected by recent PEP. Other laboratory tests, such as those for sexually transmitted diseases, may be indicated, depending on the nature of the exposure.

Table 56.10 Baseline Postexposure Laboratory Testing

Scenario	Laboratory Tests
PEP not prescribed	HIV and hepatitis B and C antibodies
Hepatitis B PEP only prescribed	HIV and hepatitis B and C antibodies
HIV PEP prescribed	HIV and hepatitis B and C antibodies
	Complete blood count with differential
	Serum chemistry/electrolytes
	Liver enzymes
Conduct pregnancy testing for women of childbearing capacity.	

PEARLS AND PITFALLS

1. Establish and maintain exposure protocols that include:

   - expedited evaluations for PEP – reduce "door-to-drug" time
   - rapid HIV testing
   - regimens available for dispensing in the ED, including starter packs of HIV PEP medications
   - patient information handouts
   - expedited consultation with blood or body fluid and prophylaxis experts
   - facilitated follow-up and referrals to social, mental health, substance abuse counseling, and sexual assault advocacy services, as appropriate

2. Remember that most potential blood or body fluid exposures are not true mucous membrane or nonintact skin exposures and thus do *not* require HIV PEP.
3. Check the hepatitis B vaccination status on all exposed patients and initiate vaccination in the ED when appropriate.
4. Do not forget to provide prophylaxis against other sexually transmitted diseases and offer emergency contraception to childbearing-age female patients with sexual exposures.
5. Prescribe antiemetics for patients who experience nausea from PEP.

PEP RESOURCES

PEPline: The National Clinicians' Post-Exposure Prophylaxis Hotline. Phone: 1-888-448-4911. Available at: http://www.ucsf.edu/hivcntr/Hotlines/PEPline.html.
National and State PEP Guidelines Websites:
CDC:
Antiretroviral postexposure prophylaxis after sexual, injection-drug use, or other nonoccupational exposure to HIV in the United States. Available at: http://www.cdc.gov/mmwr/PDF/rr/rr5402.pdf.
Sexually transmitted diseases treatment guidelines (2002). Available at: http://www.cdc.gov/std/treatment/ rr5106.pdf.
Updated U.S. Public Health Service guidelines for the management of occupational exposures to HBV, HCV, and HIV and recommendations for postexposure prophylaxis (2001). Available at: http://www.cdc.gov/mmwr/PDF/rr/rr5011.pdf.
Updated U.S. Public Health Service Guidelines for the Management of Occupational Exposures to HIV and

Recommendations for Postexposure Prophylaxis (2005). Available at: http://www.cdc.gov/mmwr/PDF/rr/rr5409.pdf.

California:

Offering HIV post-exposure prophylaxis (PEP) following non-occupational exposures: recommendations for health care providers in the state of California. Available at: http://www.dhs.ca.gov/ps/ooa/Reports/PDF/OfferingPEPFollowingNonOccupExp0604.pdf.

Massachusetts:

Clinical advisory – HIV prophylaxis for non- occupational exposures. Available at: http://www.mass.gov/dph/aids/guidelines/ca_exposure_nonwork.htm.

New York:

HIV post-exposure prophylaxis following non-occupational exposure including sexual assault. Available at: http://www.hivguidelines.org/public_html/npep/npep.pdf.

HIV post-exposure prophylaxis for children beyond the perinatal period. Available at: http://www.hivguidelines.org/public_html/p-pep/p-pep.pdf.

HIV prophylaxis following occupational exposure. Available at: http://www.hivguidelines.org/public_html/oe/oe.pdf.

Rhode Island:

Nonoccupational HIV post-exposure prophylaxis guidelines for Rhode Island healthcare practitioners. Available at: http://www.brown.edu/Departments/BRUNAP/resources.html.

REFERENCES

Busch MP, Glynn SA, Stramer SL, et al. A new strategy for estimating risks of transfusion-transmitted viral infections based on rates of detection of recently infected donors. Transfusion 2005 Feb;45(2):254–64.

Catalano SM. Criminal victimization, 2004. Washington, DC: US Department of Justice, 2005.

Centers for Disease Control and Prevention (CDC). HIV/AIDS surveillance report, 2004. Vol. 16. Atlanta, GA: Centers for Disease Control and Prevention, 2005.

Chen GX, Jenkins EL. Potential work-related exposures to bloodborne pathogens by industry and occupation in the United States [abstract M2-B1301]. Paper presented at National HIV Prevention Conference, Atlanta, GA, 2005.

Ganem D, Prince AM. Hepatitis B virus infection–natural history and clinical consequences. N Engl J Med 2004 Mar 11;350(11):1118–29.

Glynn MK, Rhodes P. Estimated HIV prevalence in the United States at the end of 2003 [Abstract T1-B1101]. Paper presented at 2005 National HIV Prevention Conference, Atlanta, GA, 2005.

Kruszon-Moran D, McQuillan GM. Seroprevalence of six infectious diseases among adults in the United States by race/ethnicity: data from the third national health and nutrition examination survey, 1988–94. Adv Data 2005 Mar 9;352:1–9.

Mast EE, Margolis HS, Fiore AE, et al. A comprehensive immunization strategy to eliminate transmission of hepatitis B virus infection in the United States: recommendations of the Advisory Committee on Immunization Practices (ACIP) part 1: immunization of infants, children, and adolescents. MMWR Recomm Rep 2005 Dec 23;54(RR-16):1–31.

Panlilio AL, Cardo DM, Grohskopf LA, et al. Updated U.S. Public Health Service guidelines for the management of occupational exposures to HIV and recommendations for postexposure prophylaxis. MMWR Recomm Rep 2005 Sep 30;54(RR-9):1–17.

Rich JD, Merriman NA, Mylonakis E, et al. Misdiagnosis of HIV infection by HIV-1 plasma viral load testing: a case series. Ann Intern Med 1999 Jan 5;130(1):37–9.

Roland ME, Elbeik TA, Kahn JO, et al. HIV RNA testing in the context of nonoccupational postexposure prophylaxis. J Infect Dis 2004 Aug 1;190(3):598–604.

Roland ME, Neilands TB, Krone MR, et al. Seroconversion following nonoccupational postexposure prophylaxis against HIV. Clin Infect Dis 2005 Nov 15;41(10):1507–13.

Sexually transmitted diseases treatment guidelines 2002. Centers for Disease Control and Prevention. MMWR Recomm Rep 2002 May 10;51(RR-6):1–78.

Smith DK, Grohskopf LA, Black RJ, et al. Antiretroviral postexposure prophylaxis after sexual, injection-drug use, or other nonoccupational exposure to HIV in the United States: recommendations from the U.S. Department of Health and Human Services. MMWR Recomm Rep 2005 Jan 21;54(RR-2):1–20.

Updated U.S. Public Health Service Guidelines for the management of occupational exposures to HBV, HCV, and HIV and recommendations for postexposure prophylaxis. MMWR Recomm Rep 2001 Jun 29;50(RR-11):1–52.

57. Postoperative Infections

Ramin Jamshidi and William Schecter

INTRODUCTION

Of the 20 million operations performed annually in the United States, a growing number are conducted with accelerated discharge, or on an outpatient basis, and many patients with postoperative infections will present to emergency departments rather than to their surgeons' clinics. Most postoperative infections are surgical site infections (SSIs) and are classified based on anatomic depth (Table 57.1). Other infections related to perioperative procedures and anesthesia include urinary tract infections, pneumonia, thrombophlebitis, and antibiotic-associated colitis.

EPIDEMIOLOGY

Even with increasing attention to proper technique and preoperative antibiotics, SSI occurs in approximately 3% of all surgical patients. Infections are considered consequent to the operation when they occur within 30 days of sugery (or within 1 year in cases where implants are placed). In certain patient subgroups such as those undergoing emergent abdominal operations, the incidence rises to 20%. A variety of risk factors have been identified including diabetes, obesity, hypothermia, lengthy operation, and steroid therapy. Degree of risk correlates well with the American Society of Anesthesiologists' patient classification and the degree of contamination inherent to the operation (Table 57.2).

CLINICAL FEATURES

The majority of infections develop between the third and 10th postoperative days, but some may manifest as late as a month after surgery.

Superficial SSIs are generally evident on direct inspection. Early signs are warmth, tenderness, and bright red coloration (due to hyperemia), that blanches with pressure. On the extremities, erythema may streak proximally (a feature of streptococcal cellulitis). Cellulitis may progress to suppuration with superficial abscess formation and skin dehiscence, or may indicate the presence of an underlying abscess. All incisions with cellulitis should be examined for associated abscess because abscesses are unlikely to respond to antibiotic therapy alone and require prompt drainage. Superficial SSIs are unusual within the first 12–48 hours postoperatively, though streptococcal and clostridial infections should be considered in this time period, because they may be rapidly progressive and have high morbidity.

Deep SSIs are very similar to their superficial counterparts, but present at a more advanced state because early development is not evident to the naked eye. As deep infection progresses to suppuration, pressure from the collecting pus increases until it dissects through the surgical wound. When this process has worked its way superficially enough to drain through the skin incision, patients usually present for medical attention. If such infection is profound or prolonged, the viability of fascial tissues can be compromised and fascial dehiscence may occur. The most serious deep SSI is a poststernotomy wound infection because of the close proximity to the heart and potential for mediastinitis.

Table 57.1 Postoperative Infection Types

Surgical Site Infections			Others
Superficial	**Deep**	**Organ/Space**	
Cellulitis	Fascial	Intracavitary	Thrombophlebitis
Subcutaneous	dehiscence	abscess	Urinary infection
abscess		Anastomotic	Pneumonia
Skin		leak	Antibiotic-associated
dehiscence			colitis

Table 57.2 Classification of Operation Sterility

	Clean	**Clean Contaminated**	**Contaminated**	**Dirty**
Description	Skin or subcutaneous tissues	Controlled opening of a luminal tract without spillage	Spillage from a luminal tract	Operation on infected tissues or major break in sterile technique
Examples	Inguinal hernia Coronary bypass	Cholecystectomy Lung resection	Colectomy Urinary diversion	Anastomotic leak repair Debridement of necrosis

Table 57.3 Risk of Anastomotic Leak

Gastric Bypass	1.7–2.7%
Appendectomy	2–3%
Small Bowel Resection	3–4%
Bronchoplastic Lung Resection	3–4%
Gastrectomy	2–5%
Pneumonectomy	4–5%
Colectomy	2.0–5.6%
Urinary Diversion	3–8%
Pancreas Resection	5–10%
Rectal Resection	6.0–13.6%
Esophagectomy	5–16%

Organ or space SSIs are the most problematic of postoperative infections because they cannot drain as easily as the superficial and deep SSIs. Spontaneous drainage and decompression occur only with fistula formation and/or fascial dehiscence. Two mechanisms account for these collections: infection of a hematoma at the operative site, and leakage of infectious fluid from an anastomosis or site of viscus closure. The likelihood of leakage from an anastomosis depends highly on the type of operation and the indications for which it was performed Table 57.3 lists approximate leakage rates for various operations.

Among the SSIs, organ or space infections generally pose the greatest risk to patients. In the abdomen they present as secondary peritonitis, with abdominal pain, tenderness, nausea, and anorexia, and may cause signs and symptoms of systemic inflammation, such as fever and chills. Organ or space infections in the chest most commonly present with pleuritic chest pain and shortness of breath, while mediastinal infections are more likely to present with tachycardia and signs of severe infection, such as altered mental status. When rapid fluid accumulation occurs, pericardial infections may progress to cardiac tamponade.

In the setting of infection, output from drainage catheters may either significantly increase (because of increased leakage from inflammation) or decrease (because catheter blockage has led to an accumulation of fluid that becomes infected).

Pneumonia

Several aspects of operative treatment increase patients' risk of pneumonia. Postoperative abdominal and thoracic pain frequently causes patients to splint and hypoventilate. Limited lung inflation leads to atelectasis and poor clearance of airway secretions, increasing the chance of pneumonia. Furthermore, tracheal intubation and prolonged use of nasogastric or orogastric tubes are increasingly recognized risk factors for pneumonia.

Urinary Infection

A vast number of hospitalized patients have urinary (Foley) catheters placed, and often left in place longer than necessary. These urethral foreign bodies increase the risk of lower urinary tract infection, with some studies documenting a 10% incidence of catheter-related urinary tract infection after abdominal and orthopedic surgery. Often, these catheters are removed within a day of discharge and patients first develop urinary symptoms at home.

Colitis

Among the untoward effects of antibiotics is alteration of the natural balance of enteric flora, which allows some pathogenic species to proliferate and cause symptomatic disease. *Clostridium difficile* is the classic offender, though other species may be involved. Extended duration or spectrum of therapy does increase the risk, but it has been shown that a single dose of any antibiotic can cause this infectious colitis. This diagnosis should be entertained in any recently discharged patient with watery, foul-smelling stools.

Thrombophlebitis

Peripheral intravenous catheters are ubiquitous in hospitalized patients. Some 5% of patients develop superficial venous thrombosis related to these catheters, and local inflammation may result. Such phlebitis is manifested by a palpable cordlike lesion with overlying warmth and erythema extending from the venipuncture site. *Septic* thrombophlebitis is characterized by purulent drainage from the site, palpable fluctuance, or associated sepsis and requires aggressive treatment.

DIFFERENTIAL DIAGNOSIS

Superficial inflammatory erythema may result from normal wound healing or seroma. Noninfectious incisional hernia may be mistaken for dehiscence. Dehiscence occurs within the few weeks after operation and denotes almost complete failure of the fascia to heal. Incisional hernia refers to isolated defects in healing that present weeks to months after the operation.

Fluid accumulated in a deep space may be a sterile hematoma or serous fluid collection. In the abdomen, bilomas and urinomas may not necessarily be infected, but should be drained and may require operative repair of the source of the leak. In the chest, a milky pleural effusion does not necessarily indicate empyema, but may be chylothorax from thoracic duct injury. This also should be drained, and if output remains high, may require surgical revision.

Dysuria may represent urinary infection though the presence of a catheter alone can cause uretheral inflammation resulting in dysuria.

LABORATORY AND RADIOGRAPHIC FINDINGS

Any patient who presents with possible infection following an operation warrants a complete blood count (CBC) to evaluate for leukocytosis and neutrophilia (though the elderly and immunosuppressed may be unable to mount such a response).

If the patient is febrile, has significant leukocytosis, or is immunosuppressed with constitutional symptoms, then peripheral blood cultures should be obtained because they may affect antibiotic therapy. Cultures from wound swabs are *not* useful and lead to diagnostic confusion because wounds are not sterile sites. Results are clouded by microbial colonizers, contaminants, and species present in low density. If drainage catheters have been recently placed in sterile cavities, this fluid may be sent for Gram stain and culture.

Fluid from drainage catheters can be sent for other assays that test for the presence of specific bodily fluids to evaluate for leakage. These include creatinine for urinary leakage, bilirubin for biliary leakage, amylase and lipase for pancreatic leakage, and triglycerides and lymphocytes for lymph (chyle) leakage.

Urine analysis can indicate hydration status as well as diagnose urinary tract infection.

Chest radiographs should be obtained in any thoracic surgery patient who presents postoperatively for evaluation and in any patient with symptoms of dyspnea or cough. Pneumonia is not uncommon, and a postoperative fluid collection may manifest on chest radiograph as a widened mediastinum or cardiomegaly.

Ultrasound is increasingly used in the ED evaluation of superficial abscess and is often the preferred first study in children, but computed tomography (CT) is the standard for the evaluation of deep fluid collections. When looking for infectious processes, intravenous (IV) contrast is ideal but must be balanced with the risk of renal dysfunction. Although the evidence is not conclusive, this risk may be offset by pretreatment intravenous fluids, *N*-acetylcysteine, or sodium bicarbonate.

Patients who have undergone abdominal operations should also be given enteral contrast. This agent should be water soluble in case of perforation. If colorectal, gynecologic, or urologic procedures were performed, then rectal contrast should also be administered. Imaging plans should be discussed with the radiologist and surgeon for highest yield, as repeat doses of intravenous contrast within a short period significantly increase renal toxicity.

TREATMENT AND PROPHYLAXIS

Prophylaxis for surgical site infections is believed to be most effective when use is limited to the immediate perioperative period. Current recommendations suggest antibiotic treatment for the duration of the operation and up to 24 hours afterward. By the time patients are discharged from the hospital, there should be no prophylactic antibiotic regimen. Postdischarge antibiotics should be prescribed as treatment for a specific infection with a defined period of therapy.

Superficial surgical site infections without associated abscess are treated primarily with antibiotics. Because the usual microbes are skin flora, antibiotics should be aimed primarily at gram-positive cocci. Although the prevalence of methicillin-resistant *Staphylococcus aureus* (MRSA) infection is increasing in urban centers, it is still a minor agent in most wound infections, and empiric treatment should be based on local prevalence. In most cases, initial treatment should consist of a first-generation cephalosporins. If there is no clinical response, vancomycin should be added to cover MRSA. Contaminated or dirty cases may have superficial infections caused by bacteria seeded during the operation, so the relevant microbes should be covered, based on the source of contamination.

Table 57.4 Antibiotics for Secondary Peritonitis

	Mild or Community-Acquired	Severe
Primary Treatment	piperacillin-tazobactam 4.5 g IV q8h *or* ampicillin-sulbactam 3 g IV q6h *or* ticarcillin-clavulanate 3.1 g IV q6h *or* ertapenem 1 g IV q24h	imipenem-cilastatin 750 mg IV q8h *or* meropenem 1 g IV q8h *or* ampicillin 500 mg IV q6h *plus* ciprofloxacin 400 mg IV q12h *plus* anti-anaerobe (clindamycin 600 mg IV q8h or metronidazole 500 mg IV q8h)
Penicillin-Allergic	ciprofloxacin 400 mg IV q12h *plus* anti-anaerobe (clindamycin 600 mg IV q8h or metronidazole 500 mg IV q8h)	aztreonam 1 g IV q12h *plus* ciprofloxacin 400 mg IV q12h *plus* anti-anaerobe (clindamycin 600 mg IV q8h or metronidazole 500 mg IV q8h)
Children	As above, but weight-based dosing and no fluoroquinolones	As above, but weight-based dosing and no fluoroquinolones

The cornerstones of managing an infected fluid collection are to establish drainage and control the source. In a superficial wound, this may simply mean probing with a blunt instrument to open the skin and allow pus to escape. Drainage of deep spaces may be accomplished operatively (especially if revision is required) or percutaneously with radiologic guidance. Until drainage can be established, broad-spectrum antibiotics should be administered (Table 57.4). Because drainage is definitive treatment, antibiotics need not be continued long-term unless there are risk factors for persistent infection, such as prosthetic material or bacteremia.

Treatment of urinary tract infections, pneumonia, infectious diarrhea, catheter-related bacteremia, and suppurative thrombophlebitis in postoperative patients is the same as that for other hospitalized patients and is addressed elsewhere.

MANAGEMENT AND ADMISSION CRITERIA

Any patient who requires a radiologic or operative drainage procedure should be managed as an inpatient. High-risk patients such as the immunosuppressed and those who have undergone reconstructive operations with soft-tissue "flaps" also require inpatient management to limit further complications.

Profound leukocytosis, metabolic acidosis, hypoxia, or inability to maintain hydration or nutrition are also indications for admission. Simple endpoints of therapy are establishment of source control and/or drainage; normalization of leukocytosis and pyrexia; and a patient's improved sense of wellness.

INFECTION CONTROL

Postoperative infections generally do not pose risks for health care workers and others in proximity to the patient. The exceptions to this are *Clostridium difficile* colitis and vancomycin-resistant *Enterococcus* infections. Contact precautions should be strictly exercised in any patient with possible antibiotic-associated colitis or any history of VRE infection. Contagious risk for the former ends after a few days of appropriate treatment, but the latter poses a risk until a series of three weekly anal swab cultures reveal no vancomycin-resistant *Enterococcus*.

PEARLS AND PITFALLS

1. Infected fluid collections cannot be treated with antibiotics alone. Drainage and/or source control is necessary and often sufficient.
2. Careful review of a patient's operative report and discharge summary can disclose useful details as to possible infectious agents and sources for a fluid collection.
3. Foreign bodies such as mesh placed during inguinal hernia repair can cause large seromas with overlying erythema, but these are generally not infected. Consider a patient's clinical wellness when deciding whether intervention is required.
4. Contact with the original surgeon will often provide valuable information and help ensure appropriate follow-up.

REFERENCES

Dellinger EP. Roles of temperature and oxygenation in prevention of surgical site infection. Surg Infect 2006;7(3):27–32.

Fry DE. Basic aspects of and general problems in surgical infections. Surg Infect 2001;2(1):3–11.

Gomes GF, Pisani JC, Macedo ED. The nasogastric feeding tube as a risk factor for aspiration and aspiration pneumonia. Curr Opin Clin Nutr Metab Care 2003;6(3):327–33.

Katz SC, Pachter HL, Cushman JG, et al. Superficial septic thrombophlebitis. J Trauma 2005;59(3):750–3.

Stephan F, Sax H, Wachsmuth M, et al. Reduction of urinary tract infection and antibiotic use after surgery: a controlled, prospective, before-after intervention study. Clin Infect Dis 2006;42(11):1544–51.

ADDITIONAL READINGS

Barie PS, Eachempati SR. Surgical site infections. Surg Clin North Am 2005;85(6):1115–35.

Loutit J. Intra-abdominal infections. In: Wilson WR, Sande MA, eds. Current diagnosis & treatment in infectious diseases 2001. New York: McGraw-Hill, 2001:164–76.

58. Postpartum and Postabortion Infections

Lisa Rahangdale

INTRODUCTION – INFECTIONS AND AGENTS

Infections prevalent in the postpartum and postabortion period include urinary tract and genital tract infections (including endometritis, septic pelvic thrombophlebitis, pelvic inflammatory disease, and tubo-ovarian abscess), as well as mastitis, pneumonia (as a complication of anesthesia), and wound infection. Approximately 6% of women develop infections after vaginal delivery or cesarean section, the majority (94%) after hospital discharge. The most common postpartum infections are mastitis and urinary tract infection. This chapter reviews genital tract infections, mastitis, and episiotomy site infections. See Chapters 32, 37, and 57 for discussions of pneumonia, urinary tract infections, and surgical wound infections.

Endometritis: Postpartum and Postabortion

Endometritis is infection of the uterus. This may include the lining of the uterus (endometrium), the muscular layer (myometrium), or the entire organ. Endometritis is a polymicrobial infection occurring either at the time of delivery or during operative procedures via exposure of the upper genital tract to vaginal flora. Pathogens include aerobic and anaerobic gram-positive cocci (group A beta-hemolytic *Streptococcus*, coagulase-positive *Staphylococcus aureus*, group B *Streptococcus*, *Streptococcus pneumoniae*, and *Enterococcus faecalis*) as well as aerobic and anaerobic gram-negative agents (*Escherichia coli*, *Gardnerella vaginalis*, and *Bacteroides fragilis*). Other pathogens include those associated with prior sexually transmitted infection such as *Chlamydia trachomatis* and *Neisseria gonorrhoeae*, and those associated with bacterial vaginosis such as *Mycoplasma hominis* and *Ureaplasma urealyticum*.

Endometritis or pelvic inflammatory disease after surgical abortion may be associated with preexisting infections such as gonorrhea, *Chlamydia*, or *Mycoplasma* that are translocated during the procedure, or related to retained products of conception or operative trauma such as perforation of the uterus. Though there have been case reports of *Clostridium sordellii* sepsis and death associated with medical abortion, the con-

nection between this mode of abortion and the organism is unclear.

Septic Pelvic Thrombophlebitis

Septic pelvic thrombophlebitis can be separated into two clinical entities: ovarian vein thrombosis and deep septic pelvic vein thrombophlebitis. Frequently, the two are difficult to distinguish and may occur simultaneously. Septic pelvic thrombophlebitis occurs in the setting of pelvic surgery and, therefore, shares common causal organisms with endometritis as above.

Mastitis

Mastitis is acute inflammation of the interlobular connective tissue within the mammary gland. It is usually the result of a polymicrobial infection by maternal skin flora and infant nasal flora. Pathogens include *Staphylococcus aureus*, coagulase-negative *Staphylococcus*, and less commonly, group A and B beta-hemolytic *Streptococcus*, *Haemophilus influenzae*, *E. coli*, *Enterococcus faecalis*, *Klebsiella pneumoniae*, *Enterobacter cloacae*, *Serratia marcescens*, *Ralstonias pickettii*, and *Candida albicans*. *Staphylococcus aureus* accounts for 40% of mastitis cases and most cases of breast abscess. Methicillin-resistant *S. aureus* (MRSA) must be considered in areas where prevalence is high and in cases of treatment failure.

Episiotomy Site Infection

The organisms associated with episiotomy site infection include the predominant flora of the vagina or cervix; hence the organisms associated with endometritis are all potential agents. Of particular concern is the potential for necrotizing fasciitis, which can rapidly spread along fascial planes to the abdominal wall, buttocks, and thigh. This infection is classically associated with group A streptococci, but a combination of aerobic and anaerobic bacteria can cause this condition as well. (See also Chapter 43, Bacterial Skin and Soft-Tissue Infections.)

EPIDEMIOLOGY

Endometritis: Postpartum and Postabortion

Postpartum uterine infections occur in approximately 5.5% of vaginal deliveries and up to 6.0–7.4% of cesarean deliveries. In the preantibiotic era, postpartum endometritis was life-threatening, particularly when caused by group A hemolytic *Streptococcus*. With the widespread use of penicillin in the 1950s, this organism was replaced by *Staphylococcus aureus* as the most common etiology. Since then, the polymicrobial nature of endometritis has been better understood, and other species, including gram-negative aerobes and anaerobes, have emerged as significant agents. In the 1980s and 1990s bacterial vaginosis and sexually transmitted infections such as *C. trachomatis* were also found to cause pelvic infection after abortion or delivery.

Approximately 0.1 to 4.7% of surgical abortions worldwide are affected by uterine infection. The rate of infection among medical abortions is estimated at 0.09% to 0.6%.

Septic Pelvic Thrombophlebitis

Septic pelvic thrombophlebitis is an unusual condition with an overall prevalence of approximately 1 in 3000 deliveries. Risk is higher with cesarean section (1 in 800) than with vaginal delivery (1 in 9000).

Mastitis

It is estimated that between 2% and 33% of breastfeeding women develop lactation mastitis. Though it can occur anytime during lactation, most cases occur in the first 12 weeks after delivery. Breast abscess is a complication of mastitis and occurs in 5–11% of mastitis cases.

Episiotomy Site Infection

Infection can occur at the site of a vaginal laceration sustained in the course of delivery or at the site of an incision made by a provider to facilitate delivery. Such infections occur in approximately 0.3% of vaginal deliveries.

CLINICAL FEATURES

Endometritis

Postpartum endometritis can develop immediately after delivery in the setting of chorioamnionitis or, more commonly, several days later (Table 58.1). Clinical signs include temperature of ≥101°F or two separate temperatures of 100.4°F at least 6 hours apart, uterine tenderness, and purulent vaginal discharge.

Risk factors for postpartum endometritis include increased duration of labor, cesarean delivery, increased duration of rupture of membranes, increased number of vaginal examinations, increased duration of internal fetal monitoring, low socioeconomic status, and diabetes. Delayed-onset endometritis may be associated with prior *Chlamydia* infection.

Women who develop infection after abortion or who are having a septic abortion usually present with fever, lower abdominal pain, vaginal bleeding, and possibly passage of products of conception (Table 58.2). Diagnosis can sometimes

Table 58.1 Clinical Features: Postpartum Endometritis

Incubation Period	• Most within first 5 days of delivery • Early onset: with 48 hours of delivery • Late onset: up to 6 weeks after delivery
Signs and Symptoms	• Temperature of ≥101°F *or* • Two separate temperatures of 100.4°F at least 6 hours apart • Uterine tenderness • Purulent vaginal discharge • Nonspecific findings (malaise, abdominal pain, chills, tachycardia)
Laboratory Findings	• WBC may be elevated • Possible bacteremia

WBC, white blood (cell) count.

Table 58.2 Clinical Features: Postabortion Endometritis

Incubation Period	Similar to postpartum endometritis
Signs and Symptoms	• Lower abdominal pain • Vaginal bleeding • Fever • Tachycardia, tachypnea • Bacteremia and blood loss puts patient at more risk for shock • Bimanual exam: Uterine tenderness, parametrial cellulitis/abscess, crepitus in pelvis consistent with gas gangrene • Lacerations to cervix or vaginal wall
Laboratory Findings	• WBC count may be elevated • Hemoglobin/hematocrit may be low • Possible bacteremia

WBC, white blood (cell) count.

be delayed in women who have undergone illegal abortion because of their reluctance to divulge history. These women are frequently at higher risk for infection that those undergoing legal abortion.

Of note, the three cases of *Clostridium sordellii* infection associated with medical abortion in the United States had unusual presentations in that the patients remained afebrile. However, all had refractory hypotension, ascites and pleural effusions, hemoconcentration, and markedly elevated white blood cell counts (WBCs) consistent with toxic shock syndrome.

Septic Pelvic Thrombophlebitis

Most women with this complication will present with findings consistent with endometritis or pelvic cellulitis. They will usually have lower abdominal pain and fevers within 48 to 96 hours of delivery (Table 58.3). Predisposing factors for development of septic pelvic thrombophlebitis include cesarean section, pelvic infection, and the hypercoagulable state of pregnancy.

Diagnosis is made based on clinical findings, although computed tomographic (CT) scan or magnetic resonance

Table 58.3 Clinical Features: Septic Pelvic Thrombosis

Incubation Period	• Immediately postpartum to 1 month • Most common within 1 week postpartum
Signs and Symptoms	Ovarian vein thrombosis: • Fever up to 103–104°F • Lower abdominal/flank pain localized to one side • Ropelike tender abdominal mass possible (more frequently on right) • Pelvic exam consistent with uterine tenderness • Nausea, ileus, other gastrointestinal symptoms possible • No improvement in fever or symptoms despite antibiotics Deep septic pelvic vein thrombophlebitis: • Fevers despite 48–72 hours of antibiotics • Pain improves and patient appears well in between fever spikes • No palpable abdominal masses
Laboratory Findings	WBC count may be elevated

Table 58.4 Clinical Features: Mastitis and Breast Abscess

Incubation Period	Mastitis: • Most common 2–3 weeks postpartum • Can occur anytime during lactation Breast abscess: • Most common in first 6 weeks postpartum • Mastitis is predisposing factor
Signs and Symptoms	Mastitis: • Systemic illness (fever, chills, malaise) • Fever ≥38.5°C (102°F) • Tender, hot, swollen wedge-shaped erythematous area of breast • Usually one breast • Nipple fissure, sharp, shooting pains (fungal infection) Breast abscess: • Fluctuant mass • Fevers despite 48–72 hours of antibiotics
Laboratory Findings	• WBC count may be elevated • Skin and milk cultures often contaminated with skin flora

imaging (MRI) can be used to attempt visualization of venous thrombosis. Complications include spread of septic emboli leading to infection of other organ systems including the lungs.

Mastitis

Mastitis is thought to be caused by stagnant milk in the breast that leaks into surrounding breast tissue (Table 58.4). The milk itself leads to an inflammatory response and also provides a medium for bacterial growth for maternal skin flora and infant nasal flora. Predisposing factors include the following: milk stasis, breast engorgement, history of mastitis, improper nursing technique, maternal stress, and local skin disruption including nipple fissures, sores, and traumatic injuries. Breast abscess is a complication in 5–11% of mastitis cases that presents as a fluctuant or indurated mass and requires drainage.

Episiotomy Site Infection

Symptoms of episiotomy infection include pain and vaginal discharge. Physical exam findings include localized edema and erythema with exudates. More extensive infection and spread to the deep perineal fascia should be suspected if there is significant surrounding tenderness outside the area of visible skin inflammation. The entire area should be evaluated for signs of necrotizing fasciitis. (See Chapter 43, Bacterial Skin and Soft-Tissue Infections.) Simple episiotomy inflammation is not usually associated with signs of systemic infection such as fever or bacteremia. It is important to obtain aerobic and anaerobic cultures of any exudates, because more aggressive treatment may be considered in the case of group A *Streptococcus* infection.

DIFFERENTIAL DIAGNOSIS

In the postpartum or postabortion patient with a fever, the following sources of infection must be considered:

- genital tract: endometritis, septic pelvic thrombophlebitis, abscess
- urinary tract infection
- mastitis or breast abscess
- anesthesia complications (including aspiration pneumonia)
- wound infection of abdominal incision or episiotomy

Endometritis

Key features that distinguish endometritis from other conditions are:

- uterine tenderness
- purulent vaginal discharge
- exclusion of other sources of fever

Other conditions to consider (if no response within 48 to 72 hours of therapy):

- pelvic abscess
- infected wound or pelvic hematoma
- extensive cellulitis
- retained placenta
- septic pelvic thrombophlebitis
- organism resistant to antibiotic choice

Septic Pelvic Thrombophlebitis

Key features that distinguish septic pelvic thrombophlebitis from other conditions are:

- tender ropelike cord in right lower quadrant
- persistent fevers despite broad-spectrum antibiotic therapy
- exclusion of other sources of fever and pain

Other conditions to consider:

- appendicitis
- urologic conditions such as kidney stone or pyelonephritis

- gynecologic conditions such as adnexal torsion or degenerating leiomyoma
- broad ligament cellulitis or hematoma
- pelvic cellulitis or abscess
- operative injury to bowel or bladder
- drug fever

Mastitis

Key features that distinguish mastitis from other conditions are:

- tender, hot, swollen wedge-shaped erythema
- fever

Other conditions to consider:

- fullness (bilateral, warmth, heavy, hard, no erythema)
- engorgement (bilateral, tender, minimal diffuse erythema, with or without low-grade fever)
- clogged milk duct (painful lump with overlying erythema, no fever, well-appearing, particulate matter in milk)
- galactocele (smooth rounded swelling or cyst)
- abscess (tender hard breast mass, with or without fluctuance, skin erythema, induration, with or without fever)
- inflammatory breast carcinoma (unilateral, diffuse and recurrent, erythema, induration)

Episiotomy Site Infection

Key features that distinguish episiotomy site infection from other conditions are:

- erythema, bilateral edema, and exudate localized to superficial layers of the perineum

Other conditions to consider:

- vulvar hematoma
- generalized edema from delivery, trauma, or preeclampsia
- allergic reaction
- necrotizing fasciitis

LABORATORY AND RADIOGRAPHIC DIAGNOSIS
Endometritis

Endometritis is generally a clinical diagnosis based on history, symptoms, and physical examination. Associated laboratory findings may include an elevated WBC and decreased hemoglobin in the setting of vaginal bleeding. However, it is important to note that postpartum women may normally have a slightly elevated WBC count. Cervical and blood cultures may grow one of the organisms associated with postpartum or postabortion uterine infection though, cervical cultures are not routinely performed because of the high likelihood of contamination and the likely polymicrobial nature of the infection.

Ultrasound is useful to evaluate for retained placenta or parametrial abscess or hematoma. Chest x-ray or abdomi-

nal/pelvic x-ray may detect air in pelvic organs or under the diaphragm in the case of uterine perforation after surgical abortion. CT scan of the pelvis is useful where extensive cellulitis, hematoma, or abscess is suspected.

Septic Pelvic Thrombophlebitis

Diagnosis of septic thrombophlebitis is based on clinical findings. Laboratory findings affected by inflammation, such as WBC, may be abnormal, though again, these findings are particularly nonspecific in the postpartum or postabortion setting. CT scan of the pelvis may reveal findings consistent with venous thrombosis such as enlargement of the vein, low-density lumen of the vessel wall, or a sharply defined vessel wall enhanced by contrast media. MRI is also useful for diagnosing septic pelvic thrombophlebitis, although it is more expensive than CT. Absence of radiographic findings does not rule out this diagnosis. Ultrasound is useful to rule out other pelvic pathology but is not sensitive for pelvic thrombosis.

Mastitis

Mastitis is generally a clinical diagnosis based on presenting signs and symptom of breast infection in the postpartum period. Obtaining cultures of milk rarely alters management, because the etiologic agents are common skin and nasal flora and are difficult to isolate from contamination by breast skin flora. Proper milk cultures are obtained by catching milk in midstream away from the skin. Milk cultures are encouraged in women with hospital-acquired mastitis or recurrent mastitis, or in women who have had not clinical improvement after 2 days of antibiotic treatment.

Breast abscess is suspected when a fluctuant or indurated mass is found on physical exam. Confirmation is made by ultrasound. When drained, abscess fluid should be sent for bacterial culture, although these cultures have the same limitations noted above.

Episiotomy Site Infection

Diagnosis is made based on physical exam findings, primarily evidence of inflammation local to the site. Aerobic and anaerobic cultures of exudate should be obtained.

TREATMENT AND PROPHYLAXIS
Endometritis

In the setting of postpartum endometritis, the most studied and effective treatment regimen is a combination of intravenous gentamicin (1.5 mg/kg every 8 hours) and clindamycin (900 mg every 8 hours). Peak and trough levels of gentamicin should be obtained to ensure therapeutic dosing. There is research that also supports the use of once-daily gentamicin and clindamycin, and alternate drugs are listed below (Table 58.5). Ampicillin can be added when there is inadequate clinical response within 40 to 72 hours, particularly if the mother is known to have clindamycin-resistant group B *Streptococcus* colonization. Additionally, metronidazole can replace clindamycin and be used in combination with ampicillin and gentamicin in these refractory cases.

In cases of treatment failure, the possibility of pelvic abscess or infected hematoma and septic pelvic

Table 58.5 Treatment of Postpartum Endometritis and Pelvic Infections

- Gentamicin 1.5 mg/kg q8h and clindamycin 900 mg q8h
- Alternative regimens to gentamicin and clindamycin:
  - ampicillin-sulbactam 3 g IV q6h
  - cefotaxime 1 g IV q8h
  - cefoxitin 2 g IV q6h
  - ceftriaxone 2 g IV every 24 hours, followed by 1 g IV q24h
  - piperacillin-tazobactam 3.375 g IV q6h
  - ticarcillin-clavulanate 3.1 g IV q4h
  - levofloxacin 500 mg IV q24h *plus* metronidazole 500 mg IV q8h*

*Use of metronidazole is controversial during lactation. Consult current guidelines prior to use.

Table 58.6 Treatment of Mastitis and Breast Abscess

	Therapy Recommendation

Mastitis	• Supportive therapy: Rest, fluids, pain medication, anti-inflammatory agents
	• Continue breastfeeding
	• Antibiotics* that cover *Staphylococcus* and *Streptococcus*
	  ○ dicloxacillin 500 mg PO qid
	  ○ cephalexin 500 mg PO qid
	  ○ erythromycin if PCN allergic
	  ○ If resistant penicillinase-producing *Staphylococcus*, then vancomycin until 2 days after infection subsides
	• Minimum treatment 10–14 days

Breast Abscess	• Same as above • Needle drainage with or without drain placement (may be ultrasound-guided)* • Incision and drainage less commonly used for treatment

*Safe in lactating women.
PCN, penicillin.

thrombophlebitis must be considered. Although similar antibiotic regimens will be used, the need for drainage in the case of pelvic abscess or anticoagulation in the case of septic pelvic thrombophlebitis must be evaluated. Endometrial curettage is performed if retained products of conception are suspected.

A first-generation cephalosporin or ampicillin can be given at the time of cesarean section as prophylaxis against postpartum endometritis. The most common choice is cefazolin 1–2 g intravenously (IV). Timing of administration is controversial (preoperative dosing versus dosing at cord clamp) because some pediatricians prefer to avoid infant exposure to prophylactic antibiotics. However, preoperative dosing is likely more effective at preventing maternal postpartum infections. Prophylaxis in the postabortion period includes doxycycline 100 mg every 12 hours for 1–3 days, though other regimens, including metronidazole, erythromycin, and ofloxacin, have also been found effective.

Septic Pelvic Thrombophlebitis

The broad-spectrum antibiotics used for treatment of endometritis are also used for the initial treatment of septic pelvic thrombophlebitis. Persistent fever and pain are criteria for switching regimens. The use of anticoagulation is controversial though, heparin is generally still used for treatment. The duration of antibiotic and heparin therapy is usually 1 week, unless signs and symptoms of infection persist. Continuation of anticoagulation beyond antibiotic treatment is unnecessary. Surgical intervention is not routinely required and should be reserved for patients with no response to medical therapy or with other findings requiring surgery.

Mastitis

The most important aspects of treatment of mastitis are supportive therapy, antibiotics, and continued breastfeeding. Medications listed in Table 58.6 are considered safe during breastfeeding, and continued breastfeeding or expression of breast milk from the affected breast(s) is essential to preventing further milk stasis.

Episiotomy Site Infection

Simple episiotomy site infection should be opened and debrided using local anesthetic. The episiotomy incision should remain open for either healing by secondary inten-

tion or repair at a later date once the infection is cleared. Timing of this repair varies, but generally, 1 week is required for healthy tissue to be available for adequate repair. Good hygiene, sitz baths, and stool softeners are useful in promoting healing.

If cellulitis is suspected or extensive infection is noted, the patient should be treated with antibiotics. Surgical exploration is indicated if the wound appearance is suspicious for necrotizing fasciitis, if inflammation extends beyond the labia, if there is significant unilateral edema, if symptoms fail to resolve in 24 to 48 hours, or if the patient shows signs of systemic toxicity.

INFECTION CONTROL

There are no data to suggest person-to-person transmission of postpartum or postabortal infections. Therefore, Standard Precautions are considered adequate for patients with postpartum or postabortal infections. Patients do not require isolation rooms. Frequent provider hand washing is essential. Mothers and infants do not require separation during treatment for infection.

PEARLS AND PITFALLS

1. Consider septic pelvic thrombophlebitis in the setting of high fevers and no response to antibiotic treatment for endometritis. However, this disorder is rare among postpartum women and other sources of infection must be ruled out.
2. It is safe and important to continue breastfeeding during treatment for mastitis.
3. Consider coverage of MRSA when treating mastitis or breast abscess without clinical improvement in 48 to 72 hours.
4. Episiotomy site infection is rare, but careful examination is important to assess for serious infections such as necrotizing fasciitis, which requires immediate surgical intervention.

REFERENCES

American College of Obstetrics & Gynecology. ACOG Educational Bulletin No. 258. Breastfeeding: maternal and infant aspects. July 2000.

American College of Obstetrics & Gynecology. ACOG Practice Bulletin No. 67. Medical management of abortion. Oct 2005.

Barbosa-Cesnik C, Schwartz K, Foxman B. Lactation mastitis. JAMA 2003;289(13):1609–12.

Brown CE, Stettler W, Twickler D, et al. Puerperal septic pelvic thrombophlebitis: Incidence and response to heparin therapy. Am J Obstet Gynecol 1999;181(1):143–8.

Centers for Disease Control and Prevention (CDC). *Clostridium sordellii* toxic shock syndrome after medical abortion with mifepristone and intravaginal misoprostol – United States and Canada, 2001–2005. MMWR 2005 July 22;54(Dispatch):1.

Centers for Disease Control and Prevention (CDC). [Title]. Available at: http://www.cdc.gov/mmwr/preview/mmwrhtml/mm54d722a1.htm.

Faro S. Postpartum endometritis. Clin Perinatol 2005;32:803–14.

Hopkins L, Smaill F. Antibiotic prophylaxis regimens and drugs for cesarean section (Review). Cochrane Library 2006;2. New York: Wiley. The Cochrane Collaboration.

Larson JW, Hager WD, Livengood CH, et al. Guidelines for diagnosis, treatment and prevention of postoperative infections. Infect Dis Obstet Gynecol 2003;11:65–70.

Ledger WJ. Postpartum endomyometritis diagnosis and treatment: a review. J Obstet Gynecol Res 2003 Dec;29(6):364–73.

Livingston JC, Llata E, Rinehart E. Gentamicin and clindamycin therapy in postpartum endometritis: the efficacy of daily dosing versus dosing every 8 hours. Am J Obstet Gynecol 2003;188(1):149–52.

Sawaya GF, Grady D, Kerlikowske K, et al. Antibiotics at the time of induced abortion: The case for universal prophylaxis based on a metaanalysis. Obstet Gynecol 1996;87:884–90.

Shannon C, Brothers LP, Phillip NM, et al. Infection after medical abortion: a review of the literature. Contraception 2004;70:183–90.

Sweet RL, Gibbs RS. Infectious diseases of the female genital tract, 4th ed. Philadelphia: Lippincott Williams & Wilkins, 2002.

Yokoe DS, Christiansen CL, Johnson R, et al. Epidemiology and surveillance for postpartum infections. Emerg Infect Dis 2001 Sept–Oct; 7(5):837–41.

Special Populations

59. The Febrile Post-Transplant Patient

Aparajita Sohoni

INTRODUCTION

In the United States, solid organ transplants and hematopoietic stem cell transplants are increasingly common forms of treatment for a variety of medical conditions. The 1- and 5-year survival rates vary depending on the organ transplanted. In general, kidney, pancreas, and liver transplants have higher survival rates (86–98% at 1 year and 73–98% at 5 years) than do heart, lung, or combined heart-lung transplants. Overall, improvements in transplant candidate selection, surgical technique, immunosuppressive regimens, and long-term medical care have resulted in high survival rates from solid organ transplants. As the number of successful transplants increases, so does the number of acute care visits made by these patients. An understanding of the differential diagnosis of fever in a post-transplant patient, of the risk of infection at different times after transplant, and of the risk associated with various levels of immunosuppression can aid in a comprehensive and cost-effective work-up.

EPIDEMIOLOGY

Infectious complications are a serious cause of morbidity and mortality in post-transplant patients, with serious infection occurring in up to two-thirds of organ transplant patients. In one study of renal transplant recipients, the incidence of infection in the first year post-transplant ranged from 25% to 80%. In a separate study of liver transplant patients, up to 67% of recipients had one serious infection, and infection factored in 53% of early post-transplant deaths. Notably, while infection must be ruled out in any febrile transplant patient, some infected patients will be afebrile because of therapeutic immunosuppression. Practitioners should have a high level of suspicion for the presence of serious infectious disease in all transplant patients.

CLINICAL FEATURES

Infections in transplant patients can best be approached by distinguishing between infections associated with solid organ transplant and those associated with hematopoietic stem cell transplant.

Infections in Solid Organ Transplantation

Solid organ transplant recipients are usually treated with multidrug prophylaxis against rejection for 3–12 months after transplant (see Treatment section below). Given that the immunosuppressive regimens are similar for all solid organ transplants, there is a general timeline for risk of infection in the post-transplant course. This can be conceptually divided into the early phase (1 month post-transplant), middle phase (1–6 months post-transplant), and late phase (more than 6 months post-transplant). Though exceptions are numerous, there is a distinct group of infectious etiologies in each phase (Figure 59.1).

EARLY PHASE (LESS THAN 1 MONTH POST-TRANSPLANT)

In the first month post-transplant, infections are similar to those in a nonimmunosuppressed host undergoing a similar surgical procedure: wound infections, infected hematomas, postsurgical pneumonia (either aspiration or due to prolonged intubation), urinary tract infections secondary to indwelling catheters, or bacteremia due to vascular access devices such as central lines. In fact, more than 95% of infections are due to such causes. The risk of infection increases with the duration of intubation or prolonged usage of catheters, vascular access devices, or with the presence of any indwelling catheters or stents. Common pathogens include gram-negative bacilli, *Staphylococcus aureus*, *Staphylococcus epidermidis*, and *Enterococcus* (Table 59.1). Opportunistic pathogens are uncommon in the first month after transplantation and, when seen, likely indicate a nosocomial exposure, a severe degree of immunosuppression prior to the transplant, or a preexisting infection in either the donor or the recipient. Although pretransplant screening of both the donors and recipients is thorough, transplantation of an infected allograft, contamination of the allograft during transplantation, or unrecognized or inadequately treated pretransplant infections in the host may occur.

MIDDLE PHASE (1 TO 6 MONTHS POST-TRANSPLANT)

The state of immunosuppression is greatest in the middle phase, as the effects of prolonged T-cell dysfunction become evident. The top four infectious causes of fever in this group

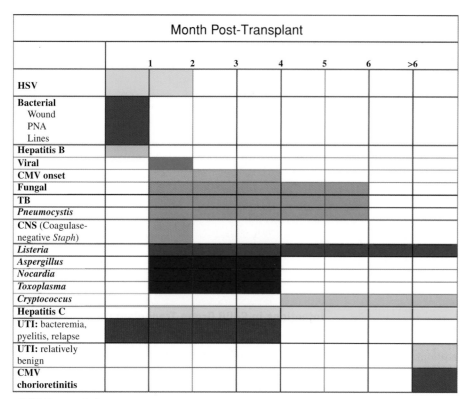

CMV, Cytomegalovirus
UTI, Urinary tract infection

Figure 59.1 Infectious etiologies in the post–solid organ transplant patient.

Table 59.1 Pathogens with Documented Transmission During Transplantation

Class	Pathogen
Bacterial	• Enteric gram-negative bacilli • *Pseudomonas aeruginosa* • *Staphylococcus aureus* • *Bacteroides fragilis*
Viral	• Cytomegalovirus • Herpes simplex virus • Hepatitis B • Hepatitis delta virus • HIV • Adenovirus • West Nile virus • Arenaviruses (new cases in Australia)
Fungal	• *Candida albicans* • *Histoplasma capsulatum* • *Cryptococcus neoformans*
Protozoal	• *Toxoplasma gondii* • *Strongyloides stercoralis*
Mycobacterial	• *Mycobacterium chelonae* • *Mycobacterium tuberculosis*

HIV, human immunodeficiency virus.

of patients are cytomegalovirus (CMV), *Listeria monocytogenes*, *Aspergillus* species, and *Pneumocystis jiroveci* (formerly *carinii*). *Nocardia asteroides*, and *Salmonella* species are also significant threats to patients in both the middle and late phases post-transplant. New infection with immunomodulatory viruses (such as CMV, Epstein-Barr virus [EBV], hepatitis C virus [HCV], hepatitis B virus [HBV], and human immunodeficiency virus [HIV]), for which these patients are also at risk, may further impair immune responses, resulting in increased susceptibility to opportunistic pathogens such as *Pneumocystis*, *Aspergillus*, and *Listeria*. The most common pathogens are discussed below, with general guidelines for treatment. Specific algorithms should be determined after reviewing individual hospital and community susceptibility patterns, discussion with infectious disease specialists, and examination of all past cultures and biopsy results.

Cytomegalovirus is a member of the Herpesviridae and is the most common viral infection in post-transplant patients. Some studies have found CMV infection present in 60–90% of all solid organ transplant patients. Infection can be asymptomatic or symptomatic. In asymptomatic patients, the disease is usually diagnosed by testing for seroconversion. In symptomatic patients, complaints often include prolonged fever, anorexia, fatigue, and myalgias. On examination, splenomegaly, elevated transaminases, thrombocytopenia, leukopenia, and atypical lymphocytosis are commonly seen. CMV can present as pneumonitis (usually bilateral), gastroenteritis, pancreatitis, encephalitis, transverse myelitis, myocarditis, skin ulcerations, or chorioretinitis (more frequently seen in the late phase). CMV may also cause allograft injury, such as chronic hepatitis in a liver transplant patient, early atherosclerosis in a heart transplant patient, or bronchiolitis obliterans in a lung transplant patient. Disease is more severe in newly infected patients than in patients who have had CMV infection prior to transplantation. Diagnosis is made via blood culture, bronchoalveolar lavage, or tissue biopsy demonstrating intranuclear inclusions. The approach to prophylaxis and treatment of CMV disease is controversial and should be discussed with transplant or infectious disease specialists.

Listeria monocytogenes is a gram-positive bacillus that can cause bacteremia, meningitis, or meningoencephalitis. This organism is one of the most common bacterial causes of central nervous system (CNS) infection in the post-transplant patient. Patients often present with a subacute onset of fever, headache, altered mental status, and sometimes seizures, though frank meningismus is less common. Lumbar puncture often shows an increased opening pressure, and cerebrospinal fluid (CSF) demonstrates a decreased glucose level, neutrophilic pleocytosis, and a negative Gram stain. The CSF and blood cultures are key to the diagnosis given that the Gram stain is often negative. Recommended treatment is with high-dose intravenous penicillin, ampicillin, or trimethoprim-sulfamethoxazole (in penicillin-allergic patients) for 21 days.

Aspergillus species is a fungus that is a common cause of pneumonia in the severely immunosuppressed patient. Common presentations include fever and nonproductive cough that may progress to pleuritic chest pain or pulmonary hemorrhage. Hematogenous dissemination to the CNS can occur, causing confusion, altered mental status, and focal neurological findings. A stroke pattern can develop, with computed tomographic (CT) scan findings of low-density lesions. CSF cultures are usually negative and diagnosis is generally made from bronchoscopy with fluid culture, or via biopsy of affected organs, including the lung, liver, or heart. Blood cultures are usually negative, even in patients with hematogenous dissemination. Whereas the mainstay of treatment used to be amphotericin B in life-threatening illnesses, or with itraconazole or voriconazole in less critical disease, recent studies suggest that combination antifungal therapy using caspofungin and voriconazole confers a higher 90-day survival rate in patients with severe infection. This mortality benefit was seen in patients with renal disease as well as those with more severe species of *Aspergillus*, such as *A. fumigatus*.

Pneumocystis jiroveci is a fungal species (previously thought to be a protozoon) that causes significant infection in post-transplant patients, especially in heart-lung and lung transplant patients, with a rate of infection as high as 88%. Patients characteristically complain of a subacute onset of a nonproductive cough, dyspnea, and fever. On examination, exertional hypoxia is seen, with variable pulmonary findings. The chest radiograph classically shows diffuse interstitial infiltrates. Diagnosis is made by examination of induced sputum, bronchoalveolar lavage fluid or tissue biopsy. First-line prophylaxis and treatment is with trimethoprim-sulfamethoxazole.

Nocardia asteroides is an aerobic, gram-positive, weakly acid-fast staining, branching filamentous bacteria that generally causes pneumonia or brain abscesses in the post-transplant patient. Symptomatic patients commonly present with fever (~67% of patients) or cough (>50% of patients). Patients with CNS infection may have fever, headache, or focal neurological signs, though CSF study results are usually nonspecific. In patients with pneumonia secondary to this organism, the chest radiograph will often show a focal cavitary or nodular lesion. *Nocardia* has a predilection for vascular sites and can form abscesses within the kidney, liver, bone, joint, eye, skin, or other sites. Blood cultures are rarely positive, and the diagnosis is often made by tissue biopsy of skin lesions, pulmonary cavities, or other affected sites. Treat-

ment is prolonged antimicrobial therapy, with up to 1 year of trimethoprim-sulfamethoxazole.

Salmonella is a gram-negative bacterium that commonly infects the gastrointestinal tract, resulting in gastroenteritis, often causing mucosal ulcerations and hemorrhagic diarrhea. These patients usually present with fever, bacteremia, or sometimes with abscesses secondary to hematogenous spread of the bacillus. Stool, blood, or tissue culture is required to diagnose this infection. Treatment consists of prolonged therapy using amoxicillin, ceftriaxone, trimethoprim-sulfamethoxazole, or ciprofloxacin, depending on the susceptibility of specific isolates.

LATE PHASE

To identify a patient's infectious disease risk at this distance from transplantation, it is best to assign patients to one of three categories based on their level of immunosuppression. Patients on minimal immunosuppressive agents (>80% of patients) with good allograft function and no active immunomodulatory virus infections are susceptible to the same infections as the general community. Opportunistic infections are rarely seen unless there has been either a direct exposure to a contagious host or a probable link to a specific environmental exposure, such as gardening and subsequent development of aspergillosis.

An additional 10% of solid organ transplant recipients have chronic or progressive infection with HBV, HCV, CMV, human papilloma virus (HPV), or EBV that can affect allograft function, cause generalized immunosuppression, and predispose to the development of cancer. In these patients, the level of suspicion for any infectious process must remain high and they should be treated aggressively.

Many of the remaining 10% of patients suffer from chronic allograft rejection, are on higher doses of immunosuppressive agents, and are more likely to become infected with opportunistic agents. Any possible source of infection should be aggressively pursued when patients in this group present with fever, given the high likelihood of serious disease.

Hematopoietic Stem Cell Transplant

In addition to the standard risks of infection from environmental exposures, catheters, tubes, and vascular access devices, patients who have undergone hematopoietic stem cell transplant also have a distinct triphasic timetable of infectious risks (Figure 59.2) determined by their degree of immune reconstitution and by the presence or absence of graft-versus-host disease (GVHD).

PHASE 1: CONDITIONING REGIMEN TO ENGRAFTMENT

The conditioning regimen refers to the chemotherapy or irradiation given immediately prior to the hematopoietic stem cell transplant. The purpose of conditioning is to eradicate as much of the patient's disease as possible prior to transplantation, and also to suppress host immune reactions to engraftment. These regimens usually cause profound granulocytopenia, and major risks during this phase include exacerbation of residual pre-transplant infections (i.e., aspergillosis), or hematogenous invasion by bacteria or yeast facilitated by breaks in the integrity of mucocutaneous surfaces. Gram-negative bacteria such as *Pseudomonas aeruginosa* and *Enterobacter* and gram-positive cocci such as *Staphylococcus*

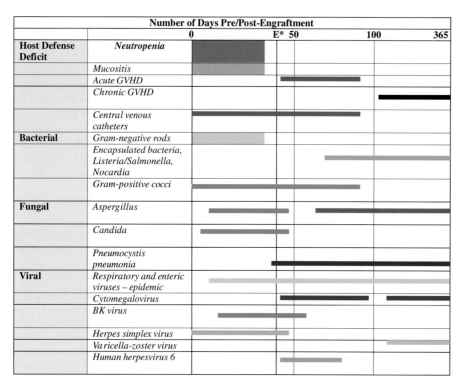

		Number of Days Pre/Post-Engraftment				
		0	E* 50		100	365
Host Defense Deficit	*Neutropenia*					
	Mucositis					
	Acute GVHD					
	Chronic GVHD					
	Central venous catheters					
Bacterial	*Gram-negative rods*					
	Encapsulated bacteria, Listeria/Salmonella, Nocardia					
	Gram-positive cocci					
Fungal	*Aspergillus*					
	Candida					
	Pneumocystis pneumonia					
Viral	*Respiratory and enteric viruses – epidemic*					
	Cytomegalovirus					
	BK virus					
	Herpes simplex virus					
	Varicella-zoster virus					
	Human herpesvirus 6					

E*, Day of engraftment

Figure 59.2   Infectious etiologies in the post–hematopoietic stem cell transplant patient.

and *Streptococcus* along with *Candida* infections are frequently seen. As the duration of neutropenia lengthens, the risk of invasive fungal infections increases. These patients are at high risk for developing sepsis, in the setting of almost complete immunocompromise.

PHASE 2: ENGRAFTMENT TO DAY 100

The major infectious risks during this phase are reactivation of the herpes viruses including CMV, varicella-zoster virus (VZV), human herpesvirus (HHV) 6, and herpes simplex virus (HSV). If engraftment was delayed, then an increased incidence of invasive fungal infections is seen.

PHASE 3: MORE THAN 100 DAYS POST-ENGRAFTMENT

In this phase, the risk of infection is determined by the presence or absence of GVHD. In the absence of GVHD, the major infectious threats include VZV, *Streptococcus pneumoniae*, and respiratory virus infection (including influenza, parainfluenza, and respiratory syncytial virus [RSV]), largely because of the functional immaturity of the reconstituted immune system. Late-onset CMV is also seen, especially in patients who have not received adequate prophylaxis. In patients who have severe GVHD, there is an increased risk of infection with CMV, *Pneumocystis*, invasive fungi, and other organisms.

DIFFERENTIAL DIAGNOSIS

The differential diagnosis, aside from infection, for fever in a post-transplant patient (either solid organ transplant or hematopoietic stem cell transplant) is:

- allograft rejection or graft-versus-host disease
- drug reaction/hypersensitivity
- thromboembolic disease
- transfusion reaction

Allograft Rejection and Graft-versus-Host Disease

Fever and isolated organ dysfunction can occur at any time post-transplant. The laboratory abnormalities will be specific to the organ transplanted (i.e., elevated creatinine in renal transplants, elevated bilirubin and alkaline phosphatase in liver recipients, hyperglycemia in pancreatic transplant patients). Pain at the site of the organ graft often occurs in kidney and liver transplant patients. Graft biopsy is necessary to diagnose rejection, and the transplant service should be consulted.

In GVHD, the immune cells generated by the "graft," or hematopoietic stem cells that were transplanted, attack host tissues. Acute GVHD generally presents 2 to 8 weeks following transplantation. The most commonly involved organs include the skin, intestine, and liver, and patients may present with fever, diarrhea, or skin findings such as bullous lesions and erythematous macules.

In chronic GVHD, attack on host tissues results in inflammation, further complicated by the development of fibrosis or scar tissue. Chronic GVHD necessitates long-term high-dose immunosuppression that predisposes patients to infection with invasive opportunistic pathogens.

Drug Reaction and Hypersensitivity

Post-transplant patients regularly take medications that can cause fever as part of a drug reaction or "drug fever."

These include antibiotics and antifungals such as the beta-lactams, sulfonamides, and amphotericin B. Other medications that can cause fever include immunosuppressants such as OKT3, azathioprine, cyclosporine, and tacrolimus (FK506). Most febrile drug reactions will present within 10 days of initial administration. Drug fever generally persists for several days after withdrawal of the offending agent. This diagnosis is difficult to make in the emergency department, especially if past medical records are unavailable. This diagnosis should be one of exclusion, as infection must be ruled out in any febrile post-transplant patient.

Thromboembolic Disease and Vascular Events

Deep venous thrombosis (DVT) and pulmonary embolus are important causes of fever in postoperative patients. Other sites of thrombosis are specific to the organ transplantation such as hepatic artery thrombosis in liver transplant patients. Thrombosis also predisposes patients to bacterial or fungal infection, and may cause infectious seeding of distant organs.

Transfusion-Related Fever

Given the high number of blood products generally required in transplant patients, post-transfusion causes of fever should also be considered. Specifically, hemolytic reactions may be seen in patients with symptoms occurring during a transfusion or with evidence of red blood cell destruction on their peripheral smear. Urticaria may accompany fever in the setting of a transfusion-related hypersensitivity. Transmission of various organisms via transfusion should also be considered, including CMV, hepatitis B and C, *Treponema pallidum*, *Plasmodium*, *Trypanosoma cruzi*, *Brucella*, *Babesia*, and *Toxoplasma*.

LABORATORY AND RADIOGRAPHIC FINDINGS

Laboratory Studies

The choice of laboratory studies should be guided by the amount of time since organ transplant and by clinical presentation. In patients who are more than 6 months post-transplant, without a significant level of immunocompromise or chronic rejection, and generally well-appearing, the laboratory work-up may be identical to that of a nontransplant patient (i.e., targeted to the chief complaint only).

However, in any post-transplant patient for whom there is concern for immunosuppression, graft function, significant infection, or who is less than 6 months post-transplant, a thorough laboratory work-up should be performed, regardless of localizing complaints. This work-up should include complete blood count with differential; chemistries including calcium, magnesium, and phosphate; renal and liver function tests; and urinalysis. These patients should be pan-cultured: send blood samples for bacterial and fungal cultures (at least two sets), urine, sputum, wound cultures, and cultures from any indwelling lines, stents, or tubes. If a lumbar puncture is performed, fluid analysis should include CMV polymerase chain reaction (PCR), culture, Gram stain, smear, fungal culture, and acid-fast bacillus (AFB) staining. Serum levels for the following immunosuppressants should be obtained when relevant: cyclosporine, azathioprine, tacrolimus, mycophenolate mofetil, or sirolimus.

Table 59.2 Treatment

Patient Category	Therapy Recommendation

Adults	**Bacterial infections:** Broad-spectrum coverage of gram-positive, gram-negative, and anaerobic infections using:
	• cefepime 1–2 g IV q8h
	  plus
	  vancomycin 1 g IV q12h
	• Consider addition of metronidazole (500 mg IV q8h) if intra-abdominal focus suspected
	Fungal infections:
	• amphotericin B 0.7 mg/kg/day IV
	• fluconazole 200–400 mg/day IV or PO
	Viral infections:
	• ganciclovir 5 mg/kg/dose IV q12h
	• foscarnet 60 mg/kg/dose IV q8h
	Pneumocystis infections:
	• trimethoprim-sulfamethoxazole 20 mg/kg IV divided 4 times per day (or 1 double-strength tablet PO bid).

Children	**Bacterial infections:** Broad-spectrum coverage of gram-positive, gram-negative, and anaerobic infections using: • ceftazidime 100–150 mg/kg/day divided every 8 hours, maximum 6 g/day • tobramycin 2.5 mg/kg IV q8h • vancomycin if documented infection with coagulase-negative *Staphylococcus*, MRSA, or other aerobic gram-positive cocci is identified, or if patient has had an infected catheter • meropenem can substitute for ceftazidime if high concern for anaerobic infection **Fungal infections:** No history of invasive fungal infections: • fluconazole 5 mg/kg/day IV, maximum dose 400 mg/day. Adjust dose based on creatinine clearance. Discontinue if LFTs are elevated to 2–3 times normal, or if itraconazole or liposomal amphotericin B (AmBisome) used. • amphotericin B 1.0–1.5 mg/kg/day IV, but if renal insufficiency or toxicity occurs, change to amphotericin B lipid complex (if serum creatinine is ≥2 mg/dL, or has doubled in absolute value, or if creatinine clearance is <25 mL/min). In patients with a history of invasive fungal infections, antifungal agent will be determined by past sensitivities. Other agents include: • voriconazole loading dose 6 mg/kg/dose IV q12h × 2 doses, then 4 mg/kg/dose q12h maintenance. Administer infusion over 1–2 hours, not to exceed 3 mg/kg/hour. • itraconazole 3–5 mg/kg/day daily • caspofungin age 2–11 years: 2 mg/kg IV loading dose, maximum 70mg, then 50 mg/m^2 IV to maximum of 50 mg once daily thereafter. If children >12 years old, give 70 mg IV loading dose on day 1, then 50 mg IV daily thereafter. **Viral infections:** • ganciclovir 5 mg/kg/dose IV q12h • foscarnet 60 mg/kg/dose every IV q8h **Pneumocystis infections:** Trimethoprim-sulfamethoxazole prophylaxis: • Pretransplant: patients >30 kg: 1 SS PO bid; <30 kg, give 5 mg/kg/day. TMP component in divided doses. Suspension is 40 mg TMP per 5 mL in divided doses. • Post-transplant: >30 kg: 1 SS PO bid twice weekly on two consecutive days. <30 kg: 5 mg/kg/day TMP component in two divided doses twice weekly on two consecutive days. Alternatives: dapsone or IV pentamidine For treatment of active infection with *Pneumocystis jiroveci*, give trimethoprim-sulfamethoxazole 15–20 mg TMP/kg/day in divided doses every 6–8 hours

LFT, liver function test; MRSA, methicillin-resistant *Staphylococcus aureus*; SS, single strength; TMP, trimethoprim.

Table 59.3 Interactions of Common Immunosuppressive Agents and Other Medications

Immunosuppressive Agent	Interacting Drug	Mechanism of Interaction	Possible Adverse Effect/Clinical Implication
Cyclosporine, Tacrolimus, Sirolimus	Diltiazem Verapamil Amiodarone Azoles (keto-, flu-, itra-) Macrolides (erythromycin, azithro-, clarithro-)	Inhibition of hepatic cytochrome P-450, causing an increased level of the immunosuppressive agent	Nephrotoxicity due to elevated cyclosporine or Tacrolimus levels; can also enhance adverse effects of each of interacting drugs
Cyclosporine, Tacrolimus, Sirolimus	Phenobarbital Phenytoin Carbamazepine Rifampin Isoniazid	Induction of hepatic cytochrome P-450, causing a decreased level of the immunosuppressive agent	Increased risk of rejection due to a lower level of the immunosuppressive agent
Cyclosporine or Tacrolimus	HMG CoA reductase inhibitors ("statins")	Level of statin increased by immunosuppressive drug	Increased risk of statin-induced rhabdomyolysis
Cyclosporine or Tacrolimus	Aminoglycosides, iodinated radiocontrast, amphotericin B	Synergistic nephrotoxicity of the immunosuppressive agent and the interacting drug	Synergistic nephrotoxicity
Azathioprine	Allopurinol	Xanthine oxidase inhibition by allopurinol causes a decreased metabolism of azathioprine, resulting in increased azathioprine levels	Increased azathioprine levels capable of causing bone marrow suppression

HMG CoA, 3-hydroxy-3-methylglutaryl coenzyme A.

Imaging Studies

A variety of imaging studies may help detect infectious processes and evaluate allografts in post-transplant patients:

- Chest radiograph: The lung is one of the most common sites of invasive infection in post-transplant patients. Given the degree of immunosuppression in these patients, there may be a significant delay in the development of radiographic findings. CT of the chest should be obtained when there is clinical concern for pneumonia and a negative or equivocal chest radiograph.
- Ultrasound of the transplanted organ: Ultrasound can be used to evaluate for adequate perfusion and drainage of the transplanted organ.
- CT scan: CT scanning may be used to rule out other pathology.

Biopsy

A tissue sample is needed to rule out rejection, and biopsy should be coordinated by the consulting transplant service.

TREATMENT AND PROPHYLAXIS

Treatment

The use of antibiotics in post-transplant patients is potentially complicated by the interaction of antibiotic agents and immunosuppressive medications (Table 59.2). In addition, the lengthy courses of antibiotics required for complete treatment may necessitate long hospital stays and heighten risk of renal or hepatic damage.

The interactions of antibiotics and other medications with the most common immunosuppressive agents are shown in Table 59.3. The clinician should use caution when initiating or altering any drug therapy in an immunosuppressed post-transplant patient.

Prophylaxis

Transplant patients are maintained on complicated antibiotic and immunosuppressive regimens for prophylaxis against infection and rejection. This section covers prophylaxis for infection, while prophylaxis against rejection is addressed in the following section.

For both solid organ transplant and hematopoietic stem cell transplant recipients, anti-infection prophylaxis includes influenza immunization and avoidance of environmental hazards including gardening, community cleaning activities, exposure to construction, travel to the developing world, and contact with infected individuals. Additionally, patients must be reimmunized after hematopoietic stem cell transplant as their immune systems have been reconstituted. Patients who have received a solid organ transplant such as liver transplant should not be exposed to anyone who may be actively shedding a virus, including those who have recently received live virus vaccines. Any exposures should be reported to the transplant service coordinator.

In solid organ transplant patients specifically, infection prophylaxis by stage includes:

First month:

- perioperative surgical wound prophylaxis
- initiation of trimethoprim-sulfamethoxazole prophylaxis

Table 59.4 Immunosuppressive Agent, Mechanism of Action, and Adverse Effects

Agent	Mechanism of Action	Usage	Adverse Effects
Corticosteroids (Prednisone, Methylprednisolone)	Decreases inflammation (suppresses migration of polymorphonuclear leukocytes), reverses increased capillary permeability, suppresses immune system, reduces activity and volume of the lymphatic system. Can cause adrenal suppression, antitumor, or antiemetic effects	Used as part of a triple-drug regimen along with azathioprine and cyclosporine	Weight gain, Cushingoid appearance, cataracts, acne, skin thinning, bruising, osteoporosis, fractures, avascular necrosis of hip or knee, upper gastrointestinal ulceration/bleeding, diabetogenicity, psychologic effects, hyperlipidemia
Cyclosporine (Gengraf, Neoral, Restasis, Sandimmune)	Inhibits production and release of interleukin-2, thereby preventing activation of resting T-cells	Used as part of a triple-drug regimen along with azathioprine and prednisone. Dosage based on trough levels	Acute and chronic nephrotoxicity, hyperkalemia, hypomagnesemia, hyperuricemia/gout, hemolytic-uremic syndrome, hypertension, hyperlipidemia, diabetogenicity, hepatotoxicity, neurotoxicity, hirsutism, gingival hyperplasia
Azathioprine (Azasan, Imuran)	Inhibits B- and T-cell proliferation	Used as part of a triple-drug regimen along with cyclosporine and prednisone	Bone marrow suppression, leukopenia, thrombocytopenia (first weeks after therapy), macrocytosis, with or without anemia, hepatotoxicity (reversible), pancreatitis
Tacrolimus/FK-506, (Prograf, Protopic)	Inhibits T-cell activation	Used either as an induction agent or as rescue therapy for refractory rejection. Dosage based on trough levels	Neurotoxicity more common than with cyclosporine (manifests as tremors, paresthesias, headache, insomnia, and seizures); nephrotoxicity, hyperkalemia, hypomagnesemia, hyperuricemia/gout, hemolytic-uremic syndrome, diabetogenicity, hepatotoxicity, hair loss; less hypertension and hyperlipidemia than with cyclosporine
Mycophenolate Mofetil (CellCept, Myfortic)	Inhibits T- and B-cell proliferation	Can be used to replace azathioprine in the triple-drug regimen	Abdominal pain, anorexia, nausea, vomiting, upper gastrointestinal bleeding, diarrhea, anemia, leukopenia, thrombocytopenia
Sirolimus (Rapamune)	Inhibits T-cell activation and proliferation, inhibits antibody production, inhibits acute rejection of allografts, prolongs graft survival	Used in combination with cyclosporine or after withdrawal of cyclosporine	Thrombocytopenia, hyperlipidemia, buccal ulceration, diarrhea, interstitial pneumonitis, less commonly leukopenia/anemia

1–6 months:

- filtered air and water supply
- low-dose trimethoprim-sulfamethoxazole prophylaxis (prophylaxis against urosepsis, *Pneumocystis*, *Listeria*, *Toxoplasma*)
- CMV prophylaxis or preemptive treatment strategy as determined by transplant service and infectious disease services

After 6 months:

- lowest risk category: no prophylaxis
- in 10% with chronic hepatitis C or B: use of hyperimmune hepatitis B immunoglobulin and antivirals such as lamivudine and adefovir
- in 10% highest risk group: lifelong trimethoprim-sulfamethoxazole and fluconazole prophylaxis

In patients who have received a hematopoietic stem cell transplant, anti-infection prophylaxis includes:

Phase 1:

- use of mask and gloves by health care workers, high-efficiency particulate air (HEPA) filters, pneumococcal polysaccharide vaccine (PPV)
- prophylactic fluoroquinolones, systemic antifungals

Phase 2:

- anti-CMV preventive strategies

Phase 3:

- treatment determined by presentation, no specific prophylaxis

Prophylaxis against rejection consists of three-drug immunosuppressive therapy for 3–12 months after transplant; subsequently one of the three drugs is removed, most commonly corticosteroids. Though a full discussion of the immunosuppressive regimens is beyond the scope of this chapter, any alterations or additions to the patient's regimen should only be made after discussion with the transplant center. Table 59.4 lists the most common immunosuppressive agents, their mechanism of action, and common adverse effects.

COMPLICATIONS AND ADMISSION CRITERIA

The major complications facing the febrile transplant patient include severe infection, sepsis, organ failure, and rejection.

Aside from obvious admission criteria, such as hemodynamic instability or sepsis, any of the following will usually necessitate admission of the febrile post-transplant patient:

- new-onset graft failure
- recent (within 1 year) transplant
- high levels of immunosuppression
- difficulty with medication compliance

INFECTION CONTROL

The key measure is early placement of these patients in reverse isolation when they are known or suspected to be significantly neutropenic or otherwise immunocompromised.

PEARLS AND PITFALLS

1. Take the risk of infection in these patients seriously. They will often have life-threatening infections and may not present with signs and symptoms typical for an immunocompetent host.
2. Be aggressive with the laboratory and radiographic workups. They are more often positive than negative in this cohort.
3. Pan-culture ideally prior to any antibiotics, but do not delay therapy in a toxic-appearing patient.
4. Consult the appropriate transplant service early and often.
5. Start empiric treatments early.
6. In a generally well-appearing patient, more than 1 year out from transplantation, and on minimal immunosuppressive therapy, consider outpatient management with close follow-up with the transplant service.

REFERENCES

Annual Report of the U.S. Organ Procurement and Transplantation Network and the Scientific Registry of Transplant Recipients: transplant data 1996–2005. Rockville, MD: Health Resources and Services Administration, Healthcare Systems Bureau, Division of Transplantation, 2006.

Fischer SA. Infections complicating solid organ transplantation. Surg Clin North Am 2006;86(5):1127–45, v–vi.

Fischer SA, Trenholme GM, Levin S. Fever in the solid organ transplant patient. Infect Dis Clin North Am 1996;10(1):167–84.

Fishman JA, Rubin RH. Infection in organ-transplant recipients. N Engl J Med 1998;338(24):1741–51.

Marty FM, Rubin RH. The prevention of infection post-transplant: the role of prophylaxis, preemptive and empiric therapy. Transpl Int 2006;19(1):2–11.

Munoz P, Singh N, Bouza E. Treatment of solid organ transplant patients with invasive fungal infections: should a combination of antifungal drugs be used? Curr Opin Infect Dis 2006;19(4):365–70.

Renoult E, Buteau C, Lamarre V, et al. Infectious risk in pediatric organ transplant recipients: is it increased with the new immunosuppressive agents? Pediatr Transplant 2005;9(4):470–9.

Rubin RH, Schaffner A, Speich R. Introduction to the Immunocompromised Host Society consensus conference on epidemiology, prevention, diagnosis, and management of infections in solid-organ transplant patients. Clin Infect Dis 2001;33(Suppl 1):S1–4.

Savitsky EA, Uner AB, Votey SR. Evaluation of orthotopic liver transplant recipients presenting to the emergency department. Ann Emerg Med 1998;31(4):507–17.

Savitsky EA, Votey SR, Mebust DP, et al. A descriptive analysis of 290 liver transplant patient visits to an emergency department. Acad Emerg Med 2000;7(8):898–905.

Slifkin M, Doron S, Snydman DR. Viral prophylaxis in organ transplant patients. Drugs 2004;64(24):2763–92.

Venkat KK, Venkat A. Care of the renal transplant recipient in the emergency department. Ann Emerg Med 2004;44(4):330–41.

60. Rabies

Amy E. Vinther and Fredrick M. Abrahamian

INTRODUCTION

In the United States, rabies is primarily a disease of animals and rarely occurs in humans. During 1980–2004, a total of 56 cases of human rabies were reported to the Centers for Disease Control and Prevention (CDC) in the United States. The majority of cases were associated primarily with silver-haired and eastern pipistrelle bats. The decline of rabies in developed countries is attributed to control of the disease in domestic animals, as well as effective pre- and postexposure vaccination programs.

EPIDEMIOLOGY

The epidemiology of human rabies for a specific geographic region is related to the prevalence of rabies in animals, and the extent of human contact with them. In the United States, rabies is most commonly reported in animals such as raccoons, skunks, bats, and foxes. Other animals that can potentially transmit the disease include bobcats, coyotes, and mongooses. Smaller mammals such as squirrels, rabbits, mice, and rats are considered to be at a lower risk for transmitting the disease. If infected, these animals often succumb to the disease, and therefore have a very limited chance of spreading the disease. Nonmammalian bites (e.g., birds and reptiles) pose no risk of rabies transmission.

In the United States, dogs, cats, ferrets, and livestock are considered to be at a lower risk of being infected with rabies virus because of effective vaccination practices. However, dogs along the U.S.-Mexico border (e.g., Texas-Mexico border) and cats that roam freely in endemic areas of terrestrial animal rabies (e.g., raccoons in northeastern United States) should be considered at higher risk.

Exposure to rabies most commonly occurs from a bite of an infected animal, which has the greatest potential for disease transmission. Bites from bats may go unnoticed because of their small, thin, and sharp teeth. In addition to a bite, other mechanisms of disease transmission from bats may include scratch or mucous membrane exposure. In contrast, nonbite exposures such as handling, petting, or contact with low-risk bodily fluids (e.g., blood, urine, stool) from terrestrial animals carry a low risk of disease transmission. Human-to-human rabies transmission has been reported in the setting of organ transplantation.

CLINICAL FEATURES

Rabies is a highly fatal disease, and yet preventable by proper wound care and timely and appropriate administration of rabies postexposure prophylaxis. Rabies virus is a single-stranded negative polarity RNA virus belonging to the genus *Lyssavirus* of the Rhabdoviridae family. Once the virus gains entry into its host, it begins to replicate within the cells of striated muscle. It then travels within the peripheral nervous system to the central nervous system, where replication occurs almost exclusively within the gray matter. From the brain through autonomic nerves, it travels to peripheral organs such as the salivary glands, heart, lungs, liver, kidneys, and skeletal muscle.

The clinical manifestation of rabies can be categorized into three distinct phases: the prodromal phase, acute neurologic phase (encephalitic), and coma (Table 60.1). The incubation period is variable and can range from 7 days to more than a year. In the majority of cases, the incubation period is 1–3 months. In comparison to bites of the extremities, bites to the head have shorter incubation periods.

The prodromal phase typically has a duration of 2–10 days, with nonspecific symptoms that include fever, headache, myalgia, malaise, fatigue, anorexia, nausea, vomiting, sore throat, nonproductive cough, irritability, agitation, or anxiety. Prodromal symptoms that are suggestive of rabies (occurring in 50–80% of patients) are paresthesia and fasciculation at or near the site of the bite.

The acute neurological (encephalitic) phase commonly lasts less than 1 week. This phase is diagnosed when there are objective signs of central nervous system disease (e.g., confusion, delirium, hallucinations, incoordination, aphasia, dysphasia, and seizures). This phase is often described in two forms: furious rabies (80%) and paralytic rabies (20%). Patients with furious rabies exhibit disorientation, hallucinations, and bizarre behavior. Early within this period, lucid and calm periods may intersperse with abnormal behavior. The majority of patients also exhibit hydrophobia and aerophobia to a variable degree. The act of swallowing liquids or inspiring

Table 60.1 Clinical Features: Rabies

Organism	Rabies virus, a single-stranded RNA virus belonging to the genus *Lyssavirus*
Incubation Period	1–3 months
Signs and Symptoms	**Prodromal phase:** Nonspecific symptoms (e.g., fever, headache, myalgia, malaise, fatigue, anorexia, nausea, vomiting, sore throat, nonproductive cough, irritability, agitation and anxiety), paresthesias or fasciculations at or near the wound site. **Acute neurologic phase (encephalitic):** Confusion, delirium, hallucinations, incoordination, excessive salivation, hydrophobia, dysphasia, aerophobia, aphasia, seizures, hyperthermia, postural hypotension, and nuchal rigidity. In the paralytic form, paralysis is the predominant clinical feature either localized to the bitten extremity or diffuse. An ascending paralysis similar to Guillain-Barré syndrome may also occur. **Coma and death**
Laboratory Findings	There are no specific laboratory findings that can reliably make the diagnosis of rabies in the emergency department
Treatment	Therapy directed at supportive measures and the prevention of complications

deeply results in violent contractions of the diaphragm and the accessory muscles of inspiration. This is due to exaggerated respiratory tract protective reflexes and is an indication of central nervous system dysfunction. The presence of these symptoms should raise a high suspicion for rabies. Other symptoms can include autonomic dysfunction (e.g., excessive salivation, hyperthermia, postural hypotension), nuchal rigidity, and convulsions. In the paralytic form of rabies, paralysis is the predominant clinical feature, which can either be localized (to the extremity that was bitten) or diffuse. The paralysis may also occur in an ascending pattern similar to Guillain-Barré syndrome.

In the final stages, the disease progresses to coma and eventually death. Death usually occurs from complications such as respiratory failure and cardiac dysfunction.

DIFFERENTIAL DIAGNOSIS

Other conditions to consider include:

- encephalitis from other pathogens (e.g., herpesviruses)
- meningitis
- poliomyelitis
- Guillain-Barré syndrome
- transverse myelitis
- intracranial mass lesions (e.g., brain abscess)
- cerebrovascular accident
- tetanus
- severe alcohol withdrawal
- adrenergic or cholinergic poisoning

Key features that may help to distinguish rabies are:

- Prodromal symptom, including paresthesia and fasciculation at or near the site of the bite.
- The majority of patients with rabies exhibit hydrophobia and aerophobia, symptoms that should raise a high suspicion for rabies.
- In comparison to rabies, patients with tetanus most often have normal mental status and normal cerebrospinal fluid.

LABORATORY DIAGNOSIS

There are no specific laboratory findings that can reliably make the diagnosis of rabies in the emergency department. Similar to other viral infections, the cerebrospinal fluid may demonstrate mild pleocytosis with lymphocytosis, mildly elevated protein, and a normal glucose. The ultimate antemortem diagnosis of rabies rests on the isolation of the organism from bodily fluids (e.g., saliva, cerebrospinal fluid) or an infected tissue sample (e.g., nape of the neck). Other diagnostic tools include the demonstration of the viral antigen or nucleic acid in the patient's saliva or tissue sample. Additionally, the discovery of a specific antibody in the serum of a previously unvaccinated person or cerebrospinal fluid may be helpful.

TREATMENT

Once a patient develops signs and symptoms consistent with clinical rabies, there is no specific therapy. To reduce the potential for precipitating agitation, it is best to place patients in rooms that are quiet, limit procedures, and minimize patient manipulation and stimulation. Interventions are directed at supportive measures and the prevention of complications.

COMPLICATIONS

Death from rabies occurs from complications of the disease such as respiratory failure (e.g., acute respiratory distress syndrome, hypoxia) and cardiac dysfunction (e.g., arrhythmias). Other complications can include pituitary dysfunction, ileus, gastrointestinal bleeding, thrombocytopenia, and secondary bacterial infections.

POSTEXPOSURE PROPHYLAXIS

When evaluating a patient who has potentially been exposed to rabies, it is imperative to gather the following information: type of animal exposure, whether the animal is available for brain testing, vaccination history (both for the patient and the animal), when and where the exposure occurred, and whether the attack was provoked or unprovoked (Figure 60.1).

Rabies postexposure prophylaxis includes administration of rabies vaccine and, depending on the patient's immunization history, rabies immunoglobulin (RIG). If indicated, pregnant women may receive rabies postexposure prophylaxis. Rabies vaccine provides active immunity, whereas RIG provides passive immunity. Individuals who have not been previously immunized should receive rabies vaccine on days 0, 3, 7, 14, and 28. Previously vaccinated patients should receive the vaccine only on days 0 and 3. In adults and older children, rabies vaccine should be administered intramuscularly (IM) in the deltoid area. In young children, the preferred injection

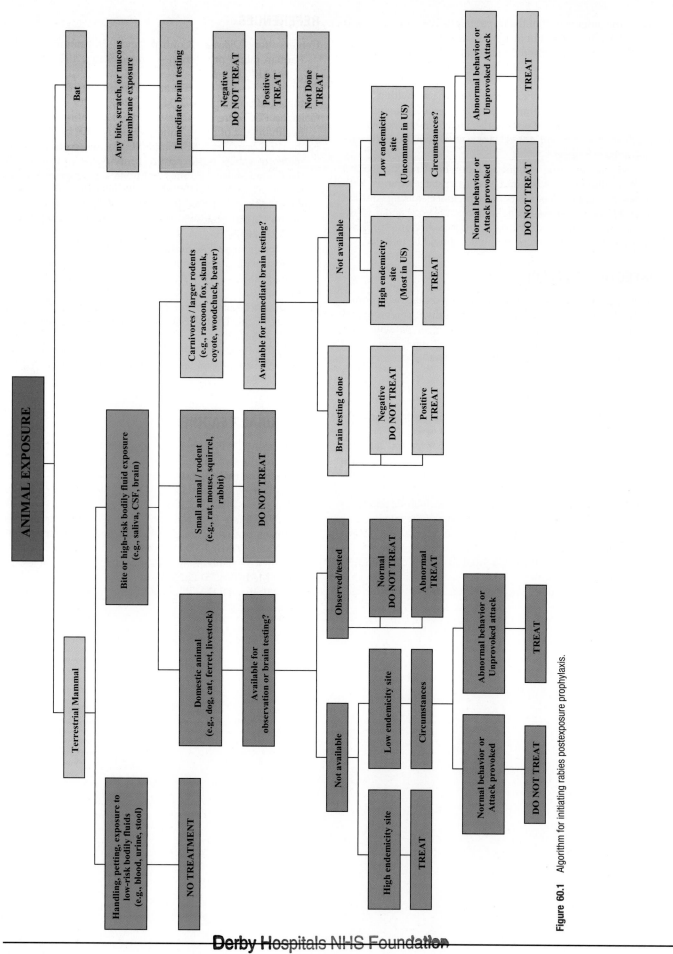

Figure 60.1 Algorithm for initiating rabies postexposure prophylaxis.

site is the outer aspect of the upper thigh. The vaccine should never be administered in the gluteal area.

RIG is only administered to patients who have never been vaccinated against rabies. It is administered only once on the initial visit (day 0) at a dose of 20 international units/kg. If not given during the initial visit, it can be given once within 7 days of the rabies vaccine administration. If possible, the full dose should be infiltrated IM around the bite wounds. The remaining dose should be infiltrated IM at a site distant from the vaccine administration.

Local wound care should include cleansing the wound with a solution of soap and water. Irrigate wounds with copious amounts of iodine-based virucidal cleansing solution (e.g., diluted povidone-iodine solution). Necrotic and devitalized tissues should be debrided. As indicated, tetanus prophylaxis and administration of antibiotics should be initiated.

INFECTION CONTROL

Standard precautions aimed at preventing contact with potentially infectious bodily fluids such as saliva, cerebrospinal fluid, and tears are adequate for the care of patients with rabies. Blood and feces are not considered infectious. These patients do not require respiratory isolation.

PEARLS AND PITFALLS

1. In the United States, animal rabies is most commonly reported in raccoons, skunks, bats, and foxes.
2. Dogs along the United States-Mexico border and cats that roam freely in endemic areas of terrestrial animal rabies should be considered at higher risk of being infected with rabies virus.
3. Prodromal symptom suggestive of rabies include paresthesias and fasciculation at or near the site of the bite.
4. Hydrophobia and aerophobia should raise a high suspicion for rabies.
5. Consider rabies in the differential diagnosis of ascending paralysis.
6. Patients previously vaccinated for rabies should not receive RIG.

REFERENCES

Centers for Disease Control and Prevention (CDC). Human rabies prevention – United States, 1999. MMWR 1999;48(RR-1):1–21.

Centers for Disease Control and Prevention (CDC). Human rabies, Mississippi, 2005. MMWR 2006;55:207–8.

Coleman PG, Fevre EM, Cleaveland S. Estimating the public health impact of rabies. Emerg Infect Dis 2004;10:140–2.

Krebs JW, Long-Marin SC, Childs JE. Causes, costs and estimates of rabies postexposure prophylaxis treatments in the United States. J Public Health Manage Pract 1998;4:56–62.

Krebs JW, Mandel EJ, Swerdlow DL, et al. Rabies surveillance in the United States during 2004. J Am Vet Med Assoc 2005;227:1912–25.

McQuiston J, Yager PA, Smith JS, et al. Epidemiologic characteristics of rabies virus variants in dogs and cats in the United States, 1999. J Am Vet Med Assoc 2001;218:1939–42.

Noah DL, Drenzek CL, Smith JS, et al. Epidemiology of human rabies in the United State, 1980–1996. Ann Intern Med 1998;128:922–30.

Weiss HB, Friedman DI, Coben JH. Incidence of dog bite injuries treated in emergency departments. JAMA 1998;279:51–3.

ADDITIONAL READINGS

Chutivongse S, Wilde H, Benjavongkulchai M, et al. Postexposure rabies vaccination during pregnancy: effect on 202 women and their infants. Clin Infect Dis 1995;20:818–20.

Dreesen DW. A global review of rabies vaccines for human use. Vaccine 1997;15:S2–S6.

Moran GJ, Talan DA, Mower W, et al. Appropriateness of rabies postexposure prophylaxis treatment for animal exposures. JAMA 2000;284:1001–7.

Rupprecht CE, Gibbons RV. Prophylaxis against rabies. N Engl J Med 2004;351:2626–35.

Warrell MJ, Warrell DA. Rabies and other lyssavirus diseases. Lancet 2004;363:959–69.

61. Septic Shock

Clement Yeh and Robert Rodriguez

Outline   Introduction

INTRODUCTION

The term *sepsis* describes a spectrum of pathophysiologic responses to infection. In the setting of advanced antibiotic therapies, sophisticated respiratory and cardiovascular support, and improved diagnosis, sepsis-associated mortality has declined in recent years, though it remains greater than 50% in some groups. Early recognition and aggressive management are critical to reducing morbidity and mortality.

EPIDEMIOLOGY

The causative organisms implicated in sepsis have changed over time, and many cases have nondiagnostic or negative cultures. The identified sites of primary infection are predominantly lung (47%), followed by unknown/other (28%), peritoneum (15%), and urinary tract (10%). Prior to 1987, gram-negative organisms were the predominant organisms identified. In the past 20 years, however, sepsis caused by gram-positive organisms has increased markedly, and gram-positives are now the predominant etiologic agents. Additionally, over the same time period, the incidence of fungal sepsis has increased by over 200%. These changes likely reflect the increased numbers of immunocompromised patients and debilitated surgical patients, and the increased use of indwelling catheters and devices.

CLINICAL FEATURES

The American College of Chest Physicians and the Society of Critical Care Medicine have developed standardized diagnostic criteria for sepsis, severe sepsis, and septic shock to describe the continuum of evolving physiologic derangement (Table 61.1). Categorization of patients in this system provides vital prognostic information and guides critical disposition and treatment decisions. There is a clear incremental increase in mortality associated with sepsis (16%), severe sepsis (20%), and septic shock (46%).

Septic patients often survive the acute septic shock state, only to die later from multiple organ failure and its complications (Table 61.2). Nearly all organ systems may be affected by the hyperinflammation, hypercoagulation, and hypoperfusion states of severe sepsis, and prompt recognition and early, aggressive resuscitation decrease the likelihood of organ dysfunction and death.

DIFFERENTIAL DIAGNOSIS

Many entities can mimic the presentation of severe sepsis (Table 61.3). Acute coronary syndrome, pancreatitis, medication reactions, and many other conditions can result in systemic inflammatory response and end-organ hypoperfusion that may be difficult to differentiate from severe sepsis.

LABORATORY AND RADIOGRAPHIC FINDINGS

No single laboratory study confirms or excludes the diagnosis of sepsis. Sepsis can present as a spectrum of laboratory and radiographic study derangements related to primary infection, systemic inflammatory response, or response to end-organ hypo-perfusion (Table 61.4).

Table 61.1 Sepsis Definitions

SIRS (Systemic Inflammatory Response Syndrome)	• Hyperthermia: temperature >38.0°C *or* • Hypothermia: temperature <36.0°C • Tachycardia: heart rate >90 bpm • Tachypnea: respiratory rate >20 breaths/min or PCO_2 <32 mm Hg • Leukocytosis/leukopenia: WBC >12K or <4K/mm^3 or >10% immature neutrophils
Sepsis	• SIRS *and* • Suspected or documented infectious process
Severe Sepsis	• Sepsis *and* • Hypotension or hypoperfusion
Septic Shock	• Severe sepsis *and* • Persistent hypotension/hypoperfusion despite adequate fluid resuscitation
SIRS, systemic inflammatory response syndrome; WBC, white blood (cell) count.	

Table 61.2 Major Organ Dysfunction in Severe Sepsis

Organ	Complications	Clinical Signs and Symptoms
Pulmonary	• ARDS	Tachypnea Hypoxia Respiratory failure
Cardiovascular	• Myocardial depression • Disseminated vasodilation	Tachycardia Hypotension Poor capillary refill Edema
Renal	• Acute renal failure	Oliguria
GI	• Ileus • Hepatic ischemia • Mesenteric ischemia	Abdominal pain or tenderness Decreased bowel sounds Constipation or diarrhea Bleeding
CNS	• Altered mental status	Disorientation Agitation
Hematologic	• DIC • Anemia • Thrombocytopenia • Leukopenia	Bleeding Bruising Petechiae Immunosuppression
Endocrine	• Relative adrenal insufficiency	Hypo/hyperglycemia Persistent hypotension

ARDS, acute respiratory distress syndrome; CNS, central nervous system; DIC, disseminated intravascular coagulation; GI, gastrointestinal.

Table 61.3 SIRS and Hypoperfusion Differential Diagnosis

Diagnosis	Features
Severe sepsis	Suspected infectious source
Tumor lysis syndrome	Large tumor burden, chemotherapy
Jarisch-Herxheimer reaction	Release of endotoxin following microbial cell death in response to antibiotics
Pulmonary infarction	Dyspnea, pleuritic chest pain, risk factors for pulmonary embolism
ARDS	Hypoxia, bilateral infiltrates on chest radiograph
Pancreatitis	Abdominal pain, elevated lipase or amylase
Myocardial infarction	ECG changes, elevated serum cardiac biomarkers
Thyrotoxicosis or thyroid storm	Thyromegaly, elevated serum thyroid function tests
Drug fever	New medication initiation, urticarial rash
Neuroleptic malignant syndrome or malignant hyperthermia	Muscular rigidity, general anesthesia or dopaminergic medications
Alcohol withdrawal	Tremulousness, chronic alcohol use
Acute adrenal insufficiency	Chronic steroid use

ARDS, acute respiratory distress syndrome; ECG, electrocardiogram.

TREATMENT AND PROPHYLAXIS

Early Goal Directed Therapy

The landmark study in which a protocol of early goal-directed therapy (EGDT) reduced mortality by 16% established the ED as a focal point for resuscitation of the septic patient. Goals in this treatment strategy refer to hemodynamic and perfusion-related targets (central venous pressure 8–12 mm Hg, mean arterial pressure 65–90 mm Hg, and central venous oxygenation >70%) to be achieved rapidly and sequentially using fluids, vasopressors, blood transfusions, and occasionally ventilatory support with sedation (Table 61.5; Figure 61.1).

Emergency departments not enacting a formal EGDT protocol should nonetheless consider two points. (1) Primary hemodynamic therapy for septic patients must occur in the ED. (2) Prompt aggressive fluid resuscitation is the mainstay of therapy.

RESPIRATORY SUPPORT

The hypoxic patient should be given oxygen and the patient who is obtunded and unable to protect his or her airway should be intubated. Many septic patients have very high work of breathing that can lead to respiratory failure, exhaustive energy expenditure, and lactic acidosis. Many patients with septic shock require respiratory support at some point during hospitalization, and preemptive intubation with ventilatory support should be considered.

If mechanical ventilation is initiated, a "lung protective" strategy should be used (Table 61.6). Lower tidal volumes (6 mL/kg vs. 10–12 mL/kg) and lower plateau pressure goals ($\leq$30 cm H_2O) may decrease barotrauma and ongoing inflammatory lung damage. This low tidal volume strategy improves survival and decreases ventilator-associated complications of sepsis.

FLUID RESUSCITATION

Crystalloid fluids are the intravenous fluids of choice for septic patients. They should be delivered in bolus form (500–1000 mL per dose), targeted to a central venous pressure (CVP) greater than 8 mm Hg, and guided by indices of perfusion, especially urine output. Bicarbonate administration for sepsis-induced lactic acidosis has not been shown to be beneficial and is not recommended.

VASOPRESSORS

Vasopressors should be initiated promptly in patients who have hypoperfusion despite volume resuscitation. All of the vasopressors in Table 61.7 have been shown to be capable of increasing blood pressure in patients with septic shock. Dopamine is used commonly, although putative improved splanchnic blood flow and renal protective effects remain unproven. Norepinephrine is an effective first-line agent because of its predominantly vasoconstrictive effects and may be superior in patients who cannot tolerate the tachycardia and dysrhythmias associated with agents such as dopamine and epinephrine. Initiation of any vasopressor should be viewed as a therapeutic trial. Selection and titration of the agent should be guided by indices of end-organ perfusion.

Table 61.4 Common Laboratory and Radiographic Findings in Sepsis

Study	Finding
Complete blood count	• Leukocytosis >12 K/mm^3 WBC • Leukopenia <4 K/mm^3 WBC • Left shift/bandemia $>10\%$ immature neutrophils
Chemistry panel	• Acidosis • Renal failure • Hypo/hyperglycemia
Coagulation	• Elevated INR • Elevated PTT • DIC
Lactate	• Hyperlactemia (>5 mmol/L with septic shock)
Cultures: blood urine cerebrospinal fluid wound	• May identify infection source • Microbial susceptibilities guide antibiotic treatment • Blood cultures frequently negative*
Urine	• Oliguria • Pyuria/urinary tract infection
Chest Radiograph	• Diffuse bilateral infiltrates, ARDS • Focal infiltrate, pneumonia

*Negative blood cultures in 31% with septic shock.
ARDS, acute respiratory distress syndrome; DIC, disseminated intravascular coagulation; INR, international normalized ratio; PTT, partial thromboplastin time; WBC, white blood (cell) count.

Table 61.5 Hemodynamic Goals of EGDT

Parameter	Goal	Intervention
1. CVP	8–12 mm Hg	Infuse intravenous bolus either crystalloid or colloid for CVP <8 mm Hg
2. MAP	65–90 mm Hg	Initiate pressors for MAP <65 mm Hg
3. ScvO$_2$ Central Venous Oxygen Saturation	$>70\%$	Transfuse packed cells to HCT above 30 and initiate inotropic agents for ScvO$_2$ $<70\%$

CVP, central venous pressure; HCT, hematocrit; MAP, mean arterial pressure.

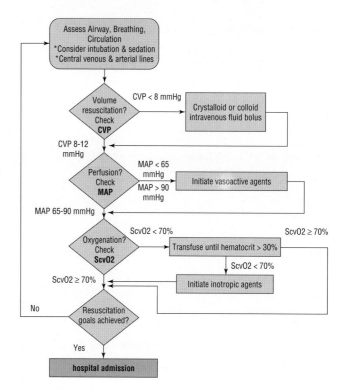

Figure 61.1 Early goal-directed therapy algorithm. Adapted from Rivers et al. (2001).

Table 61.6 Ventilation Parameters

	Traditional	Lung Protective
Ventilator Mode	Volume assist-control	Volume assist-control
Initial Tidal Volume	12 mL/kg	6 mL/kg
Plateau Pressure	≤50 cm H$_2$O	≤30 cm H$_2$O
Rate Settings	6–35 breaths/min	6–35 breaths/min
Inspiratory: Expiratory Ratio	1:1 to 1:3	1:1 to 1:3
Oxygenation Goal	PaO$_2$ 55–88 mm Hg SpO$_2$ 88–95%	PaO$_2$ 55–88 mm Hg SpO$_2$ 88–95%

bial sensitivities, broad-spectrum antibiotic coverage of likely pathogens is favored.

ANTIBIOTICS

The ED physician must initiate prompt and appropriate empiric antibiotic coverage. The Surviving Sepsis Campaign guidelines recommend that empiric antibiotics be given within 1 hour of the diagnosis of severe sepsis and that they should be active against likely pathogens with adequate penetration into presumed sites of infection (Table 61.8). ED protocols with standardized regimens of premixed antibiotics for common infection sites can facilitate adherence to these guidelines. The specific choice of antibiotic coverage should be guided by suspected source and community resistance patterns, but in the absence of confirmed infections and micro-

PHYSIOLOGIC STEROID THERAPY FOR RELATIVE ADRENAL INSUFFICIENCY

Three randomized controlled trials of patients with refractory (vasopressor requiring) septic shock demonstrated marked shock reversal with corticosteroid infusions. One of these studies also showed a remarkable decrease in mortality. Thus, for patients with persistent septic shock despite pressors and fluid resuscitation, administration of hydrocortisone 100 mg every 8 hours for 7 days is recommended. The practice of testing for relative adrenal insufficiency by performing a cosyntropin stimulation test or a random pretreatment cortisol level remains controversial.

Table 61.7 Common Vasopressors in Septic Shock

Agent	Action	Dosage Range
Norepinephrine	Alpha and beta	1–30 µg/min
Dopamine	Beta Alpha Dopamine	6–25 µg/kg/min
Phenylephrine	Alpha	40–180 µg/min
Epinephrine	Beta, alpha	1–10 µg/min
Vasopressin	V1	0.01–0.04 units/min

Table 61.8 Common Empiric Antibiotic Regimens for Severe Sepsis

Class	Example
Extended-spectrum penicillin	piperacillin-tazobactam 3.375 g IV q6h
Carbapenem	imipenem-cilastin 500 mg IV q6–8h
Third- or fourth-generation cephalosporin	cefepime 1–2 g IV/IM q8–12h
Beta-lactam plus anti-pseudomonal aminoglycoside	ceftriaxone 1 g q24h *plus* gentamicin* 5 mg/kg q24h
Beta-lactam allergic	vancomycin 1 g IV q12h *plus* ciprofloxacin 400 mg IV q12h
Anti-MRSA agent[†]	vancomycin 1 g IV q12h
Antifungal agent[‡]	caspofungin 70 mg IV loading dose × 1, then 50 mg IV q24h maintenance dose

*Contraindicated in renal failure.
[†]Recommended in most U.S. communities, where prevalence of MRSA is high.
[‡]Recommended if patient at high risk for invasive candidiasis because of risk factors such as immunocompromise, recent surgery, indwelling catheters or devices, diabetes, parenteral nutrition, or recent broad-spectrum antibiotic use.
MRSA, methicillin-resistant *Staphylococcus aureus*.

ACTIVATED PROTEIN C

The hyperinflammatory pathophysiology of sepsis led to a multitude of trials aimed at suppressing the inflammation cascade; essentially all reported negative results until a large, randomized, controlled trial of recombinant activated protein C (APC) showed a decrease in mortality. APC functions in shock because of its fibrinolytic and anti-inflammatory properties. However, APC therapy benefits only those with overt septic shock, acute respiratory distress syndrome (ARDS), multiple organ failure, or Acute Physiology and Chronic Health Evaluation (APACHE) II scores above 25. The primary adverse event seen with APC is bleeding that usually resolves with discontinuation of the infusion.

EUGLYCEMIA

Glucose control also improves outcome in sepsis. In diabetic patients, the increased metabolic demands of infection can cause both hyper- and hypoglycemia. However, even in the non-diabetic patient, glucose control by insulin drips titrated to 80–110 µg/dL decreases mortality. The mechanism for this benefit may be related to antiapoptotic effects of insulin, as well as the impaired phagocytosis in hyperglycemia.

Table 61.9 Acute Respiratory Distress Syndrome Criteria

Acute onset
Bilateral infiltrates on chest radiography
Pulmonary capillary wedge pressure <18 or absence of clinical evidence for left atrial hypertension
Acute lung injury (ALI) is characterized by PaO_2/FiO_2 of $\leq$300 mm Hg
ARDS is characterized by PaO_2/FiO_2 $\leq$200

COMPLICATIONS AND ADMISSION CRITERIA

All patients with severe sepsis should be admitted to an intensive care unit (ICU). In addition to early resuscitation, septic patients require continuous monitoring for the development of end-organ complications.

Acute Respiratory Distress Syndrome

The most common of the organ dysfunctions associated with sepsis, ARDS is characterized by persistent arterial hypoxemia despite treatment with supplemental oxygen (Table 61.9). The presence of bilateral pulmonary infiltrates and severe hypoxia (defined as $PaO_2/FiO_2 \leq 200$) in the absence of left atrial hypertension is a currently accepted diagnostic standard for ARDS. Additional features of ARDS include decreased lung compliance and an interstitial, centrally located pattern of opacities.

Although ARDS may be the most evident dysfunction seen in sepsis, it does not confer as grave a prognosis as does failure of other organ systems. Renal failure, central nervous system (CNS) dysfunction, and thrombocytopenia correlate more closely with mortality. This underrecognized point forms part of the basis for current resuscitation protocols in sepsis. Aggressive fluid resuscitation to improve perfusion and prevent renal failure is now favored over cautious fluid support aimed at decreasing pulmonary interstitial fluid.

Myocardial Depression

Severe sepsis may be associated with myocardial depression. Many inflammatory mediators have been implicated and the mechanism remains controversial. Unlike acute coronary syndrome, this dysfunction is not believed to be caused by myocardial hypoperfusion and ischemia. Patients who survive severe sepsis associated with cardiac dysfunction usually regain normal cardiac function in 7–10 days. However, patients with underlying coronary artery disease are at risk for acute ischemia from increased cardiac workload, and sepsis may precipitate myocardial infarction.

Renal Failure

Renal failure in sepsis may acutely manifest as oliguria. In severe sepsis this may reflect decreased renal perfusion due to systemic hypotension. Persistent renal hypoperfusion may result in acute tubular necrosis and renal failure, though, as with sepsis-associated cardiac depression, the majority of survivors recover baseline renal function. This may suggest the involvement of inflammatory mediators in temporarily decreasing kidney function without causing irreversible injury.

INFECTION CONTROL

Universal precautions should be observed in all cases. Contact precautions should be observed if the primary source of infection is due to soft-tissue infections or skin sources. Cases with suspected high-risk pulmonary sources require respiratory precautions as per organism-specific institutional protocols.

PEARLS AND PITFALLS

1. The first goals in sepsis care are early recognition and aggressive resuscitation.
2. In patients with severe sepsis or septic shock of unclear etiology, broad-spectrum antibiotics should be administered as soon as possible.
3. Early aggressive intravenous fluid resuscitation is critical. Titrate fluids to perfusion parameters such as CVP, blood pressure, heart rate, and urine output.
4. Septic shock may induce relative adrenal insufficiency. Consider replacement therapy (hydrocortisone 100 mg IV every eight hours) in cases of refractory hypotension.
5. Intubate early using lung-protective ventilator settings.
6. Do not withhold fluid resuscitation out of concern for possible respiratory compromise.

REFERENCES

Angus DC, Laterre P, Helterbrand J, et al. The effect of drotrecogin alfa (activated) on long term survival after severe sepsis. Crit Care Med 2004;32:2199–206.

Angus DC, Wax RS. Epidemiology of sepsis: An update. Crit Care Med 2001;29:S109–16.

Annane D, Sebille V, Charpentier C, et al. Effect of treatment with low doses of hydrocortisone and fludrocortisone of mortality in patients with septic shock. JAMA 2002;288:862–71.

Bernard GR. Drotrecogin alfa (activated) (recombinant human activated protein C) for the treatment of severe sepsis. Crit Care Med 2003;31:S85–93.

Bochud PY, Bonten M, Marchetti O, et al. Antimicrobial therapy for patients with severe sepsis and septic shock: an evidence-based review. Crit Care Med 2004;32:S495–512.

Centers for Disease Control and Prevention (CDC). Increase in national hospital discharge survey rates for septicemia: United States, 1979–1987. MMWR 1990;39:31–4.

Dellinger RP, Carlet JM, Masur H, et al. Surviving Sepsis Campaign guidelines for management of severe sepsis and septic shock. Crit Care Med 2004;32:858–73.

Forsythe SM, Schmidt GA. Sodium bicarbonate for the treatment of lactic acidosis. Chest 2000;117:260–7.

Hotchkiss RS, Karl IE. The pathophysiology and treatment of sepsis. N Engl J Med 2003;342:138–50.

Krisnagopalan S. Myocardial dysfunction in the patient with sepsis. Curr Opin Crit Care 2002;8:376–88.

Mitchell MM, Fink MP, Marshall JC, et al. 2001 SCCM/ESICM/ACCP/ATS/SIS International Sepsis Definitions Conference. Crit Care Med 2003;31:1250–6.

Rangel-Frausto M, Pittet D, Costigan M, et al. The natural history of the systemic inflammatory response syndrome (SIRS): a prospective study. JAMA 1995;273:117–23.

Rivers E, Nguyen B, Havstad S, et al. Early goal-directed therapy in the treatment of severe sepsis and septic shock. N Engl J Med 2001;345:1368–77.

Santacruz JF, Zavala ED, Arroliga AC. Update in ARDS management: recent randomized controlled trials that changed our practice. Cleve Clin J Med 2006; 217–36.

The Acute Respiratory Distress Syndrome Network. Ventilation with lower tidal volumes as compared with traditional tidal volumes for acute lung injury and the acute respiratory distress syndrome. N Engl J Med 2000;342: 1301–8.

Van den Berghe G, Wilmer A, Milants I, et al. Intensive insulin therapy in mixed medical/surgical intensive care units. Diabetes 2006;55:3151–9.

Ware LB, Matthay MA. The acute respiratory distress syndrome. N Engl J Med 2000;342:1334–49.

ADDITIONAL READINGS

Bernard GR, Wheeler AP, Russell JA, et al. The effects of ibuprofen on the physiology and survival of patients with sepsis. N Engl J Med 1997;336:912–8.

Dellinger RP. Cardiovascular management of septic shock. Crit Care Med 2003;31:946–55.

Vincent JL, Fink MP, Marini JJ, et al. Intensive care and emergency medicine: progress over the last 25 years. Chest 2006;129:1061–7.

62. Sickle Cell Disease

Suzanne Lippert

INTRODUCTION

Sickle cell hemoglobinopathy results from the substitution of a valine for glutamic acid as the sixth amino acid of the beta globin chain. Sickle cell disease (SCD) includes the most severe and most common form, homozygous sickle cell anemia (Hb SS), as well as the heterozygous condition of intermediate severity, S combined with hemoglobin C (Hb SC). Hemoglobin S is also seen in combination with beta thalassemia producing the more severe form, HbS-β^0 thalassemia, and the less severe HbS-β^+ thalassemia. The heterozygous (carrier) form in which hemoglobin S combines with normal hemoglobin A (Hb AS) is usually asymptomatic.

The sickling of erythrocytes that results from the deoxygenation-induced deformation of the hemoglobin S molecule causes erythrostasis, thrombosis, and ultimately infarction in the spleen of affected patients. SCD patients develop early functional asplenia, usually by 2–4 years of age, which leads to susceptibility to encapsulated organisms: *Streptococcus pneumoniae, Haemophilus influenzae, Mycoplasma pneumoniae, Chlamydia pneumoniae*. Prophylactic penicillin, given as 125 mg orally twice a day until 2–3 years of age and 250 mg twice daily until at least 5 years of age, is recommended as prevention against invasive pneumococcal disease.

EPIDEMIOLOGY

According to a World Health Organization report from 2005, "Sickle cell anemia affects millions throughout the world. In the United States, it affects around 72,000 people. The disease occurs in about 1 in every 500 African-American births and 1 in every 1000 to 1400 Hispanic-American births. About 2 million Americans, or 1 in 12 African Americans, carry the sickle cell allele."

Infection is the primary cause of death in sickle cell patients during childhood, while chronic organ failure from vaso-occlusive disease becomes an equally important cause of mortality in adulthood.

Differential Diagnosis

In adult sickle cell patients, it is imperative to consider infectious and noninfectious causes of fever, including:

- vaso-occlusive crisis
- bone infarction
- pulmonary fat embolism
- ischemic cerebrovascular accidents
- hepatic or mesenteric infarction
- infection with encapsulated organisms including bacteremia, pneumonia, meningitis, osteomyelitis, and septic arthritis

History and Physical Examination

The history and physical exam should include a thorough review of systems in an attempt to elicit complaints that might localize the source of fever. In particular, the patient should be explicitly questioned about symptoms characteristic of meningitis or stroke, pneumonia, bone or joint infections, urinary tract infections, cholecystitis or cholangitis, viral hepatitis, and mesenteric ischemia.

Initial Diagnostic Approach

The initial work-up of all SCD adults with nonlocalizing fever includes complete blood count with differential, reticulocyte count, lactate dehydrogenase (LDH), urinalysis, blood and urine cultures, and a chest radiograph (CXR). Further work-up, which may include lumbar puncture (LP), arthrocentesis, and abdominal imaging, is based on signs and symptoms elicited during the history and physical exam as detailed in the subsequent sections on specific infections.

BACTEREMIA AND SEPSIS

Several recent studies have shown bacteremia to be a relatively rare event in SCD adults, on the order of 1.2 episodes per 100 patient-years. Bacteremia in adults is most commonly associated with severe underlying disease and central venous catheters. The most commonly isolated organisms, in contrast to *Streptococcus pneumoniae* in children, are *Staphylococcus aureus* including methicillin-resistant *S. aureus* (MRSA) and coagulase-negative staphylococci, followed by gram-negative bacilli, such as *Escherichia coli* and *Klebsiella*.

Bacteremia in children with SCD is most commonly caused by *S. pneumoniae*; however, with widespread use of daily prophylactic penicillin regimens and the pneumococcal vaccine, the incidence of pneumococcal bacteremia has markedly decreased. Similarly, the incidence of *Haemophilus influenzae* bacteremia, which previously accounted for up to 25% of childhood episodes of SCD bacteremia, has declined since the introduction of the *Haemophilus influenzae* type B (HIB) vaccine.

Clinical Features

Sepsis may present with a myriad of symptoms and signs, most commonly fever or hypothermia, hyperventilation, chills, rigors, diffuse purpuric rash, tachycardia, delirium, decreased urine output, and/or hypotension (Table 62.1).

Table 62.1 Clinical Features: Bacteremia and Sepsis

	Children	Adults
Organisms	• *Streptococcus pneumoniae* • *Haemophilus influenzae* • *Salmonella* • *Escherichia coli, Klebsiella*	Community acquired: • *E. coli, Klebsiella* • *Staphylococcus aureus* • *S. pneumoniae* • *Salmonella* Hospital acquired: • *S. aureus*, including MRSA
Risks and Associations	• Noncompliance with penicillin prophylaxis • Unvaccinated for *Streptococcus pneumoniae* and *Haemophilus influenzae*	• Severe immunosuppression • Venous catheter-associated • High frequency of bone and joint infections
Signs and Symptoms	• Fever or hypothermia • Chills, rigors • Tachycardia, hypotension • Confusion, delirium • Decreased urine output	
Laboratory and Radiographic Tests	• CBC: leukocytosis, left shift • Reticulocyte count: aplastic or hypoproliferative crisis • Blood cultures • CXR to rule out ACS • UA with urine culture • Consider LP • Consider abdominal imaging	
Treatment	ceftriaxone 75 mg/kg/day IV q24h	vancomycin 1 g IV q12h *plus* ceftriaxone 1 g IV q24h *or* (as single agent) levofloxacin 750 mg IV q24h

ACS, acute chest syndrome; CBC, complete blood count; UA, urinalysis.

Differential Diagnosis

Differential diagnosis includes:

- vaso-occlusive crisis
- acute chest syndrome (ACS)
- aplastic crisis secondary to viral infection (parvovirus B19)
- meningitis
- osteomyelitis
- cholecystitis
- intra-abdominal catastrophe (i.e., mesenteric infarction, perforation)

Laboratory and Radiographic Findings

When bacteremia or sepsis is suspected, blood and urine cultures should be sent and a search for the source of infection initiated. The white blood cell count (WBC) is neither sensitive nor specific for serious infection in this setting. Patients with SCD are also at risk of a hypoplastic or aplastic red blood cell (RBC) crisis in the setting of severe infection, manifesting in a low reticulocyte count and dropping hemoglobin levels. Severe sepsis commonly results in increasing lactate levels and, secondary to disseminated intravascular coagulation (DIC), low fibrinogen and prolonged prothrombin time (PT) and partial thromboplastin time (PTT). To ensure that an occult source of bacteremia is not overlooked, at a minimum, urinalysis (UA), urine culture, and chest radiography should be obtained. Lumbar puncture and abdominal ultrasound (US) or computed tomographic (CT) scan should be obtained based on clinical suspicion for meningitis or intra-abdominal pathology, respectively.

Treatment

Because bacteremia in adult SCD patients is associated with venous catheters 41–80% of the time in various studies, immediate removal of central lines should be considered. Initial antibiotic therapy in children with SCD is a parenteral third-generation cephalosporin to cover *S. pneumoniae*. Empiric antibiotics for hospitalized adults or those with venous catheters should cover *S. aureus*, including MRSA, whereas community-acquired bacteremia in SCD adults should initially be treated with antibiotics covering *E. coli*, *S. aureus*, and *S. pneumoniae*. Initial parenteral empiric therapy in adults should begin with vancomycin and ceftriaxone. Levofloxacin may be substituted for ceftriaxone in beta-lactam allergic patients.

PNEUMONIA AND ACUTE CHEST SYNDROME (ACS)

Bacterial pneumonia in sickle cell disease is clinically indistinguishable from ACS, which is defined by a new alveolar consolidation involving at least one complete lung segment and associated with acute respiratory symptoms, fever, or chest pain. ACS results when a precipitating etiology initiates a proinflammatory cascade causing increasingly severe sickling, thrombosis, and lung injury. The trigger may be a combination of infectious causes (bacterial, viral, or mixed infection) and noninfectious causes (pulmonary fat embolism and pulmonary infarction).

The incidence of ACS is age and genotype dependent, with rates of 24.5 events per 100 patient-years in HbSS children ages 2–4 years, decreasing to 8.8 events per 100 patient-years in HbSS adults more than 20 years old. Infection is the most frequent cause of ACS in young children. Vascular occlusion and pulmonary fat embolism are thought to be more frequent causes of ACS in adults because there is less frequent identification of microbial infection and a strong association with bone pain.

Clinical Features

Fever above 38.5°C and cough are the most common presenting symptoms in all age groups, though these are more common in children than in adolescents and adults (Table 62.2). Dyspnea is variably present in all age groups, whereas chest, rib, and extremity pain are more commonly seen in adolescents and adults. On physical exam, children are more likely than adults to exhibit signs of bronchospasm, wheezing, and tachypnea.

Presenting symptoms observed during a patient's first episode of ACS are predictive of symptoms during subsequent events. Nevertheless, clinical assessment alone is unreliable in diagnosing ACS.

Differential Diagnosis

In the Cooperative Study of Sickle Cell Disease (CSSCD) trial, adult patients who were eventually diagnosed with ACS during the same hospitalization most commonly presented with complaints of extremity pain and no evidence of ACS on initial exam. Febrile illness in children and vaso-occlusive pain crises in adults are viewed as precursors to ACS. The differential includes bacterial pneumonia and noninfectious causes of ACS, such as:

- pulmonary fat embolism
- pulmonary infarction
- pulmonary edema
- rib or sternal infarction

Characteristics that may help to distinguish the etiology of ACS:

- Fat embolism syndrome classically presents with a triad of hypoxemia, neurologic abnormalities and a petechial rash.
- Pulmonary infarction usually results from in-situ thrombosis secondary to sickling rather than embolic events; therefore, these patients are no more likely to have identifiable deep venous thrombosis (DVT).
- Positive blood cultures in the setting of ACS should be treated as infectious pneumonia until proven otherwise.

Laboratory and Radiographic Findings

Children younger than 10 years old have a higher frequency of upper and middle lobe disease, whereas adults more often have isolated lower lobe infiltrate or multilobar disease. Pleural effusions are seen in more than half of all episodes of ACS, but occur more frequently in adults. In direct comparison with simultaneous high-resolution CT scan, chest radiograph has been shown to underestimate the degree of pulmonary disease in patients presenting with ACS.

Table 62.2 Clinical Features: Bacterial Pneumonia and ACS

	Age <10	Age >10
Organisms	• Viral: RSV, rhinovirus • *Mycoplasma pneumoniae* • *Clamydophila pneumoniae*	• *C. pneumoniae* • *M. pneumoniae* • *Staphylococcus aureus* • *Streptococcus pneumoniae*
Signs and Symptoms	• Fever >38.5°C • Cough • Bronchospasm, wheezing • Tachypnea • Dyspnea • Hypoxia	• Fever >38.5°C • Cough • Chest pain • Dyspnea • Extremity pain • Hypoxia
Laboratory and Radiographic Findings	• Hb decrease by 0.7 g/dL • WBC increase of 70% • Bacteremia • Secretory phospholipase A₂ dramatically increased • CXR: variable with isolated upper and middle lobe disease with or without pleural effusions	• Hb decrease by 0.7 g/dL • WBC increase of 70% • Secretory phospholipase A₂ dramatically increased • CXR: variable with lower lobe or multilobar disease with or without pleural effusions
Treatment	• Third-generation cephalosporin (cefotaxime 1 g IV q8h or ceftriaxone 2 g IV q24h) *plus* macrolide (azithromycin 500 mg IV q24h or erythromycin). • Add vancomycin (15 mg/kg IV q12h) for large or progressing infiltrates. • Pain control: PCA narcotics, intercostal nerve block • Bronchodilator therapy if reactive airway disease (empiric trial) • Oxygen supplementation • Maintain euvolemia: hypotonic IV fluids at 1.5–2× maintenance • Incentive spirometry • RBC transfusion if respiratory compromise, significant anemia, clinical deterioration	

PCA, patient-controlled analgesia; RSV, respiratory syncytial virus.

At diagnosis, hypoxemia to a mean oxygen saturation of 92% is common. Hemoglobin and white blood cell counts differ markedly from steady-state values. Hemoglobin declines by approximately 0.7 g/dL while white blood cells increase by an average of 70% in ACS. Platelet counts often decrease throughout the course of the illness, with platelets below 200,000/mm³ as a strong predictor of morbidity and mortality. The average forced expiratory volume (FEV) is 53% of the predicted value, with approximately 25% of patients showing improvement with bronchodilators.

Despite the historically low yield, sputum and blood cultures should be obtained. Bronchoalveolar lavage (BAL) is preferred as it provides higher quality specimens for culture and allows examination for the fat-laden macrophages characteristic of pulmonary fat embolism. Serologic studies for *Mycoplasma*, *Chlamydophila*, and parvovirus and, in children especially, nasopharyngeal samples for viral cultures should be obtained.

Treatment

The treatment of ACS should address the causative agent as well as the host response in order to prevent further pulmonary injury and respiratory compromise. Broad-spectrum antibiotics, proper pain management, alleviation of bronchospasm, oxygen therapy, cautious intravenous fluids (IVF) administration, incentive spirometry, transfusion, and, in severe cases, mechanical ventilation are the fundamentals of therapy in ACS.

There is a lack of data on the appropriate use of antibiotics in ACS. Broad-spectrum antibiotics that cover common community-acquired and atypical pathogens, and a macrolide to cover *M. pneumoniae*, are generally given in all patients. Therapy should begin with a third-generation cephalosporin, cefotaxime or ceftriaxone, in conjunction with a macrolide. The CSSD study identified more than 27 unique infectious pathogens as causative agents in ACS; therefore, patients that are rapidly deteriorating should have antibiotic coverage broadened. Local pathogen predominance and sensitivity patterns in community-acquired pneumonia (CAP) should be used to guide initial antibiotic therapy.

Pain management should include patient-controlled analgesia (PCA) and intercostal nerve blocks to minimize narcotic-induced hypoventilation. The use of adrenergic bronchodilators should be attempted in all ACS patients, using caution in adults because of the hypertensive and cardiac effects. Oxygen should be administered in all hypoxic patients and has questionable benefit in other patients presenting with pain. Intravenous fluid administration should be limited to a rate of 1.5–2 times maintenance, in order to avoid pulmonary edema from overly aggressive hydration. A hypotonic solution, one-half normal saline (NS) in adults and one-quarter NS in children, should be considered because the primary goal is hydration of erythrocytes. Incentive spirometry, used at least every 2 hours, is recommended in all patients.

Transfusion therapy is recommended if there is clinical deterioration, multilobar infiltrates, or a history of underlying pulmonary or cardiac disease. Exchange transfusion is preferred, though simple transfusion should be used for patients with significant anemia. Leukocyte-poor packed red blood cells matched for Rh, C, E, and Kell antigens should be used to minimize erythrocyte antibody formation. Mechanical ventilation is indicated for respiratory failure.

OSTEOMYELITIS AND SEPTIC ARTHRITIS

Because of their overall increased susceptibility to bacterial infection and bone infarction, patients with SCD have a greater risk of osteomyelitis than the general population. SCD patients with a history of osteonecrosis were shown to have a 2.5- to 3.8-fold greater risk of developing bone and joint infections after bacteremia. The organisms most commonly isolated in SCD-related osteomyelitis are *Salmonella*, *Staphylococcus aureus*, and, less commonly, aerobic gram-negative rods. Despite this increased risk of infection, however, once patients reach adolescence, vaso-occlusive crisis is up to 50 times more likely than osteomyelitis to be the cause of bone pain. Patients with sickle cell disease are also susceptible to septic arthritis, although it occurs less frequently than osteomyelitis. Septic arthritis is generally caused by the same organisms as osteomyelitis, as well as *Streptococcus pneumo-*

Table 62.3 Clinical Features: Osteomyelitis

Organisms	• *Salmonella* • *Staphylococcus aureus* • Gram-negative enteric bacilli: *Escherichia coli*, *Enterobacter*
Risks and Associations	• Areas of previously infarcted bone
Signs and Symptoms*	• Fever • Localized tenderness and swelling • Limitation of movement of joint (septic arthritis) • Commonly involves femur, tibia, humerus
Laboratory and Radiographic Tests	• ESR elevated • Blood and stool cultures for *Salmonella* • Plain radiographs: nonspecific periostitis and osteopenia, lucent areas characteristic of osteomyelitis appear 10–14 days into the course of the illness • CT, MRI, US: locates area of focus for aspiration and identifies possible presence of abscess • Culture of bone aspirate or biopsy remains the gold standard
Treatment	• IVF • Adults: vancomycin 1g IV q12h *plus* ceftriaxone 2g IV q24h • Children: oxacillin 100–200 mg/kg/day in three to four divided doses *plus* (in areas of high MRSA prevalence) vancomycin 15 mg/kg/dose q8h (target trough level 5–15 mg/L) • Aggressive pain control

*Signs and symptoms are indistinguishable from acute infarction.
ESR, erythrocyte sedimentation rate.

niae, and tends to occur in association with vaso-occlusive crisis.

Clinical Features

Osteomyelitis often presents with fever; persistent and severe bone pain commonly involving the femur, tibia, or humerus; and localized swelling and tenderness over the involved bone (Table 62.3). Septic arthritis usually presents in the setting of a vaso-occlusive crisis, with fever, swelling, and tenderness of a joint, and a dramatically limited range of motion of the involved joint.

Differential Diagnosis

Bone infarction is extremely difficult to distinguish from osteomyelitis because both present with fever, bone pain, and soft-tissue swelling.

Key features that distinguish bone infarction from osteomyelitis include:

* a history of recurrent bone infarction
* multifocal rather than unifocal bone pain

Pain with joint motion raises suspicion for joint involvement and requires an arthrocentesis to rule out septic arthritis. Plain films, although expected to reveal only nonspecific changes, are helpful in excluding pathologic fractures or bone tumors.

Ultrasonography may help diagnose osteomyelitis by demonstrating:

- periosteal elevation
- subperiosteal or intramedullary abscesses
- cortical erosions

Laboratory and Radiographic Findings

In both infarction and osteomyelitis, the complete blood count usually shows leukocytosis, and the erythrocyte sedimentation rate (ESR) is usually elevated. Blood and stool cultures should be obtained because *Salmonella* has been identified as the most prevalent pathogen in osteomyelitis. Plain films may be normal or show the nonspecific periostitis and osteopenia consistent with the early stages of both osteomyelitis and bone infarction. The destructive changes of osteomyelitis, appearing as lucent areas on plain radiographs, do not appear until 10–14 days after onset. CT, MRI, and bone scintigraphy may help in localizing the area of activity and following the course of the disease; however, no single radiographic modality has shown sufficient specificity to differentiate between infarction and osteomyelitis. There is also significant overlap in the US findings characteristic of infarction and infection; nevertheless, US provides an accessible, noninvasive means of evaluating for obvious elements of infection, such as subperiosteal or intramedullary abscesses. Cultures of the blood, stool, and bone aspirate or biopsy remain the gold standard in the diagnosis of osteomyelitis.

In the case of joint involvement, arthrocentesis with synovial fluid analysis for cell count, Gram stain, and culture should be done to rule out septic arthritis.

Treatment

Empiric parenteral antibiotics covering *Salmonella* and *Staphylococcus aureus* should be initiated in the emergency department for any patient with SCD and strongly suspected osteomyelitis. Recommended initial therapy in adults is vancomycin plus ceftriaxone, and in children is oxacillin plus (in areas of high MRSA prevalence) vancomycin. In cases of confirmed osteomyelitis, antibiotic treatment tailored to the specific organism and sensitivities should continue for 4 to 6 weeks. Patients not responsive to antibiotics may require surgical debridement and drainage.

CHOLECYSTITIS AND CHOLANGITIS

Excessive production of bilirubin caused by RBC hemolysis in sickle cell patients often results in pigmented gallstone formation. The incidence of cholelithiasis in sickle cell patients increases with age and corresponds to the rate of hemolysis. One study revealed the prevalence of cholelithiasis to be 58% in HbSS patients aged 10–50 years and 17% in HbSC and sickle-thalassemia patients. This increased propensity to form gallstones increases the risk of cholecystitis and, to a lesser degree, cholangitis, in sickle cell patients.

Differential Diagnosis

Abdominal pain is a common component of vaso-occlusive crisis and is thought to result from infarcts of the mesentery or abdominal viscera. Although the majority of abdominal pain in sickle cell patients remains idiopathic and resolves spontaneously, acute intra-abdominal infection must be excluded in any sickle cell patient presenting with fever and abdominal pain, or new abdominal symptoms.

Abdominal pain in the sickle cell patient has a broad differential, including acute sickle hepatic crisis, hepatic sequestration and infarction, transfusion-related viral hepatitis and iron overload, and disease resulting from pigmented gallstone formation: cholelithiasis, cholecystitis, and cholangitis. Rarely, acute pancreatitis results from biliary obstruction or ischemic pancreatic injury. Acute splenic sequestration, although primarily a complication in infants, can occur in adults and carries a high mortality. Common causes of abdominal pain, including appendicitis, should not be overlooked.

Laboratory and Radiographic Findings

See Chapter 14, Infectious Biliary Diseases, for the standard laboratory and radiographic work-up. Additional laboratory tests for SCD patients include reticulocyte count, LDH, UA, and blood and urine cultures.

COMPLICATIONS AND ADMISSION CRITERIA

Adult SCD patients with a history of osteonecrosis were shown to have a 2.5- to 3.8-fold greater risk of developing bone and joint infections 1–6 months after suffering a *S. aureus* bacteremia. SCD patients suspected of having bacteremia should be admitted to the hospital for broad-spectrum parenteral antibiotics. Patients exhibiting signs of sepsis should be treated with goal-directed therapy and admitted to the intensive care unit (ICU).

Adults with SCD who are diagnosed with ACS are more likely than children to have complications such as respiratory failure and neurologic complications, as well as prolonged hospital stays and death. Mortality was 4- to 9-fold greater in adults older than 20 years. Neurologic complications increased with age and included coma, seizures, anoxic brain injury, and stroke. Febrile illness in children and vaso-occlusive pain crises in adults are viewed as precursors to ACS; therefore, all patients presenting with fever and pain crisis should undergo chest radiography, and patients who exhibit any of the signs or symptoms of ACS should be admitted for serial CXR exams. Febrile sickle cell patients with severe, persistent musculoskeletal pain should be admitted for diagnostic work-up of osteomyelitis.

PEARLS AND PITFALLS

1. Adults with SCD are asplenic and at high risk of fulminant sepsis from encapsulated bacteria.
2. Sepsis is more common in SCD children than adults.
3. Initiate a thorough search for a source of bacteremia.
4. Rapidly institute broad-spectrum antibiotics for all SCD patients with bacteremia, and goal-directed therapy for septic patients.
5. ACS results from infectious and noninfectious causes.
6. ACS in adults is commonly characterized by extremity pain.
7. Platelet count below 200,000/mm^3 is a strong predictor of morbidity and mortality.

8. Febrile illness in children and vaso-occlusive pain crises in adults may be precursors to ACS.
9. Pulmonary infarction usually results from in-situ thrombosis secondary to sickling rather than embolic events; therefore, these patients do not have an increased prevalence of identifiable DVT.
10. Bone infarction and osteomyelitis are extremely difficult to distinguish.
11. Routine laboratory work, plain radiographs, and even CT, MRI, and US are unlikely to help distinguish bone infarction from osteomyelitis.
12. A diagnosis of osteomyelitis is supported by stool and blood cultures positive for *Salmonella*.
13. A diagnosis of bone infarction is supported by a history of recurrent infarction and multifocal bone pain.
14. Perform arthrocentesis and admit all patients with suspected joint involvement.
15. For any patient with strongly suspected osteomyelitis and intractable pain, admission, parental antibiotics, and cultures of bone aspirate are essential.
16. Because of the broad differential in SCD, febrile patients with abdominal complaints will likely need to undergo abdominal CT scan.

REFERENCES

Ahmed S, Shahid RK, Russo LA. Unusual causes of abdominal pain: sickle cell anemia. Best Pract Res Clin Gastroenterol 2005;19(2):297–310.

Almeida A, Roberts I. Bone involvement in sickle cell disease. Br J Haematol 2005;129(4):482–90.

Ashley-Koch A, Yang Q, Olney RS. Sickle Hemoglobin (HbS) allele and sickle cell disease: A HuGE REview. Am J Epidemiol 2000;151(9):839–45.

Bond LR, Hatty SR, Horn ME, et al. Gall stones in sickle cell disease in the United Kingdom. Br Med J (Clin Res Ed) 1987;295(6592):234–6.

Burnett MW, Bass JW, Cook BA. Etiology of osteomyelitis complicating sickle cell disease. Pediatrics 1998;101(2):296–7.

Castro O, Brambilla DJ, Thorington B, et al. The acute chest syndrome in sickle cell disease: incidence and risk factors. The Cooperative Study of Sickle Cell Disease. Blood 1994;84(2):643–9.

Chulamokha L, Scholand SJ, Riggio JM, et al. Bloodstream infections in hospitalized adults with sickle cell disease: a retrospective analysis. Am J Hematol 2006;81(10):723–8.

Johnson CS. The acute chest syndrome. Hematol Oncol Clin North Am 2005;19(5):857–79.

Leikin SL, Gallagher D, Kinney TR, et al. Mortality in children and adolescents with sickle cell disease. Cooperative Study of Sickle Cell Disease. Pediatrics 1989;84(3):500–8.

Lottenberg R, Hassell KL. An evidence-based approach to the treatment of adults with sickle cell disease. Hematology 2005;2005(1):58–65.

Morris C, Vichinsky E, Styles L. Clinician assessment for acute chest syndrome in febrile patients with sickle cell disease: is it accurate enough? Ann Emerg Med 1999;34(1):64–9.

Piehl FC, Davis RJ, Prugh SI. Osteomyelitis in sickle cell disease. J Pediatr Orthop 1993;13(2):225–7.

Vichinsky EP, Neumayr LD, Earles AN, et al. Causes and outcomes of the acute chest syndrome in sickle cell disease. National Acute Chest Syndrome Study Group. N Engl J Med 2000;342(25):1855–65.

Vichinsky EP, Styles LA, Colangelo LH, et al. Acute chest syndrome in sickle cell disease: clinical presentation and course. Cooperative Study of Sickle Cell Disease. Blood 1997;89(5):1787–92.

William RR, Hussein SS, Jeans WD, et al. A prospective study of soft-tissue ultrasonography in sickle cell disease patients with suspected osteomyelitis. Clin Radiol 2000;55(4):307–10.

Wong AL, Sakamoto KM, Johnson EE. Differentiating osteomyelitis from bone infarction in sickle cell disease. Pediatr Emerg Care 2001;17(1):60–3.

Wong WY, Powars DR, Chan L, et al. Polysaccharide encapsulated bacterial infection in sickle cell anemia: a thirty year epidemiologic experience. Am J Hematol 1992;39(3):176–82.

Zarrouk V, Habibi A, Zahar JR, et al. Bloodstream infection in adults with sickle cell disease: association with venous catheters, *Staphylococcus aureus*, and bone-joint infections. Medicine (Baltimore) 2006;85(1):43–8.

ADDITIONAL READINGS

Alexander N, Higgs D, Dover G, Serjeant GR. Are there clinical phenotypes of homozygous sickle cell disease? Br J Haematol 2004;126(4):606–11.

Bunn HF. Pathogenesis and treatment of sickle cell disease. N Engl J Med 1997;337(11):762–9.

Neumayr L, Lennette E, Kelly D, et al. Mycoplasma disease and acute chest syndrome in sickle cell disease. Pediatrics 2003;112(1 Pt 1):87–95.

Styles LA, Aarsman AJ, Vichinsky EP, Kuypers FA. Secretory phospholipase A(2) predicts impending acute chest syndrome in sickle cell disease. Blood 2000;96(9):3276–8.

63. Tetanus

Heather K. DeVore and Fredrick M. Abrahamian

INTRODUCTION

Clostridium tetani is an obligatory anaerobic spore-forming microorganism. Spore germination and proliferation occurs in environments with low oxygen tension (e.g., necrotic tissue, frostbite, crush injuries). The two main toxins released by *C. tetani* are tetanospasmin and tetanolysin. Tetanospasmin, also known as tetanus toxin, is the neurotoxin that is responsible for the clinical manifestations of tetanus. It enters the nervous system through the neuromuscular junctions of alpha motor neurons. Tetanospasmin travels to the motor neuron body by retrograde axonal transport and then spreads transsynaptically to other neurons preventing the release of inhibitory neurotransmitters such as glycine and gamma-aminobutyric acid (GABA). Uninhibited motor neuron firing results in sustained muscular contractions and rigidity. Tetanolysin damages cell membranes and lowers the oxygen content of tissue, providing a favorable environment for proliferation of the organism.

EPIDEMIOLOGY

Tetanus is rare in the developed world, but remains widespread in developing countries. Large-scale immunization protocols, especially for infants and school-aged children, have significantly reduced the number of cases worldwide. Other factors such as availability of tetanus immunoglobulin, improved wound care management and childbirth practices, and advances in supportive care and airway management have also resulted in a decline in tetanus-associated morbidity and mortality.

Neonatal tetanus accounts for the majority of cases worldwide. However, in the United States, tetanus occurs primarily in adults, with the majority of cases reported in older adults and injection drug users (IDUs).

Other at-risk populations include immigrants from outside North America or Western Europe and persons lacking a formal education past grade school.

CLINICAL FEATURES

Clinically, tetanus is classified into generalized, neonatal, local, and cephalic tetanus.

Generalized tetanus, the most common form of the disease, results from the hematogenous spread of the toxin to myoneural junctions throughout the body (Table 63.1). A common symptom at presentation is trismus or "lockjaw," which is due to masseter muscle contraction and rigidity. Other initial symptoms can include dysphagia and neck, back, and shoulder pain and stiffness. As the disease progresses, patients develop generalized muscle rigidity and spasms, which may occur spontaneously or be precipitated by some external stimulus such as touch, light, or noise. A sardonic smile (risus sardonicus) occurs from sustained contraction and rigidity of facial muscles. Opisthotonos, where the head and feet are drawn backward and the spine arches forward, is another classical finding. Elevated levels of catecholamines lead to a hypersympathetic state and autonomic dysfunction. This typically occurs around the second week of the disease

Table 63.1 Clinical Features: Generalized Tetanus

Organisms	*Clostridium tetani*
Incubation Period	Variable (3–21 days); majority of cases occur within 14 days.
Signs and Symptoms	Trismus, dysphagia, neck, back, and shoulder pain and stiffness, risus sardonicus, opisthotonos
Laboratory Findings	There are no specific laboratory findings that can reliably make the diagnosis of tetanus.
Treatment	• Stabilization of the airway • Aggressive control and management of muscle spasms and rigidity with benzodiazepines • Passive immunization with human tetanus immune-globulin, 500 units IM • Active immunization with age-specific tetanus toxoid–containing vaccine • Antibiotics (metronidazole 1 g IV every 12 hours) • Control of autonomic instability • General wound care (e.g., debridement, incision and drainage of abscesses) and supportive measures

with clinical manifestations including fever, blood pressure extremes, and cardiac arrhythmias.

Neonatal tetanus occurs in newborns of mothers who are unvaccinated or inadequately vaccinated for tetanus. The most common source of infection is the umbilical stump, through either contamination from nonsterile delivery or improper umbilical cord care practices. Clinical manifestations occur within 10 days of birth and include generalized weakness, inability to suck, and irritability. The mortality rate is high, and survivors are often afflicted with mental and growth retardation.

Local tetanus manifests with rigidity and muscular spasms around the inciting wound and has the potential to become generalized. Affected muscles are painful at rest and during contractions, and deep tendon reflexes are pronounced. These symptoms may persist for weeks to months. Local tetanus has a better prognosis than other forms of tetanus.

Cephalic tetanus is a specific type of local tetanus that affects the cranial nerves. It is usually associated with ear infections or traumatic head wounds. The initial presentation typically includes trismus and cranial nerve palsy, most commonly of the facial nerve. Cephalic tetanus is considered a severe form of tetanus because of its potential for rapid progression to the generalized form.

DIFFERENTIAL DIAGNOSIS

Other conditions to consider include:

- generalized convulsive seizures
- extrapyramidal reaction
- hypocalcemic tetany
- hyperventilation syndrome
- black widow spider bite
- strychnine poisoning
- drug withdrawal
- peritonitis
- temporomandibular joint dislocation
- rabies
- progressive fluctuating muscular rigidity (stiff-man syndrome)
- conversion reaction

Key features that may help to distinguish tetanus are:

- generalized muscle rigidity and spasms precipitated by some external stimulus such as touch, light, or noise
- history of wound or injection drug use
- development of trismus, risus sardonicus, or opisthotonos

LABORATORY DIAGNOSIS

There are no specific laboratory findings that can reliably make the diagnosis of tetanus. C. tetani is rarely isolated from wounds, and as a result, the diagnosis does not depend on bacterial confirmation. Even with isolation of the organism, routine bacteriologic studies cannot determine whether that strain possesses the plasmid required for tetanospasmin production.

The tetanus toxoid antibody titer is potentially helpful in assessing susceptibility of a patient, but is not diagnostic.

There have been case reports of tetanus occurring in individuals with high serum tetanus antibody titers that are assumed to be in the "protective" range.

Electromyographic studies may be helpful in documenting denervation and lack of intraspinal inhibition, and for tracking the progress of reinnervation in individual patients.

TREATMENT

All patients with tetanus should initially be managed in an intensive care unit. Stabilization and control of the airway should be a priority, and the patient should be intubated at the first sign of airway compromise. Environmental triggers should be minimized by creating a dark, quiet room, and limiting procedures and patient manipulation.

Muscle spasms and rigidity are controlled with benzodiazepines. In addition, benzodiazepines also provide sedative, amnestic, and anxiolytic effects. Patients typically require large doses of intravenous (IV) benzodiazepines to achieve control of the muscle spasms. At these high doses, there have been reports of patients developing metabolic acidosis secondary to the accumulation of propylene glycol, a solvent vehicle. To avoid this complication, a constant infusion of midazolam, a water-soluble agent that does not contain propylene glycol, is recommended. Other drugs, such as propofol, intrathecal baclofen, dantrolene, magnesium, chlorpromazine, and barbiturates, have also been used to treat tetanus-induced muscle spasms. When muscle spasms are refractory to the above-mentioned medications, prolonged neuromuscular blockade is recommended to prevent rhabdomyolysis. Nondepolarizing neuromuscular blocking agents (e.g., vecuronium or pancuronium) are preferred because of their minimal cardiovascular effects. Benzodiazepines should be continued alongside neuromuscular blockade to ensure adequate sedation.

Human tetanus immune globulin (HTIG) passively immunizes patients by neutralizing unbound circulating tetanospasmin. In adults, HTIG should be administered intramuscularly (IM) into the deltoid muscle, and in infants and children into the anterolateral aspect of the upper thigh muscles. HTIG should be given on the opposite side from the tetanus toxoid. Muscle spasms should be controlled prior to the administration of HTIG, because IM injections may precipitate additional spasms. The recommended dosage of HTIG for the *treatment of active tetanus* ranges from 250 to 500 units with no definitive consensus on an optimal dose. HTIG does not cross the blood-brain barrier and has no effect on intraneural bound toxin. There is no advantage of directly injecting HTIG into the wound, and because of its long half-life (~23 days) there is no need for repeated injections. Weight adjusting the dose is also not necessary, as the amount of toxin produced in the body is independent of the patient's body mass. Dosage adjustments are not necessary in patients with renal failure. HTIG may be administered to pregnant patients when indicated (Pregnancy Category C).

Active immunization with tetanus toxoid containing vaccine is also necessary because the disease does not confer immunity. The first two doses are given 4–6 weeks apart, and the third dose is given 6–12 months after the second dose. Tetanus toxoid should not be administered in the same syringe or at the same site as HTIG.

Local wound care (e.g., debridement, incision and drainage of abscesses, removal of foreign bodies) and antibiotics are routinely given in an attempt to eliminate the source of toxin production. It is essential that HTIG be given prior to wound manipulation and antibiotic administration because these interventions have the potential to release additional free toxin into the bloodstream. Recommended antibiotics include metronidazole (1 g IV every 12 hours), penicillin G (24 million units per day in divided doses), or doxycycline (100 mg IV every 12 hours) for 7–10 days. Penicillin is not preferred by some authorities because of its centrally acting GABA antagonist activity and the potential to amplify the effects of tetanospasmin.

Autonomic instability may result in hemodynamic failure and unexpected cardiac arrest. There is no consensus as to a drug of choice for the sympathetic overactivity associated with tetanus. In hypertensive crisis, esmolol is preferred by some authorities because of its short duration of action. Bradydysrhythmias are less common and may require cardiac pacing.

COMPLICATIONS

A shorter incubation period (<7 days), treatment delay greater than 24 hours, and early signs suggestive of autonomic dysfunction are factors commonly associated with poor prognosis. The incubation period is defined as the time from initial injury to the first symptom (e.g., trismus). It has a variable range from a few days to weeks with the majority of cases occurring within 14 days. Tetanus associated with wound types such as burns, surgical procedures, umbilical stump infections, and septic abortions also carries a poor prognosis.

Hemodynamic failure may result from poorly controlled autonomic instability and nosocomial infections. Currently these are the leading causes of mortality associated with tetanus. Respiratory failure used to be the leading cause of death before the ability to paralyze and mechanically ventilate patients, but is now less common. However, several respiratory complications still contribute to the morbidity and mortality of the disease (e.g., aspiration, pneumonia, acute respiratory distress syndrome). Prolonged muscle spasms may lead to rhabdomyolysis and subsequent hyperkalemia and renal failure.

POSTEXPOSURE PROPHYLAXIS

Postexposure prophylaxis is based on the wound type and the patient's vaccination history (Table 63.2). Wounds are classified as either low- or high-risk for tetanus. Clean, superficial (≤1 cm in depth), minor, acute (≤6 hours) wounds are considered to be at low risk for harboring *C. tetani*. High-risk wounds for tetanus, although not limited, include deep wounds (>1 cm in depth); puncture wounds; wounds contaminated with dirt, feces, soil, and saliva; and wounds associated with missiles, avulsions, crush injuries, devitalized or necrotic tissue, burns, and frostbite.

There are two important points to consider in the patient's vaccination history. First is whether or not the patient has received a primary immunization series, which consists of at least three doses of tetanus toxoid-containing vaccine. The second is the time elapsed from the last tetanus booster to possible exposure. Many people do not recall whether they have completed a primary series of tetanus immunization. All individuals who have served in the military or who went to

Table 63.2 Current Summary Guide to Tetanus Prophylaxis in Routine Wound Management

History of Adsorbed Tetanus Toxoid (Doses)	Clean, Minor Wounds		All Other Wounds*	
	Tdap or Td† (0.5 mL IM)	TIG (250 units IM)	Tdap or Td† (0.5 mL IM)	TIG (250 units IM)
Unknown or <3	Yes	No	Yes	Yes
Three or more	No‡	No	No§	No

*Such as, but not limited to, wounds contaminated with dirt, feces, soil, or saliva; puncture wounds; avulsions; and wounds resulting from missiles, crushing, burns, or frostbite.

†Tdap is preferred to Td for adolescents aged 11–18 years and adults aged 19–64 years who have never received Tdap. The preferred tetanus toxoid-containing vaccine for children aged <7 years is the pediatric diphtheria and tetanus toxoids and acellular pertussis vaccines (DTaP). Minimum age for DTaP administration is 6 weeks and maximum age is 6 years.

‡Yes, if ≥10 years have elapsed since the last tetanus toxoid-containing vaccine dose.

§Yes, if ≥5 years have elapsed since the last tetanus toxoid-containing vaccine dose.

Tdap, Tetanus-diphtheria-acellular pertussis vaccine adsorbed formulated for use in adolescents and adults ≤ 64 years of age (Boostrix approved for use in persons aged 10–18 years; Adacel approved for use in persons aged 11–64 years); Td, Adult diphtheria-tetanus vaccine adsorbed (minimum age: 7 years); TIG, tetanus immunoglobulin.

elementary school in North America or Western Europe after 1950 are most likely to have received their primary immunization series. Conversely, immigrants from outside North America or Western Europe, and immigrants or older persons uneducated beyond elementary school are more likely to lack the tetanus primary immunization series.

Primary immunization should begin in infancy with IM injections of diphtheria-tetanus-acellular pertussis vaccine adsorbed (DTaP) at 2, 4, and 6 months of age. The first and second boosters with DTaP should occur at 15–18 months and 4–6 years of age, respectively. The next tetanus booster is recommended at age 11–12 years with Tdap (tetanus-diphtheria-acellular pertussis vaccine adsorbed formulated for use in adolescents and adults ≤64 years of age). Subsequent routine vaccinations are recommended with Td (adult tetanus and diphtheria toxoids vaccine adsorbed) every 10 years. For adults aged 19–64 years who require tetanus toxoid-containing vaccine, a single dose of Tdap is preferred to Td if they have not previously received Tdap. Adults older than 65 years should not receive Tdap, and Td is the recommended tetanus toxoid-containing vaccine within this age group. The most current recommended immunization schedule can be obtained through the Centers for Disease Control and Prevention National Immunization Program website at http://www.cdc.gov/vaccines.

Additional important vaccination history includes the time elapsed between the last tetanus booster and possible exposure. For low-risk tetanus wounds, it is recommended that a patient receive tetanus prophylaxis if it has been 10 or more years since the last tetanus toxoid-containing vaccine dose. This time span decreases to 5 years when a high-risk wound is involved.

Postexposure prophylaxis with HTIG is recommended for patients with high-risk wounds who have missed their primary immunization series (i.e., history of <3 doses of adsorbed tetanus toxoid-containing vaccine) or for patients who are unaware of their vaccination history. The dose for *postexposure prophylaxis* is 250 units IM into the deltoid muscle or anterolateral aspect of the upper thigh muscles (preferred site for infants and small children). HTIG will provide adequate antitoxin levels from 2 days to 4 weeks following administration.

Immunosuppressed individuals may receive tetanus toxoid, although there is some question as to whether these patients mount an adequate immunologic response to the vaccine.

Both Td and Tdap are categorized as Pregnancy Category C, though because of a lack of safety data, Tdap is not recommended for administration in pregnant patients.

There is no evidence that Td is teratogenic, and it is the recommended tetanus toxoid-containing vaccine in pregnant patients (preferred to be given during the second or third trimester of pregnancy). Both Td and Tdap are acceptable for administration during breastfeeding.

INFECTION CONTROL

Standard contact precautions are adequate for the care of patients with tetanus. These patients do not require isolation.

PEARLS AND PITFALLS

1. Populations at higher risk for developing tetanus in the United States include elderly, immigrants, IDUs, persons uneducated beyond grade school, and those with inadequate vaccination history.
2. A patient's tetanus vaccination history should include whether or not the patient has received a primary immunization series and the time elapsed from the last tetanus booster to possible exposure.
3. Postexposure prophylaxis is based on the wound type and the patient's vaccination history.
4. For low-risk tetanus wounds, it is recommended that a patient receive tetanus prophylaxis if it has been 10 or more years since the last tetanus toxoid-containing vaccine dose. This time span decreases to 5 years when a high-risk tetanus wound is involved.
5. For adults aged 19–64 years who require tetanus toxoid-containing vaccine, a single dose of Tdap is preferred to Td if they have not previously received Tdap.
6. To reduce the potential for precipitating muscle spasms and rigidity, it is best to place patients in rooms that are quiet, to limit procedures, and to minimize patient manipulation.

REFERENCES

Abrahamian FM. Management of tetanus: a review. Curr Treat Options Infect Dis 2001;3:209–16.

Abrahamian FM, Pollack CV, LoVecchio F, et al. Fatal tetanus in a drug abuser with "protective" antitetanus antibodies. J Emerg Med 2000;18:189–93.

Centers for Disease Control and Prevention (CDC). Diphtheria, tetanus, and pertussis: recommendations for vaccine use and other preventive measures. MMWR 1991;40(RR-10):1–28.

Centers for Disease Control and Prevention (CDC). Recommended adult immunization schedule – U.S., October 2006–September 2007. MMWR 2006;55(40):1–4.

Centers for Disease Control and Prevention (CDC). Recommended immunization schedules for persons aged 0–18 years – U.S., 2007. MMWR 2007;55(51&52):1–4.

Centers for Disease Control and Prevention (CDC). Update on adult immunization – recommendations of the Immunization Practices Advisory Committee (ACIP). MMWR 1991;40(RR-12):1–94.

Centers for Disease Control and Prevention (CDC). Update: vaccine side effects, adverse reactions, contraindications, and precautions. MMWR 1996;45(RR-12):1–35.

Cook TM, Protheroe RT, Handel JM. Tetanus: a review of the literature. Br J Anaesth 2001;87:477–87.

Ernst ME, Klepser ME, Fouts M, et al. Tetanus: pathophysiology and management. Ann Pharmacother 1997;31:1507–13.

Gergen PJ, McQuillan GM, Kiely M, et al. A population-based serologic survey of immunity to tetanus in the United States. N Engl J Med 1995;332:761–6.

Hsu SS, Groleau G. Tetanus in the emergency department: a current review. J Emerg Med 2001;20:357–65.

Santos ML, Mota-Miranda A, Alves-Pereira A, et al. Intrathecal baclofen for the treatment of tetanus. Clin Infect Dis 2004;38:321–8.

Trujillo MH, Castillo A, Espana J, et al. Impact of intensive care management on the prognosis of tetanus. Chest 1987;92:63–5.

ADDITIONAL READINGS

Abrahamian FM. Tetanus: an update on an ancient disease. Infect Dis Clin Pract 2000;9:228–35.

Attygalle D, Rodrigo N. New trends in the management of tetanus. Expert Rev Anti-Infect Ther 2004;2:73–84.

Centers for Disease Control and Prevention (CDC). Preventing tetanus, diphtheria, and pertussis among adults: use of tetanus toxoid, reduced diphtheria toxoid and acellular pertussis vaccine. MMWR 2006;55(RR-17):1–37.

Centers for Disease Control and Prevention (CDC). Preventing tetanus, diphtheria, and pertussis among adolescents: use of tetanus toxoid, reduced diphtheria toxoid and acellular pertussis vaccine. MMWR 2006;55(early release):1–43.

Talan DA, Abrahamian FM, Moran GJ, et al. Tetanus immunity and physician compliance with tetanus prophylaxis practices among emergency department patients presenting with wounds. Ann Emerg Med 2004;43:305–14.

PART IV

Current Topics

64. Anthrax

David M. Stier, Jennifer C. Hunter, Olivia Bruch, and Karen A. Holbrook

INTRODUCTION

Anthrax is an acute infection caused by *Bacillus anthracis*, a large, gram-positive, spore-forming, aerobic, encapsulated, rod-shaped bacterium. Spores germinate and form bacteria in nutrient-rich environments, whereas bacteria form spores in nutrient-poor environments. The anthrax bacillus produces high levels of two toxins: Edema toxin causes massive edema at the site of germination, and lethal toxin leads to sepsis. Severity of anthrax disease depends on the route of infection and the presence of complications, with case fatality ranging from 5% to 95% if untreated.

The Working Group for Civilian Biodefense considers *B. anthracis* to be one of the most serious biological threats. Anthrax has been weaponized and used. It can be fairly easily disseminated and causes illness and death. Of the ways that *B. anthracis* could potentially be used as a biological weapon, an aerosol release would be expected to have the most severe medical and public health outcomes.

EPIDEMIOLOGY

Anthrax as a Biological Weapon

Anthrax was successfully used as a biological weapon in the United States in October 2001. Cases resulted from direct or indirect exposure to mail that was deliberately contaminated with anthrax spores. In total, 22 cases were identified, 11 with inhalational (five fatal) and 11 with cutaneous anthrax (seven confirmed, four suspected).

Several countries, including the United States, have had anthrax weaponization programs in the past. In 1979 an outbreak of anthrax in the Soviet Union resulted from accidental release of anthrax spores from a facility producing weaponized anthrax. Of 77 reported human cases, all but two were inhalational, and there was an 86% fatality rate.

Experts believe that an aerosol release of weapons-grade spores is the most likely mechanism for use of anthrax as a biological weapon in the future. Anthrax spores could also be used to deliberately contaminate food and water. Spores remain stable in water for several days and are not destroyed by pasteurization.

Disease caused by an intentional release of anthrax may have the following characteristics:

- Multiple similarly presenting cases *clustered in time*:
  Severe acute febrile illness or febrile death
  Severe sepsis not due to predisposing illness
  Respiratory failure with a widened mediastinum on CXR
- Atypical host characteristics: unexpected, unexplained cases of acute illness in previously healthy persons who rapidly develop a progressive respiratory illness
- Multiple similarly presenting cases *clustered geographically*: Acute febrile illness in persons who were in close proximity to a deliberate release of anthrax
- Absence of risk factors: patients lack anthrax exposure risk factors (e.g., veterinary or other animal handling work, meat processing, work that involves animal hides, hair, or bones, or agricultural work in areas with endemic anthrax)

Intentionally released anthrax spores may be altered for more efficient aerosolization and lethality (e.g., highly concentrated, treated to reduce clumping and reduce particle size, genetically modified to increase virulence, resist antimicrobials and reduce vaccine efficacy).

Naturally Occurring Anthrax

RESERVOIR

The natural reservoir for *B. anthracis* is soil, and the predominant hosts are herbivores (e.g., cattle, sheep, goats, horses, pigs, and others) that acquire infection from consuming contaminated soil or feed. Anthrax spores can persist in soil for years and are resistant to drying, heat, ultraviolet light, gamma radiation, and some disinfectants. Anthrax in animals is endemic in many areas of the world and anthrax outbreaks in animals occur sporadically in the United States.

MODE OF TRANSMISSION

Anthrax is generally a zoonotic disease. Humans become infected through contact with infected animals and animal products through several mechanisms:

- contact with infected animal tissues (e.g., veterinarians, animal handlers, meat processors, and other processes that involve animal hides, hair, and bones) or contaminated soil
- ingestion of contaminated, undercooked meat from infected animals
- inhalation of infectious aerosols (e.g., those generated during processing of animal products, such as tanning hides, processing wool or bone)

Person-to-person transmission of *B. anthracis* does not occur with gastrointestinal (GI) or inhalational anthrax, but has been reported rarely with cutaneous anthrax.

WORLDWIDE OCCURRENCE

Worldwide, approximately 2000 cases are reported annually. Anthrax is more common in developing countries with less rigorous animal disease control programs. Cases of human anthrax are most often reported in South and Central America, Southern and Eastern Europe, Asia, Africa, the Caribbean, and the Middle East. The largest reported outbreak of human anthrax occurred in Zimbabwe (1979–1985), which involved more than 10,000 individuals and was associated with anthrax disease in cattle.

UNITED STATES OCCURRENCE

Naturally occurring anthrax is rare in the United States, with approximately 1–2 cases reported each year. The majority of anthrax cases in the United States are cutaneous and acquired occupationally in workers who come in contact with animals or animal products. Only 19 cases of naturally occurring inhalational anthrax have been reported since 1900, and there have been no confirmed gastrointestinal cases. Recent cases of naturally occurring anthrax include:

- In 2007, two people in Connecticut acquired cutaneous anthrax after exposure to untanned animal hides.
- In 2006, a New York City resident contracted inhalational anthrax while making drums from goat hides imported from Africa. The untanned hides were contaminated with anthrax spores, which may have been aerosolized during removal of hair. The CDC believes that this was an isolated case and considers handling animal skins or making drums to be a low risk for cutaneous anthrax and extremely low risk for inhalational anthrax.
- In 2002, two cases of cutaneous anthrax were reported. A laboratory worker from a Texas lab that processed environmental *B. anthracis* specimens contracted cutaneous anthrax through direct contact with a contaminated surface. The second case occurred in a veterinarian who contracted the infection from a cow during necropsy.
- Two cases of human cutaneous anthrax were reported following epizootics in North Dakota (2000) and southwest Texas (2001). Both cases resulted from exposure during disposal of infected animal carcasses.

CLINICAL FEATURES

There are three primary clinical types of anthrax disease, inhalational, cutaneous, and gastrointestinal, which result from the way infection is acquired. Anthrax meningitis, which generally occurs as a complication of these primary forms of disease, is most likely to be seen with inhalational anthrax.

Anthrax infection is a severe clinical illness and can be life-threatening. Case fatality varies by the clinical type of disease. Overall case-fatality rates have declined because of more prompt administration of antibiotics and improved supportive care. Compared to historical rates, mortality has decreased from 86–95% to 45% for inhalational anthrax, 5–20% to less than 1% for cutaneous anthrax, and 25–60% to 12% for gastrointestinal anthrax. Anthrax meningitis case-fatality rates approach 95% even with antibiotic treatment.

In the event of bioterrorism, the method of dissemination would influence the type of clinical disease that would be expected. Following an aerosol release, the majority of cases would be inhalational with some cutaneous cases, whereas use of a small volume powder could result in both inhalational and cutaneous anthrax cases (as seen in the 2001 attacks). Gastrointestinal cases might occur following contamination of food or water.

Inhalational Anthrax

Inhalational anthrax is caused by inhalation of spores that reach the alveoli, undergo phagocytosis and travel to regional lymph nodes. The spores then germinate to become bacterial cells, which multiply in the lymphatic system and cause lymphadenitis of the mediastinal and peribronchial lymph nodes. The bacteria release toxins that cause hemorrhage, edema, and necrosis. Bacteria entering the bloodstream can lead to septicemia, septic shock, and death. Systemic infection following inhalational anthrax is almost always fatal.

One of the key clinical features of inhalational anthrax is evidence of pleural effusion and mediastinal widening on CXR (Figure 64.1) or chest computed tomographic (CT) scan (Table 64.1). Based on experience from the 2001 attacks, chest CT (without contrast) was found to be more sensitive than CXR for identification of mediastinal widening typical of inhalational anthrax.

Cutaneous Anthrax

In cutaneous anthrax, spores or bacilli are introduced through cuts or breaks in the skin (Table 64.2). Spores germinate at the site of contact and release toxins, causing development of a lesion and edema (Figure 64.2). Organisms may be carried to regional lymph nodes and cause painful lymphadenopathy and lymphangitis. Septicemic complications of cutaneous anthrax occur in 10–20% of untreated cases.

Pediatric considerations: A case of cutaneous anthrax occurred in a 7-month-old during the anthrax attack of 2001. This case was difficult to recognize and rapidly progressed to severe systemic illness despite timely antibiotic treatment. Clinical features included painless draining lesion with edema that developed into an eschar, fever, leukocytosis, severe microangiopathic hemolytic anemia, renal failure, and coagulopathy.

Gastrointestinal Anthrax

Gastrointestinal (GI) anthrax results from ingestion of *B. anthracis* bacteria, such as may be found in poorly cooked meat from infected animals. The incubation period for GI anthrax is 1–7 days. Two clinical presentations have been described: intestinal and oropharyngeal.

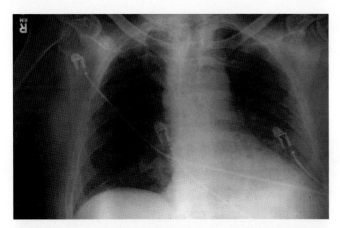

Figure 64.1 Anthrax chest x-ray with mediastinal widening and pleural effusion. (From: Jernigan JA, Stephens DS, Ashford DA, et al., Bioterrorism-related inhalational anthrax: the first 10 cases reported in the United States. Emerg Infect Dis 2001;7(6):933–44. Available at: http://www.cdc.gov/ncidod/eid/vol7no6/jernigan.htm.)

With *intestinal anthrax*, intestinal lesions occur in the ileum or cecum and are followed by regional lymphadenopathy. Symptoms of intestinal anthrax are initially nonspecific and include low-grade fever, malaise, nausea, vomiting, anorexia and fever. As disease progresses, abdominal pain, hematemesis, and bloody diarrhea develop. The patient may present with findings of an acute abdomen. After 2–4 days, ascites develops and abdominal pain lessens. Hematogenous spread with resultant septicemia can occur. Mesenteric adenopathy on CT scan is likely, and mediastinal widening on CXR is possible.

Table 64.1 Clinical Features: Inhalational Anthrax

Incubation Period	1–6 days (range <1 day to 8 weeks)
Transmission	Inhalation of aerosolized spores
Signs and Symptoms	• Initial presentation: Nonspecific symptoms (low-grade fever, chills, nonproductive cough, malaise, fatigue, myalgias, profound sweats, chest discomfort) • Intermediate presentation: Abrupt onset of high fever, dyspnea, progressive respiratory distress, confusion, nausea or vomiting • Fulminant disease progression, if untreated
Progression and Complications	• Severe respiratory distress (dyspnea, stridor, cyanosis), which may be preceded by 1–3 days of improvement • Pleural effusions • Meningitis • Shock
Laboratory and Radiographic Findings	• Chest CT or radiograph: Mediastinal widening (often), pleural effusions that are commonly hemorrhagic (often), infiltrates (rare) • Gram-positive bacilli on unspun peripheral blood smear or CSF • Elevated transaminases • Hypoxemia • Metabolic acidosis • Total WBC count normal or slightly elevated with elevated percentage of neutrophils or band forms

CSF, cerebrospinal fluid; WBC, white blood (cell) count.

Table 64.2 Clinical Features: Cutaneous Anthrax

Incubation Period	3–4 days (range 1–12 days)
Transmission	• Direct skin contact with spores; in nature, contact with infected animals or animal products (usually related to occupational exposure) • Bite of infective arthropod (rare)
Signs and Symptoms	• Local skin involvement after direct contact with spores or bacilli (commonly seen on hands, forearms, head, and neck) • Skin lesion with the following progression: (1) development of a papular lesion and localized itching, (2) papule turns into vesicular or bulbous lesion accompanied by painless edema, (3) lesion becomes necrotic and vesicles may surround the ulcer, and (4) lesion develops painless black eschar within 7–14 days of initial lesion • Lymphadenopathy and lymphangitis • Fever and malaise (common)
Progression and Complications	• Bacteremia • Meningitis • Extensive edema causing airway compression • Sepsis
Laboratory Findings	Bacilli may be seen on Gram stain of subcutaneous tissue

In *oropharyngeal anthrax*, a mucosal ulcer occurs initially in the mouth or throat, associated with fever, throat pain, and dysphasia (Figure 64.3). This is followed by cervical edema and regional lymphadenopathy. Ulcers may become necrotic with development of a white patch covering the ulcer. Swelling can become severe enough to affect breathing. Hematogenous spread, septicemia, and meningitis can occur.

Gram stain of ascitic fluid, oropharyngeal ulcers, or unspun peripheral blood may show gram-positive rods. Leukocytosis with left shift may be present. *B. anthracis* can be cultured from oropharyngeal swabs and stool specimens.

Anthrax Meningitis

Anthrax meningitis can occur as a complication of cutaneous, inhalational, or GI anthrax, but is most commonly seen with inhalational anthrax (up to 50%). Patients may or may not present with symptoms of the primary site of infection. In addition to typical symptoms of bacterial meningitis, anthrax meningitis may involve hemorrhage or meningoencephalitis. Case fatality with anthrax meningitis is greater than 90%. Even one case of anthrax meningitis should alert public health authorities to identify the source of exposure and investigate the possibility of bioterrorism.

Anthrax and Pregnant Women

Maternal and perinatal complications are not well understood, because anthrax infection during pregnancy is rare. Preterm delivery may be one of the major complications.

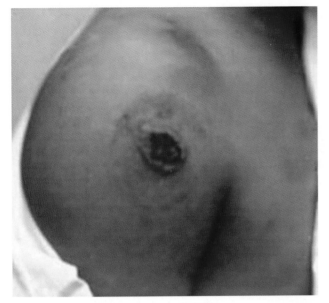
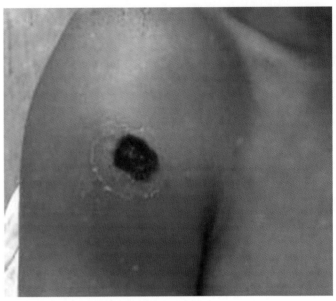

Figure 64.2 Progression of lesion caused by anthrax infection. Note the raised vesicular ring at the perimeter and subsequently the black eschar. (From the U.S. Centers for Disease Control and Prevention Emergency Preparedness and Response. Anthrax: Images: Cutaneous Anthrax. Available at: http://www.bt.cdc.gov/agent/anthrax/anthrax-images/cutaneous.asp.)

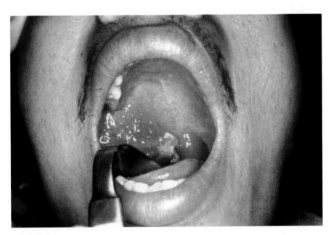

Figure 64.3 Lesion from oropharyngeal anthrax infection. (From: Sirisanthana T, Brown AE. Anthrax of the gastrointestinal tract. Emerg Infect Dis 2002;8(7): 649–51. Available at: http://www.cdc.gov/ncidod/eid/vol8no7/02-0062.htm.)

DIFFERENTIAL DIAGNOSIS

Because of its mild, nonspecific nature in the early states, a high index of suspicion is necessary to make a timely diagnosis of anthrax. Screening protocols and clinical prediction tools have been proposed and partially evaluated. Prompt administration of antibiotics can be critical to patient survival; therefore, clinicians should administer appropriate antibiotics when the diagnosis is suspected.

Differential: Inhalational Anthrax

Early disease mimics influenza and other respiratory infections. However, nasal symptoms are typically not present and rapid diagnostic tests, such as nasopharyngeal swabs for detection of respiratory virus antigens, would typically be negative.

Key features that distinguish *inhalational* anthrax from other conditions are:

- CXR is abnormal even during early stages of flulike illness
- CXR or chest CT show widened mediastinum and pleural effusion but minimal or no pneumonitis
- characteristics distinguishing inhalational anthrax from influenza:
  - neurological symptoms without headache (e.g., confusion, syncope) and nausea/vomiting are more common in inhalational anthrax
  - rhinorrhea and pharyngitis was uncommon in inhalational anthrax cases from 2001 U.S. attack

Other conditions to consider are:

- bacterial pneumonia (*Mycoplasma, Staphylococcus, Streptococcus, Haemophilus, Klebsiella, Moraxella, Legionella*)
- *Chlamydia* infection
- influenza
- other viral pneumonia (respiratory syncytial virus [RSV], cytomegalovirus [CMV], hantavirus)
- Q fever
- pneumonic plague
- tularemia
- primary mediastinitis
- ruptured aortic aneurysm
- histoplasmosis
- coccidioidomycosis
- silicosis
- sarcoidosis

Differential: Cutaneous Anthrax

Key features that distinguish *cutaneous* anthrax are:

- painlessness of the lesion itself
- large extent of local edema

Other conditions to consider:

- ecthyma gangrenosum
- ulceroglandular tularemia
- bubonic plague
- cellulitis (staphylococcal or streptococcal)
- brown recluse spider bite
- necrotizing soft-tissue infections (e.g., *Streptococcus*, *Clostridium*)
- Coumadin or heparin necrosis
- rickettsial infection
- necrotic herpes simplex infection
- orf virus infection
- glanders
- cutaneous leishmaniasis
- cat scratch fever
- melioidosis

Differential: Gastrointestinal Anthrax

The differential diagnosis for the *intestinal* form of the disease includes:

- typhoid fever
- intestinal tularemia
- acute bacterial gastroenteritis (e.g., *Campylobacter*, *Shigella*, toxicogenic *Escherichia coli*, *Yersinia*)
- bacterial peritonitis
- peptic or duodenal ulcer
- any other causes of acute abdomen

The differential diagnosis for the *oropharyngeal* form of the disease includes:

- streptococcal pharyngitis
- infectious mononucleosis
- diphtheria
- pharyngeal tularemia
- other causes of pharyngitis (e.g., enteroviral vesicular, herpetic, anaerobic or Vincent's angina, *Yersinia enterocolitica*)

Differential: Anthrax Meningitis

A key feature that distinguishes anthrax meningitis is bloody cerebrospinal fluid (CSF) containing gram-positive bacilli. Other conditions to consider are:

- subarachnoid hemorrhage
- bacterial meningitis
- aseptic meningitis

LABORATORY AND RADIOGRAPHIC FINDINGS

Diagnosis of anthrax requires a high index of suspicion because the disease often presents with nonspecific symptoms. Routine laboratory and radiographic findings for specific clinical presentations of anthrax are listed in the clinical features tables.

Initial identification and diagnosis of the organism relies on evaluation of infected tissue (blood, sputum, CSF, fluid collected from an unroofed vesicle, ulcer, eschar, skin lesion scraping, or stool). The gold standard for anthrax diagnosis is direct culture of clinical specimens onto blood agar with demonstration of typical Gram stain, motility, and biochemical features. Blood cultures, which are positive nearly 100% of the time in inhalational anthrax, should be obtained prior to antibiotic administration because there is rapid sterilization of blood after a single dose of antibiotics. Because laboratories may view gram-positive bacilli as contaminants and because *B. anthracis* may be a risk to laboratory personnel, clinicians should notify the laboratory when anthrax is suspected.

Although rapid diagnostic tests are not widely available, the public health laboratory system may be able to provide this testing on clinical specimens. Other tests available through the Centers for Disease Control and Prevention (CDC) or the public health laboratory system include polymerase chain reaction (PCR), serologic tests, and immunohistochemistry. Nasal swab cultures have been used to study environmental exposure to aerosolized anthrax; however, they are not recommended for use in the clinical setting. The sensitivity, specificity, and predictive value of nasal swab cultures are not known.

TREATMENT AND PROPHYLAXIS

Treatment of Confirmed or Suspected Anthrax

This section refers to individuals with suspected or confirmed anthrax disease.

The basic components of treatment for anthrax consist of hospitalization with intensive supportive care and IV antibiotics. After obtaining appropriate cultures, antimicrobials should be started *immediately* on suspicion and prior to confirmation of the diagnosis. Patients with inhalational anthrax who received antibiotics within 4.7 days of exposure had a 40% case fatality, compared to a 75% case fatality in those with treatment initiated after 4.7 days.

Because susceptibility data will be delayed, initial antibiotics must be chosen empirically (Table 64.3). Recommendations for initial empiric therapy of suspected or confirmed anthrax disease are described below. Empiric therapy with at least two agents is recommended because of the potential for infection with strains of *B. anthracis* engineered to be penicillin- and/or tetracycline-resistant. Engineered resistance to amoxicillin is believed to be more likely than resistance to doxycycline or ciprofloxacin; therefore, amoxicillin is not recommended as a first-line agent unless the strain has been proven susceptible. Therapy may be switched to oral antimicrobials when clinically indicated. Therapy should be continued for a total duration of 60 days because spores can persist and then germinate for prolonged periods. There is a possibility that spores could germinate and cause illness up to 100 days after exposure.

Contained casualty setting: Parenteral antimicrobial therapy with at least two agents is recommended for *inhalational and GI anthrax* when individual medical management is available (Table 64.3). After clinical improvement is noted, treatment can be switched to oral therapy with ciprofloxacin or doxycycline, based on susceptibilities and clinical considerations.

Cutaneous anthrax can be treated with oral antibiotics. If in addition to cutaneous lesions there are signs of systemic disease or extensive edema, or if lesions are present on

Table 64.3 Anthrax: Treatment and Postexposure Prophylaxis Recommendations[1]

	Initial IV Therapy[2,3] for Inhalational, GI Anthrax, or Cutaneous Anthrax with Complications[4]	Initial Therapy for Cutaneous anthrax[2,4]	Therapy for Anthrax in the Mass Casualty Setting, or Postexposure Prophylaxis, or After Clinical Improvement on IV Therapy[5,6]
Adult	**ciprofloxacin**, 400 mg IV q12h *or* **doxycycline**,[7] 100 mg IV q12h *and* one or two additional antimicrobials (agents with in vitro activity include rifampin, vancomycin, penicillin, ampicillin, chloramphenicol, imipenem, clindamycin, and clarithromycin)[8]	**ciprofloxacin**, 500 mg PO bid for 60 days *or* **doxycycline**, 100 mg PO bid for 60 days	**ciprofloxacin**,[9] 500 mg PO bid for 60 days *or* **doxycycline**,[10] 100 mg PO bid for 60 days
Children	**ciprofloxacin**,[11,12] 10 mg/kg IV q12h (max 400 g/dose) *or* **doxycycline**[7,12,13]: ≥45 kg, 100 mg IV q12h <45 kg, give 2.2 mg/kg IV q12h (max 200 mg/day) *and* one or two additional antimicrobials (agents with in vitro activity include rifampin, vancomycin, penicillin, ampicillin, chloramphenicol, imipenem, clindamycin, and clarithromycin)[8]	**ciprofloxacin**, 15 mg/kg PO bid (max 500 mg/dose) for 60 days *or* **doxycycline**[7,12,13]: ≥45 kg, give 100 mg PO bid for 60 days <45 kg, give 2.2 mg/kg PO bid (max 200 mg/day) for 60 days	**ciprofloxacin**,[9] 15 mg/kg PO bid (max 500 mg/dose) for 60 days *or* **doxycycline**[10]: ≥45 kg, give 100 mg PO bid for 60 days <45 kg, give 2.2 mg/kg PO bid (max 200 mg/day) for 60 days *or* **amoxicillin**[14]: >20 kg, give 500 mg PO tid daily for 60 days ≤20 kg, give 80 mg/kg/day PO in three divided doses every 8 hours for 60 days
Pregnant Women	Same as for nonpregnant adults[15]	Same as for nonpregnant adults[15]	Same as for nonpregnant adults *or* **amoxicillin**[14] 500 mg PO tid daily for 60 days
Immunocompromised Persons	Same as for nonimmunocompromised persons	Same as for nonimmunocompromised persons	Same as for nonimmunocompromised persons

Adapted from: Centers for Disease Control and Prevention (CDC). Investigation of bioterrorism-related anthrax and interim guidelines for exposure management and antimicrobial therapy. MMWR 2001;50(42): 909–19; and Centers for Disease Control and Prevention (CDC). Update: Investigation of anthrax associated with intentional exposure and interim public health guidelines. MMWR 2001;50(41):889–93.

[1] The treatment recommendation included in this table are adapted from guidance during the 2001 anthrax outbreaks. Therapy recommendations in other situations should be guided by antimicrobial susceptibility.

[2] Ciprofloxacin or doxycycline should be considered an essential part of first-line therapy for inhalational anthrax.

[3] Steroids may be considered an adjunct therapy for patients with severe edema and for meningitis based on experience with bacterial meningitis of other etiologies.

[4] Cutaneous anthrax cases with signs of systemic involvement, extensive edema, or lesions on the head or neck require intravenous therapy, and a multidrug approach is recommended.

[5] Initial therapy may be altered based on clinical course of patient; one or two antimicrobial agents (e.g., ciprofloxacin or doxycycline) may be adequate as patient improves.

[6] If pharmaceutical resources permit in a mass casualty setting, therapy with at least two agents is recommended over monotherapy.

[7] If meningitis is suspected, doxycycline may be less optimal because of poor central nervous system penetration.

[8] Because of concerns of constitutive and inducible beta-lactamases in *Bacillus anthracis* isolates, penicillin and ampicillin should not be used alone. Consultation with an infectious disease specialist is advised.

[9] In vitro studies suggest that ofloxacin (400 mg orally every 12 hours) or levafloxacin (500 mg orally every 24 hours) could be used in place of ciprofloxacin – if supplies were limited in a mass casualty or postexposure prophylaxis situation.

[10] In vitro studies suggest that 500 mg of tetracycline orally every 6 hours could be used in place of doxycycline – if supplies were limited in a mass casualty or postexposure prophylaxis situation.

[11] If intravenous ciprofloxacin is not available, oral ciprofloxacin may be acceptable because it is rapidly and well absorbed from the gastrointestinal tract with no substantial loss by first-pass metabolism. Maximum serum concentrations are attained 1–2 hours after oral dosing but may not be achieved if vomiting or ileus is present.

[12] Tetracycline and quinolone antibiotics are generally not recommended during pregnancy or childhood; however, their use may be indicated for life-threatening illness. Ciprofloxacin may be preferred in pregnant women and children up to 8 years of age because of the known adverse event profile of doxycycline (e.g., tooth discoloration). Doxycycline may be preferred in children 8 years and older because of the adverse event profile of ciprofloxacin (e.g., arthropathies).

[13] American Academy of Pediatrics recommends treatment of young children with tetracyclines for serious infections (e.g., Rocky Mountain spotted fever).

[14] Amoxicillin is not approved by the FDA for postexposure prophylaxis or treatment of anthrax. However, CDC has indicated that if the isolate is determined to be susceptible to amoxicillin, it could be used for pregnant women and children for postexposure prophylaxis or for completion of 60 days antibiotic therapy after initial treatment with ciprofloxacin or doxycycline. Amoxicillin resistance to anthrax is of greater concern than that of doxycycline or ciprofloxacin, and amoxicillin is not recommended as a first-line agent unless the isolate is proven to be susceptible.

[15] Although tetracyclines are not recommended for pregnant women, their use may be indicated for life-threatening illness. Adverse effects on developing teeth and bones are dose-related; therefore, doxycycline might be used for a short time (7–14 days) before 6 months of gestation.

the head or the neck, then the multidrug IV regimen is recommended (Table 64.3).

Mass casualty setting: Use of oral antibiotics may be necessary if the number of patients exceeds the medical care capacity for individual medical management (Table 64.3). If pharmaceutical resources permit, therapy with at least two agents is recommended over monotherapy.

Draining of pleural effusions has also been associated with reduced mortality.

Anthrax meningitis can be treated using the inhalational anthrax guidelines; however, IV treatment with a fluoroquinolone plus 1–2 antimicrobials with good central nervous system (CNS) penetration and activity against *B. anthracis* (i.e., rifampin, vancomycin, penicillin, ampicillin, meropenem) is recommended. The addition of corticosteroids may help manage cerebral edema.

Prophylaxis of Persons Exposed but Without Symptoms

Postexposure prophylaxis (PEP) is the administration of antibiotics, with or without vaccine, after suspected exposure to anthrax has occurred but before symptoms are present. (If symptoms are present, see section on treatment, above.) In general, PEP is recommended for persons exposed to an air space or package contaminated with *B. anthracis*. Unvaccinated laboratory workers exposed to *B. anthracis* cultures should also receive PEP. As there is no known person-to-person transmission of inhalational anthrax, prophylaxis should not be offered to contacts of cases, unless also exposed to the original source.

Postexposure prophylaxis of potential inhalational anthrax consists of oral administration of either ciprofloxacin or doxycycline (Table 64.3). Therapy should be continued for 60 days. Patients treated for exposure should be informed of the importance of completing the full course of antibiotic prophylaxis regardless of the absence of symptoms. The Food and Drug Administration (FDA) has also approved levofloxacin and penicillin G procaine for PEP of inhalational anthrax. Because of concerns about use of doxycycline or ciprofloxacin in children and about doxycycline use in pregnant women, the CDC has indicated that for prophylaxis, therapy can be switched to amoxicillin in these groups if the isolate is determined to be susceptible. Amoxicillin may also be considered for patients allergic to both ciprofloxacin and doxycycline.

The Advisory Committee on Immunization Practices recommends the use of combined antimicrobial prophylaxis and vaccine [Biothrax (formerly Anthrax vaccine absorbed, AVA)]. Biothrax is not licensed for this use by the FDA and would need to be given under an Investigational New Drug (IND) application. The recommended regimen is three vaccine doses (given at 0, 2, and 4 weeks after exposure) and at least a 30-day course of antimicrobial therapy. The CDC does not recommend vaccination in pregnant women given lack of data.

Following the 2001 attacks, exposed persons were given the option of (1) 60 days of antibiotic prophylaxis; (2) 100 days of antibiotic prophylaxis, and (3) 100 days of antibiotic prophylaxis, plus anthrax vaccine (under IND protocol).

Anthrax Vaccine

The anthrax vaccine Biothrax (formerly Anthrax vaccine absorbed, AVA) is available but only in limited supply that is controlled by federal authorities. It is an inactivated cell-free filtrate of an avirulent strain of *B. anthracis*. Local reactions and mild systemic reactions are common. Severe allergic reactions are rare (<1 per 100,000).

The anthrax vaccine is licensed for pre-exposure use to prevent cutaneous anthrax in healthy, nonpregnant adults 18–65 years of age who have a high likelihood of coming into contact with anthrax, including certain laboratory workers and animal processing workers. Biothrax is not currently licensed for postexposure use and must be given in this context under an FDA investigational drug protocol. The CDC may recommend its use for PEP under some circumstances. Research is underway on new anthrax vaccines.

DEVELOPMENTAL ANTHRAX THERAPEUTICS

Additional therapeutic candidates for treatment and prophylaxis of anthrax are currently under development. The Department of Health and Human Services announced plans to purchase the antibody-based therapeutic candidates immune globulin (AIG) and ABthrax (raxibacumab) for the strategic national stockpile. These therapeutic approaches use antibodies to neutralize anthrax toxin. Neither AIG nor ABthrax is FDA approved, but either may be authorized for use as an investigational new drug in an emergency. Studies are still in progress to determine efficacy of these therapeutics in anthrax treatment and prophylaxis.

COMPLICATIONS AND ADMISSION CRITERIA

Without early antibiotic treatment, inhalational anthrax progresses to pneumonitis marked by severe respiratory distress and cyanosis, and often accompanied by pleural effusion. Patients with anthrax pneumonitis are particularly likely to develop septicemia and septic shock due to hematogenous dissemination of the bacteria. Sepsis may develop as a complication of cutaneous anthrax or gastrointestinal anthrax as well. Anthrax meningitis may occur as a consequence of hematogenous dissemination.

Patients with suspected or confirmed inhalational, gastrointestinal, or meningeal anthrax, as well as those with cutaneous anthrax who exhibit head or neck lesions, extensive edema, or systemic signs of illness, require admission for intravenous antibiotic therapy and supportive care.

INFECTION CONTROL

Clinicians should notify local public health authorities, their institution's infection control professional, and their laboratory of any suspected anthrax cases. Public health authorities may conduct epidemiologic investigations and implement disease control interventions to protect the public. Both HICPAC (Hospital Infection Control Practices Advisory Committee) of the CDC and the Working Group for Civilian Biodefense recommend Standard Precautions for anthrax patients in a hospital setting without the need for isolation. Person-to-person transmission has only rarely been reported for patients with cutaneous anthrax and Standard Precautions are considered adequate. Routine laboratory procedures should be carried out under Biosafety Level 2 (BSL-2) conditions.

DECONTAMINATION

Contaminated surfaces can be disinfected with commercially available bleach or a 1:10 dilution of household bleach and water. All persons exposed to an aerosol containing *B. anthracis* should be instructed to wash body surfaces and clothing with soap and water.

PEARLS AND PITFALLS

1. The initial (prodromal) phase of inhalational anthrax resembles an influenza-like syndrome and can be difficult to distinguish from seasonal respiratory illnesses. Nasal congestion and rhinorrhea, however, are common features of seasonal influenza-like syndromes and are unusual with pulmonary anthrax.
2. The classic radiographic findings of inhalational anthrax – CXR showing a widened mediastinum (due to hilar lymphadenopathy) and pulmonary effusion – although not unique to anthrax, should nonetheless prompt a high level of clinical suspicion.
3. The necrotic, edematous, eschar-covered skin lesion of cutaneous anthrax is usually painless, which is an important differentiating feature from a brown recluse spider bite.

REFERENCES

Bales ME, Dannenberg AL, Brachman PS, et al. Epidemiologic response to anthrax outbreaks: field investigations, 1950–2001. Emerg Infect Dis 2002;8(10):1163–74.

Bell DM, Kozarsky PE, Stephens DS. Clinical issues in the prophylaxis, diagnosis, and treatment of anthrax. Emerg Infect Dis 2002;8(2):222–5.

Centers for Disease Control and Prevention (CDC). Additional options for preventive treatment for persons exposed to inhalational anthrax. MMWR 2001;50(50):1142.

Centers for Disease Control and Prevention (CDC). Anthrax Q and A: Anthrax and animal hides. 2006. Available at: http://www.bt.cdc.gov/agent/anthrax/faq/pelt.asp.

Centers for Disease Control and Prevention (CDC). Emergency preparedness and response. anthrax: images: cutaneous anthrax. Available at: http://www.bt.cdc.gov/agent/anthrax/anthrax-images/cutaneous.asp.

Centers for Disease Control and Prevention (CDC). Inhalation anthrax associated with dried animal hides – Pennsylvania and New York City, 2006. MMWR 2006;55(10):280–2.

Centers for Disease Control and Prevention (CDC). Investigation of anthrax associated with intentional exposure and interim public health guidelines, October 2001. MMWR 2001;50(41):889–93.

Centers for Disease Control and Prevention (CDC). Investigation of bioterrorism-related anthrax and interim guidelines for exposure management and antimicrobial therapy, October 2001. MMWR 2001:50(42):909–19.

Centers for Disease Control and Prevention (CDC). Suspected cutaneous anthrax in a laboratory worker – Texas 2002. MMWR 2002;51(13):279–81.

Centers for Disease Control and Prevention (CDC). Use of anthrax vaccine in response to terrorism: supplemental recommendations of the Advisory Committee on Immunization Practices. MMWR 2002;51(45):1024–6.

Food and Drug Administration (FDA). Levaquin (levofloxacin) information. 2005. Retrieved March 20, 2007, from http://www.fda.gov/cder/drug/infopage/levaquin/default.htm.

Freedman A, Afonja O, Chang MW, et al. Cutaneous anthrax associated with microangiopathic hemolytic anemia and coagulopathy in a 7-month-old infant. JAMA 2002;287(7):869–74.

Holty JE, Kim RY, Bravata DM Systematic review: a century of inhalational anthrax cases from 1900 to 2005. Ann Intern Med 2006;144(4):270–80.

Howell JM, Mayer TA, Hanfling D, et al. Screening for inhalational anthrax due to bioterrorism: evaluating proposed screening protocols. Clin Infect Dis 2004;39(12):1842–7.

Jernigan JA, Stephens DS, Ashford DA, et al., Bioterrorism-related inhalational anthrax: the first 10 cases reported in the United States. Emerg Infect Dis 2001;7(6):933–44.

Kadanali A, Tasyaran MA, Kadanali S. Anthrax during pregnancy: case reports and review. Clin Infect Dis 2003;36(10):1343–6.

Meyerhoff A, Murphy D. Guidelines for treatment of anthrax. JAMA 2002;288(15):1848–9; author reply 1848–9.22.

Sejvar JJ, Tenover FC, Stephens DS. Management of anthrax meningitis. Lancet Infect Dis 2005;5(5):287–95.

Sirisanthana T, Brown AE. Anthrax of the gastrointestinal tract. Emerg Infect Dis 2002;8(7):649–51.

Swartz MN. Recognition and management of anthrax – an update. N Engl J Med 2001;345(22):1621–6.

ADDITIONAL READINGS

Center for Infectious Disease Research and Policy. Anthrax: Current, comprehensive information on pathogenesis, microbiology, epidemiology, diagnosis, treatment, and prophylaxis. 2006. CIDRAP. Retrieved January 17, 2007, from http://www.cidrap.umn.edu/cidrap/content/bt/anthrax/biofacts/anthraxfactsheet.html.

Dixon TC, Meselson M, Guillemin J. et al. Anthrax. N Engl J Med 1999;341(11):815–26.

Inglesby TV, O'Toole T, Henderson DA, et al. Anthrax as a biological weapon, 2002: updated recommendations for management. JAMA 2002;287(17):2236–52.

Lucey D. Chapter 205 – *Bacillus anthracis* (Anthrax). In: Mandell GL, Bennett JE, Dolin R, eds, Principles and practice of infectious diseases (6th ed). New York: Churchill Livingstone, 2005.

Lucey D. Chapter 324 – Anthrax. In: Mandell GL, Bennett JE, Dolin R, eds, Principles and practice of infectious diseases (6th ed). New York: Churchill Livingstone, 2005.

65. Botulism

David M. Stier, Nikkita Patel, Olivia Bruch, and Karen A. Holbrook

INTRODUCTION

Botulism is a disease caused by exposure to botulinum toxin produced from *Clostridium* species, mainly *Clostridium botulinum*. Clinical forms of the disease include foodborne, inhalational, wound, infant, adult intestinal toxemia, and iatrogenic. *C. botulinum* is a gram-positive, strictly anaerobic, spore-forming bacillus naturally found in soil and aquatic sediments. There are seven types of the toxin based on antigenic differences, labeled A through G. Types A, B, and E (and rarely, F) are pathogenic in humans. Types C, D, and E cause illness in other mammals, birds, and fish. Botulinum toxin lacks color, odor, and taste and is the most lethal toxin known. Death is caused by doses of less than 1 μg. Antibiotics have no activity against the toxin itself.

In response to unfavorable environmental conditions (changes in pH, temperature, and water or nutrient availability), *C. botulinum* bacteria "sporulate." *C. botulinum* spores are hardy, resistant to desiccation, heat, ultraviolet (UV) light, and alcohols, and can survive boiling for up to 4 hours; however, they are readily killed by chlorine-based disinfectants. Once spores encounter more favorable conditions, such as are found in human tissues, they "germinate," producing growing cells that are capable of reproducing and elaborating toxin.

The Working Group for Civilian Biodefense considers botulism to be a dangerous potential biological weapon because of the pathogen's "extreme potency and lethality; its ease of production, transport, and misuse; and the need for prolonged intensive care among affected persons." Use of botulism as a biological weapon would be expected to produce severe medical and public health outcomes.

EPIDEMIOLOGY

Botulinum Toxin as a Biological Weapon

State-sponsored military programs researched and weaponized botulinum toxin as early as the 1930s. Botulism has also been used as a weapon by a terrorist group. Unfortunately, botulism is ubiquitous in nature and access to it cannot be easily controlled.

Likely modes of dissemination for toxin used as a weapon include:

- **Contamination of food or beverages**. Possible food or beverage vehicles for botulism toxin include any that are not heated to 85°C (185°F) for 5 minutes before consumption or those that are contaminated after appropriate heating. Typical pasteurization does not remove all toxins.
- **Dispersion of aerosolized toxin**. Animal studies and rare cases of laboratory accidents have confirmed the pathogenicity of aerosolized toxin. One study estimates that aerosolizing 1 g of botulinum toxin could kill up to 1.5 million people; another estimates that a point source exposure could kill 10% of the population 500 meters downwind. Technical factors make such dissemination difficult.
- **Contamination of a water supply**. This is possible, though unlikely because of the quantity of toxin needed to effectively contaminate a water supply. Additionally, standard drinking water treatment inactivates the toxin quickly and, in fresh water, it is inactivated through natural decay in 3 to 6 days.

An outbreak of disease caused by the intentional release of botulinum toxin would have the following characteristics:

- Clustering in time: multiple cases presenting with rapidly progressing acute flaccid symmetric paralysis with prominent bulbar palsies, generally 12–36 hours after release
- Atypical host characteristics: cases of unusual botulinum toxin type (C, D, F, G, and possibly E) *or* cases without typical gastrointestinal symptoms of nausea, vomiting, and diarrhea
- Unusual geographic clustering: cases in geographic proximity during the week before symptom onset, but lack common food exposure (aerosol exposure) *or* toxin type outside of typical geographic range
- Affected patients with no exposure risk factors, or multiple outbreaks without an association with a common food source

Naturally Occurring Botulism

RESERVOIRS

The sporulated form of the bacterium is commonly found in soils and aquatic sediments. Cistern water, dust, and foods, including honey, can become contaminated from contact with the soil.

MODE OF TRANSMISSION

Botulism is caused by exposure to botulinum toxin. Humans can be exposed to toxin in a number of ways:

- inhalation of toxin (inhalational)
- consumption of toxin (foodborne)
- consumption of *C. botulinum* spores (infant; adult intestinal toxemia)
- contamination of a tissue with *C. botulinum* spores (wound)
- contamination of a tissue with toxin (iatrogenic)

WORLDWIDE OCCURRENCE

In the late 1700s, botulism emerged as a disease because of changes in sausage production in Europe. In fact, *botulus* means sausage. Soon thereafter in the early 1800s, botulism associated with consumption of fermented fish was recognized in Russia. Wound and infant botulism were discovered much later in the mid to late 1900s. In 1999–2000, more than 2500 cases of foodborne botulism were reported in Europe. The highest incidence is found in countries of the former Soviet Union and in Asia and is related to improper food handling. Type B is more common in Europe, whereas type E is more common in Scandinavia and Canada and is frequently linked to improper storage of fish and marine mammals.

OCCURRENCE IN THE UNITED STATES

In the United States, naturally occurring botulism is a rare disease with an annual incidence of approximately 140 cases (infant, 85; food, 20; and wound, 35). More than half of foodborne cases occur in the Western states of California, Oregon, Washington, Alaska, and Colorado. Type E is more common among Alaskan natives because of their diet of fermented meat from aquatic mammals and fish. Type A is found mainly in Western states and type B is more common in the East. Most cases of wound botulism result from injection drug use with black tar heroin, which is more common in the Western states.

CLINICAL FEATURES

Regardless of the route of intoxication, the same clinical neurologic syndrome develops (Table 65.1). Botulism is an afebrile descending symmetric paralytic illness. Disease generally begins with absorption of toxin by mucosal surfaces in the gastrointestinal system, the eye, or nonintact skin. Cranial nerve dysfunction ensues, followed by muscle weakness beginning with the proximal muscle groups. Severity of disease is variable, ranging from mild cranial nerve dysfunction to flaccid paralysis (Figure 65.1). Both the severity of disease and the rapidity of onset correlate with the amount of toxin absorbed into the circulation.

Botulinum toxin blocks acetylcholine release at the neuromuscular junction of skeletal muscle neurons and peripheral muscarinic cholinergic autonomic synapses. It binds irreversibly to presynaptic receptors to inhibit the release of acetylcholine and cause neuromuscular weakness and autonomic dysfunction. The effect lasts weeks to months, until the synapses and axonal branches regenerate. Death from botulism results acutely from airway obstruction or paralysis of respiratory muscles.

Table 65.1 Clinical Features: Botulism

Incubation Period	12–80 hours (range 2 hours to 8 days)
Transmission	• Inhalation of toxin • Consumption of toxin or *C. botulinum* spores • Contamination of a tissue with toxin or *C. botulinum* spores
Signs and Symptoms	**Cardinal signs:** • Afebrile • Symmetrical neurological manifestations • Normal mental status, though may appear lethargic and have difficulty with communication • Normal to slow heart rate without the presence of hypotension • Normal sensory nerve function, other than vision **Early presentation – cranial nerve abnormalities:** • Fatigue and vertigo • Double and blurred vision, intermittent ptosis and disconjugate gaze • Difficulty swallowing food **Later presentation – descending paralysis:** • Difficulty moving eyes and mild pupillary dilation and nystagmus • Tongue weakness, decreased gag reflex, indistinct speech, dysphagia, dysphonia • Symmetrical, descending progressive muscular weakness, especially arms and legs • Unsteady gait • Extreme weakness, including postural neck muscles and occasional mouth breathing • Autonomic nerve dysfunction; may include urinary retention, orthostasis • Constipation **Ingestional:** • Dry mouth and dysarthria • Nausea and vomiting, except when exposure is purified toxin **Inhalational:** • Mucus in throat • Serous nasal discharge, salivation **Infant:** • Inability to suck and swallow • Constipation • Weakened voice • Floppy neck
Progression and Complications	• Respiratory failure and possible aspiration pneumonia • Residual fatigue, dry mouth or eyes, dyspnea on exertion several years later
Laboratory and Radiographic Findings	• Normal CSF values • Normal CBC • Normal imaging of brain and spine (CT scan or MRI) Characteristic EMG findings include: • Decremented response to repetitive nerve stimulation at low frequency (3 Hz) • Facilitated response to repetitive nerve stimulation at high frequencies (10–50 Hz) • Low compound muscle action potential

CBC, complete blood count; CSF, cerebrospinal fluid; CT, computed tomographic; EMG, electromyogram; MRI, magnetic resonance imaging.

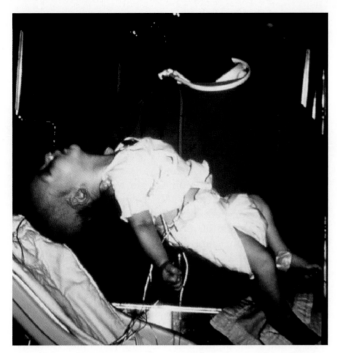

Figure 65.1 Infant with botulism. (From the U.S. Centers for Disease Control and Prevention Public Health Image Library at http://phil.cdc.gov/phil/home.asp.)

The case fatality rate was close to 60% prior to the advent of critical care. Even today, the mortality rate is high if treatment is not immediate and proper. In an outbreak setting, the mortality rate for the first case is 25% and for subsequent cases is 4%. A shorter incubation period has been linked to higher mortality, possibly reflecting a dose-dependent response. Fatality doubles in persons above the age of 60.

Foodborne botulism occurs from the consumption of preformed botulinum toxin in food. Waterborne botulism has not been seen. Toxin types A, B, and E account for most cases of foodborne botulism. Minute amounts of toxin can cause disease. A case in which a contaminated potato was spit out before being swallowed resulted in 6 months of hospitalization.

In order for foodborne botulism to occur:

- *C. botulinum* spores must contaminate the food
- anaerobic, nonacidic, low sugar and salt, and warm conditions are necessary for spores to survive, germinate, and produce toxin
- the food must not be reheated enough to inactivate the heat-labile toxin (≥85°C for 5 minutes) before consumption.

Inhalational botulism does not occur in nature; however three human cases occurred in 1962 in lab technicians working with aerosolized botulinum toxin. It has also been produced experimentally in laboratory animals.

Wound botulism is caused by toxin absorbed into the circulation through a wound. Most cases are related to injection drug use, especially in association with use of black tar heroin being injected into soft tissue ("skin popping"; see Chapter 55, Infectious Complications of Injection Drug Use).

Infant botulism occurs from the consumption of *C. botulinum* spores. The spores invade the gastrointestinal tract, replicate, and release toxin, which is absorbed into the circulation. The source of spores typically is unknown, although ingestion of corn syrup or raw honey accounts for some cases.

Adult intestinal toxemia (or undefined) botulism occurs from the consumption of *C. botulinum* spores. Characteristics include unknown source of toxin, presence of toxin in stool, and abnormal gastrointestinal pathology (e.g., Billroth surgery, Crohn's disease, and peptic ulcer disease) or antimicrobial drug use.

Iatrogenic botulism been noted very rarely after medical use or misuse of the botulinum toxin. Purified, highly diluted, injectable botulinum toxin is used to treat a range of spastic or autonomic muscular disorders. Toxin type A (Botox) is used in extremely minute doses for the treatment of facial wrinkles and blepharospasm, cervical dystonia, strabismus, glabellar lines, and primary axillary hyperhidrosis. Toxin type B (Myobloc, Neurobloc) is used to treat cervical dystonia. Dysphagia, limited paresis, and other neuromuscular impairment have been seen.

DIFFERENTIAL DIAGNOSIS

Diagnosis of botulism during the initial stages requires a high index of suspicion because of the lack of readily available rapid confirmatory tests.

Important questions to ask include:

- recent history of eating any home-canned or home-prepared vegetables or fruit, foil-wrapped baked potato, or lightly preserved or fermented meat and fish products, including seafood products from Alaska, Canada, or the Great Lakes
- other known individuals with similar symptoms
- recent history of injection drug use, particularly with black tar heroin or cocaine

Key features that distinguish botulism are the constellation of:

- afebrile illness
- normal mental status
- cranial nerves prominently involved
- descending paralysis
- symmetric bilateral impairment
- absence of paresthesias
- normal cerebrospinal fluid (CSF) studies
- characteristic electromyogram (EMG) findings

Other conditions to consider are:

- Guillain-Barré syndrome (especially Miller-Fisher syndrome)
- myasthenia gravis
- stroke or CNS tumor
- CNS infections (particularly of brainstem)
- Lambert-Eaton syndrome
- tick paralysis
- sudden infant death syndrome
- hyperemesis gravidarum
- saxitoxin (paralytic shellfish poisoning)
- tetrodotoxin (puffer fish poisoning)
- laryngeal trauma
- diabetic neuropathy
- poliomyelitis

- West Nile acute flaccid paralysis
- psychiatric illness (i.e., conversion paralysis)
- inflammatory myopathy
- streptococcal pharyngitis
- viral syndrome
- hypothyroidism
- overexertion
- diphtheria
- Wernicke's encephalopathy
- intoxication with CNS depressants (atropine, aminoglycoside, magnesium, ethanol, organophosphates, nerve gas, carbon monoxide)

LABORATORY AND RADIOGRAPHIC FINDINGS

Routine laboratory and radiographic findings for specific clinical presentations of botulism are listed in Table 65.1.

Although laboratory confirmation should be initiated as soon as possible if testing facilities are available, the clinical presentation should guide clinical management and public health interventions. Laboratory confirmation is challenging, but can be achieved in most cases by detection of botulinum toxin in serum, respiratory secretions, and stool via mouse bioassay, in which mice are injected with the patient sample and observed for the development of characteristic symptoms. Serum specimens must be taken *before* antitoxin treatment to demonstrate the presence of botulinum toxin. The test requires 1–4 days to complete and is performed only at reference laboratories. Electromyography provides diagnostic information more rapidly. Repetitive nerve stimulation at 20–50 Hz differentiates between various etiologies of acute flaccid paralysis. Electromyography is not recommended for infants.

Because the laboratory diagnosis of botulism may take several days to complete, health department officials can authorize the release of antitoxin prior to laboratory confirmation on the basis of clinical findings and may be able to provide other rapid detection tests that are currently investigational (e.g., time-resolved fluorescence assay, toxin micronanosensor, ganglioside-liposome immunoassay, enzyme-linked immunosorbent assay [ELISA]).

TREATMENT AND PROPHYLAXIS

Treatment

Outcome is based on early diagnosis and treatment. Supportive care (including airway protection, mechanical ventilation, and feeding by central tube or parenteral nutrition) and timely administration of equine botulinum antitoxin are keys to the successful management of botulism. Establish a means of communication early, because sometimes symptoms such as debilitating headaches cannot be communicated after the onset of paralysis.

ANTITOXIN

Antitoxin administration should not be delayed for laboratory confirmation, because antitoxin does not reverse disease or existing paralysis, but only stops progression of disease.

Patients given antitoxin within the first 24 hours after symptom onset had shorter hospital stays, shorter duration of ventilatory support, and a lower fatality rate (10%) than those given antitoxin more than 24 hours after onset (15%) or those who did not receive antitoxin at all (46%).

Antitoxin is provided by the Centers for Disease Control and Prevention (CDC) but is available for release only by state or local health departments. Delivery can be expected within 12 hours of request.

Consult public health authorities regarding dosage, because recommendations change. Currently, the CDC recommends immediate intravenous administration of the trivalent antitoxin (one vial diluted 1:10 over 30 minutes). If it is suspected that the exposure was to an extremely high dosage of toxin, the serum may be tested after treatment for the presence of remaining toxin.

Because antitoxin is of equine origin, hypersensitivity reactions can occur. From 1967 to 1977, 9% of persons treated with botulinal antitoxin had a nonfatal hypersensitivity reaction. In recent years, since the recommended dosage decreased 2- to 4-fold, less than 1% of patients have experienced hypersensitivity reactions. Although recommended, skin test for hypersensitivity prior to administration is not predictive of serum sickness reactions. A skin test may be valuable in patients with allergies, previous anaphylaxis, or prior receipt of equine antitoxins. If skin testing is positive, consider desensitizing over several hours before administering the complete dose of antitoxin or pretreat with antihistamines, steroids, and epinephrine infusions. Diphenhydramine, epinephrine, and airway equipment should be easily accessible during any administration.

Human botulism immune globulin is used to treat infants and is administered intravenously.

SUPPORTIVE CARE

Ventilatory support may be required for several weeks or more. One study found the mean time on a ventilator for botulism cases was 58 days.

With modern intensive care methods, case-fatality rates for botulism in the United States have dropped to less than 10%. In a mass casualty setting, measurement and management of ventilatory function may pose challenges because of limited ventilator capacities. Local health departments can request supplemental laryngoscopes, endotracheal tubes, and Ambu bags from the CDC. If personnel are limited, consider recruiting healthy civilians for bag ventilation.

A reverse Trendelenburg positioning with cervical vertebral support has been beneficial in terms of respiratory mechanics and airway protection in nonventilated infants with botulism, but has not been tested in adults (Figure 65.2).

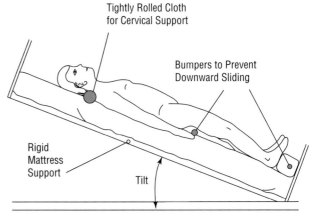

Figure 65.2   Bed position that is best for botulism patients with respiratory muscle weakness. (Aron et al., JAMA 2001;285:1059–70.)

In adults, especially those with obesity, a 20- to 25-degree angle may be beneficial.

Utilize physical therapy and physical turning to minimize intensive care complications.

SECONDARY INFECTIONS

Antibiotics may be used for treatment of secondary infections; however, aminoglycosides and clindamycin are contraindicated because they may exacerbate the neuromuscular blockade.

Postexposure Prophylaxis

There is currently no available postexposure prophylaxis for asymptomatic exposed persons. Such persons should be educated regarding the signs and symptoms of clinical botulism and instructed to seek medical care immediately if symptoms occur. Not all exposed persons will develop clinical symptoms. Exposed persons and their families may experience anxiety and/or somatic symptoms that may include neurologic symptoms. These patients should be carefully assessed. Antitoxin supplies are limited, and therapy will be reserved for patients with compatible neurological findings.

Vaccine

Preexposure immunization with botulinum toxoid is restricted to certain laboratory and military personnel. Supplies are extremely limited and are not be available for the public.

COMPLICATIONS AND ADMISSION CRITERIA

In patients with botulism, cranial nerve dysfunction progresses inexorably to a symmetric, descending muscle weakness or paralysis. Respiratory failure occurs in 40–70% of botulism patients because of declining upper airway and ventilatory muscle strength. Additional complications of botulism include secondary infection of the respiratory system and sequelae related to intubation and mechanical ventilation, prolonged immobilization, and autonomic dysfunction. Diminished respiratory muscle function and easy fatigability were described by botulism patients 2 years after recovery.

Hospital admission is required for protection of the airway, mechanical ventilatory support, and fluid and nutritional management until normal muscular function returns.

INFECTION CONTROL

Clinicians should notify local public health authorities and their laboratory of any suspected botulism case. Health authorities may conduct epidemiologic investigations and implement disease control interventions to protect the public. Both HICPAC (Hospital Infection Control Practices Advisory Committee) of the CDC and the Working Group for Civilian Biodefense recommend Standard Precautions for botulism patients in a hospital setting without the need for isolation. Person-to-person transmission does not occur.

Decontamination

After exposure to toxin, wash clothes and skin with soap and water. Inactivation of the toxin in the environment can take 2 days; however, changes in temperature and humidity can affect the rate of decomposition. Contaminated surfaces and spills of cultures or toxin can be disinfected with sodium hypochlorite (0.1% which is a 1:50 dilution of household bleach) or sodium hydroxide (0.1 N), which inactivates the toxin. Moist heat at 120°C for at least 15 minutes destroys spores.

PEARLS AND PITFALLS

1. Botulism is often misdiagnosed as a polyradiculopathy (Guillain-Barré syndrome or Miller-Fisher syndrome), myasthenia gravis, or other diseases of the central nervous system. Botulism is distinguished from other flaccid paralyses by its initial presentation with prominent cranial neuropathy, its subsequent descending, symmetrical paralysis, and the lack of sensory nerve deficits.
2. In the United States, botulism is more likely to cause a cluster of cases of acute flaccid paralysis than Guillain-Barré syndrome, chemical poisoning, or poliomyelitis.
3. Botulism antitoxin neutralizes freely circulating toxin but does not dislodge toxin already bound to presynaptic receptors. Early administration of antitoxin can help to inhibit further paralysis, but does not reverse paralysis that has already occurred.
4. Botulism antitoxin is limited in quantity and is available only through public health authorities. Because the laboratory diagnosis of botulism requires an in vivo assay and may take several days to complete, health department officials often authorize the release of antitoxin prior to laboratory confirmation, on the basis of clinical findings.

REFERENCES

Black RE, Gunn RA. Hypersensitivity reactions associated with botulinum antitoxin. Am J Med 1980;69:567–70.

Centers for Disease Control (CDC). Botulism: diagnosis and laboratory guidance for clinicians. Retrieved October 6, 2006, from http://www.bt.cdc.gov/agent/Botulism/clinicians/diagnosis.asp.

Centers for Disease Control (CDC). Drug service: General information. Retrieved April 16, 2007, from http://www.cdc.gov/ncidod/srp/drugs/formulary.html#1a.

Chertow DS, Tan ET, Maslanka SE, et al. Botulism in 4 adults following cosmetic injections with an unlicensed, highly concentrated botulinum preparation. JAMA 2006;296(20):2476–9.

Chin J. Control of communicable diseases manual (17th ed.). Washington, DC: American Public Health Association, 2000.

Franz DR, Jahrling PB, Friedlander AM, et al. Clinical recognition and management of patients exposed to biological warfare agents. JAMA 1997;278(5):399–411.

Horowitz BZ. Botulinum toxin. Crit Care Clin 2005;21:825–39.

Kongsaengdao S, Samintarapanya K, Rusmeechan S, et al. An outbreak of botulism in Thailand: clinical manifestations and management of severe respiratory failure. Clin Infect Dis 2006;43:1247–56.

Middlebrook JL, Franz DR. Botulinum toxins. In: Sidell FR, Takafuji ET, Franz DR, eds, Medical aspects of chemical and biological warfare (Textbook of military medicine, part I, vol 3). Washington, DC: Office of the Surgeon General, 1997:643–54.

Nishiura H. Incubation period as a clinical predictor of botulism: analysis of precious izushi-borne outbreaks in Hokkaido, Japan, from 1951 to 1965. Epidemiol Infect 2006;1–5.

Peck MW. *Clostridium botulinum* and the safety of minimally heated, chilled foods: an emerging issue? J Appl Microbiol 2006;101:556–70.

Shapiro RL, Hatheway C, Becher J, et al. Botulism surveillance and emergency response: a public health strategy for a global challenge. JAMA 1997;278(5):433–5.

Sobel J. Botulism. Clin Infect Dis 2005;41:1167–73.

Sobel J, Tucker N, McLaughlin J, et al. Foodborne botulism in the United States, 1990–2000. Emerg Infect Dis 2004 Sep;10(9):1606–11.

ADDITIONAL READINGS

Arnon SS, Schechter R, Inglesby TV, et al. Botulinum toxin as a biological weapon: medical and public health management. Working Group on Civilian Biodefense. JAMA 2001;285(8):1059–70.

Bleck TP. Botulinum toxin as a biological weapon. In: Mandell GL, Bennett JE, Dolin R, eds, Principles and practice of infectious diseases (6th ed). New York: Churchill Livingstone, 2005.

Bleck TP. *Clostridium botulinum*. In: Mandell GL, Bennett JE, Dolin R, eds, Principles and practice of infectious diseases (6th ed). New York: Churchill Livingstone, 2005.

Center for Infectious Disease Research and Policy (CIDRAP). Botulism: current, comprehensive information on pathogenesis, microbiology, epidemiology, diagnosis, and treatment. Retrieved March 5, 2007, from http://www.cidrap.umn.edu/cidrap/content/bt/botulism.

66. Plague

David M. Stier, Nikkita Patel, Olivia Bruch, and Karen A. Holbrook

INTRODUCTION

Plague is an acute bacterial infection caused by *Yersinia pestis*, a member of the family Enterobacteriaceae. *Y. pestis* is a pleomorphic, nonmotile, nonsporulating, intracellular, gram-negative bacillus that has a characteristic bipolar appearance on Wright, Giemsa, and Wayson's stains. There are three virulent biovars – *antiqua, mediaevalis,* and *orientalis* – and a fourth avirulent biovar, *microtus*. The *orientalis* biovar is thought to have originated in southern China and caused the most recent pandemic.

The Working Group for Civilian Biodefense considers plague to be a potential biological weapon because of the pathogen's availability "around the world, its capacity for its mass production and aerosol dissemination, and the difficulty in preventing such activities, high fatality rate of pneumonic plague, and potential for secondary spread of cases during an epidemic." Of the potential ways in which *Y. pestis* could be used as a biological weapon, aerosol release would be most likely. This method has been successfully demonstrated to cause disease in *Rhesus* macaques.

EPIDEMIOLOGY

Plague as a Biological Weapon

In the 20th century, countries including the United States, the former Soviet Union, and Japan developed ways for using *Y. pestis* as a weapon. Creating aerosolized plague is technically challenging; however, if an intentional release of aerosolized plague were to take place, an outbreak of pneumonic plague would be likely. This would be of serious concern because of the high case-fatality rate and the potential for person-to-person transmission.

An outbreak of disease caused by an intentional release of *Y. pestis* would have the following characteristics:

- Clustering in time: multiple similarly presenting cases of severe, progressive multilobar pneumonia, generally 2–4 days after release (range of 1–6 days)
- Atypical host characteristics: unexpected, unexplained cases of acute illness in previously healthy persons who rapidly develop severe, progressive multilobar pneumonia with hemoptysis and gastrointestinal symptoms
- Unusual geographic clustering: multiple cases in an urban area where naturally occurring plague is not endemic
- Absence of risk factors: patients lack plague exposure risk factors (e.g., recent flea bite; exposure to rodents, especially rabbits, squirrels, wood rat, chipmunk, or prairie dogs; scratches or bites from infected domestic cats)

Intentionally released *Y. pestis* strains may be altered to have enhanced virulence, antimicrobial resistance, or increased ability to evade vaccines and diagnostic tests.

Naturally Occurring Plague

RESERVOIRS

The natural reservoir for *Y. pestis* is primarily wild rodents. Around the world, the domestic rat has been associated with the most human cases; however, in the western United States, burrowing rodents (e.g., ground squirrels, rock squirrels, and prairie dogs) are the most important reservoir. Mammals that act as hosts include cats, goats, sheep, camels, and humans. Human plague cases often follow epizootics in local rodent populations.

MODE OF TRANSMISSION

Humans can become infected in a number of ways:

- bite of infected rat flea
- direct contact with infected draining buboes
- direct contact (including bites or scratches) with infected animals
- inhalation of respiratory droplets from pneumonic plague-infected humans or animals (within 2 meters)
- ingestion of bacteria (e.g., eating infected meat)

Human plague cases in nature are most commonly acquired from animal reservoirs via bites of the Oriental rat flea.

WORLDWIDE OCCURRENCE

The first recorded plague pandemic was the Justinian plague (541–767 AD), which caused approximately 100 million deaths and is thought to have contributed to the demise of the Roman Empire. The second pandemic, also known as the Black Death, lasted from the 14th to the 19th centuries and is estimated to have killed between a third and a half of Europe's population. The third and most recent pandemic began in 1894 in China and caused an estimated 12 million deaths. Recent outbreaks in humans have occurred in India (1994), Zambia (1996), Indonesia (1997), Algeria (2003), Uganda (2004), and the Congo (2005). Approximately 1800 worldwide cases of plague are reported annually to the World Health Organization (WHO), from all continents except Europe and Australia.

OCCURRENCE IN THE UNITED STATES

Ships carrying infected rats introduced plague to the Americas via the ports on the Pacific Ocean and Gulf of Mexico in the early 1900s. In San Francisco, urban rats passed along the disease to native rodent populations. Eventually, plague spread across the western half of the United States and has been found in the native rodent population, their fleas, and their predators. Naturally occurring plague generally occurs during the summer months in persons exposed to the reservoir. The last urban plague outbreak in the United States occurred in Los Angeles in 1925.

From 1990 to 2005, a median of 7 cases of plague per year were reported in the United States. In 2006, based on provisional data, there were 16 cases.

CLINICAL FEATURES

Human plague occurs in many forms, determined primarily by the route of infection. The most common forms of plague in humans are bubonic plague, septicemic plague, and pneumonic plague. These are presented in detail below.

Plague infection is a severe clinical illness that can be life-threatening. Case fatality rates vary based on the route of infection. Mortality was historically much higher with nearly 100% mortality for untreated septicemic and pneumonic plague and 50–60% mortality for untreated bubonic plague cases. Administration of appropriate antibiotic treatment within the first 18 to 24 hours has decreased mortality rates to 30–50% for septicemic plague, 5–15% for pneumonic plague, and less than 5% for bubonic plague. Thus, early administration of appropriate antibiotic treatment is critical, because poor outcomes occur with delays in seeking care and/or instituting effective antimicrobial treatment.

Pneumonic Plague

Primary pneumonic plague (Table 66.1) occurs when the organism is inhaled in respiratory droplets from infected humans or animals or in infectious aerosols accidentally or intentionally produced (e.g., spilled lab specimen or bioterrorism related release). Secondary pneumonic plague occurs when there is hematogenous spread of the organism to the lung. Primary pneumonic plague causes a more acute and fulminant disease. Pneumonic plague is not highly contagious, but transmission can occur with prolonged close contact (within 2 meters) with a coughing patient in the end stage of illness. In a recent outbreak in Uganda, 1.3 pneumonic plague transmissions per pneumonic plague case were reported. If untreated, pneumonic plague can spread and progress to septicemic plague.

Table 66.1 Clinical Features: Pneumonic Plague

Incubation Period	1–4 days, with a maximum of 6 days
Transmission	• Inhalation of contaminated aerosol • Inhalation of respiratory droplets from pneumonic plague-infected humans or animals (within 2 meters) • Secondary hematogenous spread to the lung
Signs and Symptoms	• Acute fever, chills, malaise, myalgia, headache • Productive cough, with sputum becoming more and more bloody • Chest pain, dyspnea, cyanosis • Tachypnea in children • Gastrointestinal symptoms
Progression and Complications	• Refractory pulmonary syndrome • Adult respiratory distress syndrome • Septicemia
Laboratory and Radiographic Findings	• Leukocytosis with left shift • Gram-negative bipolar bacilli on sputum smear • Elevated creatinine and abnormally high liver enzymes • CXR findings include alveolar infiltrates progressing to lobar consolidation, pleural effusion • Rarely, mediastinal widening on CXR due to adenopathy

CXR, chest x-ray.

Bubonic Plague

Yersinia pestis can cause bubonic plague (Table 66.2) in humans via the bite of an infected rodent flea. *Y. pestis* survives in the flea midgut after a blood meal from an infected host. The organism is transmitted to a new host when the flea regurgitates during its next feeding. *Y. pestis* migrates to regional lymph nodes where it causes hemorrhagic lymphadenitis, creating the swollen, painful buboes that are characteristic of bubonic plague (Figures 66.1 and 66.2). The organisms often enter the bloodstream, causing hemorrhagic lesions in distant lymph nodes and organs. If untreated, bubonic plague can spread and progress to pneumonic or septicemic plague. Approximately 80% of cases develop bacteremia, 25% develop clinical septicemia, and 10% develop pneumonia as a complication.

Septicemic Plague

In primary septicemic plague there is systemic sepsis caused by *Y. pestis*, but without noticeable, preceding lymph node or pulmonary involvement. Up to 25% of naturally occurring plague cases may present with primary septicemic plague (Figures 66.3 and 66.4). Secondary septicemic plague occurs commonly with either bubonic or pneumonic plague.

Septicemic plague causes a gram-negative sepsis syndrome with multiorgan involvement, disseminated intravascular coagulation (DIC), and shock (Table 66.3). In the late stages of infection, high-grade bacteremia often occurs, with identifiable organisms on peripheral blood smear. Meningitis can occur and is characterized by purulent cerebrospinal fluid (CSF).

Table 66.2 Clinical Features: Bubonic Plague

Incubation Period	1–8 days
Transmission	• Bite of infected rat flea • Direct contact with infected draining buboes • Direct contact (including bites or scratches) with infected animals
Signs and Symptoms	**Major:** • Sudden onset of chills, high fever, headache, lethargy • Buboes – swollen, red, painful lymph nodes in areas proximal to the inoculation site (e.g., inguinal, axillary or cervical areas) • Rapid pulse • Hypotension **Other:** • Gastrointestinal discomfort • Restlessness, confusion, lack of coordination • Skin lesion at the site of the flea bite occur in <10% of cases • Buboes may rupture and suppurate in second week
Progression and Complications	• Septicemia • Secondary pneumonic plague • Meningitis (rare)
Laboratory Findings	• Leukocytosis with left shift • Gram-negative bipolar bacilli on bubo aspirate smear • Elevated creatinine and abnormally high liver enzymes

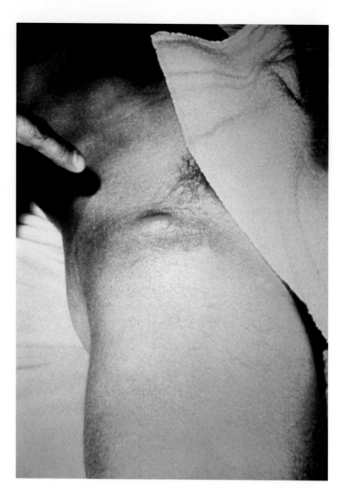

Figure 66.2 Inguinal bubo caused by plague infection. (From the U.S. Centers for Disease Control and Prevention Public Health Image Library at http://phil.cdc.gov/phil/home.asp.)

Other syndromes caused by *Y. pestis* infection include:

- **Plague meningitis**. Although it is generally a complication of other forms of plague, it can be the presenting clinical syndrome. Plague meningitis results from hematogenous spread of *Y. pestis* organisms and is characterized by purulent CSF exudates.
- **Plague pharyngitis**. Plague pharyngitis generally results from direct inoculation of the pharynx. Eating raw infected meat is a risk factor. Clinically, plague pharyngitis presents as a severe pharyngitis or tonsillitis with cervical adenitis.
- **Pestis minor**. Pestis minor is a milder form of bubonic plague. Lymph nodes drain and patients convalesce without treatment.

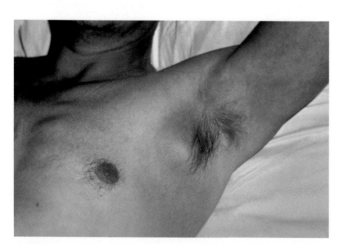

Figure 66.1 Axillary lymphadenopathy, or bubo, and edema caused by plague infection. (From the U.S. Centers for Disease Control and Prevention Public Health Image Library at http://phil.cdc.gov/phil/home.asp. Photograph taken in 1962 by Margaret Parsons and Dr. Karl F. Meyer.)

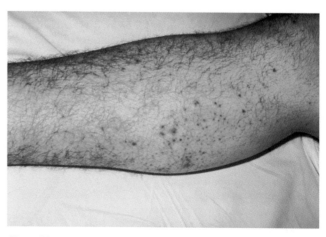

Figure 66.3 Skin hemorrhages due to capillary fragility on the leg of a person with plague. (From the U.S. Centers for Disease Control and Prevention Public Health Image Library at http://phil.cdc.gov/phil/home.asp.)

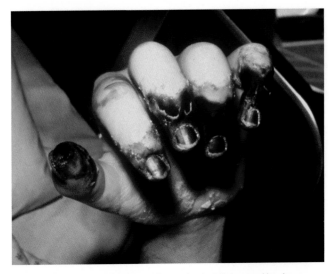

Figure 66.4 Acral necrosis due to abnormal coagulation caused by plague septicemia. (From the U.S. Centers for Disease Control and Prevention Public Health Image Library at http://phil.cdc.gov/phil/home.asp. Photograph taken in 1975 by Dr. Jack Poland.)

Table 66.3 Clinical Features: Septicemic Plague

Incubation Period	1–4 days
Transmission	Site of primary infection may be unknown
Signs and Symptoms	• Acute fever, chills, weakness, malaise • Gastrointestinal symptoms • Purpuric skin lesions and gangrene of the distal digits
Progression and Complications	• Disseminated intravascular coagulation • Shock • Multi-organ failure
Laboratory Findings	• Leukocytosis with left shift and toxic granulation • Gram-negative bipolar bacilli on blood smear • Disseminated intravascular coagulation • Elevated creatinine and abnormally high liver enzymes

DIFFERENTIAL DIAGNOSIS

The diagnosis of plague during the initial stages requires a high index of suspicion because of the nonspecific, flulike picture early in the course of disease. Early diagnosis is critical because prompt administration of antibiotics can decrease mortality.

Differential: Pneumonic Plague

Consider pneumonic plague in any case of severe gram-negative pneumonia.

Key features that may help to distinguish plague pneumonia are:

Primary pneumonic plague:

• rapid onset and rapid progression

Secondary pneumonic plague:

• presence of painful adenitis (buboes)

Primary or secondary pneumonic plague:

• no response to typical antibiotic therapy for community-acquired pneumonia
• hemoptysis in late stages of disease

Other conditions to consider are:

• bacterial pneumonia (*Mycoplasma, Legionella, Staphylococcus, Streptococcus, Haemophilus, Klebsiella, Moraxella*)
• viral pneumonia (influenza, respiratory syncytial virus [RSV], cytomegalovirus [CMV], hantavirus, severe acute respiratory syndrome [SARS])
• *Chlamydia* infection
• Q fever
• inhalation anthrax
• tularemia
• ricin
• rickettsial infections
• aerosolized exposure to staphylococcal enterotoxin B

Differential: Bubonic Plague

Key feature that may help to distinguish bubonic plague are:

• Presence of painful adenitis (buboes) progressing to systemic disease

Other conditions to consider are:

• cat scratch disease (*Bartonella*)
• ulceroglandular tularemia
• adenitis due to staphylococcal, streptococcal, or filarial infection
• tuberculosis
• nontuberculosis mycobacterial infection
• lymphogranuloma venereum
• capnocytophaga canimorsus infection
• chancroid
• primary genital herpes
• primary or secondary syphilis
• appendicitis
• strangulated inguinal or femoral hernia
• lymphadenopathy (secondary lymphoma, Kikuchi's lymphadenitis, systemic lupus erythematosus, toxoplasmosis, infectious mononucleosis)

Differential: Septicemic Plague

Key features that may help to distinguish septicemic plague are:

Primary septicemic plague:

• absence of painful adenitis (buboes) or pulmonary involvement

Secondary septicemic plague:

• presence of painful adenitis (buboes)

Other conditions to consider are:

• other gram-negative sepsis
• gram-positive sepsis (*Staphylococcus*)

- meningococcemia
- rickettsial infections
- malaria
- louse-borne relapsing fever
- appendicitis

LABORATORY AND RADIOGRAPHIC FINDINGS

Routine laboratory and radiographic findings for specific clinical presentations of plague are listed in the clinical features tables.

Initial identification of the organism relies on microscopic evaluation of infected tissue (blood, sputum, cerebrospinal fluid [CSF], or fluid aspirated from a bubo or skin lesion scraping). Staining of the infected tissue may reveal gram-negative bacilli (Gram stain) and bipolar staining (Wright, Giemsa, or Wayson stain).

Although recommended, culture and isolation may be difficult. Blood and site-specific specimens should be collected prior to antibiotic administration as sterilization can occur rapidly. *Y. pestis* is slow-growing in culture and may not demonstrate growth until 48 hours after inoculation. Also, many commercial bacterial identification systems may misidentify *Y. pestis*. To improve yield and ensure biosafety precautions, clinicians should notify laboratory personnel when plague is suspected.

Although rapid diagnostic tests are not widely available, the public health laboratory system may have rapid diagnostic testing on clinical specimens (e.g., polymerase chain reaction [PCR] or direct fluorescent antibody testing for *Y. pestis* F1 antigen).

TREATMENT AND PROPHYLAXIS
Treatment

Supportive care and timely administration of antibiotics are the keys to successful management of plague (Table 66.4). Plague pneumonia is often fatal if antibiotics are not begun within 12–24 hours of symptoms. Many patients will require intensive care with respiratory support because of complications of gram-negative sepsis.

Resistant strains may either occur naturally or be engineered. In 1995, two distinct strains of naturally occurring antibiotic-resistant *Y. pestis* were isolated from human cases of bubonic plague in Madagascar. One strain was resistant to all drugs recommended for plague treatment and prophylaxis, and the other had high-level resistance to streptomycin. Both patients recovered with oral trimethoprim-sulfamethoxazole and intramuscular injections of streptomycin. In addition, in vitro resistance has been seen to imipenem and rifampin.

Contained casualty setting: The Working Group recommends parenteral antimicrobial therapy when individual medical management is available. Antibiotics should be administered to all patients for 10 days. Therapy may be switched to oral antimicrobials when clinically indicated.

Mass casualty setting: Replacement with oral antibiotics may be needed if the number of patients exceeds the medical care capacity for individual medical management.

Postexposure Prophylaxis

Postexposure prophylaxis is the administration of antibiotics after suspected exposure to plague has occurred but before symptoms are present. If symptoms are present, see section above on treatment. Persons thought to have had an infective exposure should receive postexposure prophylaxis. Infective exposures include household, hospital, or other close contact (less than 2 meters) with a person suspected or confirmed to have pneumonic plague who has received no treatment, less than 48 hours of antimicrobial therapy, or more than 48 hours of antimicrobial therapy without clinical improvement. Postexposure prophylaxis may be recommended for persons exposed to intentional aerosol releases. In such an event, public health authorities will provide guidance. Regardless of whether postexposure prophylaxis is recommended or taken, persons potentially exposed should be observed for fever or cough for 7 days after exposure. Any potentially exposed person who develops a fever or cough should seek prompt medical attention and begin treatment. Quarantine is not currently recommended.

Vaccination

Current killed whole cell vaccines have been in use for military personnel and have been shown to generate cell-mediated responses lasting at least 15 years; however, they require repeat dosing with adjuvants, have questionable protection against respiratory infections, and are reactogenic. Vaccine production has been discontinued in the United States. Microencapsulated subunit vaccines (of F1 and V proteins) requiring only single-dose administration are under development and show the most promise against aerosol exposures.

COMPLICATIONS AND ADMISSION CRITERIA

Whereas primary pneumonic plague results from direct inhalation of plague bacilli, secondary pneumonic plague can manifest as a complication in patients with bubonic plague. Hematogenous dissemination of *Y. pestis* results in plague septicemia, which can be complicated by septic shock, disseminated intravascular coagulation, necrosis of small vessels, and purpuric skin lesions. Plague meningitis due to hematogenous seeding of the meninges occurs infrequently.

Patients with suspected or confirmed pneumonic or bubonic plague require hospitalization for intravenous antibiotics, supportive care, and close monitoring for decompensation and signs of toxemia.

INFECTION CONTROL

Clinicians should notify local public health authorities, their institution's infection control professional, and their laboratory of any suspected plague cases. Public health authorities may conduct epidemiological investigations and implement disease control interventions to protect the public. Infection control professionals will guide and enforce implementation of infection control precautions within the health care setting. Laboratory personnel should take appropriate biosafety precautions.

Although not highly contagious, plague can be transmitted person-to-person via respiratory droplets. Both the Healthcare

Table 66.4 Plague: Treatment and Postexposure Prophylaxis Recommendations[1]

		Contained Casualty Setting	Mass Casualty Setting	Postexposure Prophylaxis
Duration of Prescription		10 days	10 days	7 days
Adult	Preferred	streptomycin, 1 g IM q12h *or* gentamicin,[2] 5 mg/kg IM or IV q24h, or 2 mg/kg loading dose followed by 1.7 mg/kg IM or IV q8h	doxycycline, 100 mg PO bid *or* ciprofloxacin, 500 mg PO bid
	Alternative[8]		doxycycline,[5,6] 100 mg IV q12h or 200 mg IV q24h *or* ciprofloxacin, 400 mg IV q12h *or* chloramphenicol,[3] 25 mg/kg IV q6h (max 4 g/day)	chloramphenicol,[3] 25 mg/kg PO qid (max 4 g/day)
Children	Preferred	streptomycin, 15 mg/kg IM q12h (max 2 g/day) *or* gentamicin,[2] 2.5 mg/kg IM or IV q8h	doxycycline[5,6]: ≥ 45 kg, give adult dosage <45 kg, give 2.2 mg/kg PO bid (max 200 mg/day) *or* ciprofloxacin,[5,7] 20 mg/kg PO bid (max 1 g/day)
	Alternative[8]		doxycycline[5,6]: ≥ 45 kg, give adult dosage <45 kg, give 2.2 mg/kg IV q12h (max 200 mg/day) *or* ciprofloxacin,[5,7] 15 mg/kg IV q12h (max 1 g/day) *or* chloramphenicol,[3,4] 25 mg/kg IV q6h (max 4 g/day)	chloramphenicol,[3,4] 25 mg/kg PO qid (max 4 g/day)
Pregnant Women	Preferred	gentamicin,[2] 5 mg/kg IM or IV q24h or 2 mg/kg loading dose followed by 1.7 mg/kg IM or IV q8h	doxycycline,[5,6] 100 mg PO bid *or* ciprofloxacin,[5] 500 mg PO bid
	Alternative[8]		doxycycline,[5,6] 100 mg IV q12h or 200 mg IV q24h *or* ciprofloxacin,[5] 400 mg IV q12h	chloramphenicol,[3,4] 25 mg/kg PO qid

For plague meningitis, pleuritis, or myocarditis: Chloramphenicol should be used for 21 days for conditions when tissue penetration is important. Irreversible marrow aplasia is rare (1 in 40,000 patients).
[1] Treatment recommendations come from the Working Group of Civilian Biodefense and may not necessarily be approved by the U.S. Food and Drug Administration.
[2] Aminoglycoside doses must be further adjusted for newborns, and according to renal function.
[3] Therapeutic concentration is 5–20 µg/mL; concentrations >25 µg/mL can cause reversible bone marrow suppression.
[4] According to the Working Group on Civilian Biodefense, children younger than 2 years of age should not receive chloramphenicol because of risk of "gray baby syndrome"; however, the American Academy of Pediatrics has recommended chloramphenicol as the drug of choice for plague meningitis in children.
[5] Tetracycline and quinolone antibiotics are generally not recommended during pregnancy or childhood; however, their use may be indicated for life-threatening illness.
[6] Ciprofloxacin may be preferred in pregnant women and children up to 8 years of age because of the known adverse event profile of doxycycline (e.g., tooth discoloration).
[7] Doxycylcine may be preferred in children 8 years and older because of the adverse event profile of ciprofloxacin (e.g., arthropathies).
[8] Trimethoprim-sulfamethoxazole has been successfully used to treat plague; however, the Working Group considers this a second-tier choice.

Infection Control Practices Advisory Committee of the CDC and the Working Group on Civilian Biodefense recommend Droplet and Standard Precautions for patients with suspected or confirmed pneumonic plague. These precautions should be maintained until 48 hours of appropriate antibiotics have been administered *and* the patient shows clinical improvement. Close contacts of pneumonic plague patients should be identified, receive prophylaxis, and be monitored for symptoms. For patients with suspected or confirmed bubonic plague or other nonpneumonic plague syndromes, Standard Precautions are recommended. Aerosol-generating procedures should be avoided if possible. Routine laboratory procedures should be carried out under Biosafety Level-2 conditions; however, manipulation of cultures or other activities that may produce aerosol or droplets (e.g., centrifuging, grinding, vig-orous shaking, and animal studies) require Biosafety Level-3 conditions.

Decontamination

In general, environmental decontamination following an aerosol event has not been recommended, because experts have estimated that an aerosol of *Y. pestis* organism would be infectious for only about 1 hour. A recent study demonstrated that *Y. pestis* can survive on selected environmental surfaces for at least several days; however, the potential for re-aerosolization of these organisms was not addressed. Commercially available bleach or 0.5% hypochlorite solution (1:10 dilution of household bleach) is considered adequate for cleaning and decontamination. All persons exposed to an aerosol containing *Y. pestis* should be instructed to wash body surfaces and clothing with soap and water.

PEARLS AND PITFALLS

1. Bubonic plague is not transmitted directly from one human to another in the absence of lymph node suppuration and drainage. Persons with bubonic plague become more infectious as *Y. pestis* organisms reach the lungs via hematogenous spread. Once pneumonic plague develops, transmission occurs via direct contact with respiratory secretions or inhalation of respiratory droplets.
2. Clinical clues pointing toward a diagnosis of primary pneumonic plague are sudden onset of headache, malaise, and fever, fulminant pneumonitis with rapid progression from dry cough to tachypnea, dyspnea, and productive cough, and in the late stage of disease, hemoptysis with copious amounts of bright red sputum.

REFERENCES

Begier EM, Asiki G, Anywaine Z, et al. Pneumonic plague cluster, Uganda, 2004. Emerg Infect Dis 2006;12(3):460–7.

Bin Saeed AA, Al-Hamdan NA, Fontaine RE. Plague from eating raw camel liver. Emerg Infect Dis 2005;11(9):1456–7.

Brouillard JE, Terriff CM, Tofan A, et al. Antibiotic selection and resistance issues with fluoroquinolones and doxycycline against bioterrorism agents. Pharmacotherapy 2006;26(1):3–14.

Centers for Disease Control and Prevention (CDC). Human plague – four states, 2006. MMWR 2006;55(34): 940–3.

Cono J, Cragan JD, Jamieson DJ, et al. Prophylaxis and treatment of pregnant women for emerging infections and bioterrorism emergencies. Emerg Infect Dis 2006;12(11):1631–7.

Drancourt M, Houhamdi L, Raoult D. *Yersinia pestis* as a telluric, human ectoparasite-borne organism. Lancet Infect Dis 2006;6(4):234–41.

Elvin SJ, Eyles JE, Howard KA, et al. Protection against bubonic and pneumonic plague with a single dose microencapsulated sub-unit vaccine. Vaccine 2006;24(20):4433–9.

Franz DR, Jahrling PB, Friedlander AM, et al. Clinical recognition and management of patients exposed to biological warfare agents. JAMA 1997;278(5):399–411.

Galimand M, Carniel E, Courvalin P. Resistance of *Yersinia pestis* to antimicrobial agents. Antimicrob Agents Chemother 2006;50(10):3233–6.

Koirala J. Plague: disease, management, and recognition of act of terrorism. Infect Dis Clin North Am 2006;20(2):273–87, viii.

Kool JL. Risk of person-to-person transmission of pneumonic plague. Clin Infect Dis 2005;40(8):1166–72.

Mwengee W, Butler T, Mgema S, et al. Treatment of plague with gentamicin or doxycycline in a randomized clinical trial in Tanzania. Clin Infect Dis 2006;42(5):614–21.

Rose LJ, Donlan R, Banerjee SN, et al., Survival of *Yersinia pestis* on environmental surfaces. Appl Environ Microbiol 2003;69(4):2166–71.

ADDITIONAL READINGS

Borio LL. Plague as an agent of bioterrorism. In: Mandell GL, Bennett JE, Dolin R, eds, Principles and practice of infectious diseases (6th ed). New York: Churchill Livingstone, 2005.

Butler T, Dennis DT. *Yersinia* species including plague. In: Mandell GL, Bennett JE, Dolin R, eds, Principles and practice of infectious diseases (6th ed). New York: Churchill Livingstone, 2005.

Center for Infectious Disease Research and Policy (CIDRAP). Plague: current, comprehensive information on pathogenesis, microbiology, epidemiology, diagnosis, treatment, and prophylaxis. Retrieved March 5, 2007, from http://www.cidrap.umn.edu/cidrap/content/bt/plague.

Inglesby TV, Dennis DT, Henderson DA, et al. Plague as a biological weapon: medical and public health management. Working Group on Civilian Biodefense. JAMA 2000;283(17):2281–90.

67. Smallpox

David M. Stier, Nikkita Patel, Olivia Bruch, and Karen A. Holbrook

INTRODUCTION

Smallpox is caused by variola viruses, which are large, enveloped, single-stranded DNA viruses of the Poxvirus family and the *Orthopoxvirus* genus. Variola major strains cause three forms of disease (ordinary, flat type, and hemorrhagic), whereas variola minor strains cause a less severe form of smallpox. Vaccination with vaccinia virus, another member of the *Orthopoxvirus* genus, protects humans against smallpox because of the high antibody cross-neutralization between orthopoxviruses.

The Working Group for Civilian Biodefense considers smallpox a dangerous potential biological weapon because of "its case-fatality-rate of 30% or more among unvaccinated persons and the absence of specific therapy." Of the potential ways in which smallpox could be used as a biological weapon, an aerosol release is expected to have the most severe medical and public health outcomes because of the virus's stability in aerosol form, low infectious dose, and high rate of secondary transmission. A single case of smallpox would be a public health emergency.

EPIDEMIOLOGY

Smallpox as a Biological Weapon

Smallpox has been used as a biological weapon in the distant past and has recently been a focus of bioweapons research. In the 18th century, British troops in North America gave smallpox-infected blankets to their enemies, who went on to suffer severe outbreaks. Defecting Russian scientists describe covert Russian operations during the 1970s and 1980s that focused on the development of more virulent smallpox strains and of missiles and bombs that could release smallpox.

Aerosol release of virus (such as into a transportation hub) would likely result in a high number of cases. Other possibilities include use of "human vectors" (i.e., persons who have been deliberately infected with smallpox) and use of fomites (e.g., contamination of letters sent through the mail).

Smallpox is of concern as a biological weapon because:

- much of the population (80%) is susceptible to infection
- the virus has a low infectious dose and carries a high morbidity and mortality
- a vaccine without significant side effects is not yet available for general use
- experience has shown that introduction of the virus creates havoc and panic

An outbreak of disease caused by an intentional release of smallpox would likely involve multiple temporally and spatially clustered cases presenting with fever and rash on the face, arms, and legs. Onset of symptoms would be expected days after exposure to the virus.

Naturally Occurring Smallpox

RESERVOIRS

The natural reservoir for smallpox was humans with disease; there was no chronic carrier state. In 1980, the World Health Organization (WHO) declared smallpox eradicated from the world and recommended destruction or transfer all remaining stocks to one of two WHO reference labs, the Centers for Disease Control and Prevention (CDC) in Atlanta, Georgia, and the former Institute of Virus Preparations (later transferred to the Vector Institute) in Russia. Since eradication, there is no natural reservoir for smallpox. Presently, smallpox is officially found only in these designated reference laboratories.

MODE OF TRANSMISSION

Historically, humans were infected in a number of ways:

- inhalation of droplet nuclei or aerosols originating from the mouths of smallpox-infected humans
- direct contact with skin lesions or infected body fluids of smallpox-infected humans
- direct contact with contaminated clothing or bed linens

WORLDWIDE OCCURRENCE

In 1967, a WHO-led international campaign of mass vaccination, surveillance and outbreak containment was started in order to eradicate smallpox. In 1977, the last community-acquired smallpox case was reported in Somalia, and in 1978, a laboratory accident in England caused the last human case.

OCCURRENCE IN THE UNITED STATES

The last case of smallpox in the United States occurred in the Rio Grande Valley of Texas in 1949. The risk of disease was low enough to end routine vaccination of the U.S. population in 1971. Vaccination is currently required for most military personnel and is recommended for select health care and emergency workers, described below. Because of the relative frequency and seriousness of vaccine-related complications and the low risk of smallpox outbreak in the United States, routine vaccination is not recommended for the vast majority of health care workers or for the general U.S. population.

In 2002, the CDC recommended pre-event vaccination for local smallpox response teams, consisting of public health, medical, nursing, and public safety personnel, who would conduct investigation and management of initial smallpox cases. As of July 31, 2004, 39,579 health care workers and first responders had been vaccinated nationally.

CLINICAL FEATURES

Historically, smallpox has been divided into variola major and variola minor based on severity of clinical disease. Variola major was more common and more severe. The case mortality was 15–45% for variola major and 1% for variola minor.

The infectious dose for smallpox is a few virions. The virus typically enters the body via respiratory or oral mucosa and is carried by macrophages to regional lymph nodes from which a primary asymptomatic viremia develops on the 3rd or 4th day after infection. The reticuloendothelial organs are invaded and overwhelmed leading to a secondary viremia around the 8th–12th day after infection. Toxemia and fever onset follow. Seven to 17 days following infection, fever, malaise, and extreme exhaustion begin. A maculopapular rash first presents on the face, mouth, pharynx, and forearms and spreads to the trunks and legs (Figure 67.1). The rash progresses to a vesicular and pustular stage (round and deeply embedded). Scabs form on the 8th day of the rash. Scars are formed from sebaceous gland destruction and granulation tissue shrinking and fibrosis.

Although most data support communicability with rash onset, some low level of communicability is present prior to rash because viral shedding from oral lesions occurs during the 1–2 days of fever preceding rash onset. However, secondary transmission peaks 3–6 days after fever onset (1st week after rash onset), and 91.1% of secondary cases occur by the 9th day after fever onset (Figure 67.2). The period of communicability ends when all the scabs have fallen off. Scabs are not very infectious because the tight binding of the fibrin matrix retains the virions; however, secondary cases have been documented through transmission from direct contact with contaminated clothing and bedding.

Secondary bacterial infection and other organ involvement are uncommon. Encephalitis is a possible complication. Mortality is most commonly associated with toxemia of circulating immune complexes and soluble variola antigens and is seen in the second week of illness. Approximately 30–80% of unvaccinated close contacts will develop the disease. In addition, 3.5–6 transmissions per smallpox case are estimated.

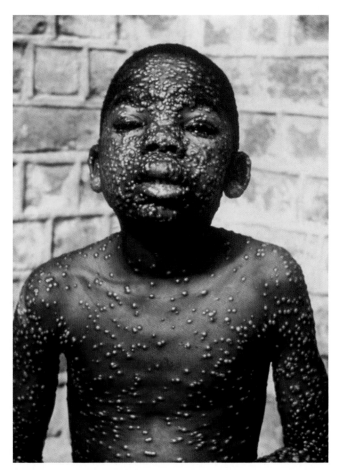

Figure 67.1 Typical distribution of smallpox, with concentration on the face and arms, is seen on this African child. From the U.S. Centers for Disease Control and Prevention Public Health Image Library.

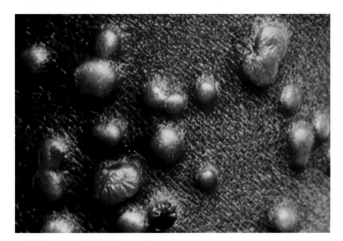

Figure 67.2 Smallpox pustules on day 6 of the rash, located on the thigh of the patient. From the U.S. Centers for Disease Control and Prevention Public Health Image Library.

Variola Major

Variola major is associated with the most severe disease and presents with distinct clinical syndromes:

- ordinary (80% or more of cases; mortality is 30% in unvaccinated and 3% in vaccinated patients; see Table 67.1)
- flat (4–6% of cases; mortality is 95% in unvaccinated and 66% in vaccinated patients)

Table 67.1 Clinical Features: Ordinary Variola Major

Incubation Period	10–13 days (range 7–19 days)
Transmission	• Inhalation of droplet nuclei or aerosols originating from the mouths of smallpox-infected humans • Direct contact with skin lesions or infected body fluids of smallpox-infected humans • Direct contact with contaminated clothing or bed linens
Signs and Symptoms	Prodromal phase: • 2–4 days of fever, chills, headache, backache, and often GI symptoms Rash phase: • Enanthem (papules, vesicles, then ulcers) of oropharyngeal mucosa beginning 1 day before skin lesions appear • First skin lesions ("herald spots") are often on the face • Lesions spread centrifugally: trunk to proximal extremities to distal extremities • Palms and soles are usually involved, and truncal rash is usually sparse • Lesion progression: maculopapular (days 1–2), vesicular (days 3–5), pustular (days 7–14) • Vesicles and pustules are frequently umbilicated • Pustules can be like small, embedded hard balls or "shotty" • Lesions tend to progress at same rate • Lesions may be discrete, semiconfluent, or confluent • Lesions are typically painful and cause pitted scars as they heal • Lesions gradually scab over during days 13–18
Progression and Complications	• Viral bronchitis or pneumonitis • Third spacing of fluid with resulting electrolyte and renal abnormalities • Skin desquamation • Secondary bacterial infection, particularly skin and pulmonary • Spontaneous abortion, stillbirth • Rarely: blindness, keratitis, corneal ulceration, encephalitis, osteomyelitis or arthritis, orchitis • Death may occur during 2nd week of illness, from high-level viremia and circulating immune complexes
Laboratory Findings	Lymphocytopenia and/or granulocytopenia

GI, gastrointestinal.

• hemorrhagic (2–3% of cases; mortality is 99% in unvaccinated and 94% in vaccinated patients)
• modified (13% of cases and low risk of death)
• variola sine eruptione (30–50% of vaccinated contacts of smallpox and low risk of death)

Other forms of smallpox caused by variola major infection include:

Flat-type smallpox (also known as *malignant smallpox*) occurred in about 4–6% of cases and more frequently in children. It is associated with a late, deficient cellular immune response. It is characterized by a short incubation period, incapacitating prodromal illness, severe systemic toxicity, and high mortality (90–97%). The lesions do not progress to the pustular stage, instead remaining soft, velvety, and flattened.

If the patient survives, the lesions will resolve by desquamation without scabs or scarring.

Hemorrhagic smallpox occurred in about 2–3% of cases. Pregnant women are highly susceptible. Similar to flat-type smallpox, it is associated with a defective immune response. It is characterized by a short incubation period, incapacitating prodromal illness, severe systemic toxicity, and high mortality (96%). The rash begins as a dusky erythema, followed by extensive petechiae, mucosal hemorrhage, and intense toxemia. Thrombocytopenia and coagulopathy may be present. These patients usually died during week 1 of illness, often before the development of the typical pox lesions.

Modified smallpox occurred in about 13% of cases. It occurred in persons with some immunity. The pre-eruptive illness is typical in duration and severity as ordinary smallpox; however, during the eruption, fever is absent and the skin lesions are superficial, pleomorphic, fewer in number, and evolve rapidly.

Variola sine eruption occurred in about 30–50% of vaccinated contacts of smallpox cases. It is characterized by a sudden onset of fever, headache, occasional backache that resolves within 48 hours, influenza-like symptoms, and no rash.

Variola Minor

Variola minor, caused by different strains of variola, is a milder form of smallpox. Compared with variola major, there are milder constitutional symptoms, discrete lesions that evolve a bit more rapidly, lower rates of hemorrhagic disease, and only rare fatal outcomes (<1%). The illness may be difficult to distinguish clinically from modified smallpox and variola without eruption. In the 1890s, variola minor spread from South Africa to Florida. In the early 1900s, variola minor became prevalent in the United States, Latin America, and Europe.

DIFFERENTIAL DIAGNOSIS

The characteristic features of smallpox need to be differentiated from other illnesses that present with vesicular or pustular rash. In particular, chicken pox (varicella) may be differentiated clinically as shown in Table 67.2.

Monkeypox may also be confused with smallpox. In 2003, an outbreak of monkeypox, associated with prairie dog contact, occurred in the midwestern United States. Monkeypox in humans presents similarly to ordinary smallpox. However, monkeypox is milder and has prominent lymphadenopathy and a shorter duration of rash.

The CDC has outlined criteria for determining the risk of smallpox when evaluating patients with generalized vesicular or pustular rash (Table 67.3): http://www.bt.cdc.gov/agent/smallpox/diagnosis/riskalgorithm/index.asp.

Additional considerations in the differential diagnosis of smallpox include:

Macular/papular stage:

• measles
• scarlet fever
• rubella

Vesicular/pustular stage:

• disseminated herpes zoster
• disseminated herpes simplex
• molluscum contagiosum

Table 67.2 Clinical Differentiation of Variola Versus Varicella

Feature	Variola	Varicella
Prodrome	• Duration: 2–4 days • Fever, chills, headache, backache, often GI symptoms	• Commonly does not occur • If present, mild symptoms and duration of 1 day
Rash Distribution	• Centrifugal: more dense on face and distal extremities • Frequently involves palms and soles • More involvement of back than abdomen	• Centripetal: more dense on trunk • Spares palms and soles • Back and abdomen equally involved
Lesion Evolution	• Usually appear on oropharyngeal mucosa first, then all over within 1–2 days • Progress at same rate; at any point in time, lesions are at same stage of evolution • Lesions progress slowly (7–14 days) from macules to papules to vesicles to pustules to scabs	• Lesions appear in crops • At any point in time, crops of lesions are at different stages of evolution • Lesions progress quickly (1–2 days) from macules to papules to vesicles to scabs
Lesion Attributes	• May be semiconfluent or confluent • Deep • May be umbilicated • Often painful; pruritic only as scabs	• Usually discrete • Superficial • Rarely found on palms and soles • Do not umbilicate or dimple • Typically painless; intensely pruritic

GI, gastrointestinal.

Table 67.3 Risk of Smallpox in Patients with Generalized Vesicular or Pustular Rash

High	All three major criteria present: a. *Febrile prodrome* 1–4 days before rash onset, with fever >101°F, plus *1 or more* of the following: weakness, headache, backache, chills, vomiting, severe abdominal pain b. *Classic smallpox lesions* present (vesicles or pustules that are deep-seated, firm or hard, round, and well-circumscribed; sharply raised and feel like BB pellets under the skin; may become umbilicated or confluent as they evolve) c. Lesions on any one part of the body are in the *same stage of development*
Moderate	Febrile prodrome as in (a) above, plus *either* (b) or (c) above *or* Febrile prodrome as in (a) above, plus *at least four* of the following minor criteria: • Centrifugal distribution • First lesions appeared on the oral mucosa/palate, face, or forearms • Patient appears toxic or moribund • Slow evolution of lesions from macules to papules to pustules over several days • Lesions on the palms and soles
Low	No viral prodrome *or* Febrile prodrome as in (a) above, plus <4 minor criteria above

Source: Centers for Disease Control and Prevention (www.bt.cdc.gov/agent/smallpox/diagnosis/rashtestingprotocol.asp).

• bullous pemphigoid
• impetigo (*Streptococcus, Staphylococcus*)
• human monkey pox

Either stage:

• erythema multiforme major (Stevens-Johnson syndrome)
• miscellaneous drug eruptions
• secondary syphilis
• enteroviral infection (hand, foot and mouth disease)
• chickenpox
• contact dermatitis
• generalized vaccinia (secondary to vaccination or exposure)
• acne
• scabies/insect bites

Hemorrhagic smallpox may resemble:

• meningococcemia
• rickettsial infections
• gram-negative septicemia

Flat-type smallpox may resemble:

• hemorrhagic chickenpox

LABORATORY AND RADIOGRAPHIC FINDINGS

The diagnosis of smallpox requires a high index of suspicion because the disease has been eradicated and its clinical presentation is similar to other pox viruses. Routine laboratory findings for specific clinical presentations of smallpox are listed in the Table 67.1. Radiographic findings do not assist in identification of smallpox.

Diagnosis of smallpox will be clinical initially, but followed by laboratory confirmation. Once smallpox has been confirmed in a geographic area, additional cases can be diagnosed clinically, and specimen testing can be reserved for specific cases in which the clinical presentation is unclear or to assist with law enforcement activities.

Clinicians should use the CDC-developed tools to assess the likelihood that patients with acute generalized vesicular or pustular rash illnesses have smallpox (above and http://www.bt.cdc.gov/agent/smallpox/diagnosis/evalposter.asp). CDC has also developed algorithms for laboratory evaluation of suspect smallpox cases based on the likelihood of disease (http://www.bt.cdc.gov/agent/smallpox/diagnosis/rashtestingprotocol.asp). If a patient is determined to be at high risk for smallpox, clinicians should call their local public health authorities immediately and obtain photos of the patient. Public health will provide guidance on specimen collection and packaging and will facilitate transport of specimens to the appropriate public health laboratory.

Multiple tests will be used to evaluate for smallpox: polymerase chain reaction (PCR) testing, electron microscopic examination of vesicular or pustular fluid or scabs, direct examination of vesicular or pustular material looking for inclusion bodies (Guarnieri's bodies), culture on egg chorioal-lantoic membrane, tissue culture, strain analysis with a restriction fragment length polymorphism assay, and serology. Definitive laboratory identification and characterization of the variola virus requires several days.

TREATMENT AND PROPHYLAXIS

Treatment

The management of confirmed or suspected cases of small-pox consists of supportive care, with careful attention to electrolyte and volume status, and ventilatory and hemodynamic support. General supportive measures include ensuring adequate fluid intake (difficult because of the enanthema), alleviation of pain and fever, and keeping skin lesions clean to prevent bacterial superinfection.

Currently there are no antiviral agents with proven activity against smallpox in humans.

Antiviral agents that have shown some activity in vitro against poxviruses may be available from the CDC under an investigational protocol. Additionally, cidofovir, a nucleoside analogue DNA polymerase inhibitor, might be useful if administered within 1–2 days after exposure; however, there is no evidence that it would be more effective than vaccination, and it has to be administered intravenously and causes renal toxicity.

Immunity from Prior Vaccination

Protection from smallpox is estimated to last between 5 and 10 years after primary vaccination and longer for variola minor than for variola major. Those who were previously vaccinated may retain some protection that could decrease the severity of the disease.

Postexposure Prophylaxis

Postexposure prophylaxis for smallpox is the administration of vaccinia vaccine after suspected exposure to smallpox has occurred but before symptoms are present. Immunity generally develops within 8 to 11 days after vaccination with vaccinia virus. Because the incubation period for smallpox averages about 12 days, vaccination within 4 days may confer some immunity to exposed persons and reduce the likelihood of a fatal outcome. Postexposure vaccination may be particularly important for those vaccinated in the past, provided that revaccination is able to boost the anamnestic immune response. In addition to vaccination, exposed persons should be monitored for symptoms. Temperature should be checked once a day, preferably in the evening, for 17 days after exposure to evaluate for fever (over 38°C).

If a case or cases of smallpox occur, public health authorities will conduct surveillance and implement containment strategies. Ring vaccination will be important and includes identification of contacts of cases and provision of prophylaxis and guidance on monitoring for symptoms. Large-scale voluntary vaccination may be offered to low-risk populations to supplement and address public concerns.

Vaccine Supply, Administration, and Efficacy

The smallpox vaccine used in the United States (formerly Dryvax, now ACAM2000) is a lyophilized (freeze-dried) preparation of live attenuated vaccinia virus, an *Orthopoxvirus* closely related to cowpox that induces antibodies that are protective against smallpox. The ACAM2000 vaccine uses vaccinia virus derived from the Dryvax vaccine via plaque purification cloning. The virus is then grown in African green monkey (Vero) cells. The ACAM2000 preparation also contains HEPES, human serum albumin, mannitol, and trace amounts of neomycin and polymixin B. The diluent contains glycerin and a phenol preservative.

Production of the Dryvax vaccine stopped in the 1980s. Acambis currently makes the ACAM2000 vaccine, which received FDA approval in September 2007. By that time 192.5 million doses of ACAM2000 vaccine were already in the U.S. stockpile. All lots of Dryvax vaccine expired February 29, 2008, and were destroyed by March 31, 2008.

Technique: The vaccine should be administered by trained, vaccinated personnel using a bifurcated needle and scarification technique. Vaccinees are instructed to keep the site dry and covered, to avoid touching the site, and to thoroughly launder or carefully discard any materials that come into contact with the site. *Should smallpox vaccination be deemed necessary, it will be coordinated by local, state, and federal health agencies.* For additional information on vaccine administration, see http://www.bt.cdc.gov/agent/smallpox/vaccination.

Vaccine Contraindications and Complications

The ACAM2000 and Dryvax vaccines have similar safety profiles. Both have serious complications. Likelihood of adverse effects is 3- to 4-fold higher in infants and in primary vaccine recipients. Based on the U.S. Vaccine Adverse Events Reporting System of recently vaccinated people, there was a rate of 26.4 serious adverse events per 10,000 vaccinees. Adverse events included the following: 33% cardiac, 25% nonspecific chest pain, 21% neurological, 14% infection, 3% malignancy, 3% pulmonary (noninfectious), and 1% normal vaccination response.

Vaccination during the pre-exposure period is contraindicated for certain persons. During a smallpox emergency, however, all contraindications would be reviewed in the context of the risk of smallpox exposure, and updated recommendations would be issued by public health authorities. Current contraindications to vaccination are as follows (see http://www.bt.cdc.gov/agent/smallpox/vaccination for further description):

- past or present eczema or atopic dermatitis (risk of eczema vaccinatum)
- other acute or chronic exfoliative skin conditions (e.g., burns, impetigo, chicken pox, contact dermatitis, shingles, herpes, severe acne, psoriasis), until the condition resolves
- immunodeficiency states, due to disease or treatment of disease
- pregnancy (vaccination may offer partial protection for mother, but increases risk of fetal vaccinia)
- breastfeeding
- hypersensitivity to vaccine components

- under 18 years of age in nonemergency situations
- having a household contact who is immunodeficient, who has past or present eczema or atopic dermatitis, or who has an acute, chronic, or exfoliative skin condition
- physician-diagnosed cardiac disease, or three or more major risk factors for cardiac disease

Well-documented *adverse reactions to vaccination* are listed below:

- tenderness, erythema, or other localized reactions at the injection site
- systemic symptoms of fever, malaise, myalgias, local lymphadenopathy
- dermatologic reactions, including erythema multiforme and Stevens-Johnson syndrome, urticaria, exanthems, contact dermatitis, and erythematous papules
- secondary bacterial infections at injection site
- focal and generalized suppurative folliculitis (without evidence of viral infection; may be mistaken for generalized vaccinia)
- inadvertent autoinoculation of another body site (most common sites are face, eyelid, nose, mouth, genitalia, rectum)
- generalized vaccinia: vesicles or pustules appearing distant from the vaccination site
- eczema vaccinatum: localized or dissemination of vaccinia virus; usually mild but may be severe and fatal
- vaccinia keratitis
- progressive vaccinia: progressive necrosis in vaccination area, often with metastatic sites; can be severe and fatal
- postvaccinial encephalitis
- fetal vaccinia: occurs when mother is vaccinated during pregnancy; usually results in premature birth or miscarriage
- myopericarditis, identified among military personnel vaccinated between December 2002 and December 2003
- death: 1.1 deaths per 1 million primary vaccine recipients
- contact vaccinia: transmission of vaccinia virus from newly vaccinated persons to susceptible unvaccinated contacts

The primary therapy for adverse reactions to smallpox vaccination is vaccinia immunoglobulin (VIG). However VIG is contraindicated in vaccinia keratitis and provides no benefit in postvaccinial encephalitis. VIG is manufactured from the plasma of persons vaccinated with vaccinia vaccine. An intravenous preparation (VIGIV) was recently licensed by the FDA. Cidofovir and topical ophthalmic antiviral agents are also recommended by some experts. Cidofovir use requires an Investigational New Drug (IND) protocol, and topical ophthalmic agent use is off-label.

COMPLICATIONS AND ADMISSION CRITERIA

Before smallpox was eradicated worldwide, viral bronchitis and pneumonitis were the most frequent complications of ordinary-type smallpox. Cutaneous complications included desquamation, massive subcutaneous fluid accumulation with electrolyte abnormalities and renal failure, or, less commonly, secondary bacterial infection of smallpox lesions. Infrequently, smallpox patients experienced encephalitis, osteomyelitis, corneal ulceration, or ocular keratitis. Ordinary-type smallpox with confluent lesions, rather than discrete lesions, carried a much higher risk of massive exfoliation, tissue destruction, bacterial sepsis, and death. Hemorrhagic-type and flat-type smallpox were nearly always fatal.

Many patients do not require hospitalization. Those with discrete lesions, nonhemorrhagic and non-flat-type, are less likely to become critically ill or require much supportive care and can be more easily managed outside the hospital. These people should be isolated and monitored at home or in a non-hospital facility, and smallpox vaccination should be provided to caregivers and household members. Patients with evidence of severe disease or presentations that suggest progression to severe disease is likely should be considered for admission to a negative-pressure environment with strict maintenance of Airborne Precautions.

INFECTION CONTROL

Clinicians should notify local public health authorities, their institution's infection control professional, and their laboratory of any suspected smallpox cases. Public health authorities may conduct epidemiological investigations and will implement disease control interventions to protect the public. Infection control professionals will implement infection control precautions within the health care setting. Laboratory personnel should take appropriate safety precautions.

Smallpox is transmissible from person to person by exposure to respiratory secretions and by direct contact with pox lesions and fomites. Airborne and Contact Precautions in addition to Standard Precautions should be implemented for patients with suspected smallpox. Health care workers caring for patients with suspected smallpox should be vaccinated immediately.

Detailed instructions on infection control practices for smallpox have been prepared by the CDC and may be found at http://www.bt.cdc.gov/agent/smallpox/response-plan/files/guide-f.doc.

Decontamination

Survival of the virus in the environment is inversely proportional to temperature and humidity. All bedding and clothing of smallpox patients should be minimally handled to prevent re-aerosolization and autoclaved or laundered in hot water with bleach. Standard disinfection and sterilization methods are deemed adequate for medical equipment used with smallpox patients and cleaning surfaces and rooms potentially contaminated with the virus. Airspace decontamination (fumigation) is not required.

PEARLS AND PITFALLS

1. The CDC has developed a number of clinical diagnostic tools to assist with the visual recognition, differential diagnosis, and initial management of suspected smallpox. These resources are available at http://www.cdc.gov/smallpox.
2. Hemorrhagic smallpox is rare but can be confused with invasive meningococcal disease, rickettsial infections, or gram-negative sepsis because of the patient's ill appearance, petechial and purpuric lesions, and hemorrhagic manifestations.

3. Smallpox is most often transmitted through direct contact with respiratory droplets as a result of close (within 2 meters) or face-to-face contact. Viruses can also travel over greater distances as airborne particles, particularly in cases with coughing. Transmission has occasionally been linked to fomites carried on clothing or bedding that has been contaminated by dried respiratory secretions or draining skin lesions.

4. Since 2003, many health departments have established smallpox preparedness teams consisting of providers who have been vaccinated against smallpox who can assist with the response to a suspected case of smallpox.

REFERENCES

Bhatnagar V, Stoto MA, Morton SC, et al. Transmission patterns of smallpox: systematic review of natural outbreaks in Europe and North America since World War II. BMC Public Health 2006;6:126.

Breman JG, Henderson DA. Diagnosis and management of smallpox. N Engl J Med 2002;346:1300–8.

Casey CG, Iskander JK, Roper MH, et al. Adverse events associated with smallpox vaccination in the United States, January–October 2003. JAMA 2005;294:2734–43.

Centers for Disease Control and Prevention (CDC). Acute, generalized vesicular or pustular rash illness testing protocol in the United States. Available at: http://www.bt.cdc.gov/agent/smallpox/diagnosis/rashtestingprotocol.asp.

Centers for Disease Control and Prevention (CDC) Poster: evaluating patients for smallpox. Available at: http://www.bt.cdc.gov/agent/smallpox/diagnosis/evalposter.asp.

Cohen HW, Gould RM, Sidel VW. Smallpox vaccinations and adverse events. JAMA 2006;295:1897–8.

Fenner F, Henderson DA, Arita I, et al. Smallpox and its eradication. Geneva: World Health Organization, 1988. Retrieved February 10, 2007, from http://whqlibdoc.who.int/smallpox/924156.pdf.

Huhn GD, Bauer AM, Yorita K, et al. Clinical characteristics of human monkeypox, and risk factors for severe disease. Clin Infect Dis 2005;41:1742–51.

Kim S-H, Bang J-W, Park K-H, et al. Prediction of residual immunity to smallpox by means of an intradermal skin test with inactivated vaccinia virus. J Infect Dis 2006;194:377–84; comments and author reply in 195:160–2.

Kiang KM, Krathwohl MD. Rates and risks of transmission of smallpox and mechanisms of prevention. J Lab Clin Med 2003;142:229–38.

Moore ZS, Seward JF, Lane JM. Smallpox. Lancet 2006;367:425–35.

Nishiura H. Smallpox during pregnancy and maternal outcomes. Emerg Infect Dis 2006;12:1119–21.

Nishiura H, Schwehm M, Eichner M. Still protected against smallpox? Estimation of the duration of vaccine-induced immunity against smallpox. Epidemiology 2006;17:576–81.

Nishiura H, Eichner M. Infectiousness of smallpox relative to disease age: estimates based on transmission network and incubation period. Epidemiol Infect 2006;1–6.

Sejvar JJ, Labutta RJ, Chapman LE, et al. Neurologic adverse events associated with smallpox vaccination in the United States, 2002–2004. JAMA 2005;294:2744–50.

ADDITIONAL READINGS

Center for Infectious Disease Research and Policy (CIDRAP). Smallpox: current, comprehensive information on pathogenesis, microbiology, epidemiology, diagnosis, treatment, and prophylaxis. Retrieved May 18, 2005, from http://www.cidrap.umn.edu/cidrap/content/bt.

Damon I. Orthopoxviruses: vaccinia (smallpox vaccine), variola (smallpox), monkeypox, and cowpox. In: Mandell GL, Bennett JE, Dolin R, eds, Principles and practice of infectious diseases (6th ed). New York: Churchill Livingstone, 2005.

Henderson DA, Inglesby TV, Bartlett JG, et al., for the Working Group on Civilian Biodefense. Smallpox as a biological weapon: medical and public health management. JAMA 1999;281(22):2127–39.

Rotz LD, Cono J, Damon I. Smallpox and bioterrorism. In: Mandell GL, Bennett JE, Dolin R, eds, Principles and practice of infectious diseases (6th ed). New York: Churchill Livingstone, 2005.

68. Tularemia

David M. Stier, Jennifer C. Hunter, Olivia Bruch, and Karen A. Holbrook

INTRODUCTION

Tularemia is a zoonotic disease caused by *Francisella tularensis*, a nonsporulating, nonmotile, aerobic, gram-negative coccobacillus. There are several subspecies of *F. tularensis*, with the biovars *tularensis* (type A) and *holarctica* (type B) occurring most commonly in the United States. The clinical syndromes caused by tularemia depend on the route of infection and subspecies of the infecting organism. Tularemia is highly infectious, requiring inhalation or inoculation of as few as 10 organisms to cause disease. Although its virulence factors are not well characterized, type A is generally thought to be the more virulent subspecies. However, the virulence of type A subspecies may vary between geographic regions within the United States, with the midwestern and eastern states having more severe infections.

The Working Group for Civilian Biodefense considers tularemia to be a dangerous potential biological weapon because of its "extreme infectivity, ease of dissemination, and its capacity to cause illness and death." Of the potential ways that *F. tularensis* could be used as a biological weapon, an aerosol release is expected to have the most severe medical and public health outcomes.

EPIDEMIOLOGY

Tularemia as a Biological Weapon

Weaponized *F. tularensis* was developed and stockpiled by the U.S. military, though the supply was destroyed in the 1970s. The Soviet Union is reported to have developed antibiotic- and vaccine-resistant strains of weaponized *F. tularensis*.

Experts believe that an aerosolized release is the most likely intentional use of *F. tularensis* organisms. Exposure to aerosolized *F. tularensis* would cause:

Via inhalation:

- primary pneumonic tularemia (majority of patients)
- typhoidal tularemia (nonspecific febrile illness of varying severity)
- oropharyngeal tularemia

Via contact with eyes:

- oculoglandular tularemia

Via contact with broken skin:

- gladular or ulcerglandular disease

An outbreak of disease caused by the intentional release of tularemia would have the following characteristics:

- Multiple cases clustering in time presenting with: acute nonspecific febrile illness with onset 3 to 5 days after the initial release (range 1–14 days) and community-acquired atypical pneumonia unresponsive to typical antimicrobials
- Atypical host characteristics: unexpected, unexplained cases of acute illness in previously healthy persons who rapidly develop pleuropneumonia and systemic infection, especially if patients develop pleural effusions and hilar lymphadenopathy
- Unusual geographic clustering: multiple cases in an urban area, where naturally occurring tularemia is not endemic
- Affected patients without exposure risk factors: e.g., outdoor field work or recreational activity, contact with tissues of potentially infected animals

Intentionally released *F. tularensis* strains may be altered to have enhanced virulence or antimicrobial resistance.

Naturally Occurring Tularemia

RESERVOIR

The natural reservoirs for *F. tularensis* are small and medium-sized mammals. In the United States these are primarily lagomorphs (rabbits, hares) but may include beavers, squirrels, muskrats, field voles, and rats. Incidental hosts include some species of mammals (e.g., humans, cats, dogs, cattle), birds, fish, and amphibians. Organisms can survive for weeks in moist environments, including water, mud, and decaying animal tissue.

MODE OF TRANSMISSION

Tularemia is not spread from person to person, and the primary vectors for infection in the United States are ticks

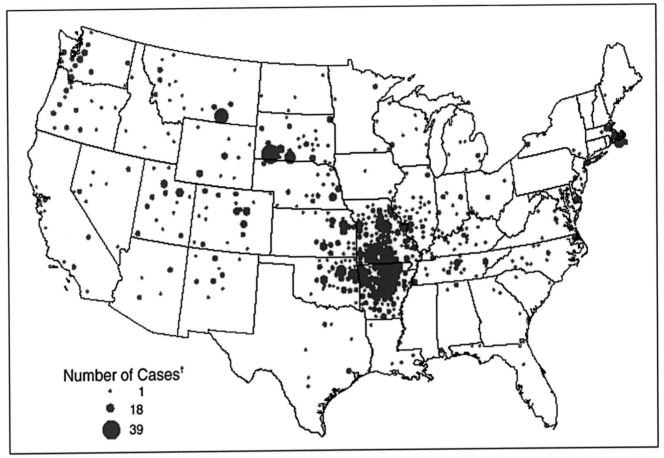

Number of Cases†
- · 1
- ● 18
- ⬢ 39

Figure 68.1 Distribution of reported cases of tularemia in the United States, 1990–2000. (From: Centers for Disease Control and Prevention (CDC), 2000. Available at: http://www.cdc.gov/mmwr/PDF/wk/mm5109.pdf.)

(dog ticks, wood ticks) and flies, such as the deerfly. Humans become infected by a number of mechanisms:

- bites by infected arthropods (majority of cases)
- contact with infectious animal tissues or fluids, during, for example, hunting or butchering
- ingestion of contaminated food, water, or soil
- inhalation of infectious aerosols, including aerosols generated during landscaping activities (e.g., lawn mowing, using a power blower, or brush cutting)
- exposure in the laboratory (accidental inhalation of aerosol, direct contact with an infectious specimen including accidental parenteral inoculation, or ingestion)

WORLDWIDE OCCURRENCE

Worldwide, human cases of tularemia occur throughout North America, Europe, and Asia. Infections with type A strain are generally only seen in North America. Within Europe and Asia, the greatest numbers of human cases are reported in Scandinavian countries and countries of the former Soviet Union. Recent significant outbreaks of tularemia in humans include Sweden (2000, 2003, 2006), Turkey (2004–2005), Kosovo (2002), and Bulgaria (1997–2005).

U.S. OCCURRENCE

Nationwide, incidence of tularemia has declined from approximately 2000 annually reported cases during the first half of the 20th century to an average of 124 cases per year during the 1990s (Figure 68.1). Most cases occur in rural or semirural environments, during the summer months, with the greatest number of cases occurring in Missouri, Oklahoma, South Dakota, Montana, and Martha's Vineyard, Massachusetts. From 1990 to 2000, incidence of tularemia in the United States was highest in children 5–9 years and adults 75 years and older. Regardless of age, males had a higher incidence of tularemia, potentially because of participation in activities more likely to cause exposures, such as hunting, trapping, butchering, and farming. Recent significant outbreaks include:

- In 1978 and 2000, outbreaks of the rare primary pneumonic tularemia occurred on Martha's Vineyard, Massachusetts. These represent the only outbreaks of primary pneumonic tularemia in the United States. Additional cases of tularemia have been reported each year in Martha's Vineyard (2000–2006). Exposure is most likely from breathing infectious aerosols generated during landscaping activities. The reservoir in these outbreaks is still unclear, but may involve skunks and raccoons.
- In 2002, tularemia was responsible for a die-off of several hundred prairie dogs caught in the wild in South Dakota and then commercially distributed widely throughout the United States. One human case occurred in an animal handler who cared for the infected animals.

Table 68.1 Clinical Features: Pneumonic Tularemia

Incubation Period	3–5 days (range 1–14 days)
Transmission	• Inhalation of contaminated aerosols • Secondary hematogenous spread to the lung
Signs and Symptoms	• Initial presentation as atypical community acquired pneumonia unresponsive to routine antibiotic therapy, which can progress slowly or rapidly to severe disease • Fever (abrupt onset), headache, cough, minimal or no sputum production, dyspnea, pleuritic chest pain, myalgias (often prominent in lower back), bronchiolitis and/or pharyngitis may be present • Generalized maculopapular rash with progression to pustules or erythema-nodosum type rash occurs in 20% • Nausea, vomiting, diarrhea is not uncommon • Hemoptysis (not common)
Progression and Complications	• Respiratory failure, ARDS • Severe pneumonia • Lung abscess or cavitary lesions • Sepsis
Laboratory and Radiographic Findings	• Leukocytosis; differential may be normal • Liver enzymes and/or CK may be abnormal • Sputum Gram stain usually nonspecific • Lobar, segmental, or subsegmental opacities on CXR, pleural effusion, pleural adhesions, hilar adenopathy

ARDS, acute respiratory distress syndrome; CK, creatine kinase; CXR, chest x-ray.

Table 68.2 Clinical Features: Glandular and Ulceroglandular Tularemia

Incubation Period	3–5 days (range 1–14 days)
Transmission	• Bite of an infected arthropod • Direct contact with infectious material (i.e., contaminated carcass, settled infectious aerosol)
Signs and Symptoms	• Ulceroglandular form – local skin involvement at site of exposure that develops into a painful cutaneous papule with subsequent ulceration within several days. Papule becomes necrotic and scars. • Glandular form – no cutaneous lesion occurs • Enlarged and tender regional lymphadenopathy that can persist for months • Fever, chills, malaise, myalgias, arthralgias, headache, anorexia, GI symptoms are common
Progression and Complications	• Lymph node suppuration • Secondary pneumonia • Hematogenous spread to other organs • Sepsis
Laboratory Findings	• Leukocytosis; differential may be normal • Liver enzymes and/or CK may be abnormal

CK, creatine kinase; GI, gastrointestinal.

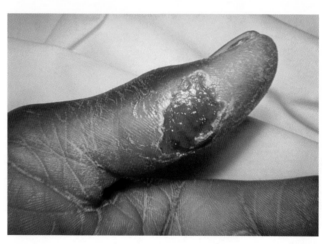

Figure 68.2 Thumb lesion caused by tularemia infection. (From the U.S. Centers for Disease Control and Prevention Public Health Image Library at http://phil.cdc.gov/phil/home.asp.)

CLINICAL FEATURES

Human tularemia occurs in six recognized forms, determined primarily by route of infection. Tularemia infection can range from mild to severe clinical illness and can be life-threatening. Overall case-fatality rates have declined from 5–15% in the preantibiotic era to approximately 2% currently. Mortality was historically much higher with pneumonic and typhoidal tularemia, with case fatality as high as 30–60% if untreated. Administration of appropriate antibiotic treatment typically leads to general symptom improvement within 24–48 hours. Recognition of tularemia as a potential etiologic agent is critical, because poor outcomes have been associated with delays in seeking care and/or instituting effective antimicrobial treatment.

Pneumonic Tularemia

Pneumonic tularemia is associated with the most severe disease and presents as a nonspecific febrile illness with progression to pleuropneumonitis and systemic infection (Table 68.1).

Glandular and Ulceroglandular Tularemia

Glandular and ulceroglandular tularemia account for the majority of naturally occurring cases of tularemia (Table 68.2). In the *ulceroglandular* form, an ulcer is formed at the site of inoculation, with subsequent lymphadenopathy in the proximal draining lymph nodes (Figures 68.2, 68.3, and 68.4). Occa-

sionally, lymphadenopathy occurs without an ulcer, leading to the designation of *glandular* disease.

Oculoglandular Tularemia

Oculoglandular tularemia results either from ocular inoculation from the hands after contact with contaminated material or from splashes or aerosols generated during handling of infective material (e.g., animal carcasses). This form of tularemia could occur in a bioterrorism setting as a result of an aerosol exposure. Organisms spread from the conjunctiva to regional nodes, where they cause focal necrosis and lesions.

After an incubation period of 3–5 (range 1–14) days, oculoglandular tularemia presents as a painful "red eye" with purulent exudation, chemosis, vasculitis, and painful regional lymphadenopathy. Additional signs and symptoms may include photophobia, lacrimation, itching, local edema, and changes in visual acuity. There is a potential for lymph

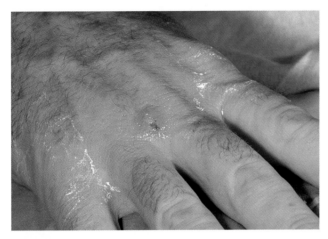

Figure 68.3 Lesion caused by tularemia infection. (From the U.S. Centers for Disease Control and Prevention Public Health Image Library at http://phil.cdc.gov/phil/home.asp.)

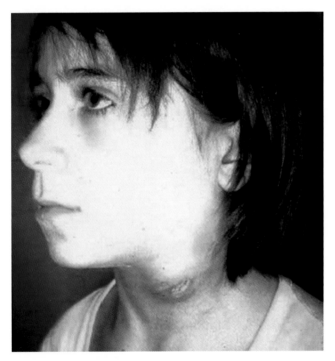

Figure 68.4 Girl with ulcerating lymphadenitis caused by tularemia infection. (From: Reintjes R, Dedusha I, Gjini A, et al. Tularemia outbreak investigation in Kosovo: case control and environmental studies. Emerg Infect Dis 2002 Jan;8(1):69–73.)

node suppuration, hematogenous dissemination, and development of sepsis.

Laboratory values are generally nonspecific, and Gram stain of conjunctival scrapings may or may not demonstrate organisms.

Oropharyngeal Tularemia

Oropharyngeal or gastrointestinal tularemia occurs via ingestion of contaminated food including undercooked meat, contaminated water or droplets, and oral inoculation from the hands after contact with contaminated material.

After an incubation period of 3–5 (range 1–14) days, oropharyngeal tularemia presents either as acute pharyngi-

Table 68.3 Clinical Features: Typhoidal Tularemia

Incubation Period	3–5 days (range 1–14 days)
Transmission	• Site of primary infection usually unknown
Signs and Symptoms	• Fever, chills, headache, malaise, weakness, myalgias, arthralgias, cough • Weakness, dehydration, hypotension, pharyngitis • Watery diarrhea, anorexia, nausea, vomiting, abdominal pain (children may have more severe GI involvement) • Generalized maculopapular rash with progression to pustules or erythema-nodosum type rash may occur • Splenomegaly and hepatomegaly (not common)
Progression and Complications	• Secondary pneumonia • Hematogenous spread to other organs – osteomyelitis, pericarditis, peritonitis, endocarditis, meningitis • Sepsis • Rhabdomyolysis • Cholestasis with jaundice • Renal failure • Debilitating illness lasting several months
Laboratory and Radiographic Findings	• Pleural effusions • Leukocytosis; differential may be normal • Liver enzymes and/or CK may be abnormal • Sterile pyuria may occur

CK, creatine kinase; GI, gastrointestinal.

tis with cervical lymphadenopathy or as ulcerative gastrointestinal lesions with fever, abdominal pain, diarrhea, nausea, vomiting, mesenteric lymphadenopathy, and gastrointestinal bleeding. Severity can range from mild diarrhea to overwhelming ulceration with frank gastrointestinal bleeding and sepsis. A large inoculum (approximately 10^8 organisms) is required to transmit disease via ingestion. There is a potential for lymph node suppuration, hematogenous dissemination, and development of sepsis.

Routine tests are generally nonspecific. Leukocytosis may or may not be present.

Typhoidal Tularemia

Typhoidal (septicemic) tularemia is an acute, nonspecific febrile illness associated with *F. tularensis* without prominent lymphadenopathy (Table 68.3).

DIFFERENTIAL DIAGNOSIS

A high index of suspicion is required to diagnose tularemia because there are no readily available rapid and specific confirmatory tests. In addition, the various forms of tularemia can have a nonspecific appearance and/or resemble a wide range of much more common illnesses.

Differential: Pneumonic Tularemia

The following are clinical syndromes that can appear similar to the pneumonic form of tularemia:

- bacterial pneumonia (*Mycoplasma, Staphylococcus, Streptococcus, Haemophilus, Klebsiella, Moraxella, Legionella*)
- *Chlamydia* infection
- Q fever
- tuberculosis
- inhalational anthrax
- pneumonic plague
- fungal pulmonary disease (histoplasmosis, coccidioidomycosis)
- severe acute respiratory syndrome (SARS)
- other causes of atypical or chronic pneumonias

Differential: Glandular and Ulceroglandular Tularemia

The following are clinical syndromes that can appear similar to the glandular and ulceroglandular forms of tularemia:

- pyogenic bacterial infections
- cat-scratch disease (Bartonella)
- syphilis
- chancroid
- lymphogranuloma venereum
- tuberculosis
- nontuberculosis mycobacterial infection
- toxoplasmosis
- sporotrichosis
- rat-bite fever
- anthrax
- plague
- herpes simplex virus infection
- adenitis or cellulitis (*Staphylococcus* or *Streptococcus*)
- *Pasteurella* infections
- rickettsial infections
- orf virus infection

Differential: Oculoglandular Tularemia

The following are clinical entities that can appear similar to the oculoglandular form of tularemia:

- pyogenic bacterial infections
- adenoviral infection
- syphilis
- cat-scratch disease
- herpes simplex virus infection
- varicella-zoster virus infection
- sporotrichosis
- coccidioidomycosis
- tuberculosis

Differential: Oropharyngeal Tularemia

The following are causes of syndromes that appear similar to the oropharyngeal form of tularemia:

- *Streptococcus* pharyngitis
- infectious mononucleosis
- adenoviral infection
- diphtheria
- GI anthrax

Differential: Typhoidal Tularemia

The following are causes of syndromes that can appear similar to typhoidal forms of tularemia:

- *Salmonella* spp. infection
- brucellosis
- *Legionella* infection
- *Chlamydia* infection
- Q fever
- disseminated mycobacterial or fungal infection
- rickettsioses
- malaria
- endocarditis
- leptospirosis
- meningococcemia
- septicemic plague
- septicemia caused by other gram-negative bacteria
- *Staphylococcus* or *Streptococcus* toxic shock syndrome
- other causes of prolonged fever without localizing signs

LABORATORY AND RADIOGRAPHIC FINDINGS

The diagnosis of tularemia requires a high index of suspicion because the disease often presents with nonspecific symptoms and nonspecific results of routine lab tests.

Although recommended, microscopy and culture are difficult and often not fruitful. The organism is rarely seen on stained clinical specimens and is difficult to isolate using routine culture media and conditions. However, isolation is possible from a variety of clinical specimens if culture conditions are optimized. Even still, some strains may require up to a week to develop visible colonies, especially if the patient has been placed on bacteriostatic antibiotic therapy. Because of the need for nonroutine laboratory methods and because *F. tularensis* is a risk to laboratory personnel, clinicians should notify the laboratory when tularemia is suspected.

Diagnosis is most commonly confirmed by serologic testing. Antibody detection assays include tube agglutination, microagglutination, hemagglutination, and enzyme-linked immunosorbent assay (ELISA). Significant antibodies appear around the end of the 2nd week of illness, peak at 4–5 weeks, and can persist indefinitely. A single titer of 1:160 or greater (by tube agglutination) or 1:128 or greater (by microagglutination) is a presumptive positive; a fourfold rise in titer is required for definitive serologic diagnosis.

Although rapid diagnostic tests are not widely available, the public health laboratory system may be able to provide polymerase chain reaction [PCR] testing on certain clinical specimens.

TREATMENT AND PROPHYLAXIS

Treatment

The treatment of choice for all forms of tularemia is streptomycin (Table 68.4). Gentamicin, which is more widely available, is an acceptable alternative. Other alternatives include tetracycline, chloramphenicol, and ciprofloxacin. Tetracyclines and chloramphenicol are bacteriostatic and their use has resulted in more relapses than treatment with

Table 68.4 Tularemia: Treatment and Postexposure Prophylaxis Recommendations[1]

		Contained Casualty Setting	Mass Casualty Setting or Postexposure Prophylaxis
Adult	Preferred	**streptomycin**, 1 g IM q12h × 10 days *or* **gentamicin**,[2] 5 mg/kg IM or IV q24h × 10 days	**doxycycline**, 100 mg PO bid × 14 days *or* **ciprofloxacin**, 500 mg PO bid × 14 days
	Alternative	**doxycycline**, 100 mg IV q12h × 14–21 days *or* **chloramphenicol**,[3] 15 mg/kg IV q6h × 14–21 days *or* **ciprofloxacin**, 400 mg IV q12h × 10 days	
Children	Preferred	**streptomycin**, 15 mg/kg IM q12h (max 2 gm/day) × 10 days *or* **gentamicin**,[2] 2.5 mg/kg IM or IV q8h × 10 days	**doxycycline**[4,5]: ≥45 kg, give adult dosage bid × 14 days <45 kg, give 2.2 mg/kg PO bid (max 200 mg/day) × 14 days *or* **ciprofloxacin**,[4,6] 15 mg/kg PO bid (max 1 g/day) × 14 days
	Alternative	**doxycycline**[4,5]: ≥45 kg, give adult dosage × 14 days <45 kg, give 2.2 mg/kg IV q12h (max 200 mg/day) × 14 days *or* **chloramphenicol**,[3] 15 mg/kg IV q6h × 14–21 days *or* **ciprofloxacin**,[4,6] 15 mg/kg IV q12h (max 1 g/day) × 10 days	
Pregnant Women	Preferred	**gentamicin**,[2] 5 mg/kg IM or IV q24h × 10 days *or* **streptomycin**,[7] 1 g IM q12h × 10 days	**doxycycline**,[4,5] 100 mg PO bid × 14 days *or* **ciprofloxacin**,[4,6] 500 mg PO bid × 14 days
	Alternative	**doxycycline**,[4,5] 100 mg IV q12h × 14–21 days *or* **ciprofloxacin**,[4,6] 400 mg IV q12h × 10 days	

[1] Treatment recommendations come from the Working Group of Civilian Biodefense and may not necessarily be approved by the U.S. Food and Drug Administration.
[2] Aminoglycoside doses must be further adjusted for newborns and according to renal function.
[3] Therapeutic concentration is 5–20 μg/mL; concentrations >25 μg/mL can cause reversible bone marrow suppression.
[4] Tetracycline and quinolone antibiotics are generally not recommended during pregnancy or childhood; however, their use may be indicated for life-threatening illness.
[5] Ciprofloxacin may be preferred in pregnant women and children up to 8 years of age because of the known adverse event profile of doxycycline (e.g., tooth discoloration).
[6] Doxycycline may be preferred in children 8 years and older because of the adverse event profile of ciprofloxacin (e.g., arthropathies).
[7] Streptomycin is not as acceptable as gentamicin for use in pregnant women because of adverse event profile of streptomycin (irreversible deafness in children exposed in utero has been reported).

aminoglycosides. Clinicians should be aware that *F. tularensis* strains released intentionally may be resistant to antimicrobials.

Supportive care, including fluid management and hemodynamic monitoring, should be considered in all patients. Intensive care with respiratory support may be necessary in patients with complications.

Contained casualty setting: The Working Group recommends parenteral antimicrobial therapy when individual medical management is available (Table 68.4). Therapy may be switched to oral antimicrobials when clinically indicated.

Mass casualty setting: Use of oral antibiotics may be necessary if the number of patients exceeds the medical care capacity for individual medical management (Table 68.4).

Postexposure Prophylaxis

Antibiotic prophylaxis should begin as soon as possible and preferably within 24 hours after exposure to an infectious aerosol containing *F. tularensis* (Table 68.4). Postexposure prophylactic treatment of close contacts of tularemia patients is not recommended because human-to-human transmission of *F. tularensis* is not known to occur.

Vaccination

A live, attenuated vaccine has been used in the United States to protect laboratory personnel who work with *F. tularensis*. This vaccine is currently under review by the Food and Drug Administration (FDA) and is unavailable. Clinical trials to develop a new tularemia vaccine are underway, but it is not likely that a vaccine will be widely available in the near future.

COMPLICATIONS AND ADMISSION CRITERIA

Disease manifestations and complications are typically related to the portal of entry of *F. tularensis*. Pneumonic tularemia may result in severe pneumonia, lung abscess, or acute respiratory distress syndrome (ARDS). Glandular and ulceroglandular tularemia may progress to lymph node suppuration and secondary pneumonia. Oculoglandular tularemia can cause localized lymph node suppuration, whereas oropharyngeal tularemia has been associated with mesenteric lymphadenitis, gastrointestinal (GI) ulceration, and GI bleeding. Typhoidal tularemia not uncommonly progresses to secondary pneumonia. All forms of human tularemia carry the potential for hematogenous dissemination of the organism to other organs such as bone, pericardium, and peritoneum, and for progression to sepsis and multiorgan failure.

Admission to the hospital is advisable for patients with any form of tularemia, to administer antibiotics intravenously and to monitor for disease progression.

INFECTION CONTROL

Clinicians should notify local public health authorities, their institution's infection control professional, and their laboratory of any suspected tularemia cases. Public health authorities may conduct epidemiologic investigations and implement disease control interventions to protect the public. Both HICPAC (Hospital Infection Control Practices Advisory Committee) of the CDC and the Working Group for Civilian Biodefense recommend Standard Precautions for tularemia patients in a hospital setting without the need for isolation. Routine laboratory procedures should be carried out under Biosafety Level 2 (BSL-2) conditions; however, manipulation of cultures or other activities that may produce aerosol or droplets (e.g., centrifuging, grinding, vigorous shaking) require BSL-3 conditions.

Decontamination

Contaminated surfaces can be disinfected with commercially available bleach or a 1:10 dilution of household bleach and water. All persons exposed to an aerosol containing *F. tularensis* should be instructed to wash body surfaces and clothing with soap and water.

PEARLS AND PITFALLS

1. The onset of tularemia is usually abrupt, with fever, headache, chills and rigors, generalized body aches, and coryza. A pulse-temperature dissociation has been noted in as many as 42% of patients.
2. Clinicians should familiarize themselves with the local epidemiology of tularemia. The occurrence of human cases may follow a local tularemia epizootic (outbreak of disease in an animal population). Occurrence of pneumonic tularemia in a low-incidence area should prompt consideration of bioterrorism.
3. The diagnosis of tularemia relies heavily on clinical suspicion. Routine laboratory tests are usually nonspecific. The organism is usually not apparent on gram-stained smears or tissue biopsies and usually does not grow on standard culture plates. However, *F. tularensis* may be recovered from blood and body fluids using special supportive media. Because of this and its potential hazards to laboratory personnel, the laboratory should be notified if tularemia is suspected.

REFERENCES

American Public Health Association. Tularemia. In: Chin J, ed, Control of communicable diseases manual. Washington, DC: Author, 2000:532–5.

Avashia SB, Petersen JM, Lindley CM, et al. First reported prairie dog-to-human tularemia transmission, Texas, 2002. Emerg Infect Dis 2004;10(3):483–6.

Barry MA. Report of pneumonic tularemia in three Boston University researchers. Boston Public Health Commission, 2005. Available at: http://www.bphc.org/reports/pdfs/report_202.pdf.

Brouillard JE, Terriff CM, Tofan A, et al. Antibiotic selection and resistance issues with fluoroquinolones and doxycycline against bioterrorism agents. Pharmacotherapy 2006;26(1):3–14.

Berrada ZL, Goethert HK, Telford SR 3rd. Raccoons and skunks as sentinels for enzootic tularemia. Emerg Infect Dis 2006;12(6):1019–21.

Centers for Disease Control and Prevention (CDC). Tularemia – United States, 1990–2000. MMWR 2002;51(9):181–4.

Centers for Disease Control and Prevention (CDC). Tularemia transmitted by insect bites – Wyoming 2001–2003. MMWR 2005;54(07);170–3.

Evans ME, Gregory DW, Schaffner W, et al. Tularemia: a 30-year experience with 88 cases. Medicine (Baltimore) 1985;64(4):251–69.

Feldman KA, Stiles-Enos D, Julian K, et al. Tularemia on Martha's Vineyard: seroprevalence and occupational risk. Emerg Infect Dis 2003;9(3):350–4.

Groseclose SL, Brathwaite WS, Hall PA, et al. Summary of notifiable diseases – United States, 2002. MMWR 2004;51(53):1–84.

Hassoun A, Spera R, Dunkel J. Tularemia and once-daily gentamicin. Antimicrob Agents Chemother 2006;50(2):824.

Johansson A, Berglund L, Sjöstedt A, et al. Ciprofloxacin for treatment of tularemia. Clin Infect Dis 2001;33(2):267–8.

Staples JE, Kubota KA, Chalcraft LG, et al. Epidemiologic and molecular analysis of human tularemia, United States, 1964–2004. Emerg Infect Dis 2006;12(7):1113–8.

World Health Organization (WHO). Biological agents. In: Health aspects of chemical and biological weapons (2nd ed). Geneva, Switzerland: Author, 2004:250–4.

ADDITIONAL READINGS

Center for Infectious Disease Research and Policy (CIDRAP). Tularemia: current, comprehensive information on pathogenesis, microbiology, epidemiology, diagnosis, treatment, and prophylaxis. Retrieved January 15, 2007, from http://www.cidrap.umn.edu/cidrap/content/bt/tularemia.

Dennis DT, Inglesby TV, Henderson DA, et al. Tularemia as a biological weapon: medical and public health management. JAMA 2001;285(21):2763–73.

Mitchell CL, Penn RL. Chapter 322 – *Francisella tularensis* (tularemia) as an agent of bioterrorism. In: Mandell GL, Bennett JE, Dolin R, eds, Principles and practice of infectious diseases (6th ed). New York: Churchill Livingstone, 2005.

Penn RL. Chapter 224 – *Francisella tularensis* (tularemia). In: Mandell GL, Bennett JE, Dolin R, eds, Principles and practice of infectious diseases (6th ed). New York: Churchill Livingstone, 2005.

69. Viral Hemorrhagic Fever

David M. Stier, Jennifer C. Hunter, Olivia Bruch, and Karen A. Holbrook

INTRODUCTION

Viral hemorrhagic fevers (VHFs) refer to a group of illnesses caused by several families of viruses, including:

- Filoviridae (Ebola and Marburg viruses)
- Arenaviridae (Lassa fever and New World hemorrhagic fever)
- Bunyaviridae (Rift Valley fever, Crimean-Congo fever, and agents of "hemorrhagic fever with renal syndrome" [HFRS])
- Flaviviridae (yellow fever, Omsk hemorrhagic fever, Kyasanur Forest disease, and dengue)

Many VHF viruses are virulent, and some are highly infectious (e.g., filoviruses and arenaviruses) with person-to-person transmission from direct contact with infected blood and bodily secretions. Effective therapies and prophylaxis are extremely limited for VHF; therefore, early detection and strict adherence to infection control measures are essential.

The Working Group for Civilian Biodefense considers some hemorrhagic fever (HF) viruses to pose a serious threat as potential biological weapons based on their risk of morbidity and mortality, feasibility of production, and their ability to cause infection through aerosol dissemination. These include Ebola, Marburg, Lassa fever, New World arenaviruses, Rift Valley fever, yellow fever, Omsk hemorrhagic fever, and Kyasanur Forest disease. This chapter will focus only on these VHF viruses and will not include a discussion of dengue fever (see Chapter 54, Fever in the Returning Traveler), hemorrhagic fever with renal syndrome (see Chapter 70, Hantavirus), and Crimean-Congo hemorrhagic fevers.

EPIDEMIOLOGY

VHF Viruses as Biological Weapons

Of the potential ways in which VHF viruses could be used as biological weapons, an aerosol release is expected to have the most severe medical and public health outcomes.

An outbreak of disease caused by the intentional release of a VHF virus would have the following characteristics:

- Multiple cases clustering in time presenting with: acute nonspecific febrile illness with onset 2 to 21 days after the initial release (may include fever, myalgias, rash, and encephalitis) and severe illness with a fever and hemorrhagic manifestations
- Atypical host characteristics: unexpected, unexplained cases of acute illness in previously healthy persons, or people with hemorrhagic symptoms who have no conditions predisposing for hemorrhagic illness
- Unusual geographic clustering: cases occurring in an area where naturally occurring VHF is not endemic
- Affected patients lacking VHF exposure risk factors: e.g., travel to a VHF endemic country such as South America, Africa, or Asia; handling animal carcasses; contact with people infected with VHF.

In the event of an intentional release, some VHFs could infect susceptible animals, potentially establishing the disease in the environment.

Naturally Occurring Viral Hemorrhagic Fever

All of the VHF agents cause sporadic disease or epidemics in areas of endemicity. The routes of transmission are variable, but most are zoonotic with spread via arthropod bites or contact with infected animals. Person-to-person spread is a major form of transmission for many of the viruses. Epidemiologic characteristics for each virus are described in Tables 69.1 and 69.2.

CLINICAL FEATURES

The clinical features of VHF vary according to the etiologic virus and are detailed by disease below. General clinical features of VHFs are provided in Table 69.3.

Ebola and Marburg

Case fatality of Ebola ranges from 50% to 90% and that of Marburg, from 23% to 70% (Table 69.4).

Table 69.1 Epidemiologic Characteristics of VHF Viruses

Virus	Worldwide Occurrence	Reservoir/ Vector Transmission	
Filoviruses			
Ebola	• Identified in 1976 during outbreaks in the Democratic Republic of Congo (formerly known as Zaire) and Sudan. Four species of Ebola virus are recognized and named after the regions where they were discovered: Ivory Coast, Sudan, Zaire, and Reston. • Reported cases of naturally occurring infections have occurred in Africa: Democratic Republic of Congo (1976, 1995), Sudan (1976, 1979, 2004), Gabon (1994, 1996, 2001–02), Ivory Coast (1994), Uganda (2000–01), Republic of Congo (2001–02, 2003–04, 2005) • Laboratory-acquired infections have occurred in England (1976) • Ebola has been introduced to quarantine facilities in United States (1989, 1990, 1996), Italy (1992), Philippines (1996)	Unknown[1]/ unknown	Person-to-person transmission[2] occurs via: • Contact with blood, secretions, or tissue of infected patient[3] (sexual transmission may occur up to 3 months after clinical illness ends) • Contact with cadaver • Airborne transmission (suspected) • Parenteral inoculation (unsterilized needles, accidental needle sticks) • Contact with blood, secretions, or tissue of infected nonhuman primate • Exposure in laboratory
Marburg	• Identified in 1967 in Germany when laboratory staff handling tissues from African green monkeys became infected • Reported cases of naturally occurring infections have occurred in: South Africa[4] (1975), Western Kenya (1987, 1980), Democratic Republic of Congo (1998–2000), Angola (2004–2005) • Laboratory-acquired infections have occurred in Germany (1967)	Unknown/ unknown	
Arenaviruses			
Lassa	• Identified in 1969 in Nigeria • Lassa fever is endemic in West African countries between Nigeria and Senegal. There are an estimated 100,000–300,000 annual infections in West Africa. Nosocomial outbreaks and endemic transmission are more common during the dry season (January – April). Outbreaks have occurred in Sierra Leone, Guinea, Liberia, and Nigeria. • Lassa fever is occasionally imported to other countries through travel.	*Mastomys*[5]/ none	• Inhalation of aerosols of rodent excreta • Ingestion of food contaminated with rodent excreta • Contact of rodents *or* rodent excreta with open skin or mucous membranes Person-to-person transmission via: • Contact with infectious blood and bodily fluids • Parenteral inoculation (unsterilized needles accidental needle sticks) • Airborne transmission (suspected) • Exposure in laboratory
New World hemorrhagic fever	• New World HFs (or South American HF) include Junin, Machupo, Guanarito, and Sabia • Reported cases of naturally occurring infections have occurred in South America: Argentina, Bolivia, Venezuela, Brazil • An additional New World HF, Whitewater Arroyo, was isolated from three cases in California	Rodents (mouse, woodrat)/ none[5]	
Bunyavirus			
Rift Valley fever	• Reported cases of naturally occurring infections have occurred in Sub-Saharan Africa, Egypt (1977–8, 1993), Kenya and Somalia (1997–8), Saudi Arabia (2000–01), Yemen (2000–01), Tanzania (2006)	Ruminants (sheep, cattle, goats, buffalo)/ mosquito	• Bite of an infected mosquito • Direct contact with infected animal tissue (ruminants) • Inhalation of aerosol from infected animal carcasses (ruminants) • Transmission by ingestion of contaminated raw animal milk (suspected) • Exposure in laboratory
Flaviviruses			
Yellow fever	Yellow fever is endemic in Sub-Saharan Africa and tropical regions of South America (mostly in forested regions). From 2000 to 2004 there were 2570 cases reported in Africa and 629 in South America. Most outbreaks occur in: • West Africa and Central Africa – in Savanna zones during the rainy season • Urban and jungle regions of sub-Saharan Africa • South America – forested areas of Bolivia, Brazil, Columbia, Ecuador, Peru, Venezuela, French Guiana, Guyana	Primate/ *Aedes* and *Haemagogus* mosquitoes[6]	• Bite of an infected mosquito • Exposure in laboratory

Table 69.1 (cont.)

Virus	Worldwide Occurrence	Reservoir/Vector	Transmission
Flaviviruses (cont.)			
Kyasanur Forest disease virus	• First identified in 1957 from a sick monkey from the Kyasanur Forest in the Karnataka State, India. Recently, a similar virus was discovered in Saudi Arabia. • Kyasanur Forest disease is only found in the Karnataka State in India, where 400–500 cases are reported annually	Vertebrates[7]/tick[8]	• Bite of an infected tick • Inhalation of aerosols by laboratory workers during cultivation of these viruses
Omsk hemorrhagic fever	• Omsk hemorrhagic fever (OHF) was first identified in 1947 in Omsk, Russia. Epizootics began occurring in western Siberia among newly introduced muskrats (for fur trade) and caused large outbreaks in humans from 1945 to 1958. • Cases of OHF have been reported in central Asia (western Siberian regions of Omsk, Novosibirsk, Kurgan, Tyumen). From 1988 to 1997, there were 165 cases of Omsk reported from these regions. Naturally occurring infections peak in spring/early summer and autumn. Few cases have occurred in recent years.	Rodents (vole, muskrat) – possibly water-borne/tick	• Bite of an infected tick • Contact with blood, secretions, or tissue of an infected animal • Inhalation of aerosols by laboratory workers during cultivation of these viruses has been reported • Ingestion of contaminated raw goat milk • Waterborne (suspected) • Airborne (suspected)

[1] Fruit bats are currently a candidate reservoir. Asymptomatic infections occur in bats within the geographical range of human Ebola outbreaks.
[2] The initial transmission of Marburg and Ebola viruses from animals to humans is not understood.
[3] Risk of transmission is greatest during the latter stages of illness when viral loads are highest, whereas transmission rarely (if ever) occurs before the onset of symptoms.
[4] Case most likely exposed in Zimbabwe; traveling nurse also became infected.
[5] No intermediate vector between rodent and human is known.
[6] While there is a sylvatic cycle, epidemic YF can circulate from human to mosquito to human.
[7] Not well understood – vertebrate hosts include rodents, bats, small mammals, monkeys.
[8] Not well understood.

Considerations for pregnant women: High mortality from Ebola infection in pregnant women (95.5%), as well as high rates of fetal and neonatal demise (100%) have been reported.

Lassa Fever

Most people infected with Lassa fever have a mild or subclinical presentation (80%) (Table 69.5). Severe disease occurs in 12–20%, with overall case fatality around 1% (10–25% mortality in hospitalized patients). During an outbreak, a clinical combination of fever, pharyngitis, retrosternal pain, and proteinuria was predictive of laboratory-confirmed disease in 70% of cases. Findings associated with death include hypotension, peripheral vasoconstriction, oliguria, edema, pleural effusions, and ascites. Lassa fever requires a high index of suspicion because clinical features are nonspecific and vary from patient to patient. Recovery generally begins around day 10 but prolonged weakness and fatigue may occur.

Considerations for children: Clinical features of Lassa fever infection in children may be even more difficult to diagnose because of heterogeneous presentation. One syndrome in children less than 2 years old is marked by severe generalized edema, abdominal distension, and bleeding (this is associated with high case fatality of 75%).

Considerations for pregnant women: Case fatality in pregnant women is higher than in nonpregnant women, and risk of death increases in the third trimester (30%). Evacuation of uterus (i.e., delivery, abortion, or evacuation of retained products of conception after spontaneous abortion) can significantly reduce risk of death in the pregnant woman. Lassa virus infection leads to a high rate of fetal and neonatal death (>80%).

New World Hemorrhagic Fevers

The New World hemorrhagic fevers (Junin, Machupo, Guanarito, Sabia) have similar clinical features and progression (Table 69.6). Mortality ranges from 15% to 30% and recovery generally takes 2–3 weeks. Sequelae are uncommon.

Considerations for pregnant women: Case fatality from New World HF infection in pregnant women is higher than in nonpregnant women. Infection also leads to a high rate of fetal death.

Rift Valley fever

Rift Valley fever (RVF) has not been documented to spread from person to person; however, low titers of virus have been isolated from throat washings. There has been one case where vertical transmission was suspected. Historically the case-fatality estimate of RVF is less than 1%; however, a recent outbreak in Saudi Arabia (2000–01) had an overall case fatality of 14–17% (33% case fatality in patients admitted to RFV unit for severe disease). Factors associated with high mortality include hepatorenal failure, severe anemia, hemorrhagic or neurological manifestations, jaundice and shock (Table 69.7).

Yellow Fever

The severity of yellow fever infection can range from subclinical (5–50% of cases) to fatal (5% overall and 50% in cases with severe disease). Mortality is highest during epidemics (20–50% case-fatality), especially in areas with a large unvaccinated population. Yellow fever may resolve after a very mild course or may progress to moderate or severe illness (15%) after a short remission (Table 69.8). In fatal cases, death occurs 7–10 days after onset of illness.

Table 69.2 Occurrence of VHF Viruses in the United States

Virus	United States Occurrence
Ebola	Ebola-Reston virus has been introduced into quarantine facilities by monkeys imported from the Philippines on three occasions. In two of the three incidents (1989, 1990), four humans were infected with Ebola-Reston but did not become ill (developed antibodies).
Marburg	No U.S. occurrences
Lassa Fever	Lassa fever is rarely encountered in the United States. In 2004, a case of imported Lassa fever occurred in a New Jersey resident who became infected while traveling in West Africa. None of the contacts of the patient developed any symptoms compatible with Lassa fever within the incubation period. This was the first reported case of Lassa fever imported into the United States since 1989.
New World Hemorrhagic Fever	Three cases of Whitewater Arroyo virus were reported in California in 1999–2000; all were fatal. Whitewater Arroyo has been isolated from woodrats in North America, but these were the first reported cases of human disease.
Rift Valley Virus	No U.S. occurrences
Yellow Fever	Virus spread from West Africa to United States through slave trade vessels caused significant outbreaks, including: • Philadelphia (1793) – 10% of population died • Mississippi (1878) – 100,000 cases Yellow fever has been imported into the United States by nonimmunized travelers to yellow-fever endemic countries three times since 1924: • 1996 (from Venezuela to Marin County, CA) • 1999 (Brazil to Tennessee) • 2002 (Brazil to Texas) All cases were fatal.
Kyasanur Forest Disease Virus	No U.S. occurrences
Omsk Hemorrhagic Fever	No U.S. occurrences

Table 69.3 Clinical Features: Viral Hemorrhagic Fever

Early Signs	• High fever, headache, malaise, fatigue, arthralgias/myalgias, prostration, nausea, abdominal pain, nonbloody diarrhea • Mild hypotension, relative bradycardia, tachypnea, conjunctival involvement, pharyngitis, rash or flushing
Progression (1–2 weeks)	• Hemorrhagic manifestations (e.g., petechiae, hemorrhagic or purpuric rash, epistaxis, hematemesis, melena, hemoptysis, hematochezia, hematuria) • CNS dysfunction (e.g., delirium, convulsions, cerebellar signs, coma) • Hepatic involvement (e.g., jaundice, hepatitis)
Complications and Sequelae	• Shock, DIC, multisystem organ failure • Illness-induced abortion in pregnant women • Transverse myelitis • Uveitis • Pericarditis • Orchitis • Parotitis • Pancreatitis • Hearing or vision loss • Impaired motor coordination • Convalescence may be prolonged or complicated by weakness, fatigue, anorexia, cachexia, alopecia, arthralgias
Laboratory Findings	• Leukopenia (except in Lassa) • Leukocytosis • Thrombocytopenia • Elevated liver enzymes • Anemia or hemoconcentration • Coagulation abnormalities (e.g., prolonged bleeding time, prothrombin time, and activated partial thromboplastin time, elevated fibrin degradation products, and increased fibrinogen) • Proteinuria, hematuria, oliguria, and azotemia

CNS, central nervous system; DIC, disseminated intravascular coagulation.

Kyasanur Forest Disease

Kyasanur Forest disease is characterized by biphasic illness; 50% of patients go on to develop the second phase with meningoencephalitis (Table 69.9). Case fatality ranges from 3% to 10%.

Omsk Hemorrhagic Fever

Omsk hemorrhagic fever (OHF) is similar to Kyasanur Forest disease. Some also characterize OHF as a biphasic illness. with the first phase lasting 5–12 days with an estimated 30–50% of patients going on to experience remission of fever, febrile illness, and more severe disease (Table 69.10). Case fatality ranges from 0.5% to 3%. Recovery may take weeks, but sequelae are not common.

DIFFERENTIAL DIAGNOSIS

A high index of suspicion is required to diagnose VHF because there are no readily available rapid and specific confirma-

tory tests. In addition, the VHF viruses can have a nonspecific appearance or resemble a wide range of much more common illnesses.

With a VHF virus used as a biological weapon, patients are less likely to have risk factors for natural infection such as travel to VHF-endemic countries (Africa, Asia, or South America), contact with sick animals or people, or arthropod bites within 21 days of symptom onset. The observation of a severe illness with bleeding manifestations as its primary feature, which develops in several related cases, should be highly suspicious for VHF.

The Working Group for Civilian Biodefense suggests considering VHF in any patient with the following clinical presentation:

• Acute onset of fever (<3 weeks duration) in severely ill patient
• Hemorrhagic manifestations (at least two of the following: hemorrhagic or purpuric rash, epistaxis, hematemesis, hemoptysis, blood in stool, or other bleeding)
• No conditions predisposing for hemorrhagic illness
• No alternative diagnosis

Table 69.4 Clinical Features: Ebola and Marburg

Incubation Period	Prominent Clinical Features	Laboratory Findings
2–21 days	• Acute onset of fever, myalgias/arthralgias, headache, weakness, fatigue (<1 week) • Nausea, vomiting, abdominal pain, diarrhea, chest pain, cough, pharyngitis, hiccups • Maculopapular rash (day 5 after symptom onset) • Hemorrhagic manifestations • Photophobia, conjunctival inflammation, lymphadenopathy, hepatitis, pancreatitis (common) • CNS dysfunction • Shock with DIC and organ failure (week 2 after symptom onset) • Complications and sequelae: arthralgias, ocular disease, parotitis, orchitis, hearing loss, pericarditis, transverse myelitis	• Leukopenia (early) • Leukocytosis (late) • Thrombocytopenia (early) • Elevated liver enzymes • Elevated amylase • Lab features of DIC

CNS, central nervous system; DIC, disseminated intravascular coagulation.

Table 69.5 Clinical Features: Lassa Fever

Incubation Period	Prominent Clinical Features	Laboratory Findings
3–16 days	• Gradual onset of fever, weakness, pain, arthralgias • Chest and back pain, exudative pharyngitis, cough, abdominal pain, vomiting (very common) • Diarrhea and proteinuria (common) • Facial and pulmonary edema, mucosal bleeding, pleural effusions, neurological involvement (encephalopathy, coma, seizures), ascites, shock (less common) • Illness-induced abortion among pregnant women • Complications and sequelae: 8th cranial nerve damage with hearing loss, pericarditis	• Leukocyte and platelet counts often normal • Elevated liver enzymes may occur

Table 69.6 Clinical Features: New World Hemorrhagic Fever

Incubation Period	Prominent Clinical Features	Laboratory Findings
7–12 days (range 5–19)	• Gradual onset of fever, malaise, myalgias (especially lower back), pharyngitis • Drowsiness, dizziness, tremor, epigastric pain and/or constipation, photophobia, retro-orbital pain, conjunctivitis, lymphadenopathy, postural hypotension • Hemorrhagic manifestations (e.g., petechial rash [oral and dermal], facial flushing, facial edema, capillary leak syndrome, membrane hemorrhage, narrowing pulse pressure, vasoconstriction) • CNS dysfunction (e.g., hyporeflexia, gait abnormalities, palmomental reflex, tremors, other cerebellar signs) • Shock, coma, seizures	• Leukopenia • Thrombocytopenia • Proteinuria • Rising hematocrit

CNS, central nervous system.

Table 69.7 Clinical Features: Rift Valley Fever

Incubation Period	Prominent Clinical Features	Laboratory Findings
2–6 days	• Fever, nausea, vomiting • Abdominal pain, diarrhea, jaundice • CNS dysfunction • Hemorrhagic disease (1–17%) • Ocular involvement (photophobia, retro-orbital pain, retinitis, vision loss, scotoma) • Renal involvement or failure • Shock	• Thrombocytopenia • Leukopenia • Severe anemia • Elevated liver enzymes • Elevated LDH and CK

CK, creatine kinase; CNS, central nervous system; LDH, lactate dehydrogenase.

Table 69.8 Clinical Features: Yellow Fever

Incubation Period	Prominent Clinical Features	Laboratory Findings
3–6 days	Prodrome: • Acute onset of fever, headache, myalgias, • Facial flushing, conjunctival injection • Illness may resolve, enter remission (lasts hours or days), or progress to: • High fever, headache, severe myalgias (especially back), nausea, vomiting, abdominal pain, weakness, fatigue, bradycardia • Hemorrhagic manifestations • Fulminant infection with severe hepatic involvement • Shock, myocardial failure, renal failure, seizures, coma • Pneumonia, sepsis	• Leukopenia (early) • Leukocytosis (late) • Thrombocytopenia • Elevated liver enzymes and bilirubin • Albuminuria • Azotemia • Alkaline phosphatase levels only slightly elevated

Table 69.9 Clinical Features: Kyasanur Forest Disease

Incubation Period	Prominent Clinical Features	Laboratory Findings
2–9 days	Phase I (6–11 days): • Acute onset of fever, myalgias, headache (6–11 days) • Conjunctival involvement, soft palate lesions, GI symptoms • Hyperemia of face and trunk (but no rash) • Lymphadenopathy • Hemorrhagic manifestations (not severe) Phase II: • Afebrile period of 9–21 days followed by meningoencephalitis (50% of patients)	• Leukopenia • Lymphopenia or lymphocytosis • Thrombocytopenia • Abnormal liver function

GI, gastrointestinal.

Table 69.10 Clinical Features: Omsk Hemorrhagic Fever

Incubation Period	Prominent Clinical Features	Laboratory Findings
3–8 days (range 1–10 days)	• Acute onset of fever, headache, myalgias • Cough, conjunctivitis, soft pallet lesions, GI symptoms • Hyperemia of face and trunk (but no rash) • Lymphadenopathy, splenomegaly • Hemorrhagic manifestations (not severe) • Pneumonia, CNS dysfunction, meningeal signs, diffuse encephalitis	• Leukopenia • Thrombocytopenia

CNS, central nervous system; GI, gastrointestinal.

Differential diagnosis of infectious conditions includes:

- gram-negative bacterial septicemia
- toxic shock syndrome (*Staphylococcus*, *Streptococcus*)
- meningococcemia
- secondary syphilis
- septicemic plague
- salmonellosis (*Salmonella typhi*)
- shigellosis
- *Chlamydia* infection
- borreliosis
- leptospirosis
- rickettsiosis
- influenza
- measles
- rubella
- dengue hemorrhagic fever
- hemorrhagic varicella
- hemorrhagic smallpox
- viral hepatitis
- hantavirus pulmonary syndrome
- malaria
- African trypanosomiasis

Noninfectious conditions are:

- thrombotic or idiopathic thrombocytopenic purpura
- acute leukemia
- hemolytic-uremic syndrome
- collagen-vascular diseases

Table 69.11 Medical Management Recommendations

Categorization	Medical Management
Exposed persons	Medical surveillance No postexposure prophylaxis is recommended[1]
Suspected VHF case of *unknown viral type*	Supportive care *plus* ribavirin therapy[2]
Suspected or confirmed VHF case known to be *caused by a flavivirus or filovirus*	Supportive care only
Suspected confirmed VHF case known to be *caused by an arenavirus or bunyavirus*	Supportive care *plus* ribavirin therapy

[1] Previous CDC recommendations state that ribavirin should be given to high-risk contacts of persons with Lassa fever. The Working Group on Civilian Biodefense recommends medical surveillance only, and notes that the CDC guidelines may be under review.
[2] Ribavirin therapy should be initiated promptly unless another diagnosis is confirmed or the etiologic agent is known to be a flavivirus or filovirus.

LABORATORY DIAGNOSIS AND RADIOGRAPHIC FINDINGS

Viral hemorrhagic fevers are a risk to laboratory personnel. Clinicians should immediately notify their laboratory, local health department, and infection control professional when VHF is suspected. In the event of an outbreak, public health authorities will provide recommendations for specimen collection based on the situation (e.g., identification of etiologic agent, laboratory capacity).

Diagnosis of VHF requires a high index of suspicion because the disease initially presents with nonspecific symptoms and nonspecific results of routine lab tests. Laboratory findings consistent with specific VHF viruses are listed in Tables 69.4–69.10.

A number of test methods can be used to diagnose VHF at specialized laboratories. These include antigen-capture testing by enzyme-linked immunosorbent assay (ELISA), IgM antibody testing, paired acute-convalescent serum serologies, reverse transcriptase polymerase chain reaction (RT-PCR), immunohistochemistry methods, and electron microscopy. Viral identification in cell culture is the gold standard of viral detection; however, this may only be attempted at a Biosafety Level 4 (BSL-4) facility. Combined ELISA Ag/IgM has high specificity and sensitivity for early diagnosis of Lassa fever and provides prognostic information (presence of indirect fluorescent antibody early in disease is associated with death).

TREATMENT AND PROPHYLAXIS

Treatment

Medical management should follow the guidelines (Table 69.11):

Medical surveillance: Persons should be instructed to record their temperature twice daily and report any temperature of 38.0°C or 100.4 °F or higher (or any other signs or symptoms) to their clinician and/or the proper public health authorities. Patients should be advised not to share ther-

mometers between family members and to properly disinfect thermometers after each use.

Supportive care: Supportive care, including careful maintenance of fluid and electrolyte balance and circulatory volume, is essential for patients with all types of VHF. Mechanical ventilation, dialysis, and appropriate therapy for secondary infections may be indicated. Treatment of other suspected causes of disease, such as bacterial sepsis, should not be withheld while awaiting confirmation or exclusion of the diagnosis of VHF. Anticoagulant therapies, aspirin, nonsteroidal anti-inflammatory medications, and intramuscular injections are contraindicated.

Ribavirin therapy: Ribavirin is recommended for (1) suspect or probable cases of *VHF of unknown viral type* or (2) suspect, probable, or confirmed cases *caused by an arenavirus or bunyavirus*. Ribavirin has shown in vitro and in vivo activity against arenaviruses (Lassa fever, New World hemorrhagic fevers) and bunyaviruses (Rift Valley fever and others). Ribavirin has shown no activity against, and is not recommended for Filoviruses (Ebola and Marburg hemorrhagic fever) or Flaviviruses (Yellow fever, Kyasanur Forest disease, Omsk hemorrhagic fever). Recommendations for intravenous (IV) ribavirin therapy are shown in Table 69.12. Use of oral ribavirin may be necessary if the number of patients exceeds the medical care capacity for individual medical management.

Passive immunotherapy with convalescent human plasma has been used in the treatment and prophylaxis of several VHFs with inconclusive results. Some suggest passive immunotherapy for treatment of New World HFs based on effectiveness in Argentine HF (Junin).

Postexposure Prophylaxis

According to the Working Group on Civilian Biodefense, exposure is defined as proximity to an initial release of VHF virus, or close or high-risk contact with a patient suspected of having VHF. *High-risk* contacts are defined as persons who "have had mucous membrane contact with a patient (such as during kissing or sexual intercourse) or have had percutaneous injury involving contact with a patient's secretions, excretions, or blood." *Close contact* is defined as "those who live with, shake hands with, hug, process laboratory specimens from, or care for a patient with VHF prior to initiation of appropriate precautions." Medical surveillance (see above) is recommended for 21 days following the potential exposure or contact with the ill person.

Previous recommendations from the Centers for Disease Control and Prevention (CDC) state that prophylaxis with ribavirin should be given to persons exposed to Lassa virus. However, because the efficacy of ribavirin prophylaxis for Lassa virus is unknown, the Working Group also recommends that persons exposed be placed under medical surveillance until 21 days after the last exposure. The CDC recommendation is under review.

Vaccine

A licensed vaccine against yellow fever is effective if given prior to exposure. It is used for travelers going to endemic areas. This vaccine does not prompt development of antibodies rapidly enough to be used in the postexposure setting. A rare but serious adverse reaction to yellow fever vaccine,

Table 69.12 Recommendations for IV Ribavirin Therapy

	IV Therapy in Contained Casualty Situation[2]	Therapy in a Mass-Casualty Setting[2]
Adult	**Ribavirin** • Loading dose 30 mg/kg (max 2 gm) IV Followed by: • 16 mg/kg (max 1 gm) IV q6h × 4 days Followed by: • 8 mg/kg (max 500 mg) IV q8h × 6 days	**Ribavirin** • Loading dose of 2000 mg PO Followed by: • (Weight >75 kg): 1200 mg/day PO in two divided doses (600 mg in am and 600 mg in pm) × 10 days[3] • (Weight <75 kg): 1000 mg/day PO in two divided doses (400 mg in am and 600 mg in pm) × 10 days[3]
Children[4]	Same as for adults	• Loading dose of 30 mg/kg PO Followed by: • 15 mg/kg/d PO in two divided doses × 10 days
Pregnant Women[5]	Same as for nonpregnant adults	Same as for nonpregnant adults

[1] Ribavirin is not labeled for use in treatment of VHF by the US Food and Drug Administration (FDA) and must be used under an Investigational New Drug (IND) protocol.
[2] Use of oral vs. parenteral treatment will depend on resource availability.
[3] The current available formulation of ribavirin is 200-mg capsules, which cannot be broken open.
[4] IV and oral ribavirin are not approved for children by the FDA; however, the benefits may outweigh the risk of ribavirin therapy.
[5] Ribavirin is contraindicated in pregnant women; however, the benefits may outweigh the fetal risk of ribavirin therapy.

viscerotropic and neurotropic disease, has recently been recognized.

There is no licensed vaccine for any of the other VHFs, though research is underway on several candidates (Table 69.13).

Developmental VHF Therapeutics

Additional therapeutic candidates for vaccine, treatment, and prophylaxis of VHFs are currently under development (Table 69.13).

COMPLICATIONS AND ADMISSION CRITERIA

Patients with filovirus infection (Ebola and Marburg viruses) often experience hemorrhagic and severe central nervous system (CNS) manifestations along with fever and jaundice during the first week of illness. In the second week patients defervesce and either improve markedly or die as a result of multiorgan dysfunction, shock, and disseminated intravascular coagulation. Survivors may develop one or more complications including arthralgia, orchitis, hepatitis, transverse myelitis, or uveitis.

Death from Lassa virus infection, when it occurs, is typically during the second week of illness and is associated with hypotension, edema, and capillary leak syndrome. Up to one-third of Lassa fever survivors develop sensorineural deafness. The arenaviruses (Lassa and New World viruses) share a propensity to cause fetal demise and high mortality rates in pregnant women.

Among the bunyavirus infections (Rift Valley fever and Crimean-Congo hemorrhagic fever), a fulminant, fatal form of the disease with hemorrhage, hepatitis, and organ failure occurs in a minority of patients. Rift Valley fever encephalitis is known to occur in a small percentage of those affected.

Table 69.13 Developmental VHF Therapeutics

Virus	Candidates for Vaccine, Treatment, and Prophylaxis
Ebola and Marburg	• A live attenuated recombinant vaccine for Ebola and Marburg HF has produced protective immune responses in nonhuman primates • A vaccine used as PEP produced some protective effect for Ebola in nonhuman primates when administered soon after infection (20–30 minutes) • A Phase I clinical trial for an Ebola DNA vaccine was safe and produced an immune response in humans • Treatment with small interfering RNAs (siRNAs) produced protective immune response for Ebola in an animal model (guinea pigs)
Lassa Fever	• An attenuated recombinant vaccine produced protective immune responses in nonhuman primates
New World Hemorrhagic Fever	• Live-attenuated vaccine available as investigational new drug in Argentine HF • Passive immunotherapy with convalescent human serum has been effective in Argentine HF
Rift Valley Virus	• Vaccine available as investigational new drug
Yellow Fever	• Licensed vaccine available (see above)
Kyasanur Forest Disease	• Formalin inactivated vaccine licensed and used in endemic areas
Omsk Hemorrhagic Fever	NA

NA, not applicable; PEP, postexposure prophylaxis.

Although many infections with yellow fever are clinically inapparent, patients may develop multisystem illness

Table 69.14 Viral Hemorrhagic Fevers: CDC Infection Control Recommendations

The following infection control recommendations should be used when caring for a person with suspected VHF:
- Patients who are hospitalized or treated in an outpatient setting should be placed in a private room and **Standard, Contact, and Droplet Precautions** should be initiated. Patients with respiratory symptoms also should wear **a face mask** to contain respiratory droplets prior to placement in their hospital or examination room and during transport.
- Caretakers should use barrier precautions to prevent skin or mucous membrane exposure with patient blood, other body fluids, secretions (including respiratory droplets), or excretions. All persons entering the patient's room should wear gloves and gowns to prevent contact with items or environmental surfaces that may be soiled. In addition, face shields or surgical masks and eye protection (e.g., goggles or eyeglasses with side shields) should be worn by persons coming within approximately 3 feet of the patient.
- Additional barriers may be needed depending on the likelihood and magnitude of contact with body fluids. For example, if copious amounts of any body fluids or feces are present in the environment, plastic apron, leg, and shoe coverings also may be needed.
- Nonessential staff and visitors should be restricted from entering the room of patients with suspected VHF. Maintain a log of persons entering the patient's room.
- Before exiting the room of a patient with suspected VHF, safely remove and dispose of all protective gear, and clean and disinfect shoes that are soiled with body fluids as described in the section on environmental infection control below.
- To prevent percutaneous injuries, needles and other sharps should be used and disposed of in accordance with recommendations for Standard Precautions.
- If the patient requires a surgical or obstetric procedure, consult your local health department regarding appropriate precautions for these invasive procedures.
- Although transmission by the airborne route has not been established, hospitals may choose to use **Airborne Precautions** for patients with suspected VHF who have severe pulmonary involvement or who undergo procedures that stimulate coughing and promote the generation of aerosols. Alert laboratory staff to the nature of the specimens prior to sending them to the clinical laboratory. Specimens should remain in the custody of designated laboratory personnel until testing is completed. Due to the potential risks associated with handling infectious materials, laboratory testing should be limited to the minimum necessary for essential diagnostic evaluation and patient care.

Environmental Infection Control Procedures
- Environmental surfaces or inanimate objects contaminated with blood, other body fluids, secretions, or excretions should be cleaned and disinfected using standard procedures.
- Disinfection can be accomplished using a U.S. Environmental Protection Agency (EPA)-registered hospital disinfectant or a 1:100 dilution of household bleach (1/4 cup bleach to 1 gallon water). For grossly soiled surfaces (e.g., vomitus or stool), use a 1:10 dilution of household bleach.
- Soiled linens should be placed in clearly labeled leak-proof bags at the site of use, transported directly to the laundry area, and laundered following routine healthcare laundry procedures. Contaminated linens should be incinerated, autoclaved, or placed in labeled, leak-proof bags at the site of use and washed without sorting in a normal hot water cycle with bleach. Hospital housekeeping staff and linen handlers should wear appropriate personal protective equipment (as outlined in the section on isolation practices above) when handling or cleaning potentially contaminated material or surfaces.
- Liquid medical waste such as feces and vomitus can be disposed of in the sanitary sewer following local sewage disposal requirements (www.cdc.gov/ncidod/hip/enviro/guide.htm). Care should be taken to avoid splashing when disposing of these materials.
- When discarding solid medical waste (e.g., needles, syringes, and tubing) contaminated with blood or other body fluids from VHF patients, contain the waste with minimal agitation during handling. Properly contained wastes should be managed according to existing local and state regulations for ensuring health and environmental safety during medical waste treatment and disposal. On-site treatment of the waste in an incinerator or a gravity-displacement autoclave for decontamination purposes will help to minimize handling of contaminated waste. Alternatively, off-site medical waste treatment resources may be used.

From CDC (2005), http://www.cdc.gov/ncidod/dhqp/bp_vhf_interimGuidance.html

dominated by an icteric hepatitis and a severe bleeding diathesis. In the latter stages of illness encephalopathy, shock, and death may ensue. Patients who recover frequently suffer from secondary bacterial infections.

The need for hospitalization and life support will be apparent in patients with bleeding diatheses, CNS dysfunction, shock, or severe hepatorenal dysfunction. Patients exhibiting milder manifestations of VHF or who appear to be in the early stages of disease could benefit from hospitalization for supportive care and close observation. Treatment with intravenous ribavirin should be initiated in patients known to have arenavirus or bunyavirus infection and in those with VHF of unknown etiology pending viral identification.

INFECTION CONTROL

Clinicians should notify local public health authorities, their institution's infection control professional, and their laboratory of any suspected VHF cases. Public health authorities may conduct epidemiologic investigations and implement disease control interventions to protect the public.

Many VHF viruses are virulent, and some are highly infectious (e.g., filoviruses and arenaviruses) with *person-to-person transmission* from direct contact with infected blood and bodily secretions. Effective therapies and prophylaxis are extremely limited for VHF; therefore, early detection and

strict adherence with infection control measures are essential (Table 69.14). Transmission rarely (if ever) occurs before the onset of symptoms. Risk of transmission is greatest during the latter stages of illness when viral loads are highest.

Among household contacts, secondary transmission for Ebola and Marburg ranges from 10% to 20%. In the 1995 Ebola outbreak in the Democratic Republic of Congo, transmission did not occur among household contacts with no direct physical contact with patients. Persons with physical contact with patients were at increased risk of transmission, and those with body fluid contact had the greatest risk.

All persons exposed to VHF should immediately wash the affected skin surfaces with soap and water. Mucous membranes should be irrigated with copious amounts of water or eyewash solution. Exposed persons should receive medical evaluation and monitoring.

PEARLS AND PITFALLS

1. Since effective postexposure prophylaxis is unavailable for VHF, strict adherence to infection control measures is essential for limiting the spread of disease.
2. The risk for person-to-person transmission of hemorrhagic fever viruses is highest during the latter phases of illness, when viral loads are high and disease manifestations are most severe.

3. VHF viruses are not endemic in the United States, with the rare exception of Whitewater Arroyo virus, which caused three cases of human disease in California in 1999–2000 and may have been related to wild rodents. Nearly all U.S. cases of VHF have been acquired by overseas travelers or by scientific research personnel.

REFERENCES

Borchert M, Mulangu S, Swanepoel R, et al. Serosurvey on household contacts of Marburg virus. Emerg Infect Dis 2006;12(3):433–9.

Centers for Disease Control and Prevention (CDC). Yellow fever vaccine recommendations of the Advisory Committee on Immunization Practices (ACIP), 2002. MMWR 2002 Nov 8;51(RR17):1–10.

Centers for Disease Control and Prevention (CDC). Factsheet: Kyasanur Forest Disease. 2002. April 6, 2007. Available at: http://www.cdc.gov/ncidod/dvrd/spb/mnpages/dispages/kyasanur.htm.

Centers for Disease Control and Prevention (CDC). Factsheet: Omsk Hemorrhagic Fever. 2002. April 6, 2007. Available at: http://www.cdc.gov/ncidod/dvrol/spb/mnpages/dispages/omsk.htm.

Centers for Disease Control and Prevention (CDC). Fatal illnesses associated with a New World arenavirus – California, 1999–2000. MMWR 2000;49(31):709–11.

Centers for Disease Control and Prevention (CDC). Fatal yellow fever in a traveler returning from Amazonas, Brazil, 2002. MMWR 2000;51(15):324–5.

Centers for Disease Control and Prevention (CDC). Fatal yellow fever in a traveler returning from Venezuela, 1999. MMWR 2000;49(14):303–5.

Centers for Disease Control and Prevention (CDC). Imported Lassa Fever – New Jersey, 2004. MMWR 2004;53(38):894–7.

Centers for Disease Control and Prevention (CDC). Interim guidance for managing patients with suspected viral hemorrhagic fever in U.S. hospitals. 2005. Available at: http://www.cdc.gov/ncidod/dhgp/bp_vhf_interimGuidence.html.

Feldmann H, Jones SM, Daddario-Dicaprio KM, et al. Effective post-exposure treatment of Ebola infection. PLoS Pathog 2007;19;3(1):e2.

Geisbert TW, Hensley LE, Kagan E, et al. Postexposure protection of guinea pigs against a lethal Ebola virus challenge is conferred by RNA interference. J Infect Dis 2006;193(12):1650–7.

Geisbert TW, Jones S, Fritz EA, et al. Development of a new vaccine for the prevention of Lassa fever. PLoS Med 2005;2(6).

Jones SM, et al. Live attenuated recombinant vaccine protects nonhuman primates against Ebola and Marburg viruses. Nat Med 2005;11(7):786–90.

Leroy EM, Kumulungui B, Pourrut X, et al. Fruit bats as reservoirs of Ebola virus. Nature 2005;438(7068):575–6.

Madani TA, et al. Rift Valley fever epidemic in Saudi Arabia: epidemiological, clinical, and laboratory characteristics. Clin Infect Dis 2003;37(8):1084–92.

Maiztegui JI, McKee KT, Barrera Oro JG, et al. Protective efficacy for a live attenuated vaccine against Argentine hemorrhagic fever. J Infect Dis 1998;177(2):277–83.

Martin JE, Sullivan NJ, Enama ME, et al. A DNA vaccine for Ebola virus is safe and immunogenic in a phase I clinical trial. Clin Vaccine Immunol 2006;13(11):1267–77.

Mupapa K, Mukundu W, Bwaka MA, et al. Ebola hemorrhagic fever and pregnancy. J Infect Dis 1999;179 Suppl 1:S11–2.

Mupapa K, Massamba M, Kibadi K, et al. Treatment of Ebola hemorrhagic fever with blood transfusions from convalescent patients. J Infect Dis 1999;179(Suppl 1):S18–23.

Pattnaik P. Kyasanur forest disease: an epidemiological view in India. Rev Med Virol 2006 May–Jun;16(3):151–65.

Peters CJ, LeDuc JW. An introduction to Ebola: the virus and the disease. J Infect Dis 1999;179(Suppl 1):ix–xvi.

Pittman PR, Liu CT, Cannon TL, et al. Immunogenicity of an inactivated Rift Valley fever vaccine in humans. Vaccine 1999;18(1–2):181–9.

ADDITIONAL READINGS

Borio L, Inglesby T, Peters CJ, et al. Hemorrhagic fever viruses as biological weapons: medical and public health management. JAMA 2002;287(18):2391–405.

Center for Infectious Disease Research and Policy (CIDRAP). Viral hemorrhagic fever (VHF): current, comprehensive information on pathogenesis, microbiology, epidemiology, diagnosis, treatment, and prophylaxis. 2006. Retrieved April 6, 2007, from http://www.cidrap.umn.edu/cidrap/content/bt/vhf/biofacts/vhffactsheet.html.

Peters CJ. Chapter 164 – Lymphocytic choriomeningitis virus, Lassa virus, and the South American hemorrhagic fevers. In: Mandell GL, Bennett JE, Dolin R, eds, Principles and practice of infectious diseases (6th ed). New York: Churchill Livingstone, 2005.

Peters CJ. Chapter 326 – Bioterrorism: viral hemorrhagic fevers. In: Mandell GL, Bennett JE, Dolin R, eds, Principles and practice of infectious diseases (6th ed). New York: Churchill Livingstone, 2005.

Tsai TF, Vaughn DW, Solomon T. Chapter 149 – Flaviviruses (yellow fever, dengue hemorrhagic fever, Japanese encephalitis, West Nile encephalitis, tick-borne encephalitis). In: Mandell GL, Bennett JE, Dolin R, eds, Principles and practice of infectious diseases (6th ed). New York: Churchill Livingstone, 2005.

70. Hantavirus

Rachel L. Chin and Deborah Colina

INTRODUCTION

Hantaviruses belong to the enveloped viruses within the family Bunyaviridae, genus *Hantavirus*, and all medically important species are carried by rodents of the family Muridae. Named for the Hantaan River in Korea, hantaviruses were first isolated in 1976, though the clinical syndrome they cause came to widespread attention in the early 1950s when more than 3000 United States and United Nations Korean War forces contracted an acute febrile illness associated with renal failure and coagulopathy. Hantaviruses are also believed to have been responsible for outbreaks of hemorrhagic fevers in Russia (1913), Scandinavia (1932–1935), and Finland (1945), though they have become clinically significant in the United States only over the past 15 years.

Hantavirus infection causes two distinct clinical syndromes characterized, respectively, by renal failure or cardiovascular collapse. The so-called "Old World" hantaviruses endemic to Asia and Europe cause hemorrhagic fever with renal syndrome (HFRS), whereas the "New World" hantaviruses endemic to North America cause hantavirus cardiopulmonary syndrome (HCPS), also known as hantavirus pulmonary syndrome (HPS). Both diseases appear to be immunopathologic.

EPIDEMIOLOGY

There are 20 distinct hantavirus species, but only 11 are associated with human disease. HFRS can be caused by any of the Old World hantavirus strains including Hantaan, Seoul, Dobrava-Belgrade, and Puumala viruses. (See Figure 70.1.) Infection with hantaviruses is associated with significant morbidity and mortality worldwide, although fewer than one-fourth of cases have a severe course. Overall mortality from HFRS varies widely, from 0.5 percent with the milder European forms of the disease, to as high as 5 to 10 percent for Korean hemorrhagic fever.

The more virulent HCPS was first recognized in 1993 in the Four Corners region of the southwestern United States, named for the intersection of the borders of Utah, New Mexico, Arizona, and Colorado. Two clusters of patients developed fever, chills, and myalgias, followed by cough and dyspnea, with rapid progression to cardiovascular collapse, respiratory failure, and death. The initial mortality rate was nearly 80%. Often referred to as the "Four Corners" virus early on, the etiologic agent isolated was finally called the "Sin Nombre" virus (SNV).

As with all viruses, the distribution of hantaviruses is dictated by the range of their natural hosts. Rodents infected with hantaviruses are chronic carriers without apparent disease, and human infection by hantavirus occurs through inhalation of aerosolized infected rodent urine, droppings, or saliva, resulting in HCPS or HFRS. Rodent reservoirs of human-pathogenic hantaviruses are not common in cities, and most cases of hantavirus disease are associated with exposure to rodents or rodent droppings in rural areas.

The deer mouse (*Peromyscus maniculatus*) is the primary reservoir of SNV and is common in rural areas throughout much of the United States. Although prevalence varies seasonally and geographically and higher rates have been documented in outbreak areas, about 10% of deer mice tested show evidence of infection with SNV. There are several hantaviruses associated with different rodent populations, such as the cotton rat (*Sigmodon hispidus*), the marsh rice rat (*Oryzomys palustris*) and the white-footed mouse (*Peromyscus leucopus*).

CLINICAL PRESENTATION OF HEMORRHAGIC FEVER WITH RENAL SYNDROME

The initial cases described in Korea were associated with renal failure, fever, hypotension, thrombocytopenia, and disseminated intravascular coagulation (DIC), a constellation of symptoms now known as HFRS. Patients with classic HFRS progress from fever with hemorrhage, to hypotension and shock, and then to oliguric renal failure. The severity of illness is related to the strain of infecting hantavirus and can be extremely variable. Infection has even been documented in asymptomatic patients (Table 70.1).

Seen mostly in Europe, the Puumala virus generally causes mild disease and can present with fever, abdominal pain, nausea and vomiting, malaise, conjunctival

Virus	Host	Localities	Distribution of Host	Disease
Hantaan	*Apodemus agrarius*	Korea	C. Europe south to Thrace, Caucasus, and Tien Shan Mountains; Amur River through Korea to E. Xizang and E. Yunnan, W. Sichuan, Fujiau, and Taiwan (China)	HFRS
Seoul	*Rattus norvegicus, R. rattus*	Korea	Worldwide; commensal rat hosts	HFRS
Dobrava/Belgrade	*A. flavicollis*	Slovenia; former Yugoslavia	England and Wales, from N.W. Spain, France, S. Scandinavia through European Russia to Urals, S. Italy, the Balkans, Syria, Lebanon, and Israel	HFRS
Puumala	*Clethrionomys glareolus*	Finland	W. Palaearctic from France and Scandinavia to Lake Baikal, south to N. Spain, N. Italy, Balkans, W. Turkey, N. Khazakhstan, Altai and Sayan Mountains, Britain and S.W. Ireland	HFRS
Sin Nombre	*Peromyscus maniculatus*	New Mexico California, United States	Alaska panhandle across N. Canada, south through most of the continental United States excluding S.E. and E. seaboard, to southernmost Baja California Sur, and to N.C. Oaxaca, Mexico.	HCPS
Black Creek Canal	*Sigmodon hispidus*	Florida, United States	S.E. United States, from S. Nebraska to C. Virginia south to S. E. Arizona and peninsular Florida; interior and E. Mexico through Middle America to C. Panama; in South America to N. Colombia and N. Venezuela	HCPS
New York	*P. leucopus*	Long Island, United States	C. and E. United States to S. Alberta and S. Ontario, Quebec and Nova Scotia, Canada; to N. Durango and along Caribbean coast to isthmus of Tehuantepec and Yucatan peninsula, Mexico	HCPS
Bayou	*Oryzomys palustris*	N. Louisiana, United States	S.E. United States, S. E. Kansas to E. Texas, eastwards to S. New Jersey and peninsular Florida	HCPS
Andes	*Oligoryzomys longicaudatus*	Patagonia, Argentina	N.C. to S. Andes, approximately to 501/S latitude, of Chile and Argentina	HCPS
Laguna Negra	*Calomys laucha*	Paraguay	N. Argentina and Uruguay, S.E. Bolivia, W. Paraguay, and W. C. Brazil	HCPS
Choclo	*Oligoryzomys fulvescens*	Panama	S. Mexico, through Mesoamerica to Ecuador, northernmost Brazil, and Guineas in South America	HCPS

Figure 70.1 Worldwide hantavirus prevalence. Reproduce with permission from: Hjelle B. Epidemiology and diagnosis of hantavirus infections. In: UpToDate, Rose BD (Ed), UpToDate, Waltham, MA, 2007. Copyright 2007 UpToDate, Inc. For more information visit www.uptodate.com.

hemorrhage, headache, and blurred vision. Dobrava infections are similar to Puumala but may also cause hemorrhagic complications.

The Asian strains cause more severe clinical symptoms with more than one-third of patients becoming hypotensive and two-thirds requiring dialysis for oliguria.

DIFFERENTIAL DIAGNOSIS FOR HEMORRHAGIC FEVER WITH RENAL SYNDROME

Given a history of exposure to rodents either due to occupation (e.g., farming, forestry, animal trapping) or recreation (e.g., camping), the possibility of HFRS should be considered in any patient with high fevers and nonspecific complaints.

The differential diagnosis in HFRS includes other infections associated with acute renal failure, as well as noninfectious causes of acute interstitial nephritis:

- murine typhus
- scrub typhus
- Colorado tick fever
- septicemia
- DIC
- hepatitis
- leptospirosis
- hemolytic uremic syndrome

- other hemorrhagic fevers: e.g., ebola, dengue fever, Lassa fever (see Chapter 69, Viral Hemorrhagic Fever)
- noninfectious acute interstitial nephritis caused by drugs (e.g., NSAIDs)

LABORATORY AND RADIOGRAPHIC FINDINGS IN HEMORRHAGIC FEVER WITH RENAL SYNDROME

Routine laboratory findings are nonspecific and include thrombocytopenia, leukocytosis, evidence of renal failure (e.g., elevated serum creatinine, proteinuria, hematuria, abnormal urinary sedimentation and reduced glomerular filtration rate), elevated C-reactive protein, and prolonged bleeding time, partial thromboplastin and prothrombin time. Chest radiograph may be normal or may show pulmonary infiltrates or edema, though this is not a defining characteristic of the illness as it is for HCPS.

Both IgM and IgG hantavirus-specific antibodies are present by the time the patient presents with symptoms. Definitive diagnosis of HFRS can easily be made by serologic assays such as enzyme-linked immunosorbent assay (ELISA), which detects IgM and IgG antibodies. Western blot and strip immunoblot assays (SIA) are most commonly used, and employ a nucleocapsid (N) antigen for the detection of hantavirus antibodies. To detect acute infection, a rapid immunoblot strip assay (RIBA) can be utilized. RIBA is a

Table 70.1 Clinical Features: Hemorrhagic Fever with Renal Syndrome

Organisms	• Hantaan • Seoul • Dobrava/Belgrade • Puumala
Incubation Period	Up to 45 days after exposure
Transmission	Aerosolized rodent urine, droppings, or saliva
Signs and Symptoms	• Fever • Abdominal pain • Nausea and vomiting • Malaise • Hemorrhage • Headache • Blurred vision • Hypotension • Shock • Oliguria • Coma
Laboratory and Radiographic Findings	• Thrombocytopenia • Leukocytosis • Renal findings (e.g. elevated serum creatinine level, proteinuria, hematuria, abnormal urinary sedimentation, and reduced glomerular filtration rate) • Prolonged bleeding time, PT, aPTT • Elevated C-reactive protein • IgM and IgG hantavirus-specific antibodies
Treatment	• Supportive care • Platelet transfusion • Renal dialysis

aPTT, activated partial thromboplastin time; PT, prothrombin time.

Table 70.2 Clinical Features: Hantavirus Cardiopulmonary Syndrome

Organisms*	• Sin Nombre virus • Black Creek Canal • New York • Bayou
Incubation Period	Up to 21 days after exposure
Transmission	Exposure to aerosolized rodent urine, droppings, or saliva
Signs and Symptoms	**Febrile prodrome:** • Sudden onset of fever, chills, malaise, weakness, myalgias, headache • Dyspnea, cough, tachypnea, tachycardia • Gastrointestinal complaints such as nausea, vomiting, abdominal pain, diarrhea • Abdominal and back pain, arthralgias • Weakness, dehydration **Progression to cardiopulmonary signs and symptoms:** • Pulmonary edema • Pleural effusions • Respiratory failure • Hypotension • Myocardial depression • Dysrhythmias
Laboratory and Radiographic Findings	**Diagnostic Triad:** • Thrombocytopenia • Increased immature granulocytes (with leukocytosis) • Atypical lymphocytes **Other laboratory findings:** • Elevated LDH • Elevated LFTs • Elevated lactate levels • Prolonged PTT and PT • IgM and IgG hantavirus-specific antibodies **Radiographic findings:** • Pulmonary edema • Bilateral interstitial infiltrates • Pleural effusions
Treatment	• Empiric therapy for possible bacterial pneumonia until diagnosis of HCPS is definitively determined • Supportive care including ICU monitoring and mechanical ventilation • Early use of vasopressors • Cautious use of IV fluids • No specific antiviral therapy is recommended • ECMO should be considered in patients with poor prognostic indicators at specialized centers

PT, prothrombin time; PTT, partial thromboplastin time.
*These hantaviruses are found in the United States. The Andes, Laguna Negra, and Choclo hantaviruses are found in South America.

dipstick-type test that detects SNV antibodies. Other tests used are indirect immunofluorescence (IFA), complement fixation, and hemagglutinin inhibition, as well as focus or plaque reduction neutralization tests to detect antibodies to hantaviruses.

TREATMENT OF HEMORRHAGIC FEVER WITH RENAL SYNDROME

There are no specific antiviral therapies for HFRS. Although one prospective double-blinded study found that intravenous ribavirin therapy resulted in a reduction in mortality, other studies did not confirm these findings.

Treatment is primarily supportive. Medications that may cause further renal injury such as NSAIDS should be avoided. Thrombocytopenia may require platelet transfusion. Renal dialysis should be provided for the usual indications such as refractory fluid overload, hyperkalemia, metabolic acidosis, and symptomatic uremia.

CLINICAL PRESENTATION OF HANTAVIRUS CARDIOPULMONARY SYNDROME

The usual incubation period for a hantavirus causing HCPS, typically SNV, is 21 days. The clinical course of HCPS advances through several stages (Table 70.2).

The Febrile Prodromal Phase

Patients with HCPS typically present with nonspecific symptoms of fevers, chills, malaise, weakness, myalgias, and headache. Other early symptoms include cough, tachycardia, gastrointestinal symptoms, abdominal and back pain, and arthralgias. Patients may also have shortness of breath and tachypnea (respiratory rate of 26–30 per minute). The physical examination is usually otherwise normal and patients are often discharged with a diagnosis of nonspecific viral syndrome. It is not uncommon for patients to return hours or a few days later extremely ill.

The Cardiopulmonary Phase

The prodrome phase is followed by the rapid onset of hypotension, non-cardiogenic pulmonary edema, and hypoxia, often requiring mechanical ventilation. Some patients develop severe myocardial depression, which can progress to sinus bradycardia with subsequent electromechanical dissociation, and ventricular tachycardia or fibrillation.

In contrast to HFRS, hemorrhage rarely occurs in HCPS. Poor prognostic indicators in HCPS include hypotension refractory to pressors, cardiac dysrhythmias, serum lactate greater than 4.0 mmol/L and a cardiac index less than 2.2 L/min/m^2. Fortunately, multiorgan failure is rarely seen, although HCPS patients may have mildly impaired renal function.

The Convalescent Phase

Survivors frequently become polyuric during the convalescent phase and improve almost as rapidly as they decompensated.

DIFFERENTIAL DIAGNOSIS FOR HANTAVIRUS CARDIOPULMONARY SYNDROME

Hantavirus cardiopulmonary syndrome is commonly confused with acute respiratory distress syndrome from other infectious causes, pyelonephritis, intra-abdominal processes, pneumonias, and systemic infections such as rickettsial disease or plague.

Key features that may help to distinguish HCPS are:

- thrombocytopenia
- history of exposure to rodents or rodent droppings
- history of travel in rural areas

Other conditions to consider in HCPS are:

- pneumonias
- influenza
- rickettsial disease
- pneumonic plague (*Yersinia pestis*)
- tularemia
- anthrax
- Colorado tick fever
- lymphocytic choriomeningitis virus infection
- dengue fever
- Rocky Mountain spotted fever
- Q fever
- Lyme disease
- rat-bite fever

Other noninfectious etiologies include diseases associated with pulmonary hemorrhage, such as Wegener's granulomatosis and Goodpasture's syndrome.

LABORATORY AND RADIOGRAPHIC FINDINGS IN HANTAVIRUS CARDIOPULMONARY SYNDROME

The classical triad of thrombocytopenia, leukocytosis with immature granulocytes (i.e., myelocytes, promyelocytes), and atypical lymphocytes is almost diagnostic of HCPS. Elevated LFT's, LDH, partial thromboplastin time (PTT) and prothrombin time (PT) are also commonly seen. Elevated hematocrit, increased lactate levels, and consequent acidosis are associated with poor prognosis.

Chest radiograph usually shows a normal caridac silhouette and evidence of interstitial pulmonary edema (Kerley B lines, peribronchial thickening). Pleural effusions are common late in the course of the disease.

Both IgM and IgG SNV-specific antibodies are present by the time the patient presents with symptoms. Definitive diagnosis of HCPS can be made by the same serologic assays described above for HFRS.

TREATMENT OF HANTAVIRUS CARDIOPULMONARY SYNDROME

Treatment for HCPS is mainly supportive. This includes intensive care unit monitoring and the use of mechanical ventilation and vasopressors as needed. Because pulmonary edema is common, crystalloid fluid resuscitation should be monitored carefully. Flow-directed pulmonary artery catheterization (PAC), or Swan-Ganz catheter, is critical in severe HCPS, and the cardiac index during the acute phase of illness has been associated with prognosis. Dobutamine is the preferred inotrope, with the addition of dopamine if necessary. Patients with HCPS may require large doses of pressors to maintain blood pressure.

Specific indicators of poor outcome include hypotension refractory to pressors, cardiac dysrhythmias, serum lactate greater than 4.0 mmol/L, and a cardiac index less than 2.5 L/min/m^2. Extracorporeal membrane oxygenation (ECMO) provides both respiratory and cardiovascular support and has resulted in better survival rates in patients with poor prognostic indicators.

Because pneumonia is in the differential diagnosis of HCPS, patients suspected of HCPS should be treated with antibiotic regimens designed to treat typical and atypical community acquired pneumonia and sepsis, until the diagnosis of HCPS is made by laboratory analysis.

COMPLICATIONS AND ADMISSION CRITERIA FOR HANTAVIRUS SYNDROMES

Hemorrhagic fever with renal syndrome is usually associated with fever, hemorrhage, hypotension, and renal failure. Patients suspected of HFRS should be admitted for supportive care and monitoring. The severity of illness is based upon the strain of infecting hantavirus and can be extremely variable.

Potential complications of HCPS include cardiovascular collapse and respiratory and renal failure. All patients suspected of HCPS should be admitted to the intensive care unit because of the high likelihood of rapid deterioration.

INFECTION CONTROL

Human infection by hantavirus most commonly occurs via inhalation of infectious, aerosolized rodent saliva or excreta. High risk of exposure has been associated with entering or cleaning rodent-infested structures. Persons have also acquired HFRS or HCPS after being bitten by rodents.

There is no need for isolation of patients with confirmed hantavirus because there is no person to person transmission. Patients should be isolated in cases of suspected hantavirus when the differential diagnosis still includes highly communicable diseases such as pneumonic plague.

PEARLS AND PITFALLS

1. The early phase of mild hantavirus infection manifests few constitutional symptoms and can be easily misdiagnosed.
2. Patients with HCPS can deteriorate quickly. Any suspected patients with HCPS should be admitted to an intensive care setting. Survival is increased with early recognition, and aggressive pulmonary and hemodynamic support.
3. Specific indicators of poor outcome include hypotension refractory to pressors, cardiac dysrhythmias, serum lactate greater than 4.0 mmol/L, and a cardiac index less than 2.5 L/min/m^2. These patients may be candidates for ECMO.

REFERENCES

Appel GB, Mustonen J. Renal involvement with hantavirus infection (hemorrhagic fever with renal syndrome). UpToDate online 15.3. Accessed February 1, 2008, from: http://www.uptodate.com.

Bharadwaj M, Nofchissey R, Goade D, et al. Humoral immune responses in the hantavirus cardiopulmonary syndrome. J Infect Dis 2000;182:43–8.

Centers for Disease Control and Prevention (CDC). Hantavirus pulmonary syndrome – United States: updated recommendations for risk reduction. MMWR Recomm Rep 2002 Jul 26;51(RR-9):1–12.

Dull SM, Brillman JC, Simpson SQ, et al. Hantavirus pulmonary syndrome: recognition and emergency department management. Ann Emerg Med 1994 Sep;24(3):530–6.

Hjelle B. Epidemiology and diagnosis of hantavirus infections. In: UpToDate, Rose BD (Ed), UpToDate, Waltham, MA, 2007. Accessed February 1, 2008, from: http://www.uptodate.com.

Hjelle B. Hantavirus cardiopulmonary syndrome. UpToDate online 15.3. Accessed February 1, 2008, from: http://www.uptodate.com.

Katai LH, Williamson MR, Telepak RJ, et al. Hantavirus pulmonary syndrome: radiographic findings in 16 patients. Radiology 1994;191(3):665–8.

Ksiazek TG, Peters CJ, Rollin PE, et al. Identification of a new North American hantavirus that causes acute pulmonary insufficiency. Am J Trop Med Hyg 1995 Feb;52(2):117–23.

Lee HW, van der Groen G. Hemorrhagic fever with renal syndrome. Prog Med Virol 1989;36:62–102.

Lumumb-Kosongo M, Gang M, Cameron S. Hantavirus cardiopulmonary syndrome. eMedicine topic 861, April 2006. Accessed January 4, 2008, from: http://www.emedicine.com/emerg/topic861.htm.

Mertz GJ, Hjelle BL, Bryan RT. Hantavirus infection. Adv Intern Med 1997;42:369–421.

Sairam V, Travis Lxxx. Hemorrhagic fever with renal failure syndrome. eMedicine, Jan 2006. Accessed January 4, 2008, from: http://www.emedicine.com/ped/topic968.htm.

Saks MA, Karras D. Emergency medicine and the public's health: emerging infectious diseases. Emerg Med Clin N Am 2006;24:1019–33.

Peters CJ, Khan AS. Hantavirus pulmonary syndrome: the new American hemorrhagic fever. Clin Infect Dis 2002;34:1224–31.

Peters CJ, Simpson GL, Levy H. Spectrum of Hantavirus infection: hemorrhagic fever with renal syndrome and hantavirus pulmonary syndrome; Annu Rev Med 1999;50:531–45.

Vapalahti O, Mustonen J, Lundkvist A, et al. Hantavirus infections in Europe. Lancet Infect Dis. 2003 Oct;3(10):653–61.

ADDITIONAL READINGS

Centers for Disease Control and Prevention (CDC). All about hantaviruses. Accessed January 1, 2008, from: http://www.cdc.gov/ncidod/diseases/hanta/hps/index.htm.

Koster F, Foucar K, Hjelle B, et al. Rapid presumptive diagnosis of hantavirus cardiopulmonary syndrome by peripheral blood smear review. Am J Clin Pathol 2001;116(5):665–72.

Mertz GJ, Miedzinski L, Goade D, et al. Placebo-controlled, double-blind trial of intravenous ribavirin for the treatment of hantavirus cardiopulmonary syndrome in Northern America. Clin Infect Dis 2004;39:1307–13.

71. Avian Influenza A (H5N1)

Timothy M. Uyeki

INTRODUCTION

Since 2003, the global panzootic of highly pathogenic avian influenza A (H5N1) among domestic poultry and wild birds has resulted in rare, sporadic, human H5N1 cases of severe respiratory disease with high mortality in Asia, Europe, the Middle East, and Africa. Family clusters of H5N1 cases have been documented, and though most transmission of H5N1 viruses to humans is believed to be directly from sick or dead birds, limited human-to-human transmission of H5N1 viruses has been reported. As H5N1 viruses continue to evolve, the concern for a global influenza pandemic rises.

EPIDEMIOLOGY

Highly pathogenic avian influenza A (H5N1) viruses are single-stranded negative-sense RNA viruses of the Orthomyxoviridae family, whose natural reservoir is in wild aquatic ducks and geese. Influenza A viruses are subtyped on the basis of the two major surface glycoproteins, hemagglutinin (HA), and neuraminidase (NA). Avian influenza A viruses include all 16 known HA and nine known NA subtypes.

Avian influenza is a disease of birds caused by infection with avian influenza A viruses that infect the respiratory and gastrointestinal tracts. Birds excrete avian influenza A viruses in feces, and the virus can remain viable for prolonged periods in the setting of low temperatures, low humidity, and abundant fecal protein matter. H5N1 virus infections of other animals, including pigs, cats, dogs, civet cats, a stone marten, tigers, and leopards have also been reported.

Two major antigenically and genetically distinct groups, or clades, of highly pathogenic H5N1 viruses have circulated among poultry and birds in different geographic areas. Clade 1 H5N1 viruses have infected poultry in Laos, Cambodia, Thailand, and Vietnam. Clade 2 H5N1 viruses include at least five antigenically and genetically distinct subclades, of which three (2.1, 2.2, 2.3) have infected humans to date. Clade 2.1 viruses are circulating among poultry in Indonesia, clade 2.2 viruses have infected poultry and wild birds in China, Europe, the Middle East, and Africa, and clade 2.3 viruses are circulating among poultry in China and Southeast Asia. As of March 2008, 10 clades of H5N1 viruses had been identified among birds, and 4 (clades 0, 1, 2, 7) had infected humans

The first known outbreak of highly pathogenic H5N1 viruses in humans occurred in Hong Kong during 1997 with 18 cases and six deaths over a wide age range. The primary risk factor was visiting a live poultry market in the week prior to illness onset. The outbreak was associated with widespread poultry deaths at live poultry markets and was controlled by the culling of 1.5 million poultry, temporary cessation of poultry importation from southern China, and implementation of improved biosecurity and other measures in poultry markets. Poultry now sold in Hong Kong live poultry markets are routinely vaccinated against H5 viruses. In February 2003, two human H5N1 cases with one death were confirmed in Hong Kong residents who had visited southern China. These cases were overshadowed by the outbreaks of severe acute respiratory syndrome (SARS) in many countries in March 2003.

During late 2003 and into early 2004, widespread poultry outbreaks of highly pathogenic H5N1 viruses occurred in Asia and Southeast Asia with associated human cases. In late 2003, human H5N1 cases were detected in Beijing, China, and in Vietnam. Waves of human H5N1 cases with high mortality followed in Vietnam, Thailand, and Cambodia between 2004 and 2005. During 2005–07, H5N1 viruses spread to poultry and birds in Europe, the Middle East, and Africa, with associated human cases documented in previously unaffected countries. Generally, human H5N1 cases have occurred during the winter months in association with poultry outbreaks, cooler temperature, and low-humidity periods. However, in countries such as Indonesia, where H5N1 is endemic among backyard poultry, human H5N1 cases have occurred in nearly every month since mid-2005. As of March 28, 2008, 373 H5N1 cases (case fatality 63%) had been reported from 14 countries since January 2004 (Vietnam, Thailand, Cambodia, Indonesia, China, Turkey, Azerbaijan, Egypt, Iraq, Djibouti, Nigeria, Laos, Burma, and Pakistan).

An analysis of 256 H5N1 cases by the World Health Organization (WHO) found an equal number of male and female cases with a median age of 18 years (range 3 months to 75 years) and approximately 90% less than 40 years of age. Overall mortality was 60%, with the highest case fatality proportion in cases aged 10–19 years (76%) and lowest in cases aged

50 years and older (40%). The median duration from illness onset to hospital admission was 4 days (range 0–18 days), and the median time from illness onset to death was 9 days (range 2–31 days). Fatal cases have included pregnant women.

Although the majority of H5N1 cases have been sporadic, clusters of at least two epidemiologically linked cases have occurred in several countries. Almost all clusters of H5N1 cases have occurred in blood-related family members. The largest family cluster to date included eight cases with seven deaths and occurred in North Sumatra, Indonesia, during May 2006. Clinically mild illness and asymptomatic H5N1 virus infections have been documented, but limited sero-surveys suggest that their frequency is very low.

TRANSMISSION AND PATHOGENESIS

Primary risk factors for H5N1 include direct or close contact (<1 meter) with infected, diseased, or dead poultry and visiting a live poultry market, but it is not clear exactly how H5N1 virus infection of the respiratory tract is initiated. The incubation period for H5N1 virus infection is not well established but is estimated at 1 week or less, somewhat longer than for human influenza virus infection. An H5N1-infected person can shed H5N1 viruses for up to 16 days after illness onset, and it is assumed, but not established, that they can shed virus 1 day prior to illness onset. Most human H5N1 cases have occurred in previously healthy children and young adults via avian-to-human transmission. Probable, limited, nonsustained, human-to-human transmission of H5N1 viruses has been documented and may be responsible for a small number of cases in clusters, usually involving blood-related family members who had very close prolonged contact with a severely ill case.

H5N1 pathogenesis appears to be mediated by high viral replication in the lower respiratory tract that stimulates a massive abnormal host inflammatory response. High H5N1 viral levels have been correlated with cytokine dysregulation in fatal human cases. H5N1 viral RNA detection or virus isolation from serum, plasma, cerebrospinal fluid, brain, placenta, and rectal swabs has been reported. Neutralizing antibodies to H5N1 virus are detectable in serum approximately 10–14 days after illness onset.

CLINICAL FEATURES

Initial signs and symptoms of H5N1 virus infection include fever and cough, with lower respiratory tract symptoms, and occasionally diarrhea (Table 71.1). Some children have had fever, cough, and upper respiratory tract symptoms. At hospital admission, most H5N1 cases have high fever, nonproductive cough, difficulty breathing, shortness of breath, and tachypnea. A smaller proportion of H5N1 cases have headache, sore throat, rhinorrhea, productive cough, hemoptysis, abdominal pain, vomiting, nonbloody diarrhea, and myalgias. Dehydration may be evident in patients with high fever, tachypnea, and diarrhea. A few atypical H5N1 cases have presented with isolated diarrhea with subsequent development of pneumonia. Nearly all H5N1 patients have pneumonia at hospital admission.

Table 71.1 Clinical Features: H5N1

Incubation Period	2–5 days (usually ≤7 days)
Signs and Symptoms	Common admission findings: • Fever ≥38°C, nonproductive cough, difficulty breathing, shortness of breath, tachypnea • Pulmonary crackles, rhonchi, diminished breath sounds, hypoxia Other findings: • Headache, rhinorrhea, sore throat, productive cough, hemoptysis, vomiting, watery diarrhea, abdominal pain, malaise, myalgias

Laboratory and Radiographic Findings	• Leukopenia, lymphopenia, mild-to-moderate thrombocytopenia, hypoalbuminemia, elevation of hepatic transaminases
	• Abnormal CXR or Chest CT scan:
	  ○ Infiltrates (patchy, interstitial, diffuse), consolidation (segmental, lobar)
	  ○ Pleural effusion

Complications	• Progression to respiratory failure and ARDS • Ventilator-associated pneumonia, pulmonary hemorrhage, pneumothorax • Multiorgan failure, cardiac compromise, renal dysfunction • Sepsis, shock, DIC • Encephalitis with seizures • Reye syndrome • Hemophagocytosis

ARDS, acute respiratory distress syndrome; CT, computed tomographic; CXR, chest x-ray.

DIFFERENTIAL DIAGNOSIS

The differential diagnosis is broad and includes pathogens that cause acute febrile influenza-like illness with lower respiratory tract disease (Table 71.2). It is essential to screen for any history of direct contact with sick or dead poultry or

Table 71.2 Differential Diagnosis: H5N1

Influenza-like illness with or without lower respiratory tract disease:
• Respiratory viruses (influenza A, influenza B, RSV, rhinovirus, parainfluenzavirus, human metapneumovirus, adenovirus, non-SARS coronavirus [CoV], bocavirus, SARS-CoV)
• Dengue
Influenza-like illness with diarrhea:
• Respiratory viruses (e.g. influenza A, influenza B, RSV)
• Enteric viruses (e.g. norovirus, rotavirus)
• Bacterial infections (e.g. ETEC, *Salmonella typhi*)
Community-acquired pneumonia:
• Bacterial (*Streptococcus pneumoniae, Haemophilus influenzae, Bordetella pertussis*)
• Secondary bacterial pneumonia (*Streptococcus pneumoniae, Haemophilus influenzae*, group A *Streptococcus pyogenes, Staphylococcus aureus*/MSSA/MRSA)
• Atypical pathogens (*Mycoplasma pneumoniae, Chlamydophila pneumoniae, Legionella pneumophila*; fungi)
Viral pneumonia:
• Influenza A, influenza B, RSV, rhinovirus, parainfluenzavirus, adenovirus, human metapneumovirus, bocavirus, CMV, hantavirus, measles, EBV, VZV, HSV, SARS-CoV

CMV, cytomegalovirus; EBV, Epstein-Barr virus; ETEC, enterotoxigenic *Escherichia coli*; HSV, herpes simplex virus; MRSA, methicillin-resistant *Staphylococcus aureus*; MSSA, methicillin-sensitive *Staphylococcus aureus*; RSV, respiratory syncytial virus; VZV, varicella-zoster virus.

Clade 2.1 H5N1 case, September 2005

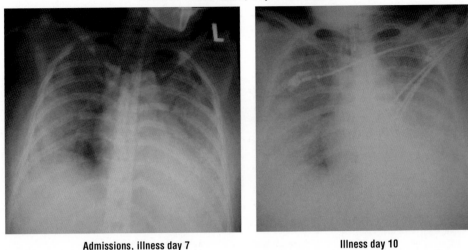

| Admissions, illness day 7 | Illness day 10 |

Figure 71.1 Clade 2.1 H5N1 case, September 2005: 37-year-old woman was admitted on illness day 7, died day 11.

Clade 2.1 H5N1 case, September 2005

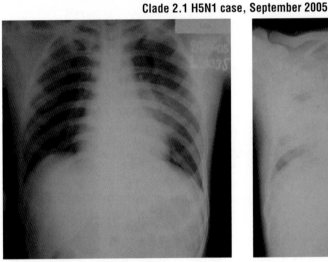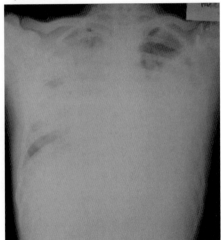

| Admission, illness day 5 | Illness day 12 |

Figure 71.2 Clade 2.1 H5N1 case, September 2005: 21-year-old man was not ventilated, fully recovered.

birds, or with a confirmed or highly suspected human H5N1 case. Some H5N1 patients have presented with fever and diarrhea with or without lower respiratory disease, and in these patients, the differential diagnosis must include locally prevalent infections that cause febrile gastrointestinal illness. Finally, community-acquired bacterial and viral pneumonias must also be considered.

LABORATORY AND RADIOGRAPHIC FINDINGS

Laboratory findings in most H5N1 cases at admission include leukopenia, lymphopenia, and mild-to-moderate thrombocytopenia. Hypoalbuminemia and moderate elevation of hepatic transaminases have been described.

Radiographic findings include diffuse, bilateral, multifocal or patchy infiltrates, interstitial infiltrates, and segmental or lobular consolidation (Figures 71.1 and 71.2). Associated pleural effusions have been reported.

H5N1 virus infection can be confirmed by detection of H5N1 viral RNA in respiratory specimens using reverse transcriptase polymerase chain reaction (RT-PCR) in a Biosafety Level 2 (BSL-2) laboratory (Table 71.3). Isolation of H5N1 virus should be attempted only under BSL-3 enhanced laboratory conditions. Proper respiratory specimen collection is essential. For nonventilated patients, nasal and throat swab specimens should be collected. Throat swabs have much higher yield for H5N1 virus than other upper respiratory tract specimens. For intubated patients, endotracheal aspirates should be collected. Pleural and bronchoalveolar lavage fluid specimens are also of great diagnostic utility. Collection and testing of multiple respiratory specimens on consecutive days can maximize detection of H5N1 viruses. The gold standard for serological testing is detection of H5N1 neutralizing antibodies by microneutralization assay using live H5N1 virus under enhanced BSL-3 laboratory conditions. Commercially available rapid influenza diagnostic tests are

Table 71.3 Laboratory Diagnosis: H5N1

Detection of H5N1 Viral RNA	Real-time or conventional reverse-transcriptase polymerase chain reaction in Biosafely Level 2 conditions Best specimens: • Endotracheal aspirate, BAL fluid, chest tube fluid, pleural fluid (from intubated patients) • Throat and nasal swabs (from nonintubated patients) • Collect specimens from multiple sites on multiple days for testing Note: Specimens should also be tested for human influenza A (H1), (H3), and B viruses.
Isolation of H5N1 Virus	Embryonated egg or tissue cell culture in Biosafely Level 3 enhanced conditions at WHO H5 Reference Laboratories Best specimens: • Endotracheal aspirate, BAL fluid, chest tube fluid, pleural fluid (from intubated patients) • Throat and nasal swabs (from nonintubated patients)
Serological Detection of H5N1 Antibodies	Microneutralization assay using live H5N1 virus in Biosafely Level 3 enhanced conditions to detect H5N1 neutralizing antibodies at WHO H5 Reference Laboratories Key issues: • Ideally paired acute (within 7 days of illness onset) and convalescent sera (collected 10–14 days later) should be collected and tested • H5N1 neutralizing antibodies may not be detectable until 14 days after illness onset • Other serological testing methods are experimental (ELISA, modified equine RBC HI assay) • Standard influenza hemagglutinin inhibition (HI) assay is inaccurate (not sensitive and not specific)
Commercially Available Rapid Influenza Diagnostic Test	Not recommended; not sensitive, not specific. False negatives are common; a positive result could indicate human influenza A virus infection, H5N1, or be falsely positive.

BAL, bronchoalveolar lavage; ELISA, enzyme-linked immunosorbent assay; RBC, red blood cell.

Table 71.4 Antiviral Treatment for H5N1

Patient Category	Therapy Recommendation*
Adults	Oseltamivir 75 mg PO bid × 5 days is recommended for seasonal influenza; initiate treatment as soon as possible. Adverse effects: nausea, vomiting. • Consider higher dosing (e.g., 150 mg PO bid; especially in patients with pneumonia, severe disease, clinical progression, or diarrhea) and longer duration (10 days) Zanamivir 10 mg (two inhalations) bid × 5 days is an option. Adverse effect: bronchospasm
Children	Oseltamivir[†] • Consider higher dosing and longer duration, especially in patients with pneumonia, severe disease, clinical progression, or diarrhea
Pregnant Women	Same as for nonpregnant adults
Immunocompromised	Same as for nonimmunocompromised persons

*Primary adverse effects of oseltamivir treatment are nausea and vomiting. H5N1 viral resistance to oseltamivir has been reported. The primary adverse effect of zanamivir treatment is bronchospasm. Amantadine and rimantadine are not recommended for primary treatment of H5N1 because of a high frequency of resistant H5N1 clade 1 (Vietnam, Thailand, Cambodia), and clade 2.1 (Indonesia) viruses. Combination antiviral treatment with a neuraminidase inhibitor (oseltamivir, zanamivir) and an adamantane drug (amantadine, rimantadine) can be considered in areas where antiviral resistance data suggests that H5N1 viruses may be susceptible to adamantanes (e.g., clade 2.2 and 2.3 H5N1 viruses).

[†]Oseltamivir is approved for treatment of influenza in persons aged ≥1 year. Dosage is based on age and weight. An oral suspension is available. Zanamivir is approved for treatment of influenza in persons aged ≥7 years. The package inserts should be consulted for the appropriate pediatric doses and contraindications.

Source: World Health Organization. Rapid Advice Guidance on pharmacological management of humans infected with avian influenza A (H5N1) virus. June 2006. Second World Health Organization Consultation on Clinical Aspects of Human Infection with Avian Influenza A (H5N1) Virus Meeting, 19–21 March 2007, Antalya, Turkey.

not recommended for detection of H5N1 virus because they have low sensitivity and specificity for H5N1. A positive rapid influenza diagnostic test result for influenza A could indicate human influenza A (H1), (H3), avian influenza (H5N1), or a different avian influenza A subtype, or be falsely positive.

TREATMENT AND CHEMOPROPHYLAXIS

Early antiviral treatment of H5N1 patients with neuraminidase inhibitor drugs (oseltamivir and zanamivir) is recommended by the WHO (Table 71.4). These medications limit the release of viral particles from infected cells. Oseltamivir is the antiviral drug of choice. The optimal dose, duration, and effectiveness of oseltamivir for H5N1 treatment are unknown. A higher dose of oseltaivir than for seasonal influenza (twice the standard dose) and treatment for 10 days (twice the standard duration) should be considered, especially for patients with pneumonia, severe disease, clinical progression, or diarrhea. Primary side effects associated with oseltamivir include nausea and vomiting. H5N1 virus resis-

tance to oseltamivir has been documented in case reports. Zanamivir is chemically similar to oseltamivir but is administered as an orally inhaled powder using an inhaler device. All H5N1 viruses to date have been susceptible to zanamivir. The primary adverse effect associated with zanamivir is bronchospasm, especially in persons with underlying chronic pulmonary disease.

Amantadine and rimantadine are not recommended because of widespread resistance in clade 1 and clade 2.1 H5N1 viruses. Combination treatment with a neuraminidase inhibitor can be considered for patients with suspected clade 2.2 and 2.3 H5N1 virus infections. Primary side effects associated with amantadine and rimantadine include vomiting, diarrhea, and central nervous system symptoms.

Additional supportive treatment includes supplemental oxygen, as well as mechanical ventilation for respiratory failure. Corticosteroid therapy is not recommended except for septic shock with adrenal insufficiency. No controlled clinical data are available for any of the H5N1 treatments.

Pre- and postexposure antiviral chemoprophylaxis should be implemented if oseltamivir is available. WHO recommends oseltamivir chemoprophylaxis for family and household members and close contacts of highly suspected and confirmed H5N1 cases for 7–10 days following the last exposure to the case. Similarly, postexposure oseltamivir chemoprophylaxis can be considered for persons with known unprotected exposures to infected poultry and birds for 7–10 days after the last exposure. The oseltamivir chemoprophylactic dose is the same as for treatment, but administered once daily.

COMPLICATIONS AND ADMISSION CRITERIA

Complications include progression to respiratory failure and acute respiratory distress syndrome (ARDS). Ventilator-associated pneumonia, pulmonary hemorrhage, and pneumothorax can occur. Sepsis-like syndrome, hypotension, hypovolemic shock, hemophagocytosis, and multiorgan failure, including renal dysfunction and cardiac compromise with dysrhythmia, can occur. One adult H5N1 patient in Thailand presented with diarrhea before developing pneumonia. One pediatric H5N1 patient in Vietnam presented with diarrhea and seizures, progressed to coma, and was clinically diagnosed with encephalitis. Another pediatric H5N1 patient in Hong Kong developed Reye syndrome after aspirin ingestion. Any patient with febrile acute respiratory illness and an epidemiological history of exposure to H5N1 virus and who is highly suspected to have H5N1 virus infection should be hospitalized for testing and clinical management.

INFECTION CONTROL

Infection control for suspected and confirmed H5N1 patients includes three key steps: isolation of the patient, use of appropriate personal protective equipment (PPE) for health care workers and visiting family members, and adherence to infection control precautions. Suspected and confirmed H5N1 patients should be isolated in a single room with a controlled entryway. Health care workers and family members should be equipped with disposable gowns, gloves, goggles, and surgical masks or, if available, fit-tested respirators (e.g., N95). Use of respirators is especially important when performing tracheal suctioning or aerosol-generating procedures such as intubation and administration of aerosolized bronchodilator medications. Standard, contact, droplet, and airborne precautions should be observed as much as possible. Negative-pressure rooms can be used if available but are not required. Proper donning and removal of contaminated PPE, safe disposal of contaminated PPE, and hand washing are essential.

PEARLS AND PITFALLS

1. Screen for any possible exposures (to sick or dead poultry, wild birds, or other animals, or to suspected or confirmed H5N1 patients) during the week prior to illness onset in suspected H5N1 patients.
2. Human influenza A and B virus infection are the most likely cause of influenza-like illness in any country and among travelers with or without poultry contact. Influenza A and B and other human respiratory viruses can cause uncomplicated influenza-like illness as well as pneumonia and severe respiratory disease.
3. Human illness from infection with highly pathogenic avian influenza A (H5N1) viruses is extremely rare, even among persons with febrile respiratory illness who had contact with sick or dead poultry.
4. Limited, nonsustained human-to-human transmission of H5N1 virus has been very rarely documented.
5. No H5N1 cases in travelers have been documented as of March 2008.
6. No human H5N1 vaccine is currently available.
7. Physicians should check the latest information about human infections with avian influenza A (H5N1) viruses, including epidemiology, clinical features, diagnosis, treatment, and H5N1 vaccines (e.g., websites of the WHO and the Centers for Disease Control and Prevention).

REFERENCES

Areechokchai D, Jiraphongsa C, Laosiritaworn Y, et al. Investigation of Avian Influenza (H5N1) outbreak in humans – Thailand, 2004. MMWR 2006;55(Suppl 1):3–6.

Chotpitayasunondh T, Ungchusak K, Hanshaoworakul W, et al. Human disease from influenza A (H5N1), Thailand, 2004. Emerg Infect Dis 2005;11:201–9.

de Jong MD, Simmons CP, Thanh TT, et al. Fatal outcome of human influenza A (H5N1) is associated with high viral load and hypercytokinemia. Nat Med 2006;12:1203–7.

Dinh PN, Long HT, Nguyen TKT, et al. Risk factors for human Infection with avian influenza A H5N1, Vietnam, 2004. Emerg Infect Dis 2006;12:1841–7.

Kandun IN, Wibisono H, Sedyaningsih ER, et al. Clustering of human H5N1 cases in Indonesia, 2005. N Engl J Med 2006;355:2186–94. (See also correspondence in N Engl J Med 2007;356:1375–7.)

Schuneman HJ, Hill SR, Kakad M et al. WHO Rapid Advice Guidelines for pharmacological management of sporadic human infection with avian influenza A (H5N1) virus. Lancet Infect Dis 2007;7:21–31.

Tran TH, Nguyen TL, Nguyen TD, et al. World Health Organization International Avian Influenza Investigative Team. Avian influenza A (H5N1) in 10 patients in Vietnam. N Engl J Med 2004;350:1179–88.

Ungchusak K, Auewarakul P, Dowell SF, et al. Probable person-to-person transmission of avian influenza A (H5N1). N Engl J Med 2005;352:333–40.

World Health Organization (WHO). Update: WHO-confirmed human cases of avian influenza A(H5N1) infection, 25 November 2003–24 November 2006. Wkly Epidemiol Re 2007;82:41–8.

Writing Committee of the Second World Health Organization (WHO) Consultation on Clinical Aspects of Human Infection with Avian Influenza A (H5N1) Virus. Update on avian influenza A (H5N1) virus infection in humans. N Engl J Med 2008;358:261–73.

ADDITIONAL READINGS

de Jong MD, Thanh TT, Khanh TH, et al. Oseltamivir resistance during treatment of influenza A (H5N1) infection. N Engl J Med 2005;353:2667–72.

Subbarao K, Luke C. H5N1 viruses and vaccines. PLoS Pathog 2007;3:e40.

World Health Organization (WHO). WHO case definitions for human infections with influenza A(H5N1) virus. 29 August 2006. Available at: http://www.who.int/csr/disease/avian_influenza/guidelines/case_definition2006_08_29/en/print.html.

World Health Organization (WHO). Avian influenza, including influenza A (H5N1), in humans: WHO interim infection control guideline for health care facilities. 24 April 2006. Available at: http://www.wpro.who.int/NR/rdonlyres/EA6D9DF3–688D-4316–91DF-5553E7B1DBCD/0/InfectionControlAIinhumansWHOInterimGuidelines-for2b_0628.pdf.

World Health Organization (WHO). Antigenic and genetic characteristics of H5N1 viruses and candidate H5N1 vaccine viruses developed for potential use as pre-pandemic vaccines. March 2007. Available at: http://www.who.int/csr/disease/avian_influenza/guidelines/summaryH520070403.pdf.

72. Pediatric and Adult SARS

Chi Wai Leung and Thomas S. T. Lai

INTRODUCTION

Severe acute respiratory syndrome (SARS) is an often fatal infectious respiratory disease with prominent systemic symptoms. It is caused by a novel coronavirus, SARS coronavirus (SARS-CoV), which was responsible for a global outbreak from November 2002 to July 2003. SARS-CoV probably has its origin in Southern China and is a zoonosis that initially affected wild animals, possibly bats, and subsequently spread to exotic animals. The virus can be identified by reverse transcriptase polymerase chain reaction (RT-PCR) in blood, plasma, respiratory secretions, and stool. Specific antibody is detected in acute and convalescent sera from patients by indirect fluorescent antibody (IFA) testing and enzyme-linked immunosorbent assay (ELISA) targeting the surface spike (S) protein.

EPIDEMIOLOGY

During the 2002–2003 SARS outbreak, a cumulative total of 8096 probable cases, with 774 deaths, were reported from 29 countries and areas. A global case-fatality rate of 9.6% was recorded at the end of the outbreak. The total number of health care workers affected was 1706 (21.1% of all probable cases). Interestingly, the severity of the syndrome appears to have been greater in adults and adolescents than in young children. No mortality was reported in children worldwide.

The incubation period of SARS generally ranged from 2 to 10 days. The primary mode of transmission appears to be direct mucous membrane (eyes, nose, and mouth) contact with infectious respiratory droplets and/or through exposure to fomites. The majority of SARS cases had a history of direct contact with another SARS case, though transmission rates were low in the community and screening for SARS-CoV antibodies in asymptomatic direct contacts showed near zero positive rates. Subclinical infection was rare even among health care workers. Nosocomial and household contacts were most common. Transmission to casual and social contacts occurred only occasionally in cases of intense exposure to an index case (in workplaces, airplanes, or taxis) or in high-risk transmission settings, such as health care institutions and patients' homes.

Children with SARS are apparently less infectious than their adult counterparts.

Risk Factors for SARS

Risk factors for SARS include:

- health care workers, especially those involved in aerosol-generating procedures
- household contact with a probable case of SARS
- increasing age
- male sex
- presence of comorbidities
- environmental contamination

CLINICAL FEATURES

Most patients infected with SARS-CoV present with sudden onset of fever, though there are cases with distinct presentations, especially among the elderly. Symptoms such as malaise, chills, myalgia, headache, and cough are common in affected adults and children (Tables 72.1 and 72.2), though cough and sputum production may be absent even with radiographic evidence of pulmonary involvement. Upper respiratory symptoms of coryza and sore throat are present in about 25% of adult patients and 40% of children. In more advanced cases, patients may present with dyspnea and/or tachypnea.

Nausea, vomiting, and diarrhea are the main gastrointestinal symptoms of SARS. Diarrhea is common during the course of illness and is reported in 38–73% of adult patients, but it is more frequent in the first week. In studies on pathologic intestinal specimens, light microscopy findings were unremarkable with minimal inflammatory changes. Electron microscopy showed virus particles in the endoplasmic reticulum and on the luminal surface of microvilli, suggesting viral shedding into the gut lumen. Diarrhea is thus a significant infection control problem.

Involvement of most organ systems has been reported with SARS-CoV infection. Reactive hepatitis is a common complication, and patients with associated severe hepatitis had

Table 72.1 Clinical Features: SARS

Organism	SARS coronavirus (SARS-CoV)
Incubation Period	2–10 days (range 1–14 days, mean 4–6 days, median 4–5 days)
Signs and Symptoms	• Fever • Malaise, chills, myalgia, headache, and dizziness • Cough, coryza (in children), sore throat, and shortness of breath • Nausea, vomiting, and diarrhea
Laboratory and Radiologic Findings	• CXR: airspace opacification in the lower zones and periphery of lungs • HRCT findings: ground glass infiltration with or without consolidation, with septal and interstitial thickening • Lymphopenia, thrombocytopenia, prolonged aPTT, and elevated ALT and D-dimer levels • As disease progresses – elevation of CK and LDH levels occur

ALT, alanine aminotransferase; aPTT, activated partial thromboplastin time; CK, creatine kinase; CXR, chest x-ray; HRCT, high-resolution computed tomography; LDH, lactate dehydrogenase.

Table 72.2 Presenting Clinical Features of SARS in Adults and Children

	Adult Series		Pediatric Series (Combined)
	Donnelly et al. (2003)	Booth et al. (2003)	Leung et al. (2004) and Chiu et al. (2003)
Number of patients	1425	144	64
Fever (%)	94	99	97
Chills (%)	65	28	33
Malaise (%)	64	NR	56
Myalgia (%)	51	49	28
Headache (%)	50	35	28
Dizziness (%)	31	NR	19
Sore throat (%)	23	13	11
Coryza (%)	25	2	41
Cough (%)	50	69	56
Sputum production (%)	28	5	30
Shortness of breath (%)	31	NR	9
Nausea with or without vomiting (%)	22	NR	20
Diarrhea (%)	27	24	17

NR, not reported.

worse clinical outcome. Subclinical diastolic cardiac dysfunction without systolic impairment has been reported in SARS patients and was reversible in those who recovered. There is one case report of generalized seizures in a pregnant woman with SARS whose cerebrospinal fluid (CSF) was positive for SARS-CoV antibody by RT-PCR.

Acute renal impairment, uncommon in SARS infection, is likely related to multiorgan failure rather than representing renal tropism of the virus. Not surprisingly, the development of acute renal impairment is a poor prognostic indicator.

PATHOGENESIS

The primary site of attack by SARS-CoV is the respiratory tract but other organs are also seeded by early viremia. Thus, SARS is a systemic disease with extrapulmonary dissemination. The tissue tropism of SARS-CoV includes the lungs, gastrointestinal tract, liver, spleen, lymph nodes, pancreas, heart, kidneys, adrenals, skeletal muscles, sweat glands, parathyroid glands, pituitary gland, and cerebrum. Viral shedding occurs in respiratory secretions, stool, urine, and possibly sweat. The tissue and organ damage is likely the result of both viral replication and host inflammatory response.

The natural history of untreated SARS in both adults and children remains unclear. SARS is probably a triphasic disease in adults. The first week of illness (viral replication phase) is characterized by fever, myalgia, and other prodromal systemic symptoms that generally improve after a few days. In the second week, the immune system attacks the virus and infected cells, releasing inflammatory cells and mediators. This immune hyperactive phase is characterized by recrudescence of fever, increasing respiratory symptoms and lung consolidation, and the development of respiratory failure and acute respiratory distress syndrome (ARDS) in many adult patients. The final pulmonary damage phase is associated with varying degrees of residual lung injury in survivors (Figure 72.1).

In children, SARS is milder and follows a biphasic pattern. The separation of prodromal and pneumonic phases of the disease may be less distinct in comparison with adults.

Tri-phasic disease course of SARS

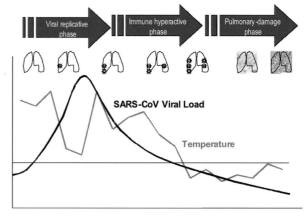

Figure 72.1 Clinical phases of SARS in adult patients. From Sung JY, Yuen KY. Clinical presentation of the disease in adults. In: Peiris M, Anderson L, Osterhaus AD, et al., eds, Severe acute respiratory syndrome. Oxford, UK: Blackwell, 2005.

Progression to ARDS is only seen in a very small number of pediatric patients, predominantly adolescents.

DIFFERENTIAL DIAGNOSIS

Early disease mimics influenza and other respiratory infections. Thus, the differential diagnosis includes most causes of community-acquired pneumonia or upper respiratory tract infections. These include:

- Acute bacterial pneumonia
- Acute viral respiratory infections:
  - influenza A virus (including avian influenza H5, H7, and H9)
  - influenza B virus
  - parainfluenza viruses 1, 2, 3, and 4
  - respiratory syncytial virus
  - adenoviruses
  - human metapneumovirus
- Community-acquired pneumonia caused by atypical respiratory pathogens:
  - *Chlamydophilae* (formerly *Chlamydia*) *pneumoniae*
  - *Chlamydophilae psittaci*
  - *Mycoplasma pneumoniae*
  - *Legionella pneumophila*

Key features that may help to distinguish SARS from other causes of pneumonia are:

- History of close contact with a patient with suspected or confirmed SARS
- Failure of clinical response after 48 hours of empiric broad-spectrum antibiotic therapy for presumed community-acquired pneumonia

LABORATORY AND RADIOGRAPHIC FINDINGS

Most SARS patients had normal or low leukocyte counts and lymphopenia at the time of presentation (Table 72.3), and lymphopenia may persist during the course of disease. Thrombocytopenia is also a common presenting feature. Prolonged activated partial thromboplastin time (aPTT) and elevated D-dimer levels were documented in one report, but were not accompanied by clinically significant bleeding.

Of adult and pediatric SARS patients, 23–35% and 10–16%, respectively, have elevated alanine aminotransferase (ALT) levels at presentation. Moreover, 76% and 24–48% of adult and pediatric patients, respectively, developed liver dysfunction during the course of illness. The peak ALT or bilirubin levels correlated with pathologic chest radiographic findings.

Elevation of creatine kinase and lactate dehydrogenase levels may occur and persist with disease progression. Three cases of acute rhabdomyolysis associated with probable SARS have been reported in adults.

The predominant chest radiographic finding is airspace opacification in the lower zones and in the periphery of the lungs (Figure 72.2). Chest radiography is the primary tool for diagnosis and for follow-up of pulmonary disease progression and response to therapy. When the initial chest radiograph is negative and clinical suspicion persists, high-resolution computed tomography (HRCT) may aid early diagnosis (Figure 72.3). Common HRCT findings include ground-glass opacification with or without consolidation, and inter-lobular, septal and intralobular interstitial thickening (Figure 72.4).

Although the Centers for Disease Control and Prevention (CDC) and World Health Organization (WHO) have promulgated clinical case definitions for SARS, final diagnosis of the disease requires laboratory confirmation. A confirmed case of SARS is a person who has a clinically compatible disease (i.e., fever with constitutional symptoms *and/or* lower respiratory symptoms *plus* an epidemiologic link) that is laboratory confirmed.

Rapid laboratory diagnosis can be accomplished by detecting the virus, viral antigens, or viral nucleic acid in respiratory secretions, blood, plasma, or stool specimens obtained during the acute illness. The most sensitive rapid diagnostic test is the real-time quantitative RT-PCR assay of either plasma or respiratory secretions (e.g., nasopharyngeal aspirate) obtained

Table 72.3 Key Laboratory Findings of SARS in Adults and Children at Presentation

	Adult Series					Pediatric Series	
	Choi et al. (2003)	Booth et al. (2003)	Lee et al. (2003)	Peiris et al. (2003)	Vu et al. (2004)	Leung et al. (2004)	Chiu et al. (2003)
Number of patients	267	144	138	75	62	44	21
Leukopenia (%)	27	NR	34	7	19	34	24
Lymphopenia (%)	73	85	70	75	79	77	57
Thrombocytopenia (%)	50	NR	45	37	40	27	24
Hyponatremia (%)	NR	NR	20	NR	30	NR	NR
Elevated ALT (%)	31	NR	23	29	35	16	10
Elevated CK (%)	19	39	32	36	NR	7	NR
Elevated LDH (%)	47	87	71	NR	NR	55	NR

ALT, alanine aminotransferase; CK, creatine kinase; LDH, lactate dehydrogenase; NR, not reported.

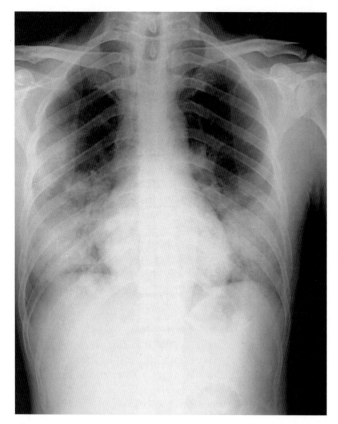

Figure 72.2 Chest radiograph showing bilateral multifocal consolidation in both lower zones.

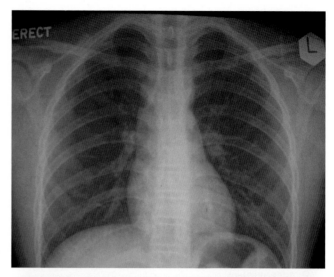

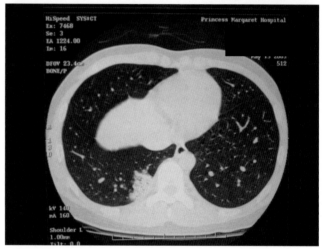

Figure 72.3 High-resolution computed tomography of thorax showing peripheral, subpleural, focal consolidation of the right lower lobe that was not evident on the admission chest radiograph.

during the first week of illness. When performed in the first 3 days of illness on nasopharyngeal aspirate, the preferred specimen, the sensitivity of RT-PCR approaches 80% and the specificity 100%. The overall diagnostic yield can be further improved to over 80% in the second week of illness when stool specimens are also examined. In the United States, the test is available from the CDC and related public health facilities, and research laboratories.

The gold standard of laboratory diagnosis is a rise in SARS-CoV specific antibody titer during illness. A negative antibody test on acute serum followed by positive antibody test on convalescent serum *or* a fourfold or greater rise in antibody titer between acute and convalescent phase sera tested in parallel is confirmatory. Seroconversion is documented by IFA or ELISA assay, and the absence of SARS-CoV specific IgG beyond 28 days from onset of symptoms practically excludes the diagnosis.

Isolation of SARS-CoV from specimens inoculated in appropriate cell cultures is hazardous, technically demanding, and limited by low sensitivity. The requirement for Biosafety Level 3 (infectious agents that may cause serious or potentially lethal diseases as a result of exposure by the inhalation route) containment precludes its application for routine clinical practice.

TREATMENT

The best treatment strategy for SARS is still unknown. Current recommendations include both anti-viral therapy and immunomodulatory agents to combat the abnormal inflammatory response (Table 72.4), though there is concern that

immunomodulation could compromise viral clearance by the host immune system. Listed below are suggested treatment regimens based on small numbers of patients. Patients and physicians should be advised that no randomized controlled studies have been performed with these agents. All regimens should include coverage for severe bacterial community-acquired pneumonia. Supportive care such as assisted ventilation is commonly required.

Antivirals

Because SARS-CoV triggers a vigorous immune response, the best approach is to halt the early viral replication to diminish the peak viral load, tissue spread, and ensuing immunopathologic damage.

Ribavirin was chosen for use empirically in the initial outbreak because of its broad-spectrum antiviral coverage. The use of ribavirin has generated considerable criticism because of its relative lack of in vitro activity against the SARS-CoV and its association with a number of adverse effects such as hemolytic anemia, bradycardia, elevated serum aminotransferase levels, and teratogenic effects. Limited studies in adult

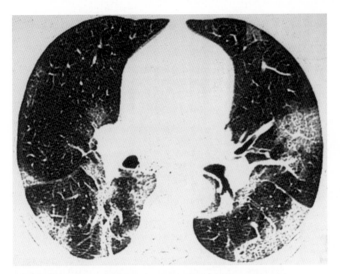

Figure 72.4 High-resolution computed tomography of thorax showing ground-glass opacification of the basal segments of both lower lobes.

Table 72.4 Treatment*

Standard Treatment for Severe Community-Acquired Pneumonia	• Broad-spectrum antibiotics (third- or fourth-generation cephalosporin plus macrolide) if not penicillin allergic (e.g., cefotaxime plus erythromycin or clarithromycin at standard dosages for adults and children) • Antipneumococcal quinolones for penicillin-allergic patients (e.g., levofloxacin at standard dosages) • General supportive care
Antiviral Treament Against SARS-CoV	Suggested regimen for adults: • Dosage of ribavirin: 2.4 g oral loading followed by 1.2 g bid orally for a total of 10 days • Dosage of Kaletra: 3 tablets bid orally (each tablet containing 400 mg of lopinavir and 100 mg of ritonavir) for a total of 10 days
Corticosteroids	Suggested regimen for adults: • Start with methylprednisolone 1 mg/kg q8h IV for 5 days, then 1 mg/kg q12h IV for 5 days, then prednisolone 0.5 mg/kg bid orally for 5 days, then 0.5 mg/kg qd orally for 3 days, then 0.25 mg/kg qd orally for 3 days • In patients suffering from "critical SARS" defined as a PaO_2/FiO_2 ratio of <200 mm Hg (<26.7 kPa) and progressive chest radiographic deterioration, the use of pulse corticosteroid and choice of regimen is at the discretion of the clinician. The suggested dosage for pulse corticosteroid therapy is methylprednisolone at 0.5 g per day IV for 3 days, followed by a tapering course starting at 3 mg/kg/day. The cumulative dose of MP should preferably not exceed 2 g.
Immunoglobulin	Salvage therapy

*The best treatment strategy for SARS is still unknown.

patients suggest that Kaletra (a mixed formulation of the protease inhibitors lopinavir and ritonavir), in combination with ribavirin, reduces the intubation and overall death rates and improves the clinical, biochemical, virologic, and radiographic parameters.

The suggested regimen for adults is:

1. Ribavirin: 2.4 g oral loading followed by 1.2 g bid orally for a total of 10 days
2. Kaletra: 3 tablets bid orally (each tablet containing 400 mg of lopinavir and 100 mg of ritonavir) for a total of 10 days

Corticosteroids

It is hypothesized that the tissue damage during SARS is caused by the exaggerated systemic inflammation or cytokine storm during the second immunopathological phase of SARS. *Corticosteroids should not be used in the early stage of SARS because they may compromise viral clearance.* They should only be considered if there is evidence of acute lung injury, defined by a PaO_2/FiO_2 ratio of 200–300 mm Hg (26.7–40.1 kPa) plus worsening chest radiographic findings not due to heart failure or other causes.

The suggested regimen for adults is:

1. Start with methylprednisolone 1 mg/kg q8h intravenously (IV) for 5 days, then 1 mg/kg q12h IV for 5 days, then prednisolone 0.5 mg/kg bid orally for 5 days, then 0.5 mg/kg qd orally for 3 days, then 0.25 mg/kg qd orally for 3 days.
2. In patients suffering from "critical SARS" defined as a PaO_2/FiO_2 ratio of less than 200 mmHg (<26.7 kPa) and progressive chest radiographic deterioration, the use of pulse corticosteroid and choice of regimen is at the discretion of the clinician. The suggested dosage for pulse corticosteroid therapy is methylprednisolone at 0.5 g per day IV for 3 days, followed by a tapering course starting at 3 mg/kg/day. The cumulative dose of methylprednisolone should preferably not exceed 2 g.

Convalescent Plasma

Convalescent plasma, obtained from patients who recovered from SARS, was used as salvage therapy in patients who deteriorated irrevocably during the SARS outbreak despite pulse methylprednisolone. Preliminary data suggest that its use may be associated with a shorter hospital stay and lower mortality but the clinical efficacy remains to be confirmed.

Immunoglobulin

Another form of salvage therapy that may be considered for patients who have a deteriorating course is intravenous immunoglobulin (IVIG). However, the use of IVIG must be balanced against the risk of hemolytic anemia and venous thrombosis.

Noninvasive Positive Pressure Ventilation

There have been anecdotal reports of the efficacy of noninvasive positive pressure ventilation (NIPPV) such as bilevel positive airway pressure (BiPAP) and continuous positive

Table 72.5 Clinical Outcome and Prognostic Factors in Adult SARS Patients

Study	Number of Patients	Median or Mean (SD) Age	Case Fatality Rate (%)	ICU Care (%)	Assisted Ventilation (%)	Adverse Outcomes	Clinical Correlates of Adverse Outcomes	Odds Ratio or Relative Risk (95% CI)
Tsui et al. (2003)	323	41 (14)	NR	21	13	Death or ICU care	Age (per 10-year increase)	1.57 (1.26–1.95)
							Admission neutrophil count (per 1×10^9/L increase)	1.28 (1.13–1.46)
							Initial LDH level (per 100 international units/L increase)	1.35 (1.11–1.64)
Choi et al. (2003)	267	39	12 (3 months)	26	21	Death	Age >60	5.1 (2.3–11.31)
							LDH > 3.8 μkat/L at presentation	2.2 (1.03–4.71)
Booth et al. (2003)	144	45	6.5 (21 days)	20	13.9	Death, ICU care, or assisted ventilation	Diabetes mellitus	3.1 (1.4–7.2)
							Other comorbid conditions	2.5 (1.1–5.8)
Lee et al. (2003)	138	39 (16.8)	3.6 (21 days)	23.2	13.8	Death or ICU care	Advanced age (per 10-year increase)	1.8 (1.16–2.81)
							High absolute neutrophil count at presentation	1.6 (1.03–2.5)
							High peak LDH level	2.09 (1.28–3.42)
Chan et al. (2003)	115	41 (14.8)	10 (21 days)	34	26	Death	Age >60	3.5 (1.2–10.2)
							Diabetes mellitus or heart disease	9.1 (2.8–29.1)
							Another coexisting condition	5.2 (1.4–19.7)
Peiris et al. (2003)	75	40 (12.2)	7 (25 days)	NR	NR	Development of ARDS	Age 60–81	28.0 (3.1–253.3)
							Positive test for hepatitis B surface antigen	18.0 (3.2–101.3)

ARDS, acute respiratory distress syndrome; CI, confidence interval; LDH, lactate dehydrogenase; NR, not reported.
From Princess Margaret Hospital SARS Study Group: Lee PO, Tsui PT, Tsang TY, et al. Severe acute respiratory syndrome: clinical features. In: Schmidt A, Wolff MH, Weber O, eds, Coronaviruses with special emphasis on first insights concerning SARS. Basel, Switzerland: Birkhäuser, 2005:71–99.

airway pressure (CPAP) in SARS patients with respiratory decompensation in China and Hong Kong. Institution of NIPPV resulted in the avoidance of intubation in 70% of treated subjects, as well as shorter length of intensive care unit (ICU) stay and lower chest radiography scores, compared with the intubated group. NIPPV initially was banned in Hong Kong because of the fear of aerosol generation and viral dissemination via mask leakage. However, evidence shows that NIPPV is a useful and safe treatment option for SARS patients with respiratory failure, and it should be considered if acute lung injury develops. The procedure must be performed under respiratory precautions with appropriate personal protective equipment in a suitable setting (single room with negative pressure and air changes of 12 cycles or more per hour).

Invasive Mechanical Ventilation

When patients fail to improve or deteriorate after 1–2 days of NIPPV, or if NIPPV is contraindicated, endotracheal intubation and mechanical ventilation must be considered. The plateau pressures are kept lower than 30 cm H_2O in intubated adults owing to the high susceptibility to barotrauma.

INFECTION CONTROL

Basic Considerations

SARS-CoV is present in respiratory secretions, blood, saliva, urine, and feces of patients. The virus is stable in the environment for up to 2 days at room temperature and longer at lower temperatures. Its survival in stool ranges from up to 4 days in alkaline, diarrheal stool to 3–6 hours in normal stool. The virus is inactivated by exposure to commonly used disinfectants (e.g., hypochlorite and alcohol) and by exposure to a temperature of at least 56°C for 15 minutes. The principal modes of transmission occur through droplets, aerosolized respiratory secretions, and direct contact with patients' secretions, excreta, and fomites.

Infection Control of SARS in the Hospital

Four specific measures are important in the infection control practice for SARS: hand washing and the wearing of masks, gowns, and gloves. The quantity of exposure is related to the duration of hospital stay of SARS patients. A longer exposure results in higher chance for procedural lapses to occur, which can result in nosocomial spread.

Specific risk assessment should include:

1. Patient-related risk (exposure to a confirmed or suspected SARS case, superspreading events, triage areas, patient with fever of unknown origin, etc.)
2. Procedure-related risk (ICU, procedure room such as bronchoscopy room or x-ray department, area serving SARS patients, dirty utility room, etc.)
3. Direct patient contact or activities with risk of exposure to blood, body fluids, secretions, excreta, and contaminated items.

In addition, procedures with high risk of generating aerosols (e.g., resuscitation, high-flow oxygen) and involving prolonged very close contact with affected patients require:

- N95 respirator (surgical mask may suffice for non-aerosol generating procedures)
- a linen or disposable gown
- full-face shield or eye shield
- latex gloves (only for procedures with exposure to blood and body fluid, secretion, excreta, and contaminated items)
- goggles (only for aerosol-generating procedures)
- disposable cap (optional)

PROGNOSIS

Young children affected by SARS generally have an excellent prognosis: respiratory failure is uncommon, and no deaths have been reported in patients under 18 years of age. The principal immediate morbidity of SARS in adults is acute respiratory failure. Some 20% of adult patients develop ARDS, while 20–34% require intensive care unit admission, and 13–26% require assisted ventilation.

The case fatality rate (CFR) is widely variable in different regions. According to WHO, the global CFR was 9.6% and ranged from 7% to 17%. The rates were between 3.6% and 12% in the major published series. The figures must be interpreted with caution. The patient population, length of follow-up, and case definition were all different in the various reports. The premorbid risk factors of patients, such as older age and multiple comorbidities, may affect the CFR substantially.

Risk stratification and management planning in SARS patients depends very much on the identification of prognostic factors. Different studies have established that advanced age, especially over 60, and concurrent medical illness, particularly diabetes mellitus, are independent prognostic indicators for adverse clinical outcomes including intensive care unit admission, need for assisted ventilation, and death (Table 72.5). In addition, high neutrophil counts, elevated initial lactate dehydrogenase level, low CD4 and CD8 lymphocyte counts, hypoxemia, and thrombocytopenia are associated with poor clinical outcomes. High initial viral load by quantitative PCR of nasopharyngeal aspirate is also a poor prognostic factor in adult patients. One report found that initial chest radiographic score was also an independent prognostic factor.

PEARLS AND PITFALLS

1. An epidemiologic link such as close contact with a SARS patient appears to be the single most important clue leading to diagnosis.
2. Though lobar pneumonia usually suggests a bacterial cause, especially pneumococcal, pneumonia in SARS may present as lobar consolidation instead of patchy infiltration.
3. SARS patients are generally most infectious shortly after hospitalization and pose significant risk to health care workers.
4. Stringent infection control measures and constant vigilance for procedural lapses are critical to preventing nosocomial transmission of SARS.
5. Chronic hepatitis B carriers should be given lamivudine to prevent the hepatitis flare that may occur on corticosteroid withdrawal.

REFERENCES

Antonio GE, Wong KT, Chu WC, et al. Imaging of severe acute respiratory syndrome in Hong Kong. AJR 2003;181:11–7.

Booth CM, Matukas LM, Tomlinson GA, et al. Clinical features and short-term outcome of 144 patients with SARS in the greater Toronto area. JAMA 2003;289: 2801–9.

Centers for Disease Control and Prevention (CDC). Severe acute respiratory syndrome: revised CSTE SARS Surveillance case definition 3 May, 2005. Retrieved October 31, 2006, from http://www.cdc.gov/ncidod/SARS/guidance/b/app1.htm.

Chan JW, Ng CK, Chan YH, et al. Short term outcome and risk factors for adverse clinical outcomes in adults with severe adult respiratory syndrome (SARS). Thorax 2003;58:686–9.

Chan KH, Poon LL, Cheng VC, et al. Detection of SARS coronavirus in patients with suspected SARS. Emerg Infect Dis 2004;10:294–9.

Chan KS, Lai ST, Chu CM, et al. Treatment of severe acute respiratory syndrome with lopinavir/ritonavir: a multicentre retrospective matched cohort study. Hong Kong Med J 2003;9:399–406.

Chau TN, Lee PO, Choi KW, et al. Value of initial chest radiographs for predicting clinical outcomes in patients with severe acute respiratory syndrome. Am J Med 2004;117:249–52.

Chiu WK, Cheung PC, Ng KL, et al. Severe acute respiratory syndrome in children: Experience in a regional hospital in Hong Kong. Pediatr Crit Care Med 2003;4:279–83.

Choi KW, Chau TN, Tsang O, et al. Outcomes and prognostic factors in 267 patients with severe acute respiratory syndrome in Hong Kong. Ann Intern Med 2003;139:715–23.

Chu CM, Cheng VC, Hung IF, et al. Role of lopinavir/ritonavir in the treatment of SARS: initial virological and clinical findings. Thorax 2004;59:252–6.

Ding Y, He L, Zhang Q, et al. Organ distribution of severe acute respiratory syndrome (SARS) associated coronavirus (SARS-CoV) in SARS patients: implications for pathogenesis and virus transmission pathways. J Pathol 2004;203:622–30.

Donnelly CA, Ghani AC, Leung GM, et al. Epidemiological determinants of spread of causal agent of severe acute respiratory syndrome in Hong Kong. Lancet 2003;361: 1761–6.

Farcas GA, Poutanen SM, Mazzulli T, et al. Fatal severe acute respiratory syndrome is associated with multiorgan involvement by coronavirus. J Infect Dis 2005;191:193–7.

Guan Y, Zheng BJ, He YQ, et al. Isolation and characterization of viruses related to the SARS coronavirus from animals in southern China. Science 2003;302:276–8.

Hui JY, Cho DH, Yang MK, et al. Severe acute respiratory syndrome: spectrum of high-resolution CT findings and temporal progression of the disease. AJR 2003;181:1525–38.

Lai ST. Treatment of severe acute respiratory syndrome. Eur J Clin Microbiol Infect Dis 2005;24:583–9.

Lai ST, Ng TK, Seto WH, et al. Low prevalence of subclinical severe acute respiratory syndrome-associated coronavirus infection among hospital healthcare workers in Hong Kong. Scand J Infect Dis 2005;37:500–3.

Lau SK, Woo PC, Li KS, et al. Severe acute respiratory syndrome coronavirus-like virus in Chinese horseshoe bats. Proc Natl Acad Sci U S A 2005;102:14040–5.

Lee N, Hui D, Wu A, et al. A major outbreak of severe acute respiratory syndrome in Hong Kong. N Engl J Med 2003;348:1986–94.

Leung CW. SARS in children. In: Peiris M, Anderson LJ, Osterhaus AD, et al., eds, Severe acute respiratory syndrome. Oxford, UK: Blackwell, 2005:30–5.

Leung CW, Chiu WK. Clinical picture, diagnosis, treatment and outcome of severe acute respiratory syndrome (SARS) in children. Paediatr Respir Rev 2004;5:275–88.

Leung CW, Kwan YW, Ko PW, et al. Severe acute respiratory syndrome among children. Pediatrics 2004;113:e535–43.

Leung GM, Chung PH, Tsang T, et al. SARS-CoV antibody prevalence in all Hong Kong patient contacts. Emerg Infect Dis 2004;10:1653–6.

Li W, Shi Z, Yu M, et al. Bats are natural reservoirs of SARS-like coronaviruses. Science 2005;310:676–9.

Ng EK, Ng PC, Hon KL, et al. Serial analysis of the plasma concentration of SARS coronavirus RNA in pediatric patients with severe acute respiratory syndrome. Clin Chem 2003;49:2085–8.

Ng PC, Leung CW, Chiu WK. SARS in paediatric patients. In: Chan JCK, Taam Wong VCW, eds, Challenges of severe acute respiratory syndrome. Singapore: Saunders, Elsevier 2006;437–49.

Ng PC, Leung CW, Chiu WK, et al. SARS in newborns and children. Biol Neonate 2004;85:293–8.

Peiris JS, Chu CM, Cheng VC, et al. Clinical progression and viral load of coronavirus pneumonia in a community outbreak: a prospective study. Lancet 2003;361:1762–72.

Poon LL, Chan KH, Wong OK, et al. Detection of SARS coronavirus in patients with severe acute respiratory syndrome by conventional and real-time quantitative reverse transcription-PCR assays. Clin Chem 2004;50:67–72.

Princess Margaret Hospital SARS Study Group: Lee PO, Tsui PT, Tsang TY, et al. Severe acute respiratory syndrome: clinical features. In: Schmidt A, Wolff MH, Weber O, eds, Coronaviruses with special emphasis on first insights concerning SARS. Basel, Switzerland: Birkhäuser 2005: 71–99.

Seto WH, Tsang D, Yung RWH, et al. Effectiveness of "droplets" and "contact precautions" in preventing nosocomial transmission of severe acute respiratory syndrome (SARS). Lancet 2003;361:1519–20.

Tsang OT, Chau TN, Choi KW, et al. Coronavirus-positive nasopharyngeal aspirate as predictor for severe acute respiratory syndrome mortality. Emerg Infect Dis 2003;9:1381–7.

Tsui PT, Kwok ML, Yuen H, Lai ST. Severe acute respiratory syndrome: clinical outcome and prognostic correlates. Emerg Infect Dis 2003;9:1064–9.

Vu HT, Leitmeyer KC, Le DH, et al. Clinical description of a completed outbreak of SARS in Vietnam, February–May 2003. Emerg Infect Dis 2004;10:334–8.

World Health Organization (WHO). Case definitions for surveillance of severe acute respiratory syndrome (SARS) 1 May 2003. Retrieved October 31, 2006, from http://www.who.int/csr/sars/casedefinition/en.

World Health Organization (WHO). Consensus document on the epidemiology of severe acute respiratory syndrome (SARS). Retrieved October 31, 2006, from http://www.who.int/csr/sars/en/WHOconsensus.pdf.

World Health Organization (WHO). Summary of probable SARS cases with onset of illness from 1 November 2002 to 31 July 2003. Retrieved October 31, 2006, from http://www.who.int/csr/sars/country/table2004_04_21/en/index.html.

ADDITIONAL READINGS

Ahuja AT, Ooi CGC, ed. Imaging in SARS. London: Greenwich Medical Media, 2004.

Chan JCK, Wong VCW, eds. Challenges of severe acute respiratory syndrome. Singapore: Saunders Elsevier, 2006.

Lau YL, Peiris JS. Pathogenesis of severe acute respiratory syndrome. Curr Opin Immunol 2005;17:404–10.

Peiris M, Anderson LJ, Osterhaus ADME, et al., ed. Severe acute respiratory syndrome. Oxford, UK: Blackwell, 2005.

Sung JJY, ed. Severe acute respiratory syndrome: from bench-top to bedside. Singapore: World Scientific, 2004.

73. West Nile Encephalitis Virus

Michael S. Diamond

INTRODUCTION

West Nile encephalitis virus (WNV) is a small, enveloped, mosquito-transmitted, positive-polarity RNA virus of the Flaviviridae family. This virus is closely related to other arthropod-borne viruses that cause human disease including dengue, yellow fever, and Japanese encephalitis viruses. WNV normally cycles in nature between mosquitoes and birds, but during epidemics will infect and cause disease in human, horses, and other vertebrate animals. Severe neurological disease in humans usually occurs within 1 to 2 weeks after mosquito inoculation and is more frequent in elderly and immunocompromised individuals.

EPIDEMIOLOGY

West Nile virus historically caused sporadic outbreaks of a mild febrile illness in regions of Africa, the Middle East, Asia, and Australia. However, in the 1990s, the epidemiology of infection appeared to change, with new outbreaks in parts of eastern Europe associated with higher rates of severe neurological disease. In 1999, WNV entered North America and caused seven human fatalities in the New York area, as well the deaths of a large number of birds and horses. Since then, WNV has spread to all 48 of the lower United States as well as to parts of Canada, Mexico, and the Caribbean. Because of the increased range, the number of human cases has continued to rise: In the United States between 1999 and 2007, there were more than 26,000 clinical cases of WNV, including nearly 1,000 deaths.

Approximately 85% of human infections in the United States occur in the late summer, with a peak in August and September, reflecting the seasonal activity of mosquito vectors and the necessity of late spring and summer virus amplification in one of several different bird hosts. In warmer parts of the country, however, virtually year-round transmission has been documented. The number of dying birds in a community in the early summer often predicts the number of human cases weeks later.

The vast majority of human cases of WNV are acquired after mosquito inoculation. Seroprevalence studies suggest that around 80% of cases are subclinical or undiagnosed. Overall, about 1 in 150 WNV infections result in the severe and potentially lethal form of the disease. During an epidemic, the seroconversion rate ranges from 3% to 20% and the attack rate for severe disease during an epidemic is approximately 7 per 100,000. The risk of severe WNV infection is greatest in the elderly, with an estimated 20-fold increased risk of neuroinvasive disease and death in those over 50 years of age. Comorbidities such as immunosuppression, diabetes mellitus, and alcohol abuse also are associated with increased risk and poor outcome.

Although most human WNV infections occur after the bite of an infected mosquito, transmission has occurred via other routes including transfusion, organ transplantation, transplacental transmission, and breastfeeding.

CLINICAL FEATURES

The clinical spectrum of WNV infection is broad and ranges from apparently asymptomatic cases, to a mild flulike illness, a more severe febrile illness, or polio-like paralysis, meningitis, and encephalitis (Table 73.1). These syndromes present within 1 to 2 weeks after mosquito inoculation or exposure. Most individuals who come to clinical attention have a self-limited West Nile fever (WNF), which is characterized by fever and some or all of the following signs and symptoms: headache, neck pain, poor concentration, myalgia, arthralgia, weakness, gastrointestinal complaints, and macular rash. This non-neuroinvasive form nonetheless can be severe: 38% of patients with WNF were hospitalized with a mean length of stay of 5 days.

Less common non-neurological clinical manifestations include hepatitis, pancreatitis, myocarditis, rhabdomyolysis, cardiac arrhythmias, orchitis, and ocular inflammation. Recent studies suggest that ocular manifestations such as chorioretinitis, vitritis, intraretinal hemorrhages, iritis, optic neuritis, and retinal artery occlusions may occur more frequently than originally perceived.

Neuroinvasive WNV disease occurs in less than 1% of infected individuals and manifests as meningitis, encephalitis, or paralysis. The clinical presentation of meningitis and encephalitis appears to differ slightly, because patients with meningitis were more likely to have nausea, vomiting, myalgia, rash, back pain, and arthralgia, whereas those with encephalitis typically had memory problems, dysarthria, dysphagia, and focal motor abnormalities. Notably, no differences in the frequency of seizure, limb weakness, or tremor were

Table 73.1 Clinical Features: West Nile Virus Infection

Organism	West Nile virus
Incubation Period	2–14 days
Transmission	• Mosquito bite • Blood transfusion • Organ recipient • Intrauterine transmission
West Nile Fever	Fever, headache, flulike illness, myalgia, arthralgia, GI complaints, macular rash, fatigue, difficulty concentrating
West Nile Meningitis	Fever, headache, myalgia, arthralgia, vomiting, back pain, macular rash, fatigue, difficulty concentrating
West Nile Encephalitis	Fever, headache, myalgia, arthralgia, vomiting, back pain, macular rash, fatigue, memory problems, dysarthria, dysphagia, focal motor exam, paralysis
West Nile Acute Flaccid Paralysis	Fever, flaccid paralysis
Post-WNV Infection Syndrome	Fatigue, weakness, difficulty concentrating, muscle weakness
Laboratory and Radiologic Findings	• Serum: leukopenia, lymphopenia, thrombocytopenia • CSF: lymphocytic pleocytosis (or early in the course, neutrophilia or absence of WBCs) • MRI: signal abnormalities in basal ganglia, thalamus, and brainstem
Laboratory Diagnosis	• Serum for anti-WNV IgM • Paired acute and convalescent serum for anti-WNV IgG (4-fold rise in titer) • Serum for WNV RT-PCR or NAAT (within first 8 days of symptoms), CSF for anti-WNV IgM
Therapy	Investigational clinical trials: • Interferon-alpha • Immune gamma-globulin

CSF, cerebrospinal fluid; GI, gastrointestinal; MRI, magnetic resonance imaging; NAAT, nucleic acid amplification test; RT-PCR, reverse transcriptase polymerase chain reaction; WBC, white blood cell.

observed in the meningitis and encephalitis patient groups. The acute paralysis that occurs with WNV infection is generally flaccid, due to infection and injury of anterior horn lower motor neurons. Because of the location and severity of neuron injury, it is referred to as a poliomyelitis-like syndrome. More rarely, inflammatory changes associated with central nervous system (CNS) infection can result in additional neuromuscular manifestations including Guillain-Barré syndrome and demyelinating neuropathies.

LABORATORY AND RADIOGRAPHIC FINDINGS

Routine clinical laboratory studies (complete blood count, serum chemistries, hepatic panels, coagulation tests) do not distinguish WNV from other viral infections. Nonspecific laboratory findings include mild leukopenia, mild to severe lymphopenia, and thrombocytopenia. In a small study, three patients with advanced encephalitis had markedly elevated serum ferritin levels (>500 ng/mL). Patients with neuroinvasive disease (meningitis or encephalitis) generally have a lymphocytic pleocytosis in their cerebrospinal fluid (CSF), although early in the course of infection, CSF findings may include neutrophilia or absence of WBCs. Notably, most transplant recipients that acquire WNV have atypical lymphocytes in their CSF. In WNV encephalitis, head computed tomography (CT) is usually normal, though magnetic resonance imaging (MRI) can show signal abnormalities in the basal ganglia, thalamus, and brainstem.

Although clinical criteria for assessment of patients with suspected WNV infection have been defined, definitive diagnosis depends on the detection of antibodies, viral nucleic acid, or infectious virus in the blood or cerebrospinal fluid (Table 73.2). Few clinical laboratories have the facilities to isolate virus directly from infected clinical samples. Because viremia is relatively transient and often precedes the severe neurological manifestations of the WNV infection, nucleic acid testing has a relatively low sensitivity, especially with delayed clinical presentation.

At present, the detection of WNV IgM in the serum or CSF by antibody capture enzyme-linked immunosorbent assay (ELISA) is the most utilized method for diagnostic confirmation. The tests, which are performed by both state and commercial laboratories, are reasonably sensitive (60 to 90%) when carried out by day 8 of illness, and are quite specific. Antibody testing within the first 72 hours of clinical presentation may yield false negative results because of the inherent delayed kinetics of the anti-WNV IgM response. Because the ELISA test also detects antibodies against related flaviviruses (e.g., St. Louis and Japanese encephalitis virus), false positives are possible, and it is thus important to obtain a history of recent vaccination (e.g., yellow fever virus) or foreign travel. Definitive serological diagnosis of WNV infection, at present, requires a comparison of antigen or neutralization activity among related flavivirus family members. Newly developed assays that utilize purified WNV proteins appear to be more specific and may allow distinction among natural infection, vaccination, and immunity. One cautionary note is that recent studies suggest that WNV IgM can persist in serum up to 500 days after onset of infection; this could confound interpretation of serologic results in patients presenting in this time frame with clinical syndromes that resemble WNV infection.

DIFFERENTIAL DIAGNOSIS

When WNV activity is present in the community and patients have had significant mosquito exposure, WNV infection should be considered in the differential diagnosis of seriously ill, febrile patients, as the burden of WNV illness is likely underestimated. Updated maps of active mosquito, animal, and human WNV transmission can be found on the Center for Disease Control and Prevention (CDC) website (http://www.cdc.gov/ncidod/dvbid/westnile). WNV infection should certainly be considered in endemic areas in elderly or immunocompromised patients with nonspecific illnesses, who lack leukocytosis, neutrophilia, or other obvious signs of bacterial infection. These patients may present in the early stages of WNV infection, which can subsequently progress to severe, life-threatening CNS disease.

The differential diagnosis of West Nile encephalitis includes both infectious and noninfectious causes. Among

Table 73.2 Interpretation of West Nile Virus Antibody Test Results*

Tests	Results	Interpretation
IgM IgG	Negative Negative	Antibody not detected (no infection, unless sample taken early in course prior to seroconversion)
IgM IgG	Negative Positive	Infection with a flavivirus at undetermined time
IgM IgG	Positive Negative	Possible evidence of recent or current infection; further confirmatory testing necessary†
IgM IgG	Positive Positive	Evidence of recent or current infection
IgM IgG	Indeterminate Negative	Inconclusive Request convalescent serum‡

*Because of heterotypic antibody responses and/or cross-reactions, serologic results should be interpreted on the basis of clinical and epidemiological information.
†False positive IgM results may occur.
‡Paired acute and convalescent serum samples may demonstrate seroconversion.

the infectious causes, several viruses can cause initial similar presentations with acute encephalopathy and fever:

- herpes simplex virus
- St. Louis encephalitis virus (which is closely related to WNV and will cross-react by serology but not by nucleic acid testing)
- equine (Eastern, Western, and Venezuelan) encephalitis viruses
- California and La Crosse encephalitis viruses
- enterovirus
- cytomegalovirus
- rabies virus
- varicella-zoster virus
- Epstein-Barr virus

In addition to the typical bacterial causes of community-acquired meningitis (which in the early stages may be difficult to distinguish from encephalitis), *Listeria*, *Legionella*, and *Mycoplasma* can cause encephalitis, especially in pregnant women and the immunocompromised.

Noninfectious causes of acute encephalopathy include toxic ingestions or exposures, metabolic causes (e.g., hyponatremia), hepatic failure, systemic lupus erythematosus, granulomatous angiitis, CNS metastatic disease, cerebrovascular accidents, and CNS hemorrhage.

TREATMENT

At present, no specific therapy has been approved for use in humans with WNV infection, and current treatment is supportive. An effective therapy must efficiently cross the blood-brain barrier into the CNS, clear virus from infected neurons, and have a beneficial effect on patient outcome. Investigational studies have begun, and the most up-to-date information on WNV therapeutic trials is available on the CDC website (http://www.cdc.gov/ncidod/dvbid/westnile/clinicalTrials.htm).

Ribavirin: Ribavirin is a broad-spectrum antiviral agent and has been used clinically to treat respiratory syncytial, hepatitis C, Lassa, Hantaan and La Crosse viruses. Ribavirin has inhibitory activity against WNV infection in cell culture. Limited *in vivo* pre-clinical studies have been performed with WNV and the results generally have not been promising. No clinical benefit of ribavirin was observed in mouse, hamster or monkey models of flavivirus infection. Finally, in a WNV outbreak in Israel in 2000, 37 patients received ribavirin and a high mortality rate (41%) was observed in this group. Thus, ribavirin is *not* recommended as therapy for WNV.

Interferon-alpha (IFN-α): IFNs comprise an important immune system control against viral infections. IFNs induce an antiviral state within cells via the up-regulation and activation of antiviral proteins and by modulating adaptive immune responses. Pretreatment of cells in vitro with IFN potently inhibits WNV. However, the inhibitory effect of IFN is markedly attenuated after viral replication has begun, as WNV specifically inhibits IFN signaling and gene transcription. Nonetheless, IFN may still have therapeutic potential. Pretreatment of rodents with IFN-α inhibited St. Louis encephalitis virus infection and resulted in decreased WNV viral loads and mortality. Treatment with IFN-α reduced complications in human St. Louis encephalitis virus cases and has been used successfully, albeit in an uncontrolled manner, to treat small numbers of human cases of WNV encephalitis.

Immune antibody: In animals, passive administration of anti-WNV antibodies is both protective and therapeutic. Passive administration of immune serum or purified immune human gamma-globulin protected rodents from WNV infection, and antibody therapy improved clinical outcome in infected rodents even after WNV had disseminated into the CNS. Small numbers of human patients have received WNV antibody therapy, and case reports have documented clinical improvement in humans with neurological infection after receiving immune gamma-globulin from Israeli donors.

Antisense technology: Antisense oligomers have been used to modulate gene expression of several viruses that are pathogenic for humans, and several are in clinical development or trials. This class of compounds inhibits viruses by binding to RNA in a sequence-specific manner, effectively blocking access to a particular region of the viral genome. Sequence-specific antisense oligomers have inhibitory activity against WNV in cell culture.

Vaccines

Significant progress has been made toward the development of an effective WNV vaccine for humans. Attenuated and heat-killed vaccines already have been developed for immunization of exotic birds and horses with varying degrees of efficacy. At present, several strategies are being used to develop vaccine candidates for preclinical and clinical assessment.

COMPLICATIONS AND ADMISSION CRITERIA

Most immunocompetent patients who present to the emergency department with WNV fever or mild meningitis will not require hospital admission. However, in specific populations (elderly, immunocompromised, pregnant women, or infants) severe, potentially life-threatening complications include aspiration pneumonia (secondary to altered mental status), respiratory failure, encephalopathy, encephalitis, seizures, paralysis, and a sepsis-like syndrome. These high-risk patients should be monitored in a hospital setting for the development of neuroinvasive disease. All patients with encephalitis and moderate to severe meningitis should be admitted.

Overall, neurological complications of WNV are common in hospitalized cases. Fulminant encephalitis can occur rapidly in at-risk populations and can result in severe long-term disability (cognitive, motor, and sensory) and death.

INFECTION CONTROL

West Nile Virus is primarily transmitted by mosquito inoculation, although other routes of transmission are possible, as described above. There is no documentation of person-to-person transmission of WNV infection. Standard precautions are adequate for patients with WNV infection, and isolation is not necessary. Articles contaminated with infected or bloody material should be bagged, labeled, and sent for decontamination by autoclave. Contaminated surfaces should be cleaned with a hospital-approved disinfectant or a 10% bleach solution.

PEARLS AND PITFALLS

1. Check the CDC website (http://www.cdc.gov/ncidod/dvbid/westnile) for current WNV activity in your area.

2. In endemic regions, consider the diagnosis of WNV in febrile patients presenting with some of the typical signs and symptoms: headache, fatigue, weakness, cognitive deficits, rash, or focal weakness.

3. CSF in WNV infection usually demonstrates lymphocytic pleocytosis but can show neutrophil predominance or no cells early in the course of disease.

4. Head CT is usually negative; MRI may have signal abnormalities in several regions of the brain.

5. Laboratory diagnosis:

   - Serum: WNV IgM
   - Serum: Nucleic acid amplification test (within 8 days of symptom onset)
   - CSF: WNV IgM

6. There are no current approved specific antiviral therapies against West Nile virus. However, this is an area of intensive research and may change in the near future. Consult the CDC website for updated information on new investigational or approved therapies:

http://www.cdc.gov/ncidod/dvbid/westnile/clinicians/treatment.htm.

REFERENCES

Bakri SJ, Kaiser PK. 2004. Ocular manifestations of West Nile virus. Curr Opin Ophthalmol 15:537–40.

Bode AV, Sejvar JJ, Pape WJ, et al. West Nile virus disease: a descriptive study of 228 patients hospitalized in a 4-county region of Colorado in 2003. Clin Infect Dis 2006;42:1234–40.

Cunha BA. Differential diagnosis of West Nile encephalitis. Curr Opin Infect Dis 2004;17:413–20.

DeSalvo D, Roy-Chaudhury P, Peddi R, et al. West Nile virus encephalitis in organ transplant recipients: another high-risk group for meningoencephalitis and death. Transplantation 2004;77:466–9.

Granwehr BP, Lillibridge KM, Higgs S, et al. West Nile virus: where are we now? Lancet Infect Dis 2004;4:547–56.

Hall RA, Khromykh AA. West Nile virus vaccines. Expert Opin Biol Ther 2004;4:1295–305.

Hayes EB, Sejvar JJ, Zaki SR, et al. Virology, pathology, and clinical manifestations of West Nile virus disease. Emerg Infect Dis 2005;11:1174–9.

Kleinschmidt-DeMasters BK, Marder BD, Levi ME, et al. Naturally acquired West Nile virus encephalomyelitis in transplant recipients: clinical, laboratory, diagnostic, and neuropathological features. Arch Neurol 2004;61:1210–20.

Leis AA, Stokic DS. Neuromuscular manifestations of Human West Nile Virus infection. Curr Treat Options Neurol 2005;7:15–22.

Monath TP, Liu J, Kanesa-Thasan N, et al. A live, attenuated recombinant West Nile virus vaccine. Proc Natl Acad Sci U S A 2006;103:6694–9.

Mostashari F, Bunning ML, Kitsutani PT, et al. Epidemic West Nile encephalitis, New York, 1999: results of a household-based seroepidemiological survey. Lancet 2001;358:261–4.

Nash D, Mostashari F, Fine A, et al. The outbreak of West Nile virus infection in the New York City area in 1999. N Engl J Med 2001;344:1807–14.

Pealer LN, Marfin AA, Petersen LR, et al. Transmission of West Nile virus through blood transfusion in the United States in 2002. N Engl J Med 2003;349:1236–45.

Sejvar JJ, Haddad MB, Tierney BC, et al. Neurologic manifestations and outcome of West Nile virus infection. JAMA 2003;290:511–5.

Watson JT, Pertel PE, Jones RC, et al. Clinical characteristics and functional outcomes of West Nile fever. Ann Intern Med 2004;141:360–5.

PART V

Overview of Antibiotics

74. Antimicrobial Overview

Conan MacDougall and B. Joseph Guglielmo

Outline Introduction – Principles of Antimicrobial Use
Properties of Antimicrobial Agents
Mechanism of Action
Differences Between Agents
Cautions
Pearls and Pitfalls
References

INTRODUCTION – PRINCIPLES OF ANTIMICROBIAL USE

Pharmacokinetics and Pharmacodynamics

Many factors affect the choice of an antimicrobial agent in the acute care setting. Selection of an agent with in vitro activity against the infecting pathogen is necessary but not sufficient. Pharmacokinetic (distribution of the drug in the body) and pharmacodynamic (effect of the drug on its target) factors must also be taken into account. The most important pharmacokinetic consideration is the concentration of the drug at the site of infection. The physicochemical properties of antimicrobials determine their distribution throughout the body, and these properties may be unfavorable for the penetration of certain tissue compartments.

Sites of particular concern for the adequate penetration of antimicrobials include bone, compartments of the eye, and the central nervous system. Additionally, abscess cavities are poorly penetrated and should be drained regardless of whether systemic antimicrobial therapy is to be used. Even treatment of pulmonary and urinary tract infections depends on site-specific penetration, and recommendations for standard therapies reflect this. Thus, clinicians should rely on standard therapy or use alternative drugs that are documented to achieve effective concentrations at the site of interest. Unfortunately, data as to the relative penetration of different drugs may be lacking, although predictions based on physicochemical characteristics (e.g., protein binding) can be made.

An important pharmacodynamic distinction is whether a drug's activity is bactericidal or bacteriostatic. Although the distinction between these is not always absolute (some drugs can be bacteriostatic against certain organisms and bactericidal against others, or bactericidal at some concentrations and bacteriostatic at others), there are a few cases in which bactericidal activity is preferred. Generally, bactericidal activity is necessary in situations where there is minimal contribution from the immune system, either because of restricted access to the tissue compartment or because of host status. Foremost among these are meningitis and endocarditis, where clinical studies have documented a lower cure rate with bacteriostatic drugs. Other conditions that generally call for bactericidal therapy include osteomyelitis, febrile neutropenia, and sepsis.

Impact of Prior Antimicrobial Use on Choice of Therapy

Prior antimicrobial use increases the risk for infection with drug-resistant organisms and leads to selection of inappropriate empiric therapy. Thus, obtaining an accurate antimicrobial history is essential. Although resistance is only one of many possible reasons for therapeutic failure, the most conservative course when a patient has failed therapy with an antimicrobial agent is to assume resistance in the infecting pathogen(s). Subsequent therapy should either move "up the ladder" to a broader-spectrum agent within the same class or, more preferably, move to a different class that is unlikely to display cross-resistance. If the previously used agent(s) is unknown or if the use of alternative agents is impractical, standard therapy with close monitoring is recommended.

Principles of Antimicrobial Allergy and Toxicity

Antimicrobials, especially beta-lactam drugs, are among the most common agents to which patients report allergies. Specific allergic reactions, however, are often poorly documented in the medical record, are subject to inaccurate recall by patients, vary greatly in their severity and clinical importance, and may change over time. A chart notation of an "allergy to penicillin," for example, is of little practical utility. Documentation of the nature and timing of the initial reaction and whether the patient has been reexposed to the agent are crucial in determining the clinical significance of an allergy. Patients inaccurately labeled with allergies face a restricted choice of antimicrobials for future infections, possibly leading to suboptimal therapy.

Complicating the matter further is the issue of cross-reactivity between drugs in similar chemical classes, the most important of which are the beta-lactam drugs. Allergies with these drugs may be due to their common pharmacophore, leading to class-wide cross-allergenicity, or to unique elements such as the side chains, which would not generally lead to cross-allergenicity. Current best estimates of the rates of cross-resistance are indicated in Figure 74.1. Note that estimates of the probability of cross-reactivity are available only for patients with known penicillin allergies who receive cephalosporins or carbapenems. For example, the likelihood of cross-reactivity between cephalosporins and carbapenems, or the probability of those with a cephalosporin allergy reacting to a penicillin, is not known. The monobactam class (aztreonam) has a unique pharmacophore and is generally considered to have no cross-reactivity with the other beta-lactams (although ceftazidime, which has an identical side chain to aztreonam, may be an exception). Cross-allergenicity with drugs in other classes (e.g., fluoroquinolones) is even less well defined.

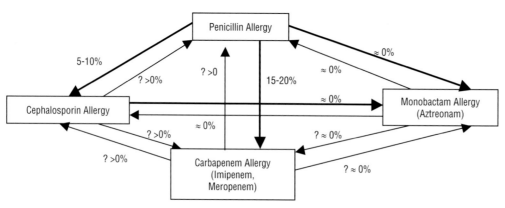

Figure 74.1 Estimated cross-reactivity between beta-lactams. Arrows denote the direction of the exposure (e.g., an arrow from a penicillin to a cephalosporin represents a patient with a penicillin allergy who receives a cephalosporin); the percentage noted indicates the estimated likelihood of a patient experiencing a reaction for that exposure direction.

Figure 74.1 provides estimates of cross-reactivity between various beta-lactams. Arrows denote the direction of the exposure (e.g., an arrow from a penicillin to a cephalosporin represents a patient with a penicillin allergy who receives a cephalosporin); the percentages noted indicate the estimated likelihood of a patient experiencing a reaction for that exposure direction.

Aside from causing allergic reactions, most antimicrobials are relatively well tolerated. Other serious toxicities that can occur with antimicrobials include nephrotoxicity (aminoglycosides), hematologic toxicity (penicillins, ganciclovir, linezolid), QT interval prolongation (macrolides, fluoroquinolones, azoles), and hepatotoxicity (macrolides, azoles). Some antimicrobials are prone to drug interactions that may enhance their own toxicity or the toxicity of coadministered drugs. The potential for administration of antimicrobials to lead to "superinfections," such as *Candida* infections or *Clostridium difficile* colitis, should also be considered a potential adverse consequence of their use.

PROPERTIES OF ANTIMICROBIAL AGENTS

The spectra of activity of commonly used antibacterial and antifungal drugs are reviewed in Table 74.1, with preferred agents highlighted. The common uses, pharmacology, and toxicity of the drugs are reviewed in the following text. Emphasis is placed on indications and agents commonly encountered in acute care settings. Important differences within a class are highlighted. General adult dosage ranges are provided with recommended adjustments for renal or hepatic dysfunction.

Beta-lactams: Penicillins, Cephalosporins, Carbapenems, and Monobactams

MECHANISM OF ACTION

Beta-lactam drugs act by disrupting the bacterial cell wall through inhibition of transpeptidases (penicillin-binding proteins, or PBPs), responsible for crosslinking peptidoglycan, the primary structural component of the cell wall. This leads to an imbalance between cell wall autolysis and synthesis. Beta-lactam drugs are generally bactericidal.

Figure 74.2 illustrates the mechanism of action of antibiotics against the bacterial cell wall. Peptidoglycan is the primary component of the bacterial cell wall, consisting of alternating units of *N*-acetylglucosamine (N-Glu) and *N*-acetylmuramic acid (N-Mur). The N-Mur units are crosslinked by polypeptide chains. Bacterial transpeptidases

(also known as PBPs) catalyze this crosslinking (as in pathway 1). Beta-lactam agents irreversibly inhibit the action of PBPs (pathway 2), preventing crosslinking. Glycopeptides (such as vancomycin) bind to the free ends of the polypeptides before crosslinking, sterically inhibiting PBP binding (pathway 3). In pathways 2 and 3 the natural autolytic activity of the bacterial cell leads to the degradation of the cell wall and cell death (beta-lactams may also enhance this autolysis).

NATURAL PENICILLINS AND AMINOPENICILLINS

See Table 74.3 for doses of natural penicillins and aminopenicillins.

DIFFERENCES BETWEEN AGENTS

The most significant differences among penicillins are in formulation (Table 74.2): penicillin G is the intravenous (IV) form, whereas penicillin V potassium is oral (PO) and benzathine penicillin G is an intramuscular (IM), long-acting depot formulation (not to be given intravenously!). Likewise, ampicillin and amoxicillin have identical spectra of activity, but ampicillin is available as an intravenous formulation while amoxicillin is orally administered (although there is an oral form of ampicillin, it is poorly absorbed). In contrast to the natural penicillins, the aminopenicillins have activity against non-beta-lactamase-producing strains of *Haemophilus influenzae* (approximately 60–80% of *H. influenzae*).

CAUTIONS

Allergic reactions are the most frequent toxicity encountered with the penicillins. These can range from mild rashes to life-threatening anaphylaxis. Depending on the severity of the reaction, patients can be challenged with a beta-lactam from another class (see Principles of Antimicrobial Allergy and Toxicity, above). A unique entity is the "amoxicillin (or ampicillin) rash," which occurs in patients receiving aminopenicillins and manifests as a self-limited, maculopapular rash. This rash is associated with concurrent infectious mononucleosis or other viral illnesses, or with allopurinol therapy, and does not appear to represent hypersensitivity in the usual sense. Patients considered to have amoxicillin rashes (and not true hypersensitivity) may be rechallenged with aminopenicillins in the future.

Neutropenia is considered to be a potential toxicity of all penicillins and is discussed in the following section.

PEARLS AND PITFALLS

1. The rise in penicillin resistance has sharply curtailed use of these agents for empiric therapy, except for selected indications (e.g., syphilis, pharyngitis, otitis media). However, if

Table 74.1 Spectra of Activity of Antibacterial Drugs

Group	Drug	S. pyogenes	S. pneumoniae (PCN-S or -I)	S. pneumoniae (PCN-R)	S. aureus (MSSA)	S. aureus[1] (MRSA)	E. faecalis[2] (VRE)	E. faecium[2]	Listeria	H. influenzae	N. meningitidis	P. mirabilis	E. coli[3]	Klebsiella[3]	P. aeruginosa	Citrobacter, Enterobacter	Serratia	B. fragilis	C. difficile	Atypicals[4]
PCNs	Penicillin G	++	++	–	–[5]	X	‡	–	++	X	++	X	X	X	X	X	X	–	–	X
PCNs	Ampicillin/amoxicillin	++	++	+	–[5]	X	++	–	++	+[6]	++	++	–	X	X	X	X	–	–	X
PCNs	Nafcillin/dicloxacillin	++	++	–	++	X	–	–	–	X	X	X	X	X	X	X	X	X	–	X
PCNs	Amoxicillin/clavulanate	++	++	–	++	X	++	–	++	++	++	++	+	+	X	X	X	‡	–	X
PCNs	Piperacillin/tazobactam	++	++	+	++	X	++	–	++	++	++	++	++	‡	‡	‡	‡	‡	–	X
Cephs	Cefazolin	++	++	+	++	X	X	X	X	X	–	++	++	+	X	X	X	X	X	X
Cephs	Cefuroxime	++	+	+	++	X	X	X	X	++	++	++	++	+	X	X	X	X	X	X
Cephs	Cefoxitin	++	+	–	++	X	X	X	X	++	++	++	+	+	X	+	X	+	X	X
Cephs	Ceftriaxone	++	++	X	++	X	X	X	X	++	++	++	++	++	X	+	‡	X	X	X
Cephs	Ceftazidime	++	+	–	–	X	X	X	X	++	++	++	++	++	++	++	++	X	X	X
Cephs	Cefepime	++	++	+	++	X	X	X	X	++	++	++	++	++	‡	‡	++	X	X	X
C/m[9]	Imipenem/meropenem	++	++	+	++	X	++	–	++	++	++	++	++	++	++	++	++	‡	–	X
C/m[9]	Aztreonam	X	X	X	X	X	X	X	X	++	++	++	++	++	++	++	++	X	–	X
FQs	Ciprofloxacin	++	+	+	+	–	+[7]	–	–	++	++	++	++	++	+	++	++	X	–	+
FQs	Levofloxacin	++	++	++	+	–	+[7]	–	–	++	++	++	++	++	+	++	++	+	–	‡
FQs	Moxifloxacin	++	++	++	+	–	–	–	–	++	++	++	++	++	–	++	++	+	–	‡
Macs	Erythromycin	+	+	–	++	–	X	X	–	X	+	X	X	X	–	X	X	X	X	‡
Macs	Azithromycin/clarithromycin	+	+	–	++	–	X	X	–	++	++	X	+/X	+/X	X	X	–	X	X	‡
Macs	Telithromycin	++	++	+	++	–	X	X	–	++	++	–	–	–	–	X	–	X	–	‡
Tets	Doxycycline	++	++	+	+	+	+	+	–	++	+	++	++	+	–	+	+	X	–	‡
Tets	Tigecycline	++	++	++	++	++	++	++	–	+	++	–	++	++	–	++	++	‡	–	‡
AGs	Gentamicin/tobramycin	–[8]	–	–	–[8]	–[8]	–[8]	–[8]	–[8]	+	–	++	++	++	++	++	++	X	X	X
AGs	Amikacin	–	–	–	–	–	X	X	–	+	–	++	++	++	++	++	++	X	X	X
Misc	TMP-SMX	–	+	+	++	++	X	X	‡	++	–	++	+	++	X	++	++	X	–	X
Misc	Clindamycin	++	++	–	++	+	X	X	–	X	X	X	X	X	X	X	X	+	X	+
Misc	Metronidazole	X	X	X	X	X	X	X	X	X	X	X	X	X	X	X	X	‡	‡	X
Misc	Linezolid	++	++	++	++	++	++	++	++	X	X	X	X	X	X	X	X	X	–	‡
Misc	Daptomycin	++	++	++	++	++	++	++	X	X	X	X	X	X	X	X	X	X	–	X
Misc	Vancomycin	++	++	‡	++	++	++	++	++	X	X	X	X	X	X	X	X	X	‡	X

++, drug of choice or >90% susceptibility; +, alternative drug or >70% susceptibility; –, minimal clinically useful activity or experience; X, intrinsically resistant.

Shaded: Preferred agent under most circumstances, although therapy should be tailored based on the susceptibility of the individual isolate.

[1] Approximately 50% of S. aureus in hospitals are MRSA; 1–50% (and increasing) of community S. aureus are MRSA.
[2] Approximately 2/3 of all enterococci are faecalis, and 1/3 are faecium (50–75% of which are vancomycin-resistant [VRE]).
[3] Does not include the approx. 1–5% of E. coli and 5–20% of Klebsiella that produce an extended-spectrum beta-lactamase, giving resistance to all beta-lactams (except carbapenems).
[4] Atypical respiratory pathogens: Legionella spp., Mycoplasma pneumoniae, Chlamydophila pneumoniae.
[5] <10% of S. aureus do not produce beta-lactamase and would be susceptible to these drugs.
[6] Non-beta-lactamase producing H. influenzae (75–90% of isolates) would be susceptible to these drugs.
[7] Fluoroquinolones are only clinically useful in the treatment of enterococcal urinary tract infections where high concentrations can be achieved (moxifloxacin would not be active).
[8] Aminoglycosides are not clinically useful as monotherapy for gram-positive infections; however they may provide synergistic killing when used in combination with a cell-wall active agent (e.g., nafcillin or vancomycin), especially in endocarditis.
[9] Carbapenems / monobactams.

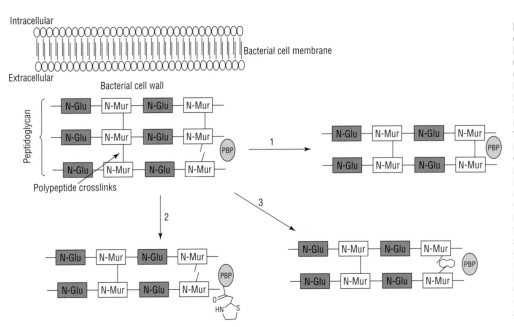

Figure 74.2 Mechanism of action of cell-wall-active antibacterials. Peptidoglycan is the primary component of the bacterial cell wall, consisting of alternating units of N-acetylglucosamine (N-Glu) and N-acetylmuramic acid (N-Mur). The N-Mur units are crosslinked by polypeptide chains. Bacterial transpeptidases (also known as penicillin-binding proteins or PBPs) catalyze this crosslinking (as in pathway 1). Beta-lactam agents irreversibly inhibit the action of PBPs (pathway 2), preventing crosslinking. Glycopeptides (such as vancomycin) bind to the free ends of the polypeptides before crosslinking, sterically inhibiting PBP binding (pathway 3). In pathways 2 and 3 the natural autolytic activity of the bacterial cell leads to the degradation of the cell wall and cell death (beta-lactams may also enhance this autolysis).

Table 74.2 Natural Penicillins and Aminopenicillins

Drug	Acute Care Uses	Toxicities
Penicillin G IV Penicillin VK PO Penicillin G benzathine IM	Syphilis Pharyngitis	*Common*: rash, diarrhea *Rare*: anaphylaxis, seizures **Drug Interactions** Minimal clinically relevant interactions
Ampicillin IV Amoxicillin PO	Pharyngitis Otitis media	

an infecting pathogen is demonstrated to be penicillin- or ampicillin-susceptible, these drugs offer many advantages for definitive therapy: they are narrow-spectrum, are inexpensive, and have rapid bactericidal activity.

2. Whereas penicillin resistance in staphylococci is essentially all-or-nothing (and more than 90% of *S. aureus* are fully penicillin resistant), resistance among streptococci tends to occur in a graded fashion. Thus, many strains have

intermediate or low-level resistance to penicillin. Because of their very high concentrations in blood and lung tissue, penicillin and amoxicillin show good cure rates for pneumonia even in the presence of low-level resistance. In cases of meningitis, however, there are documented failures of penicillins used against pneumococcal strains with intermediate resistance. Thus, penicillin resistance is much more clinically relevant in the treatment of meningitis than in treatment of pneumococcal pneumonia.

ANTISTAPHYLOCOCCAL PENICILLINS

Table 74.4 lists antistaphylococcal penicillins. See Table 74.5 for doses of antistaphylococcal penicillins.

DIFFERENCES BETWEEN AGENTS

Nafcillin is an intravenous preparation, whereas dicloxacillin is available for oral administration.

CAUTIONS

As noted above, neutropenia is considered to be a potential toxicity of all penicillins and is well documented with nafcillin therapy. Neutropenia usually manifests

Table 74.3 Dosages for Natural Penicillins and Aminopenicillins

Drug	Dosage Adjustment for Renal Function (mL/min)			Hepatic Adjust?
	CrCl >50	CrCl 10–50	CrCl <10	
Penicillin G	2–3 million units IV q4–6h	1–2 million units IV q4–6h	1 million units IV q6h	No
Penicillin VK	250–500 mg PO q6h	No adjustment	250 mg PO q8h	No
Penicillin G benzathine	1.2 million units IM × 1* 2.4 million units IM × 1†	No adjustment	No adjustment	No
Ampicillin	1–2 g IV q4–6h	1–1.5 g IV q6h	1 g IV q8–12h	No
Amoxicillin	500 mg PO q8–12h	250–500 mg PO q12h	250–500 mg PO q24h	No

*For streptococcal pharyngitis.
†For early syphilis.

Table 74.4 Antistaphylococcal Penicillins

Drug	Acute Care Uses	Toxicities
Nafcillin IV	Endocarditis	*Common*: rash
Dicloxacillin PO	Skin and soft-tissue infections	*Uncommon*: interstitial nephritis, neutropenia *Rare*: anaphylaxis, seizures **Drug Interactions** Minimal

several days into therapy and is generally considered to be reversible on cessation of the drug. This toxicity may be difficult to differentiate from progression of a severe infection with attendant neutropenia.

PEARLS AND PITFALLS

1. Nafcillin has superior bactericidal killing activity against methicillin-susceptible *Staphylococcus aureus* (MSSA), especially compared to vancomycin. It is generally the preferred therapy for invasive staphylococcal infections, such as endocarditis or osteomyelitis, due to MSSA. Nafcillin is also often preferred over cefazolin for severe MSSA infections because of its somewhat more potent activity and narrower spectrum of activity.
2. Because of the increasing incidence of community-acquired methicillin-resistant *Staphylococcus aureus* (MRSA) infections, patients with severe or unresponsive skin infections should receive drugs active against MRSA (e.g., doxycycline or vancomycin) as well as appropriate incision and drainage.

BETA-LACTAMASE INHIBITOR COMBINATIONS

See Table 74.6 for beta-lactamase inhibitor combinations. See Table 74.7 for doses of beta-lactamase inhibitor combinations.

DIFFERENCES BETWEEN AGENTS

Piperacillin-tazobactam has an enhanced gram-negative spectrum compared to the aminopenicillin drugs, with activity against *Pseudomonas* as well as enhanced activity against *Klebsiella* and *Escherichia coli*. Piperacillin-tazobactam is a more appropriate empiric choice than the aminopenicillin-based beta-lactamase inhibitor combinations for patients with severe infections, especially those of suspected nosocomial origin.

CAUTIONS

Piperacillin and other penicillins, especially at high dosages, may have qualitative effects on platelet function. These effects may predispose patients to bleeding, although direct suppression of platelets (thrombocytopenia) is not typically seen. This effect was primarily observed in older, less potent penicillins (ticarcillin, carbenicillin) that required very high doses for antipseudomonal activity. The risk with piperacillin is likely to be less, but monitoring for clinically significant bleeding, especially in patients with other risk factors for bleeding, is warranted. Hypokalemia can also occur because of the large sodium load associated with these drugs at high doses (especially with the less commonly used ticarcillin-clavulanate combination).

PEARLS AND PITFALLS

1. The beta-lactamase inhibitors (sulbactam, clavulanate, and tazobactam) serve to expand the activity of their accompanying penicillin by inhibiting bacterial beta-lactamases (enhancing activity against organisms such as *H. influenzae*, *E. coli*, *Klebsiella*, *Moraxella*, and MSSA). They do not add activity where the organism's mechanism of resistance is not beta-lactamase mediated (e.g., MRSA, *Streptococcus pneumoniae*) or where the beta-lactamases are resistant to inhibition (e.g., *Pseudomonas*).
2. The inhibitors are present in fixed ratios to the penicillin for ampicillin-sulbactam (2:1) and piperacillin-tazobactam (8:1), but vary somewhat between the different

Table 74.5 Dosages for Antistaphylococcal Penicillins

Drug	Dosage Adjustment for Renal Function (mL/min)			Hepatic Adjust?
	CrCl >50	CrCl 10–50	CrCl <10	
Nafcillin	1–2 g IV q4–6h	No adjustment	No adjustment	Possibly*
Dicloxacillin	125–250 mg PO q6h	No adjustment	No adjustment	No

*Consider reducing dose in hepatic insufficiency if concomitant renal failure.

Table 74.6 Beta-Lactamase Inhibitor Combinations

Drug	Acute Care Uses	Toxicities
Ampicillin-sulbactam IV (Unasyn) Amoxicillin-clavulanate PO (Augmentin) Piperacillin-tazobactam IV (Zosyn)	Intra-abdominal infections Diabetic foot infections Skin and soft-tissue infections Nosocomial infections* Sepsis*	*Common*: photosensitivity, headache, dizziness, GI distress (especially amoxicillin-clavulanate) *Uncommon*: platelet dysfunction, neutropenia **Drug Interactions** Minimal

*Use piperacillin-tazobactam.
GI, gastrointestinal.

Overview of Antibiotics

Table 74.7 Dosages for Beta-Lactamase Inhibitor Combinations

Drug	Dosage Adjustment for Renal Function (mL/min)			Hepatic Adjust?
	CrCl >50	CrCl 10–50	CrCl <10	
Ampicillin-sulbactam (Unasyn)	1.5–3 g* IV q6h	1.5 g IV q6–8h	1.5 g IV q12h	No
Amoxicillin-clavulanate (Augmentin)	500/125 mg† PO q8h 875/125 mg PO q12h 1000/62.5 mg PO q12h‡	250–500/125 mg PO q12h	250–500/125 mg PO q24h	No
Piperacillin-tazobactam (Zosyn)§	3.375 g‖ IV q6h/ 4.5 g IV q8h	3.375 g IV q6h/ 4.5 g IV q8h	2.25–3.375 g IV q8h	No

*1 g ampicillin/500 mg clavulanate or 2 g ampicillin/1 g clavulanate.
†Ratios are amoxicillin to clavulanate (e.g., 500 mg amoxicillin to 125 mg clavulanate).
‡Extended-release formulation.
§For documented or suspected *Pseudomonas* infections, use 4.5 g IV q6h for CrCl <20 mL/min.
‖3 g piperacillin/0.375 g tazobactam.

preparations of amoxicillin-clavulanate (from 4:1 to 16:1). The rationale for the higher amoxicillin:clavulanate ratios is that this preparation is often used for respiratory tract infections where *S. pneumoniae* is a concern; increasing the amoxicillin component may overcome low-level penicillin resistance, whereas additional clavulanate will not add activity.

3. Beta-lactamase inhibitor combinations are excellent drugs for mixed infections (e.g., aspiration pneumonia, intra-abdominal infections, diabetic foot infections) by virtue of their coverage of gram-positive, gram-negative, and anaerobic pathogens.

FIRST-GENERATION CEPHALOSPORINS

Table 74.8 lists first-generation cephalosporins. See Table 74.9 for doses of first-generation cephalosporins.

DIFFERENCES BETWEEN AGENTS

Cephalexin's spectrum of activity is similar to that of cefazolin, making it essentially an oral equivalent of cefazolin.

CAUTIONS

Although these drugs are frequently used for skin and soft-tissue infections, they are not recommended for bite infections because of their lack of activity against *Pasteurella multocida* (dog, cat) and *Eikenella* (human). Because of the increasing incidence of community-acquired MRSA infections, patients with severe or unresponsive skin infections should receive drugs active against MRSA (e.g., vancomycin) as well as appropriate incision and drainage.

Table 74.8 First-Generation Cephalosporins

Drug	Acute Care Uses	Toxicities
Cefazolin IV (Kefzol) Cephalexin PO (Keflex)	Skin and soft-tissue infections Urinary tract infections	*Uncommon*: rash *Rare*: anaphylaxis **Drug Interactions** Minimal

PEARLS AND PITFALLS

1. For serious infections due to MSSA (endocarditis, osteomyelitis), nafcillin is preferred by most experts, although it requires more frequent dosing than cefazolin (q4–6h vs. q8h). Cefazolin also has poor central nervous system (CNS) penetration and should not be used in treatment of MSSA meningitis (nafcillin is preferred).

SECOND-GENERATION CEPHALOSPORINS

Table 74.10 lists second-generation cephalosporins. See Table 74.11 for doses of second-generation cephalosporins.

DIFFERENCES BETWEEN AGENTS

Within the second generation of cephalosporins, there are two groups: drugs such as cefuroxime and cefprozil, which are primarily active against respiratory tract organisms (such as *S. pneumoniae* and *H. influenzae*) and drugs such as cefoxitin, which have activity primarily against gram-negatives and anaerobes.

CAUTIONS

The second-generation cephalosporins are frequently employed for upper and lower respiratory tract infections. However, their potency against *S. pneumoniae* is less than that of amoxicillin or ceftriaxone. Thus, their use in more severe infections such as community-acquired pneumonia should be restricted to geographic areas where pneumococcal resistance is low.

PEARLS AND PITFALLS

1. Cefoxitin is used primarily for surgical prophylaxis in gastrointestinal procedures. Although it has activity against gram-negative aerobic and anaerobic organisms, susceptibility rates among *Bacteroides fragilis*, the primary anaerobic pathogen, are unpredictable. Thus, agents such as ampicillin-sulbactam or piperacillin-tazobactam, or combinations such as ceftriaxone and metronidazole, are usually preferred for empiric therapy of intra-abdominal infections.

Table 74.9 Dosages for First-Generation Cephalosporins

Drug	Dosage Adjustment for Renal Function (mL/min)			Hepatic Adjust?
	CrCl >50	CrCl 10–50	CrCl <10	
Cefazolin	1–2 g IV q8h	1–2 g IV q12h	0.5–1 g IV q24h	No
Cephalexin	500 mg PO q6–8h	250–500 mg PO q8h	250 mg PO q12h	No

Table 74.10 Second-Generation Cephalosporins

Drug	Acute Care Uses	Toxicities
Cefuroxime IV, PO (Ceftin) Cefprozil PO (Cefzil) Cefoxitin IV (Mefoxin)	Sinusitis* Otitis media* Intra-abdominal infections†	*Uncommon*: rash *Rare*: anaphylaxis **Drug Interactions** Minimal clinically relevant interactions

*Use cefuroxime or cefprozil.
†Use cefoxitin.

THIRD- AND FOURTH-GENERATION CEPHALOSPORINS

Table 74.12 lists third- and fourth-generation cephalosporins. See Table 74.13 for doses of third- and fourth-generation cephalosporins.

DIFFERENCES BETWEEN AGENTS

Third-generation cephalosporins share excellent activity against Enterobacteriaceae (e.g., *E. coli, Klebsiella, Serratia, Proteus*) but differ somewhat in their activity against gram-positive and more-resistant gram-negative rods (*Pseudomonas, Enterobacter, Citrobacter*). Ceftriaxone, cefotaxime, and cefepime have potent activity against *S. pneumoniae* and to a lesser extent MSSA, whereas ceftazidime's activity is much less reliable against these organisms. In contrast to ceftriaxone and cefotaxime, ceftazidime and cefepime provide coverage against *Pseudomonas*. Cefepime improves somewhat on ceftazidime's spectrum by virtue of better coverage of *Enterobacter* and *Citrobacter*.

CAUTIONS

Exposure to third-generation cephalosporins has been demonstrated to be a risk factor for acquisition of a number of resistant bacteria, including vancomycin-resistant *Enterococcus* (VRE), *Clostridium difficile*, and extended-spectrum beta-lactamase-producing *Klebsiella*. When possible, more narrow-spectrum drugs should be substituted when susceptibility data have been obtained.

PEARLS AND PITFALLS

1. Dosing of these agents varies by indication, as noted in the dosage table below. Most importantly, for meningitis higher doses are indicated to compensate for reduced penetration into the central nervous system.
2. All available cephalosporins (with the exception of cefoxitin) have poor activity against important gram-negative anaerobes such as *B. fragilis*. When cephalosporins are used for empiric therapy of intra-abdominal infections, a drug with anaerobic coverage (preferably metronidazole) should be added.

CARBAPENEMS AND MONOBACTAMS

Table 74.14 lists acute care uses, toxicities, and drug interactions. See Table 74.15 for doses of carbapenems and monobactams.

DIFFERENCES BETWEEN AGENTS

The most important differences among the carbapenems are between ertapenem and the others (imipenem and meropenem). Ertapenem, unlike imipenem and meropenem, lacks clinically significant activity against *Pseudomonas, Acinetobacter*, and *Enterococcus*, making it a less attractive choice when these pathogens are a concern. There is little difference in spectrum of activity between imipenem and meropenem. However, meropenem has a lower seizure risk than imipenem (see below) and therefore is the carbapenem of choice for treatment of meningitis or in patients with preexisting seizure disorders.

CAUTIONS

Carbapenems as a class are associated with a risk of seizures, although it should be noted that other beta-lactam drugs have also caused seizures, especially at high doses. Imipenem appears to be the most epileptogenic of the class, with an incidence of seizure possibly in the range of 1–7%. Seizure risk is increased in patients with preexisting seizure disorders, or with elevated drug levels such as are seen in renal failure without dose adjustment. Meropenem, conversely, has shown to have a low incidence of drug-related seizures and is approved by the Food and Drug Administration (FDA) for the treatment of meningitis. There is less clinical experience with ertapenem; its seizure risk appears to be less

Table 74.11 Dosages for Second-Generation Cephalosporins

Drug	Dosage Adjustment for Renal Function (mL/min)			Hepatic Adjust?
	CrCl >50	CrCl 10–50	CrCl <10	
Cefuroxime	0.75–1.5 g IV q8h 500 mg PO q12h	0.75–1.5 g IV q12–24h 500 mg PO q12–24h	0.5 g IV q24h 250–500 mg PO q24h	No
Cefoxitin	1 g IV q6–8h	1 g IV q8–12h	1 g IV q24h	No

Table 74.12 Third- and Fourth-Generation Cephalosporins

Drug	Acute Care Uses	Toxicities
Ceftriaxone IV, IM (Rocephin) Cefotaxime IV, IM (Claforan) Ceftazidime IV (various) Cefepime IV (Maxipime)	Community-acquired pneumonia Acute bacterial meningitis Endocarditis Nosocomial infections Sepsis	*Uncommon*: rash, biliary sludging (ceftriaxone) *Rare*: anaphylaxis **Drug Interactions** Minimal

Table 74.14 Carbapenems and Monobactams

Drug	Acute Care Uses	Toxicities
Imipenem IV* (Primaxin) Meropenem IV* (Merrem) Ertapenem IV* (Invanz)	Nosocomial infections Sepsis Intra-abdominal infections	*Uncommon*: rash *Rare*: anaphylaxis, seizures **Drug Interactions** Minimal
Aztreonam IV† (Azactam)	Nosocomial infections Acute bacterial meningitis	

*Carbapenems.
†Monobactam.

than that of imipenem, but it is unclear whether it is as low as that of meropenem.

PEARLS AND PITFALLS

1. The carbapenems are the most broad-spectrum agents currently in clinical use. To preserve their activity, they should be reserved for use against organisms resistant to other agents.

2. Aztreonam's spectrum of activity and pharmacokinetics are similar to those of ceftazidime (although it lacks ceftazidime's weak gram-positive activity). Its primary role in therapy has been in patients with severe beta-lactam allergies, where it is generally safe to administer because of its minimal to absent cross-reactivity. For example, aztreonam would be a reasonable choice for the coverage of *Neisseria meningitidis* in a patient with suspected meningitis and a documented anaphylactic reaction to beta-lactams. Note, however, that cases of cross-allergenicity have been noted if a patient's previous reaction was to ceftazidime, because aztreonam and ceftazidime share an identical side chain.

Glycopeptides

Table 74.16 lists acute care uses, toxicities, and drug interactions. See Table 74.17 for doses of glycopeptides.

MECHANISM OF ACTION

Inhibition of cell wall synthesis at a different step from beta-lactams. Slowly bactericidal, time-dependent killing.

DIFFERENCES BETWEEN AGENTS

Although only a single agent in the glycopeptide class is currently approved in the United States, there is a large distinction between intravenous and oral administration of vancomycin. All indications for vancomycin other than treatment of *C. difficile* diseases should use intravenous vancomycin. Oral vancomycin is not appreciably absorbed and is used only for its intracolonic effects in cases of *C. difficile* colitis; note that intravenous vancomycin does not achieve adequate levels in the colon and is insufficient for treatment of *C. difficile* infection.

CAUTIONS

The most commonly observed adverse effect of vancomycin is "Red man's" (or "Red neck") syndrome, a syndrome of flushing, pruritis, and hypotension (usually mild). The reaction is thought to be the result of histamine release, is reversible on drug discontinuation, and can be reduced or eliminated by slowing the rate of infusion (to >1 hour per gram of drug administered). Premedication with a histamine antagonist may be useful in difficult cases. "Red man's syndrome" is not a contraindication to future vancomycin courses, although efforts should be made to differentiate from (much rarer) true hypersensitivity reactions.

Table 74.13 Dosages for Third- and Fourth-Generation Cephalosporins

Drug	Dosage Adjustment for Renal Function (mL/min)			Hepatic Adjust?
	CrCl >50	CrCl 10–50	CrCl <10	
Ceftriaxone	1 g IV q24h* 2 g IV q24h† 2 g IV q12h‡	No adjustment	No adjustment	No
Cefotaxime	1–2 g IV q8h* 2 g IV q4–6h‡	1–2 g IV q8–12h	1 g IV q24h	No
Ceftazidime	2 g IV q8h	2 g IV q12–24h	0.5 g IV q24h	No
Cefepime	2 g IV q8–12h§	1–2 g IV q12–24h	0.5 g IV q24h	No

*Dose for most indications.
†Dose for endocarditis or osteomyelitis.
‡Dose for meningitis.
§q8h dosing for febrile neutropenia or *Pseudomonas* infections.

Table 74.15 Dosages of Carbapenems and Monobactams

Drug	Dosage Adjustment for Renal Function (mL/min)			Hepatic Adjust?
	CrCl >50	CrCl 10–50	CrCl <10	
Imipenem	500 mg IV q6–8h	500 mg IV q8h	250–500 mg IV q12h	No
Meropenem	1–2 g IV q8h	0.5–1 g IV q12h	0.5 g IV q24h	No
Ertapenem	1 g IV q24h	0.5 g IV q24h*	0.5 g IV q24h	No
Aztreonam	2 g IV q8h	2 g IV q12h	1 g IV q12h	No

* For CrCl <30 mL/min.

Table 74.16 Glycopeptides

Drug	Acute Care Uses	Toxicities
Vancomycin IV, PO (various)	Skin and soft-tissue infections Endocarditis Osteomyelitis Meningitis Nosocomial infections *Clostridium difficile* disease	*Uncommon*: "Red man's syndrome" (histamine release) *Rare*: nephrotoxicity, neutropenia, ototoxicity **Drug Interactions** *Aminoglycosides*: possible increase in ototoxicity and nephrotoxicity

PEARLS AND PITFALLS

1. Vancomycin dosing is based on total body weight. In overweight patients or those with severe infections, dosing should follow a mg/kg approach in order to ensure optimal concentrations, rather than giving a standard 1 g IV q12h dose. Vancomycin levels may be monitored and should be 10–15 mg/dL for most indications, with higher levels (in the 15–20 mg/dL range) for severe infections (e.g., meningitis, endocarditis, and osteomyelitis).

2. Vancomycin is an important component of empiric therapy because of its activity against MRSA and penicillin-resistant *S. pneumoniae*. However, it has slower bacterial killing compared to the beta-lactam drugs. Thus, beta-lactam agents are preferred for the treatment of infections due to susceptible organisms when intravenous therapy is necessary, despite the dosing convenience offered by vancomycin (bid for vancomycin vs. tid or qid for many beta-lactam drugs).

Fluoroquinolones

Table 74.18 lists acute care uses, toxicities, and drug interactions. See Table 74.19 for doses of fluoroquinolones.

MECHANISM OF ACTION

Inhibition of DNA topoisomerases leading to strand breaks and replication failure. Bactericidal, concentration-dependent activity.

DIFFERENCES BETWEEN AGENTS

Ciprofloxacin has less potent gram-positive activity than levofloxacin or moxifloxacin and should not be used for community-acquired pneumonia. Both ciprofloxacin and levofloxacin have antipseudomonal activity (at higher doses), but moxifloxacin does not.

CAUTIONS

Fluoroquinolones are popular drugs for the treatment of respiratory tract infections in the elderly, because they are often at higher risk for resistant respiratory pathogens. However, the elderly may be more predisposed to some of the adverse effects of the fluoroquinolones. Confusion, headache, and dizziness are reported with the fluoroquinolones; the elderly may be at increased risk because of underlying dementias and because of age-related decreases in renal function leading to accumulation of drug to toxic levels. Careful attention should be paid to appropriate dosing. Older patients with heart disease, especially those on antiarrhythmic drugs (such as amiodarone), may be susceptible to the QT-prolonging effects of the fluoroquinolones. Fluoroquinolones should be used carefully or avoided in these patients. Finally, several studies have reported dysglycemias (hypo- and hyperglycemias) in patients, often elderly, receiving fluoroquinolones. The effect was most pronounced with gatifloxacin, which has subsequently been removed from distribution; however, clinicians should be aware of the possibility with the other fluoroquinolones (especially when the drugs are used in diabetic patients).

PEARLS AND PITFALLS

1. Resistance to fluoroquinolones is rapidly increasing; already these drugs cannot be considered reliable empiric

Table 74.17 Dosages for Vancomycin

Drug	Dosage Adjustment for Renal Function (mL/min)			Hepatic Adjust?
	CrCl >50	CrCl 10–50	CrCl <10	
Vancomycin	10–15 mg/kg IV q12–24h	10–15 mg/kg IV q12–24h	5–10 mg/kg IV q24–48h	No

Table 74.18 Fluoroquinolones

Drug	Acute Care Uses	Toxicities
Ciprofloxacin IV, PO (Cipro) Levofloxacin IV, PO (Levaquin) Moxifloxacin IV, PO (Avelox)	Urinary tract infections* Community-acquired pneumonia[†] Bacterial sinusitis[†] Acute exacerbations of chronic bronchitis[†] Nosocomial infections Biliary tree infections Anthrax	*Uncommon*: photosensitivity, headache, dizziness, arthralgias, confusion *Rare*: Achilles tendon rupture, seizures, QT prolongation, dysglycemias **Drug Interactions** *Oral cations (Ca, Mg, Fe)*: reduced absorption of oral fluoroquinolones

*Use levofloxacin or ciprofloxacin.
[†]Use levofloxacin or moxifloxacin.
As of 2007, fluoroquinolones are no longer recommended for the treatment of gonorrhea.

Table 74.20 Aminoglycosides

Drug	Acute Care Uses	Toxicities
Gentamicin IV (various) Tobramycin IV (various) Amikacin IV (various)	Endocarditis Nosocomial infections Urinary tract infections	*Common*: acute renal insufficiency *Uncommon*: ototoxicity (vestibular and cochlear) *Rare*: neuromuscular blockade **Drug Interactions** *Other nephrotoxins*: additive nephrotoxicity

monotherapy for *Pseudomonas* infections. Increasing resistance among *E. coli* threatens their role in urinary tract infections. In patients with urosepsis or pyelonephritis, clinicians might consider third- or fourth-generation cephalosporins as empiric therapy instead, especially if patients have prior exposure to fluoroquinolones or if local resistance to fluoroquinolones is known to be high.

2. Fluoroquinolones have excellent oral bioavailability, making them good drugs for outpatient therapy. However, their absorption is markedly decreased with coadministration of divalent and trivalent cations (calcium, iron, magnesium, etc.). Separate administration of these drugs (as well as multivitamins) by at least 2 hours; or, have the patient stop cation-containing drugs for the duration of fluoroquinolone use.

3. Moxifloxacin, by virtue of its nonrenal clearance, achieves low urinary concentrations and is thus not indicated for the treatment of urinary tract infections.

Aminoglycosides

Table 74.20 lists acute care uses, toxicities, and drug interactions. See Table 74.21 for doses of aminoglycosides.

MECHANISM OF ACTION

Ribosomal binding leading to inhibition and mistranslation of bacterial protein synthesis. Bactericidal, concentration-dependent killing.

DIFFERENCES BETWEEN AGENTS

Tobramycin has slightly more potent activity against *Pseudomonas* than gentamicin, whereas gentamicin has somewhat more potent activity against *Serratia*. Amikacin has activity against some gentamicin- and tobramycin-resistant isolates of *E. coli*, *Klebsiella*, *Pseudomonas* and *Acinetobacter* and is a second-line agent for mycobacterial infections. Only gentamicin has been widely studied as synergistic combination therapy with other drugs against gram-positive organisms.

CAUTIONS

Aminoglycosides are among the most predictably toxic antimicrobials in widespread use. Careful dosing and frequent monitoring are necessary to reduce the risk of irreversible nephro- and ototoxicity. The risk-benefit ratio dictates that these drugs should generally not be used for nonsevere infections.

PEARLS AND PITFALLS

1. "Once-daily" or "extended-interval" aminoglycoside dosing leverages the concentration-dependent killing of the drugs to create an equally effective, more convenient, and possibly safer dosing regimen compared to traditional dosing methods. However, there are many populations in which once-daily dosing has been minimally studied, including the pregnant, the critically ill, those with

Table 74.19 Dosages for Fluoroquinolones

Drug	Dosage Adjustment for Renal Function (mL/min)			Hepatic Adjust?
	CrCl >50	CrCl 10–50	CrCl <10	
Ciprofloxacin	400 mg IV q12h 500 mg PO q12h 400 mg IV q8h 750 mg PO q12h*	200–400 mg IV q12h 250–500 mg PO q12h 200–400 mg IV q8h 500–750 mg PO q12h*	200 mg IV q12h 250 mg PO q12h	No
Levofloxacin	500 mg IV/PO q24h 750 mg IV/PO q24h*	250 mg IV/PO q24h 750 mg IV/PO q48h	500 mg IV/PO q24h 500 mg IV/PO q48h[†]	No
Moxifloxacin	400 mg IV/PO q24h	No adjustment	No adjustment	Possibly

*For proven or suspected *Pseudomonas* infections.
[†]After 750 mg loading dose.

Table 74.21 Dosages for Aminoglycosides

Drug	Dosage Adjustment for Renal Function (mL/min)			Hepatic Adjust?
	CrCl >50	CrCl 10–50	CrCl <10	
Gentamicin or tobramycin	*Traditional:* 1.7 mg/kg IV q8h *Extended-interval:* 5–7 mg/kg IV q24h *Gram-positive synergy:* 1 mg/kg IV q8h	*Traditional:* 1.2–1.5 mg/kg IV q12–24h *Extended-interval:* not recommended	1.2–1.5 mg/kg IV q24–48h	No
Amikacin	*Traditional:* 7.5 mg/kg IV q12h *Extended-interval:* 15 mg/kg IV q24h	*Traditional:* 5–7.5 mg/kg IV q12–24h *Extended-interval:* not recommended	5 mg/kg IV q24–48h	No

Aminoglycoside dosing should be based on ideal or adjusted body weight, not total body weight, in obese patients (>120% of their ideal body weight).

Table 74.22 Macrolides and Ketolides

Drug	Acute Care Uses	Toxicities
Azithromycin IV, PO (Zithromax) Clarithromycin PO (Biaxin) Erythromycin IV, PO (various) Telithromycin PO (Ketek)	Community-acquired pneumonia Bacterial sinusitis Acute exacerbations of chronic bronchitis Otitis media Sexually transmitted diseases (*Chlamydia trachomatis*)	*Common*: gastrointestinal upset *Rare*: hepatotoxicity, QT prolongation **Drug Interactions** *Substrates of CYP P450 enzymes*: increased levels of substrate drugs (erythromycin ~ clarithromycin ~ telithromycin >> azithromycin)

significant renal dysfunction, and the morbidly obese. Use this dosing method with caution, if at all, in these populations.

2. Aminoglycosides are not clinically useful as single-drug therapy for gram-positive organisms but may provide synergistic activity against these organisms when used in combination with cell-wall active agents (such as a beta-lactam or glycopeptides). The dosing for gram-positive synergy uses a smaller total daily dose than traditional dosing. The primary established indications are for staphylococcal prosthetic valve endocarditis or severe enterococcal infections. Outside of these indications, the toxicity risk of the aminoglycosides should be weighed carefully against the possible benefit of synergistic activity.

3. Aminoglycosides continue to be one of the most active classes of drugs against many gram-negative organisms. For patients with sepsis potentially due to gram-negative organisms (e.g., urosepsis), addition of an aminoglycoside to an empiric regimen will improve the likelihood of covering organisms resistant to other classes. When culture and susceptibility data are available, the aminoglycoside can usually be discontinued and treatment completed with a less toxic drug. Such a strategy balances the excellent coverage of aminoglycosides and their risk of toxicity.

Macrolides and Ketolides

Table 74.22 lists acute care uses, toxicities, and drug interactions. See Table 74.23 for doses of macrolides and ketolides.

MECHANISM OF ACTION
Binding to 50S ribosome with inhibition of protein synthesis. Bacteriostatic.

DIFFERENCES BETWEEN AGENTS
Erythromycin has fallen out of favor because of its poor tolerance, frequent dosing, drug interactions, and poor coverage of *H. influenzae*. Azithromycin and clarithromycin have similar spectra of activity, although the long half-life of azithromycin allows for once-daily, short-course therapy (e.g., 3 days for sinusitis). Telithromycin is a ketolide and has activity against macrolide-resistant *S. pneumoniae*; however, there are concerns over cases of fatal hepatotoxicity associated

Table 74.23 Dosages for Macrolides and Ketolides

Drug	Dosage Adjustment for Renal Function (mL/min)			Hepatic Adjust?
	CrCl >50	CrCl 10–50	CrCl <10	
Azithromycin	500 mg IV/PO q24h	No adjustment	No adjustment	No
Clarithromycin	500 mg PO q12h	No adjustment	250 mg PO q12h	No
Erythromycin	500–1000 mg IV q6h 250–500 mg PO q-12h	No adjustment	250–500 mg IV q6h	No
Telithromycin	800 mg PO q24h	600 mg PO q24h	600 mg PO q24h	Possibly*

*For patients with combined renal and hepatic failure, give 400 mg PO q24h.

Table 74.24 Tetracyclines and Glycylcyclines

Drug	Acute Care Uses	Toxicities
Doxycycline IV, PO (various) Tigecycline IV (Tygacil)	Community-acquired pneumonia Anthrax Rickettsial diseases Skin and soft-tissue infections	*Uncommon*: photosensitivity, nausea, diarrhea *Rare*: esophagitis **Drug Interactions** *Oral cations (Ca, Mg, Fe)*: reduced absorption of oral fluoroquinolones

Table 74.26 Lincosamides

Drug	Acute Care Uses	Toxicities
Clindamycin IV, PO (Cleocin)	Skin and soft-tissue infections Aspiration pneumonia	*Uncommon*: diarrhea, *C. difficile* colitis *Rare*: Pseudomembranous colitis **Drug Interactions** Minimal

with this drug, leading to a strong FDA warning to avoid use of the drug in patients with underlying hepatic dysfunction.

CAUTIONS

Other than azithromycin, the macrolides and ketolides are potent inhibitors of human drug-metabolizing enzymes (primarily the cytochrome P-450 system), with many possible drug interactions. Patients on multiple medications should be screened for potential interactions when non-azithromycin macrolides are prescribed. Of particular concern is coadministration with drugs that prolong the QT interval, possibly leading to arrhythmias. The macrolides themselves have modest effects on the QT interval; however, when administered with drugs that also prolong the QT interval and are metabolized through enzyme pathways inhibited by the macrolides, the risk of arrhythmias increases substantially.

PEARLS AND PITFALLS

1. Macrolide resistance in *S. pneumoniae* has become increasingly common, with a number of documented treatment failures, especially in bacteremic disease. Macrolides are generally not recommended as initial monotherapy in patients with severe pneumonia (e.g., those requiring hospitalization).

Tetracyclines and Glycylcyclines

Table 74.24 lists acute care uses, toxicities, and drug interactions. See Table 74.25 for doses of tetracyclines and glycylcyclines.

MECHANISM OF ACTION

Binding to 30S ribosome with inhibition of protein synthesis. Bacteriostatic.

DIFFERENCES BETWEEN AGENTS

Doxycycline is generally favored over other tetracycline formulations (tetracycline, minocycline) because of its more convenient dosing and lower incidence of adverse effects. Tigecycline is technically a glycylcycline, a modified version of tetracyclines that evades most tetracycline resistance mechanisms. Thus, tigecycline has a broader spectrum of activity than the traditional tetracyclines, including activity against many gram-negative aerobic and anaerobic organisms (except for *Pseudomonas* and *Proteus*) as well as staphylococci and enterococci. However, it is only available as an intravenous preparation.

CAUTIONS

Tetracyclines are contraindicated in pregnancy and children under 8 years of age because of their effects on tooth development. However, in the setting of proven or highly probable rickettsial disease, the benefits of a course of tetracyclines are thought to outweigh the risks.

PEARLS AND PITFALLS

1. As with the fluoroquinolones, tetracyclines have excellent oral bioavailability but are chelated by divalent and trivalent cations (Ca, Fe, Mg, etc.). Separate administration of these agents by several hours from oral tetracyclines.
2. Tetracyclines have displayed good activity (>90%) against community-acquired MRSA isolates and are an option for oral therapy in skin and soft-tissue infections documented or suspected to be due to MRSA. However, they have relatively poor activity against group A streptococci and should not be used empirically if the likelihood of streptococcal infection is high (e.g., cellulitis).

Lincosamides

Table 74.26 lists acute care uses, toxicities, and drug interactions. See Table 74.27 for doses of lincosamides.

Table 74.25 Dosages for Tetracyclines and Glycylcylines

Drug	Dosage Adjustment for Renal Function (mL/min)			Hepatic Adjust?
	CrCl >50	CrCl 10–50	CrCl <10	
Doxycycline	100 mg IV/PO q12h	No adjustment	No adjustment	No
Tigecycline	100 mg IV × 1, then 50 mg IV q12h	No adjustment	No adjustment	Yes*

*For severe hepatic disease, loading dose of 100 mg, then 25 mg IV q12h.

Table 74.27 Dosages for Clindamycin

Drug	Dosage Adjustment for Renal Function (mL/min)			Hepatic Adjust?
	CrCl >50	**CrCl 10–50**	**CrCl <10**	
Clindamycin	600–900 mg IV q8h 300–450 mg PO q6–8h	No adjustment	No adjustment	No

MECHANISM OF ACTION

Binds to 50S ribosome, with inhibition of protein synthesis. Bacteriostatic.

DIFFERENCES BETWEEN AGENTS

Not applicable.

CAUTIONS

Diarrhea is one of the most common adverse effects associated with clindamycin. Clindamycin can itself cause a relatively benign, self-limiting diarrhea or can result in more severe diarrhea resulting from superinfection with *Clostridium difficile*. *C. difficile*-associated diarrhea and colitis can occur during or after therapy with any antibacterial agent and can be life-threatening. Clindamycin may be associated with a higher risk of *C. difficile* disease relative to other antibacterials. Patients with diarrhea, especially if it is severe, associated with fever, or persists after the end of clindamycin therapy, need evaluation for *C. difficile* disease.

PEARLS AND PITFALLS

1. Clindamycin's inhibition of protein synthesis and activity against organisms in stationary-phase growth has been utilized in the treatment of necrotizing fasciitis and other toxin-mediated diseases. Consider the addition of clindamycin to beta-lactam based therapy when treating these types of serious infections.
2. Clindamycin has good activity against most staphylococci (MRSA and MSSA). However, some strains of staphylococci possess "inducible resistance": that is, the organisms appear susceptible to clindamycin in initial in vitro susceptibility testing but have a high propensity to mutate to a resistant form during therapy. These isolates occur among strains that possess erythromycin resistance; the microbiology lab can perform a screening test (called a "D-test") on erythromycin-resistant, clindamycin-susceptible isolates to determine whether inducible resistance is likely to occur.

Trimethoprim-Sulfamethoxazole

Table 74.28 lists acute care uses, toxicities, and drug interactions. See Table 74.29 for dosing of trimethoprim-sulfamethoxazole.

MECHANISM OF ACTION

Trimethoprim and sulfamethoxazole (TMP-SMX) inhibit sequential steps in the folate biosynthesis pathway. The synergistic combination of the two agents generally results in bactericidal activity.

DIFFERENCES BETWEEN AGENTS

Trimethoprim is available as a single agent and may be used for acute cystitis.

CAUTIONS

TMP-SMX is a frequent cause of rash, most commonly due to the sulfamethoxazole component. Interestingly, the frequency of rash is increased in patients with human immunodeficiency virus (HIV) or acquired immunodeficiency syndrome (AIDS). Life-threatening reactions such as toxic epidermal necrolysis and Stevens-Johnson syndrome have been documented, and patients with a history of rash due to TMP-SMX should generally not be rechallenged because of the risk of severe reactions.

PEARLS AND PITFALLS

1. For years, TMP-SMX was considered standard first-line therapy for treatment of acute uncomplicated cystitis in women. Recent guidelines suggest, however, that in areas with local resistance rates greater than 15–20% in *E. coli*, an alternative drug (e.g., ciprofloxacin or nitrofurantoin) should be used. This recommendation is somewhat controversial because of the relatively low failure rate even with resistant organisms, as well as the increasing rate of fluoroquinolone resistance. At a minimum, TMP-SMX should not be used for empiric therapy of complicated urinary tract infection (e.g., pyelonephritis or urosepsis).
2. TMP-SMX comes in a fixed, 5:1 ratio of the two components. The intravenous form is dosed based on the TMP component. The oral form comes in two strengths: single-strength (80:400 mg TMP:SMX) and double-strength (160:800 mg TMP:SMX). TMP-SMX has excellent oral bioavailability, allowing for conversion to oral therapy when patients are tolerating oral medications.
3. Similar to the tetracyclines, TMP-SMX has excellent activity (>95% susceptibility in most series) against community-acquired MRSA but poor activity against group A streptococci.

Nitroimidazoles

Table 74.30 lists acute care uses, toxicities, and drug interactions. See Table 74.31 for doses of nitroimidazoles.

Table 74.28 Trimethoprim-Sulfamethoxazole

Drug	Acute Care Uses	Toxicities
Trimethoprim-sulfamethoxazole IV, PO (Bactrim, Septra)	Urinary tract infections *Pneumocystis* pneumonia *Stenotrophomonas* infections *Nocardia* infections *Listeria* (PCN allergic)	*Uncommon*: rash, hyperkalemia, neutropenia, pseudo-renal failure (asymptomatic increase in SCr) *Rare*: acute renal failure **Drug Interactions** *Warfarin*: increased INR
INR, international normalized ratio; PCN, penicillin.		

Table 74.29 Dosages for Trimethoprim-Sulfamethoxazole

Drug	Dosage Adjustment for Renal Function (mL/min)			Hepatic Adjust?
	CrCl >50	CrCl 10–50	CrCl <10	
TMP-SMX	10–20 mg TMP/kg/day IV divided q6–12h* 1 DS tab PO q12h†	5–15 mg TMP/kg/day IV divided q12–24h 1 SS PO q12h	2.5–10 mg TMP/kg/day IV q24h 1 SS PO q24h	No

*Higher end of IV dosing range should be used for *Pneumocystis* infections; dosing is based on TMP component.
†Dose for uncomplicated cystitis; oral dose for more severe infections should be based on mg/kg dosing.
DS, double-strength tablet; SS, single-strength tablet.

Table 74.30 Nitroimidazoles

Drug	Acute Care Uses	Toxicities
Metronidazole IV, PO (Flagyl) Tinidazole PO (Tindamax)	*Clostridium difficile* disease Trichomoniasis Giardiasis Amebiasis Intra-abdominal infections, in combination with other agents	*Uncommon*: nausea, vomiting, metallic taste *Rare*: peripheral neuropathy **Drug Interactions** *Warfarin*: increased INR *Alcohol*: disulfiram-like reaction

INR, international normalized ratio.

MECHANISM OF ACTION

Nitroreductases (present only in anaerobic bacteria) activate nitroimidazoles to highly reactive, cytotoxic metabolites. Bactericidal.

DIFFERENCES BETWEEN AGENTS

Although the spectrum of activity of the two drugs is similar, clinical efficacy data for tinidazole is available only for its use in parasitic infections. For such infections (including giardiasis, amebiasis, and trichomoniasis), single-dose or short-course therapy appears to be more effective and better tolerated than metronidazole, albeit at a higher cost.

CAUTIONS

Nitroimidazoles have a reputation for causing a disulfiram (Antabuse)-like reaction with the consumption of alcohol, because of their inhibition of aldehyde dehydrogenase. It

is recommended to have patients abstain from alcohol while taking nitroimidazoles. Also well-described is the interaction with warfarin, in which warfarin's metabolism is inhibited, leading to an increase in anticoagulation. Careful monitoring and warfarin dose reduction may be necessary.

PEARLS AND PITFALLS

1. Metronidazole is generally considered to be the first-line treatment for initial episodes of *Clostridium difficile* disease, based on its equivalent success rates with oral vancomycin in a clinical trial, and metronidazole's lower cost and lower risk of selecting for vancomycin-resistant enterococci. Unlike intravenous vancomycin, intravenous metronidazole does have some role in treatment of patients with *C. difficile* who cannot take oral medications. In severe or treatment-refractory cases, oral vancomycin may be used instead of metronidazole or as adjunctive therapy.

Nitrofurans

Table 74.32 lists acute care uses, toxicities, and drug interactions. See Table 74.33 for doses of nitrofurans.

MECHANISM OF ACTION
Not clear.

DIFFERENCES BETWEEN AGENTS

There are two preparations of nitrofurantoin: a crystalline form (Macrodantin) and a macrocrystalline/monohydrate form (Macrobid). The former is dosed four times daily for the treatment of cystitis, the latter twice daily.

Table 74.31 Dosages for Nitroimidazoles

Drug	Dosage Adjustment for Renal Function (mL/min)			Hepatic Adjust?
	CrCl >50	CrCl 10–50	CrCl <10	
Metronidazole	500–750 mg IV/PO q8h2 g PO × 1 dose*	No adjustment	500 mg IV q12h†	Possibly‡
Tinidazole	2 g PO × 1 dose§ 2 g PO q24h × 3–5 days‖	No adjustment	No adjustment	Possibly‡

*For trichomoniasis.
†Dose adjustment required only for patients with CrCl <10 mL/min and not on hemodialysis.
‡Consider dose reduction in severe hepatic impairment.
§For trichomoniasis or giardiasis.
‖For intestinal amebiasis or amebic liver abscess.

Table 74.32 Nitrofurans

Drug	Acute Care Uses	Toxicities
Nitrofurantoin PO (Macrobid, Macrodantin)	Lower urinary tract infection	*Uncommon*: nausea/vomiting *Rare*: pulmonary fibrosis
		Drug Interactions
		Minimal

Table 74.34 Oxazolidinones and Lipopeptides

Drug	Acute Care Uses	Toxicities
Linezolid IV, PO (Zyvox)	Skin and soft-tissue infections	*Uncommon*: thrombocytopenia *Rare*: optic neuritis, peripheral neuropathy
		Drug Interactions
		Antidepressants: risk of serotonin syndrome
Drug	**Acute Care Uses**	**Toxicities**
Daptomycin IV (Cubicin)	Skin and soft-tissue infections Endocarditis	*Uncommon*: myopathy *Rare*: rhabdomyolysis
		Drug Interactions
		Statins: possible increased risk of myopathy

CAUTIONS

Although generally well-tolerated (outside of gastrointestinal upset), there are rare but serious pulmonary adverse effects associated with nitrofurantoin use. These manifest either as an acute pneumonitis or a chronic pulmonary fibrosis. The acute presentation occurs within several days of initiation of the drug and subsides quickly after drug discontinuation. The chronic form is usually associated with long-term nitrofurantoin therapy (as in UTI prophylaxis) and can lead to permanent loss of pulmonary function and death. Patients receiving the drug for prophylaxis should be informed of the need to report any respiratory symptoms immediately.

PEARLS AND PITFALLS

1. Nitrofurantoin has good (>90% in most studies) activity against *E. coli* as well as adequate coverage of other common community-acquired UTI pathogens. However, its utility is limited to infections of the lower urinary tract, because the drug requires high concentrations for antimicrobial activity, and these are only reached when it concentrates in the urine. Thus, nitrofurantoin should not be used for more severe infections such as pyelonephritis and urosepsis. Also, in patients who have significant renal dysfunction (e.g., a creatinine clearance of <50 mL/min), there is insufficient accumulation of the drug in the urine for activity.

Oxazolidinones and Lipopeptides

Table 74.34 lists acute care uses, toxicities, and drug interactions. See Table 74.35 for doses of oxazolidinones and lipopeptides.

MECHANISM OF ACTION

The oxazolidinones such as linezolid are bacteriostatic inhibitors of protein synthesis, similar to tetracyclines. Daptomycin, a lipopeptide, acts on the bacterial cell membrane to produce a bactericidal effect.

DIFFERENCES BETWEEN AGENTS

Although pharmacologically and mechanistically distinct, these classes are grouped together here because of their similar spectrum of activity and clinical use. These drugs are active against gram-positive organisms, including those such as MRSA and VRE that are resistant to many other drugs. Linezolid has the advantage of having a highly bioavailable oral formulation, whereas daptomycin is rapidly bactericidal in vitro (as opposed to the bacteriostatic linezolid).

CAUTIONS

Linezolid has been associated with more adverse effects when given for extended periods of time (>14 days). Most frequent is a reversible thrombocytopenia, although neutropenia and anemia can be seen. Patients receiving long-term linezolid should have regular complete blood cell counts performed. Recently cases of peripheral and optic neuropathy associated with long-term linezolid have been described; this effect may be due to inhibition of mitochondrial protein synthesis.

PEARLS AND PITFALLS

1. Linezolid is a moderate inhibitor of monoamine oxidase (MAO) and can cause potentially fatal serotonin syndrome when given concurrently with serotonergic agents such as selective serotonin reuptake inhibitors (SSRIs) – avoid concurrent use if possible. If a patient already on an SSRI

Table 74.33 Dosages for Nitrofurans

Drug	Dosage Adjustment for Renal Function (mL/min)			Hepatic Adjust?
	CrCl >50	CrCl 10–50	CrCl <10	
Nitrofurantoin macrocrystals	100 mg PO q6h	Do not use	Do not use	No
Nitrofurantoin macrocrystal/ monohydrate	100 mg PO q12h	Do not use	Do not use	No

Overview of Antibiotics

Table 74.35 Dosages for Oxazolidinones and Lipopeptides

Drug	Dosage Adjustment for Renal Function (mL/min)			Hepatic Adjust?
	CrCl >50	CrCl 10–50	CrCl <10	
Linezolid	600 mg IV/PO daily	No change	No change	No
Daptomycin	4–6 mg/kg IV q24h*	4–6 mg/kg IV q48h	4–6 mg/kg IV q48h	No

*4 mg/kg for skin and soft-tissue infections; 6 mg/kg for bacteremia and endocarditis.

requires treatment with linezolid, it may not be feasible to discontinue the SSRI for a short course of linezolid therapy (<10–14 days), because SSRIs generally requiring tapering rather than abrupt discontinuation. Vigilant monitoring for signs and symptoms of serotonin syndrome should be performed in this case.

2. Linezolid has excellent penetration into pulmonary tissue, and preliminary evidence suggests that it is equal to vancomycin for pneumonia due to MRSA. In contrast, daptomycin has been shown to have poor activity in the lung and should not be used for pneumonia caused by any pathogen.

3. Both of these drugs are extremely expensive and in most cases have not been proven to be superior to standard therapy.

Antifungals: Azoles

Table 74.36 lists acute care uses, toxicities, and drug interactions. See Table 74.37 for doses of azoles.

MECHANISM OF ACTION

Azoles inhibit fungal P-450 enzymes, preventing the synthesis of ergosterol, a crucial component of the fungal cell membrane. These agents are generally fungistatic against yeasts, but voriconazole may be fungicidal against *Aspergillus*.

Table 74.36 Antifungals: Azoles

Drug	Acute Care Uses	Toxicities
Fluconazole IV, PO (Diflucan) Itraconazole IV, PO (Sporanox) Voriconazole IV, PO (Vfend) Posaconazole PO (Noxafil)	Fungal infections	*Common*: visual disturbances (voriconazole) *Uncommon*: rash, elevated transaminases *Rare*: hepatitis
		Drug Interactions
		Substrates of CYP P450 enzymes: increased levels of substrate drugs (voriconazole ~ itraconazole ~ posaconazole >> fluconazole)

DIFFERENCES BETWEEN AGENTS

Fluconazole, itraconazole, voriconazole, and posaconazole all have activity against *Candida* species, with voriconazole and posaconazole having the most activity against non-*albicans* species (such as *krusei* and *glabrata*) that may be fluconazole-resistant. Fluconazole has no activity against *Aspergillus* species, itraconazole has moderate activity, posaconazole has good activity (but little clinical data), and voriconazole is the gold standard therapy for *Aspergillus*. Fluconazole is cleared renally, whereas the other azoles undergo hepatic metabolism.

CAUTIONS

Similar to many of the agents in the macrolide class, drug interactions are a major concern with the azole antifungals. Voriconazole, itraconazole, and posaconazole are potent inhibitors of drug-metabolizing enzymes, with fluconazole substantially weaker. Voriconazole and itraconazole are also substrates of these enzymes and can have their concentrations affected by other drugs (i.e., there can be two-way interactions). Another similarity to the macrolides is an effect on the QT interval, warranting caution when using these drugs in patients with underlying arrhythmias. Careful screening of these drugs against a patient's current medication list is required to avoid potentially dangerous interactions.

PEARLS AND PITFALLS

1. Visual disturbances, primarily manifesting as altered color perception, are common with voriconazole administration. The effects generally occur within an hour after dosage administration and subside within an hour or so. They also tend to become less pronounced over longer durations of treatment. Patients should be warned of these effects and should not perform activities such as driving until they become used to the effects of the drug.

2. The intravenous preparations of itraconazole and voriconazole are solubilized with a cyclodextran ether that accumulates in renal failure. Although the deleterious effects of this agent are poorly characterized, the manufacturer recommends avoiding use of the intravenous formulations in patients with CrCl less than 50 mL/min. The oral formulation does not have this issue.

Antifungals: Echinocandins

Table 74.38 lists acute care uses, toxicities, and drug interactions. See Table 74.39 for doses of echinocandins.

Table 74.37 Dosages for Azoles

Drug	Dosage Adjustment for Renal Function (mL/min)			Hepatic Adjust?
	CrCl >50	**CrCl 10–50**	**CrCl <10**	
Fluconazole	400 mg IV/PO q24h	100–200 mg IV/PO q24h	50–100 mg IV/PO q24h	No
Itraconazole	200 mg IV/PO q12h × 4 doses, then 100–200 mg PO q24h	Avoid intravenous preparation	Avoid intravenous preparation	Possibly
Voriconazole	6 mg/kg IV × 2 doses, then 4 mg/kg IV q12h 400 mg PO × 2 doses, then 200 mg PO q12h	Avoid intravenous preparation	Avoid intravenous preparation	Yes*

*For moderate hepatic dysfunction, reduce maintenance dose by 50%.

Table 74.38 Echinocandins

Drug	Acute Care Uses	Toxicities
Caspofungin IV (Cancidas) Micafungin IV (Mycamine) Anidulafungin IV (Eraxis)	Fungal infections	*Uncommon*: phlebitis, elevated transaminases *Rare*: hepatitis
		Drug Interactions
		Rifampin, phenytoin: reduced levels of caspofungin

MECHANISM OF ACTION

Echinocandins inhibit the synthesis of beta-glucan, an important component of the fungal cell wall. They appear to have fungicidal activity against yeasts and fungistatic activity against molds.

DIFFERENCES BETWEEN AGENTS

All three echinocandins have similar spectra of activity and excellent safety profiles. The newer agents (micafungin and anidulafungin) are slightly more potent than caspofungin and have fewer drug interactions, but there is more clinical experience with caspofungin.

CAUTIONS

Unlike azoles and polyenes, echinocandins lack activity versus *Cryptococcus* species and have no role in the treatment of cryptococcal meningitis.

PEARLS AND PITFALLS

1. By virtue of their broad spectrum of activity against *Candida* species, echinocandins are a reasonable choice for empiric therapy when these organisms are suspected. If culture results indicate a species of *Candida* that is reliably fluconazole-susceptible (e.g., *C. albicans*), switching to fluconazole may be a cost-effective option because echinocandins have a high acquisition cost.

Antifungals: Polyenes

Table 74.40 lists acute care uses, toxicities, and drug interactions. See Table 74.41 for doses of polyenes.

MECHANISM OF ACTION

Polyenes disrupt the fungal cell membrane and are generally fungicidal.

DIFFERENCES BETWEEN AGENTS

In addition to "conventional" amphotericin B deoxycholate, three lipid-associated forms of amphotericin are available. Associating amphotericin with a lipid carrier alters the distribution of amphotericin in the body and reduces nephrotoxicity. The lipid complex and liposomal formulations also reduce the incidence of infusion-related reactions, although the colloidal dispersion product does not. The lipid-associated products are all substantially more expensive than conventional amphotericin B.

Table 74.39 Dosages for Echinocandins

Drug	Dosage Adjustment for Renal Function (mL/min)			Hepatic Adjust?
	CrCl >50	**CrCl 10–50**	**CrCl <10**	
Caspofungin	70 mg IV × 1, then 50 mg IV q24h	No adjustment	No adjustment	Yes
Micafungin	100–150 mg IV q24h	No adjustment	No adjustment	No
Anidulafungin	200 mg IV × 1, then 100 mg IV q24h	No adjustment	No adjustment	No

Table 74.40 Antifungals: Polyenes

Drug	Acute Care Uses	Toxicities
Amphotericin B deoxycholate IV (various) Amphotericin B colloidal dispersion IV (Amphotec) Amphotericin B lipid complex IV (Abelcet) Liposomal amphotericin B IV (AmBisome)	Fungal infections	*Common*: infusion-related toxicities, nephrotoxicity, hypokalemia *Uncommon*: hepatitis
		Drug Interactions
		Aminoglycosides: enhanced nephrotoxicity

Table 74.42 Anti-Herpesvirus Drugs

Drug	Acute Care Uses	Toxicities
Acyclovir IV, PO (Zovirax) Valacyclovir PO (Valtrex) Famciclovir PO (Famvir) Ganciclovir IV, PO (Cytovene) Valganciclovir PO (Valtrex)	Herpesvirus infections	*Uncommon*: headache; neutropenia (ganciclovir, valganciclovir) *Rare*: seizures, nephrotoxicity
		Drug Interactions
		Additive bone marrow suppression: other drugs causing marrow suppression (ganciclovir, valganciclovir)

CAUTIONS

Amphotericin frequently causes dose- and duration-dependent nephrotoxicity. Renal dysfunction is often reversible on discontinuation of amphotericin, but may result in permanent renal failure. Although the lipid-associated forms of amphotericin attenuate this nephrotoxicity somewhat, the risk is not eliminated. Patients receiving any amphotericin product should have frequent monitoring of their renal function, adequate hydration, and, when possible, discontinuation of other potentially nephrotoxic drugs.

PEARLS AND PITFALLS

1. Although amphotericin has a broad spectrum of antifungal activity and decades of clinical experience, the availability of newer, less toxic antifungals has diminished its role as the "gold standard." Amphotericin continues to be the drug of choice for selected indications such as cryptococcal meningitis and is a reasonable choice for empiric therapy for suspected fungal infections.

Antivirals: Anti-Herpesvirus Drugs

Table 74.42 lists acute care uses, toxicities, and drug interactions. See Table 74.43 for doses of anti-herpesvirus drugs.

MECHANISM OF ACTION

These drugs are nucleoside analogues that inhibit viral DNA synthesis.

DIFFERENCES BETWEEN AGENTS

All these agents have good activity against herpes simplex viruses (HSV) and useful but lower activity against varicella-zoster virus. Only ganciclovir has clinically useful activity against cytomegalovirus (CMV). Because of ganciclovir's greater toxicity, the other agents are preferred for treatment of herpes simplex and varicella-zoster infections. The valine-esterified forms valacyclovir and valganciclovir are oral prodrugs designed to enhance the absorption of the parent drugs. After absorption, the valine portions are hydrolyzed and acyclovir and ganciclovir are released into the circulation.

CAUTIONS

Ganciclovir (and, by extension, valganciclovir) can cause profound, reversible, dose-related bone marrow suppression. Careful dosing of this drug according to the patient's renal function and avoidance, when possible, of other bone marrow-suppressive drugs is necessary. Nephrotoxicity due to crystallization of acyclovir can be seen when the intravenous formulation is given in doses too high for the patient's renal function, especially if the patient does not receive adequate hydration.

Table 74.41 Dosages for Polyenes

Drug	Dosage Adjustment for Renal Function (mL/min)			Hepatic Adjust?
	CrCl >50	CrCl 10–50	CrCl <10	
Amphotericin B deoxycholate	0.7–1.5 mg/kg IV q24h	No adjustment*	No adjustment*	No
Lipid formulations	3–6 mg/kg IV q24h	No adjustment*	No adjustment*	No
*Although the elimination of amphotericin is unaffected by renal dysfunction, because of the drug's nephrotoxicity consideration should be given to reducing or holding the dose in the setting of renal impairment.				

Table 74.43 Dosages for Anti-Herpesvirus drugs

Drug	Dosage Adjustment for Renal Function (mL/min)			Hepatic Adjust?
	CrCl >50	CrCl 10–50	CrCl <10	
Acyclovir	5–10 mg/kg IV q8h* 400 mg PO q8h†	5–10 mg/kg IV q12–24h No adjustment	2.5–5 mg/kg IV q24h 200 mg PO q8h	No
Valacyclovir	500–1000 mg PO q12h†	500–1000 mg PO q12–24h	500 mg PO q24h	No
Famciclovir	500 mg PO q12h†	500 mg PO q12–24h	250 mg PO q24h	No
Ganciclovir	5 mg/kg IV q12h†	1.25–2.5 mg/kg IV q12h-24h	1.25 mg/kg IV q24h	No
Valganciclovir	900 mg PO q12h‡	450 mg PO q12–24h	Not recommended	No

*Use higher end of dosing range for herpes encephalitis or varicella-zoster infections.
†Treatment of recurrent genital herpes in HIV-negative adults.
‡Induction doses for severe CMV disease.

PEARLS AND PITFALLS

1. Acyclovir (and valacyclovir) and famciclovir have good activity against herpes simplex virus but poor activity against cytomegalovirus. Ganciclovir (and valganciclovir) have good activity against both HSV and CMV; however, because of their greater toxicity, these drugs are not preferred for the treatment of HSV infections. Among acyclovir, valacyclovir, and famciclovir, the choice of drug for oral treatment of HSV infections is generally based on cost and frequency of administration (acyclovir is inexpensive but requires frequent dosing compared to the more expensive valacyclovir and famciclovir).

2. There are number of different dosing regimens for genital herpes simplex infections, according to whether it is the patient's first or a recurrent episode, whether the drug is being used for suppressive therapy, and whether the patient is HIV-infected. Dosing regimens are also different for herpes zoster infections.

Antivirals: Anti-Influenza Drugs

Table 74.44 lists acute care uses, toxicities, and drug interactions. See Table 74.45 for doses of anti-influenza drugs.

MECHANISM OF ACTION

Oseltamivir and zanamavir inhibit neuraminidase, which is necessary for the release of virions from infected cells. Amantadine and rimantadine (adamantanes) inhibit the viral M2 protein responsible for viral uncoating.

DIFFERENCES BETWEEN AGENTS

The neuraminidase inhibitors (oseltamivir and zanamavir) are active against both influenza A and B strains, whereas the adamantanes are active only against influenza A. The adamantanes are generally more toxic than the neuraminidase inhibitors and are more prone to lead to the development of viral resistance. Indeed, because of increased resistance, *amantadine and rimantadine are currently not recommended by the CDC* for treatment or prophylaxis of influenza. Oseltamivir is available as an oral agent, whereas zanamavir is inhaled.

CAUTIONS

Zanamavir, which is administered via a dry-powder inhaler, has caused bronchospasm in some patients with underlying asthma or chronic obstructive pulmonary disease. For these patients, oseltamivir is preferred.

PEARLS AND PITFALLS

1. The clinical benefit of neuraminidase inhibitor therapy is time-sensitive; efficacy is greatest when given as near to the start of symptoms as possible, becoming minimal after 48 hours have elapsed. Neuraminidase inhibitors may also be used for influenza prophylaxis in unvaccinated patients.

2. Oseltamivir and zanamavir have a broader spectrum (covering influenza B as well as A) and are better tolerated than older anti-influenza drugs such as amantadine and rimantadine; however, they are significantly more expensive.

3. Oseltamivir has been used for the treatment of avian influenza (at doses up to 150 mg q12h) and could be used for mass prophylaxis in the event of an outbreak. However, strains of avian influenza with oseltamivir resistance have been described.

Table 74.44 Anti-Influenza Drugs

Drug	Acute Care Uses	Toxicities
Oseltamivir PO (Tamiflu) Zanamavir inhalation (Relenza) Amantadine PO (Symmetrel) Rimantadine PO (Flumadine)	Influenza	*Uncommon*: bronchospasm (zanamavir), nausea/vomiting *Rare*: confusion
		Drug Interactions
		Minimal

Table 74.45 Dosages for Anti-Influenza Drugs

Drug	Dosage Adjustment for Renal Function (mL/min)			Hepatic Adjust?
	CrCl >50	CrCl 10–50	CrCl <10	
Oseltamivir	75 mg PO q12h 75 mg PO q24h*	75 mg PO q24h 75 mg PO q48h	No data	No
Zanamavir	2 inhalations q12h 2 inhalations q24h*	No adjustment	No adjustment	No

*Prophylaxis dose.

4. Resistance to anti-influenza agents is evolving. During the 2005–06 influenza season, the primary circulating influenza strains in North America were resistant to amantadine and rimantadine. Strains of avian influenza (H5N1) with resistance to the neuraminidase inhibitors have been isolated. Clinicians should keep abreast of the most updated recommendations for treatment and prophylaxis of influenza for every season (available at www.cdc.gov/flu).

REFERENCES

Kucers A, Crowe S, Brayson ML, Hoy J, eds. The use of antibiotics. Boston: Butterworth-Heinemann, 1997.

Mandell GL, Bennett JE, Dolin R, eds. Principles and practice of infectious diseases (6th ed). New York: Churchill Livingstone, 2005.

Yu VL, Weber R, Raoult D, eds. Antimicrobial therapy and vaccines (vol. II). Pittsburgh: ESun Technologies, 2005.

PART VI

Microbiology/Laboratory Tests

75. Microbiology Laboratory Testing for Infectious Diseases

Barbara L. Haller

INTRODUCTION

Clinicians can often recognize specific infectious disease syndromes based on clinical presentation and, based on experience, strongly suspect a particular etiology. For example, cellulitis, skin abscesses, and sinusitis are typically associated with bacteria, whereas measles, chickenpox, zoster, croup, and bronchiolitis are caused by viruses. In many cases, identification of the specific causative microorganism by the microbiology laboratory is very important:

- some infectious disease syndromes such as pneumonia, diarrhea, and sepsis can be caused by various classes of organisms (bacteria, viruses, fungi, parasites)
- identification of the microorganism allows selection of targeted antimicrobial agents, thereby decreasing use of broad-spectrum antibiotics, the occurrence of adverse effects from antimicrobial agents, and the risk that resistant organisms will emerge
- an organism may be resistant to a given antimicrobial therapy, requiring a change in antimicrobial regimen
- an unexpected organism that might not otherwise be treated may be identified, such as *Entamoeba histolytica* causing diarrhea.

Effective use of the clinical microbiology laboratory requires collection of appropriate specimens and knowledge of the tests offered by the laboratory.

SPECIMEN COLLECTION

General Collection Procedures

1. Refer to laboratory collection guidelines for descriptions of available collection devices and instructions for proper specimen collection.
2. Talk to microbiology laboratory staff about complex cases before collecting specimens.
3. Collect specimens before antimicrobial therapy is started.
4. Because many body sites harbor commensal or normal flora, cleanse lesions with sterile saline or debride wounds before collecting specimens.
5. Clearly label specimens with patient information.
6. The requisition form or computer order should contain the following information: patient name, medical record number, patient age and sex, patient location, ordering physician name with phone or pager number, specific anatomic site, date and time of specimen collection, name of person collecting specimen.

   - Clearly describe the body site source for each specimen on the laboratory requisition, because plating methods and organism work-up are determined by the source.
   - Include clinical information to help guide culture work-up.

7. Transport specimens to the microbiology laboratory as soon as possible (usually within 2 hours of collection) and maintain proper storage temperature.

   - Organisms sensitive to environmental changes include *Shigella* spp., *Neisseria gonorrhoeae*, *Neisseria meningitidis*, and *Haemophilus influenzae*.
   - Do not refrigerate spinal fluid, genital, eye, or internal ear specimens or specimens suspected to harbor the sensitive organisms listed above.

8. Notify the microbiology laboratory immediately if a highly infectious pathogen is suspected from the patient's clinical presentation. Laboratory personnel will take special precautions when working with these organisms to prevent laboratory-acquired infections. Highly infectious pathogens include *Coccidioides immitis*, *Mycobacterium tuberculosis*, *N. meningitidis*, *Brucella* spp., *Francisella tularensis* (tularemia), *Bacillus anthracis*, severe acute respiratory syndrome (SARS) coronavirus, avian influenza (H5N1), and bioterrorism agents.

Specific Collection Procedures

1. **Blood culture:**
   a. Proper skin antisepsis with chlorhexidine or povidone-iodine is critical to prevent contamination by skin flora.
   b. Blood volume collected is also critical to optimize recovery of bacteria from blood (8–10 mL/bottle or 20 mL/set recommended for adults; 1–5 mL per bottle for neonates/infants/children).
   c. Collect two blood culture sets (one aerobic and one anaerobic bottle each set) from two different sites prior to starting antibiotics in a febrile patient. Label the site of collection on the culture bottle.

d. Collection of two to three blood culture sets in a 24-hour period detects virtually all bloodstream infections.

e. Avoid drawing blood through catheters, because contaminating organisms can make culture interpretation difficult.

f. Collection of only one blood culture set is discouraged because the significance of a possible contaminant such as coagulase-negative *Staphylococcus* in one set is difficult to interpret.

g. To increase recovery of organisms from blood, laboratories with automated blood culture systems may have a blood culture bottle available that contains a resin or activated charcoal designed to remove antibiotics from blood specimens collected from patients who are on antibiotics at presentation.

h. Request that blood cultures be incubated longer than the standard 5 days if a patient is suspected to have culture-negative endocarditis or brucellosis, which can require 21 days of incubation for growth.

2. **Urine for culture:**
   a. Instruct patients carefully on procedure for collection of clean-catch urine.
   b. Indicate the type of collection on requisition – that is, clean catch, indwelling catheter, in-and-out catheter, or suprapubic aspirate – because collection method determines the extent of organism work-up.
   c. For mycobacteria culture, collect first morning urine on 3 consecutive days.

3. **Cerebrospinal fluid (CSF):**
   a. Be sure CSF tubes are labeled with patient name and a second identifier.
   b. It may be necessary to prioritize requested tests on CSF if volume collected is not adequate for all testing.

4. **Tissue/biopsy specimens**: collect in sterile container on moistened gauze pad (do not float specimen in saline).

5. **Anaerobic culture:**
   a. Collect specimens with needle and syringe (aspirated fluid) or debride wounds, abscesses, or decubitus ulcers and send tissue from debrided lesion in a sterile cup on a pad moistened with sterile saline.
   b. The microbiology laboratory will provide an anaerobic transport device or tube that can be used for collection of aspirated fluid or tissue.
   c. Do not use swabs for collection of specimens for anaerobic culture because exposure to air and drying compromise the specimen.

6. **Sputum for mycobacterial culture:** Collect first morning sputum on 3 consecutive days.

7. **Stool for culture:**
   a. Collect in preservative vials if transportation to laboratory is delayed.
   b. Specifically request isolation of *Vibrio* spp., *Yersinia enterocolitica*, and *Escherichia coli* 0157, because these organisms are typically not included in routine culture.

8. **Stool for ova and parasite (O&P) exam:**
   a. Collect in preservative vials provided by the laboratory in order to preserve the morphology of trophozoites that may be present.
   b. Because parasites are intermittently shed in stool, collect three specimens on nonconsecutive days within a 10-day period.

9. **Viral culture:**
   a. Use viral transport swabs/media provided by the laboratory.
   b. Nasopharyngeal aspirate or wash is more sensitive than nasopharyngeal swab for detection of respiratory viruses (influenza viruses and respiratory syncytial virus).

TEST ORDERING AND SPECIMEN PROCESSING

On receipt in the microbiology laboratory, Gram stains are made and specimens are plated onto appropriate plates depending on body site and type of culture requested. In most hospitals, some tests can be ordered "stat," which usually means results will be available within 1 hour after receipt in the laboratory – for example, stat Gram stain, cryptococcal antigen latex agglutination test on CSF, and rapid tests for group A *Streptococcus* or influenza viruses. Most laboratories screen sputum specimens for the presence of excessive epithelial cells, which would indicate that the specimen was not from a deep respiratory source. Specimens with excess epithelial cells are rejected for culture unless many polymorphonuclear neutrophil leukocytes (PMNs) are present.

INTERPRETATION OF THE GRAM STAIN

Gram-positive organisms have a thick peptidoglycan layer in the cell wall while gram-negative organisms have a thin peptidoglycan layer. When organisms are stained with crystal violet and then decolorized with acid/alcohol, the gram-positive organisms resist decolorization (and appear purple) because of the thick cell wall. Gram-negative organisms are initially decolorized and appear pink as a result of subsequent application of a safranin counterstain.

The Gram stain result includes an estimate of the quantity of organism present (rare, few, moderate, many), as well as a description of the shape and distribution of organisms on the smear, which may be characteristic of a particular class (Table 75.1).

Table 75.1 Interpretation of the Gram Stain

Gram stain result . . .	May suggest . . .
Gram-positive cocci in clusters	*Staphylococcus* spp. (*S. aureus* or coagulase-negative staphylococci)
Gram-positive cocci in pairs and chains	*Streptococcus* spp. (*S. pneumoniae* or viridans streptococci) or *Enterococcus* spp.
Pleomorphic gram-positive bacilli	Coryneform bacteria (diphtheroids)
Gram-negative diplococci	*Neisseria* spp.
Thick gram-negative bacilli	Enteric-like organism (*E. coli*, *Klebsiella* spp.)
Thin gram-negative bacilli	Pseudomonas-like organism
Gram-negative coccobacilli	*Haemophilus* spp.
Oval budding yeast	*Candida* spp.
Round budding yeast	*Cryptococcus* spp.

Table 75.2 Blood Agar Hemolysis Patterns for Streptococci

Gram-Positive Organisms	Organisms	Clinical Diseases	Comments
Alpha-hemolytic streptococci	*Streptococcus pneumoniae* Viridans group streptococci	Bacteremia, pneumonia, otitis media, meningitis Bacteremia, endocarditis	Most common cause of community-acquired pneumonia Can colonize oropharynx Normal flora mouth, GI tract, female genital tract Identification to species level usually not clinically useful
Beta-hemolytic streptococci	Group A *Streptococcus* (*Streptococcus pyogenes*)	Pharyngitis, necrotizing fasciitis, toxic shock syndrome	Nonsuppurative sequelae include rheumatic fever and acute glomerulonephritis
Beta-hemolytic streptococci	Group B *Streptococcus* (*Streptococcus agalactiae*)	Neonatal sepsis and meningitis, bacteremia, endocarditis, skin and soft-tissue infections, osteomyelitis	Screen pregnant women at 35–37 weeks gestation
Beta-hemolytic streptococci	Groups C, F, G	Bacteremia, endocarditis, meningitis, septic arthritis, pharyngitis	Can be commensals in pharynx

It is extremely important to understand that the Gram stain result is meant only as a guide to help clinicians initiate appropriate empiric therapy and may not correlate with the final organisms identified by culture. A number of variables can make Gram stains difficult to read and interpret, including specimen debris, mixtures of organisms, and the administration of antibiotics prior to specimen collection.

INTERPRETATION OF CULTURE RESULTS

Characteristics used to identify bacterial colonies include Gram stain of organisms in the colony, colony morphology, growth pattern on different media, oxidative or fermentative use of carbohydrates (glucose, lactose), and biochemical tests for enzymes. Many gram-positive organisms also cause characteristic patterns of hemolysis on 5% sheep blood agar. Alpha-hemolysis is partial hemolysis of red blood cells that produces a greening of the colonies, whereas beta-hemolysis is complete hemolysis of the sheep red blood cells resulting in complete clearing of the agar around the bacterial colonies. The lack of hemolysis is termed gamma-hemolysis. Examples of organisms demonstrating characteristic hemolysis patterns are shown in Table 75.2.

The coagulase test can be performed to distinguish *Staphylococcus aureus* from the coagulase-negative *Staphylococcus* spp. A latex agglutination test is performed to detect the bound form of coagulase, and if this test is positive with typical colony morphology, the bacterial isolate is called a *S. aureus*. If the latex agglutination test is negative, a tube coagulase test is set up to detect bound and free coagulase with overnight incubation. If a clot does not form in the overnight tube coagulase test, the bacterial isolate is called a coagulase-negative *Staphylococcus* (CNS). Further identification of *Staphylococcus* spp. included in the coagulase-negative group can be difficult and is usually not clinically useful except in the case of *S. saprophyticus*, a cause of urinary tract infections, or *S. lugdunensis*, a rare cause of severe endocarditis. Coagulase-negative staphylococci are often considered culture contaminants because they are normal flora on skin and mucous membranes.

Characteristics used to identify gram-negative organisms include an ability to grow on MacConkey agar, fermentation of lactose, oxidase reaction, carbohydrate utilization, and presence of enzymes.

If cultures have many colony types, laboratory technologists will identify pathogens, or if no frank pathogens are present, the report may indicate "mixed gram-positive flora" or "normal oral flora" or "normal GU (genitourinary) flora." This usually reflects the presence of commensal organisms in the culture. Culture plates are usually held for 3–7 days after the final report so clinicians can request more work-up if necessary.

It is important to keep in mind that the anticoagulant sodium polyanetholesulfonate (SPS) in blood culture bottles can inhibit growth of *N. gonorrhoeae*, *N. meningitidis*, *Streptobacillus moniliformis* (the cause of rat-bite fever), *Peptostreptococcus anaerobius*, and *Moraxella catarrhalis*.

SEROLOGY

Evidence of an acute infection by serological testing can often be demonstrated by the presence of IgM specific for an organism or by demonstrating seroconversion, defined as a fourfold increase in antibody titer between an acute serum and a convalescent serum collected 14–21 days after symptom onset. Commonly ordered serology tests are shown in Table 75.3.

FECAL LEUKOCYTES

Results of standard stool tests, such as stool cultures and *Clostridium difficile* toxin assays, are rarely available to guide decisions about antibiotic therapy for patients presenting to the Emergency Department with acute diarrhea. The detection of fecal leukocytes (FLs) in stool using a methylene blue stain is an inexpensive, rapid test that has been used to identify patients with inflammatory diarrhea caused by invasive *E. coli*, *Shigella* spp., *Salmonella* spp., or *Campylobacter jejuni*. However, recent studies have documented the poor sensitivity (14–68%) of the FL test and questioned its use to predict the presence of *C. difficile* toxin or a positive stool culture. A study by Savola et al evaluated the FL method for inpatients and outpatients. They report that use of the FL method was a poor predictor of *C. difficile* infection and that the FL test was a poor predictor of positive stool cultures for inpatients. Among the outpatients, however, the presence of one or more white blood cells per high-power field (WBC/hpf) was positive

Table 75.3 Infections Diagnosed by Serology Testing

Test for ...	Organisms	Serology Test	Signs and Symptoms
Bartonella	*Bartonella henselae*	IgM, IgG by EIA	Cat scratch disease, bacteremia, endocarditis, bacillary angiomatosis and peliosis
	Bartonella quintana	IgM, IgG by EIA	Bacteremia, trench fever, endocarditis, bacillary angiomatosis and peliosis
Blastomycosis	*Blastomyces dermatitidis*	ID, CF	Self-limited or localized pulmonary lesions. Chronic, progressive disease involving lungs, skin, GU tract, bone, or CNS in immunocompromised patients
Cytomegalovirus (CMV)	Human cytomegalovirus	IgM, IgG by EIA	Asymptomatic to mononucleosis-like symptoms Severe systemic illness, pneumonitis, retinitis in immunocompromised patients
Coccidioidomycosis	*Coccidioides immitis*	ID, CF	Self-limited or localized pulmonary infection Pulmonary nodules, progressive pneumonia in immunocompromised patients Dissemination to extrapulmonary sites with osteomyelitis, arthritis, meningitis
Dengue Fever	Dengue fever virus	IgM, IgG by EIA	Febrile illness Hemorrhagic fever
Mononucleosis	Epstein-Barr virus	Monospot test (heterophile antibodies) IFA or EIA Antibody panel including VCA-IgM, VCA-IgG, EBNA-IgG	Fever, pharyngitis, lymphadenopathy, atypical lymphocytes For children <5 years old, immunocompromised patients, nasopharyngeal carcinoma
Helicobacter pylori	*Helicobacter pylori*	IgG by EIA	Peptic ulcer disease and GI cancers
Hepatitis A	Hepatitis A virus	IgM and Total antibody	Mild, anicteric illness to severe, prolonged hepatitis with jaundice
Hepatitis B	Hepatitis B virus	HBsAg	Positive in acute illness; if present >6 months, chronic hepatitis
		HBsAb	Appearance indicates convalescence or vaccination
		Anti-HBcore IgM	Positive in acute hepatitis
		Anti-HBcore Total	Positive indicates acute or past infection
		HBeAg	Indicates active viral replication
		Anti-HBeAg	Inicates convalescence
Hepatitis C	Hepatitis C virus	EIA	Asymptomatic acute infection with 85% developing chronic infection – can lead to cirrhosis and hepatocellular carcinoma
Herpes	Herpes simplex virus 1 and 2	IgG by EIA IgM EIA tests do not distinguish HSV-1 and HSV-2 Demonstrate seroconversion for acute disease	HSV-1 gingivostomatitis HSV-2 genital lesions
Histoplasma	*Histoplasma capsulatum*	ID, CF	Pulmonary, extrapulmonary, or disseminated infection
HIV	Human immunodeficiency virus	Conventional EIA with confirmatory IFA or Western blot Rapid HIV antibody test with confirmatory IFA or Western blot	Opportunistic infections, low CD4 counts Report "preliminary positive" or "negative" for rapid HIV antibody test
HTLV-1 and HTLV-2	Human T-cell leukemia virus type 1 and 2	EIA does not distinguish types 1 and 2	HTLV-associated myelopathy or tropical spastic paraparesis, uveitis, adult T-cell leukemia or lymphoma
Lyme Disease	*Borrelia burgdorferi*	EIA with confirmatory Western blot	Erythema migrans, arthritis Tick bite transmission
Measles	Rubella virus Rubeola virus	IgM and IgG EIA IgG test for immunity	Subclinical infection or characteristic rash, fever
Mumps	Mumps virus	IgM and IgG EIA or IFA IgG test for immunity	Slightly elevated temperature with enlargement of one or both parotid glands

Table 75.3 (*cont.*)

Test for . . .	Organisms	Serology Test	Signs and Symptoms
Mycoplasma	*Mycoplasma pneumoniae*	Cold agglutinins nonspecific so not recommended IgM or IgG EIA	Hoarseness, fever, cough, sore throat, headache, chills, pneumonia
Parvovirus	Parvovirus B19	IgM and IgG EIA	Asymptomatic, aplastic crisis, erythema infectiosum (fifth disease with "slapped cheeks" rash), hydrops fetalis, arthropathy, acute and/or chronic
Q fever	*Coxiella burnetii*	IFA	Exposure to carrier animals (sheep, cattle, goats) especially during parturition Acute form with fever, headache, sweats, shaking chills, myalgia Chronic form can manifest as endocarditis, fatigue
Syphilis	*Treponema pallidum*	Nonspecific treponemal antibody tests for screening (RPR, VDRL) Confirmatory treponemal-specific tests (FTA-ABS or TP-PA)	Determine titer for RPR and VDRL because it should decrease fourfold within 6 months for treated primary or secondary syphilis Decrease in titer more gradual for latent or late syphilis In second and latent stages, treponemal-specific tests 100% sensitive and stay positive for life in most cases
Toxoplasmosis	*Toxoplasma gondii*	Test IgG for immune status Testing variability in performance of available IgM assays coupled with the finding that *Toxoplasma*-specific IgM can persist up to 18 months after acute infection limits usefulness of IgM assays Perform IgG avidity assay for pregnant women and send to reference lab prior to intervention in pregnant woman	Generally asymptomatic in immunocompetent persons CNS disease, myocarditis or pneumonitis in immunodeficient patients Congenital infection from an acute primary infection in a pregnant woman can be devastating Ocular toxoplasmosis cause of chorioretinitis
Varicella (Chickenpox) or Zoster (Shingles)	Varicella-zoster virus	IgM or IgG EIA	Varicella in children with fever and vesicular exanthem Zoster in adults or immunocompromised patients with painful, circumscribed vesicular lesions

CF, complement fixation; CMV, cytomegalovirus; CNS, central nervous system; EBNA, Epstein-Barr virus nuclear antigen; EIA, enzyme immunoassay; FTA-ABS, fluorescent treponemal antibody absorbed; GI, gastrointestinal; HIV, human immunodeficiency virus; HSV, herpes simplex virus; HTLV, human T-cell leukemia virus; ID, immunodiffusion; IFA, indirect fluorescence assay; RPR, rapid plasma reagin; TP-PA, *Treponema pallidum* particle agglutination; VDRL, venereal disease research laboratory.

in greater than 50% of the specimens with positive culture results. If a clinician suspected bacterial diarrhea and the FL test was positive, this suggested that the stool culture would most likely be positive. In most studies, the negative predictive value of the FL test was high (87–98%), so a negative FL result may support a decision to wait for culture results before instituting therapy.

TESTING FOR *NEISSERIA GONORRHOEAE* AND *CHLAMYDIA TRACHOMATIS*

Nucleic acid amplification testing (NAAT) for *N. gonorrhoeae* and *C. trachomatis* in urine specimens and urethral or cervical specimens has become the routine screening method for detection of infections due to these sexually transmitted organisms. A recent review by Cook et al. pooled data from 29 studies of one to three commercially available NAAT tests to evaluate test performance for urine specimens. The results shown in Table 75.4 were comparable to results documented in the literature for cervical and urethral specimens.

Based on the data presented in the table, the authors recommended that polymerase chain reaction (PCR) not be used to detect *N. gonorrhoeae* (GC) in urine specimens from women because of the low sensitivity. Limitations of the NAAT testing for these sexually transmitted infections include lack of the ability to do antibiotic susceptibility testing, occasional problems with reproducibility, and the lack of a reference standard for testing, because NAAT testing is more sensitive than culture in most studies. One exciting development in NAAT testing for *Chlamydia* and GC is the recent approval by the Food and Drug Administration (FDA) of clinician-collected vaginal swabs for the transcription-mediated amplification (TMA) assay. A study by Schachter et al. demonstrated equivalent results with self-collected and clinician-collected swabs as well as urine and cervical swabs. Specificities were greater than 99%, and among culture-positive women, NAAT sensitivity with the vaginal swab (93%) was as high or higher than sensitivity with cervical swabs (91%) or urines (80.6%). The movement toward self-collected screening swabs for women should increase testing and have a beneficial effect on control efforts in sexually transmitted diseases.

Table 75.4 Comparative Sensitivity of Nucleic Acid Amplification Tests for Chlamydia and *Neisseria gonorrhea*

Urine Specimens	PCR	TMA	SDA	Organism	Patients
Pooled sensitivity (%)	98	98	94	*Chlamydia*	Women
	84.0	87.7	93.1	*Chlamydia*	Men
	55.6	91.3	84.9	GC	Women
	90.4			GC	Men
Pooled specificity (%)	>97	>97	>97	Both *Chlamydia* and GC	Both men and women

GC, *N. gonorrhoeae*; PCR, polymerase chain reaction; SDA, strand displacement amplification; TMA, transcription-mediated amplification. Adapted from Cook et al. (2005).

TESTS AVAILABLE BY SPECIMEN AND SYSTEM

Cerebral Spinal Fluid

- Cytospin Gram stain
- Bacterial culture
- PCR for viruses (herpes simplex virus, varicella-zoster virus, cytomegalovirus, enteroviruses, JC virus)
- Viral culture (herpes simplex virus, enteroviruses, varicella-zoster virus)
- Fungal culture
- Mycobacterial culture or molecular assay (tuberculosis meningitis)
- *Cryptococcus* latex agglutination test
- Bacterial latex agglutination tests

Blood

- Culture (bacterial, fungal)
- Gram stain of positive blood culture bottles
- Smear analysis for organisms such as malaria, as well as cell count and morphology
- Organism-specific serologic testing

Bone

- Culture of bone scrapings (osteomyelitis)

Respiratory Tract

- Gram stain and culture (bacterial, fungal and viral cultures usually ordered separately) of:
  ○ Sputum
  ○ Tracheal aspirate
  ○ Bronchoalveolar lavage
- Mycobacterial cultures of respiratory secretions
- *Legionella* urine antigen
- *Histoplasma* urine antigen
- *Mycoplasma* serum antibodies

- Smear of induced sputum or bronchoalveolar lavage for *Pneumocystis*

Gastrointestinal Tract

- Stool culture (culture for *Vibrio* spp., *Y. enterocolitica*, and *E. coli* 0157 usually requires special request)
- Ova and parasite exam
- Rapid Immunoassays for *Giardia* and *Cryptosporidium*
- *C. difficile* toxin assay
- Microsporida stain
- Pinworm (*Enterobius vermicularis*) examination
- Fecal leukocytes

Urinary Tract

- Urinalysis
- Culture (bacterial, fungal)
- Nucleic acid assays of urine for gonorrhea and *Chlamydia trachomatis*

Ear, Eye, Nose, Throat

- Posterior pharyngeal swabs for culture or rapid streptococcal assays
- Nasopharyngeal aspirate for *Bordetella pertussis* culture or PCR
- Nasopharyngeal aspirate for respiratory virus assays
- Nasal swab culture for *S. aureus*
- Ear or eye drainage for culture

Body Fluids (Other Than CSF)

- Culture and Gram stain of:
  ○ Peritoneal fluid
  ○ Pleural fluid
  ○ Synovial fluid
  ○ Pericardial fluid

Skin (Wounds, Abscesses, Pustular Lesions)

- Aspirated fluid or excised tissue for bacterial, fungal, or viral culture
- Direct fluorescent antibody (DFA) test for herpes simplex virus or varicella-zoster virus
- For insect infestations (ticks, fleas, lice, scabies) send insect specimens to laboratory for identification

Genitourinary Tract and Sexually Transmitted Diseases

- Culture or NAAT of urethral or cervical swab or urine for gonorrhea and *Chlamydia*
- DFA assay, viral culture of swabs for herpes simplex virus
- Dark field microscopy of genital swabs or serum RPR or VDRL (confirmed with treponemal-specific antibody assay for syphilis

REFERENCES

Cook RL, Hutchison SL, Ostergaard L, et al. Systematic review: noninvasive testing for *Chlamydia trachomatis* and *Neisseria gonorrhoeae*. Ann Intern Med 2005;142:914–25.

Detrick B, Hamilton RG, Folds JD, eds. Manual of molecular and clinical laboratory immunology (7th ed.). Washington, DC: ASM; 2006.

Miller JM. Specimen management in clinical microbiology. Washington, DC: ASM; 1999.

Murray PR, Baron, EJ, Jorgensen JH, et al. Manual of clinical microbiology. Washington, DC: ASM; 2003.

Savola KL, Baron EJ, Tompkins LS, Passaro DJ. Fecal leukocyte stain has diagnostic value for outpatients but not inpatients. J Clin Microbiol 2001;39:266–9.

Schachter J, McCormack WM, Chernesky MA, et al. Vaginal swabs are appropriate specimens for diagnosis of genital tract infection with *Chlamydia trachomatis*. J Clin Microbiol 2003;41:3784–9.

PART VII

Infection Control Precautions

Yeva Johnson and Pancy Leung

Outline   Standard Precautions
                 Droplet Precautions
                 Contact Precautions
                 Airborne Precautions
                 References

Material from this chapter has been adapted from guidance provided by the Centers for Disease Control and Prevention (CDC).

STANDARD PRECAUTIONS

Use Standard Precautions, or the equivalent, for the care of all patients.

Standard Precautions apply to (1) blood; (2) all body fluids, secretions, and excretions except sweat, regardless of whether or not they contain visible blood; (3) nonintact skin; and (4) mucous membranes. Standard Precautions are designed to reduce the risk of transmission of microorganisms from both recognized and unrecognized sources of infection in hospitals.

Hand Hygiene/Hand Washing/Hand Decontamination

Wash with soap and water when hands are visibly dirty or visibly soiled with blood or other body fluids. If hands are not visibly soiled, hand sanitizer with at least 60% alcohol content may be used.

Perform hand hygiene/decontaminate hands *before*:

- having direct contact with patients
- donning sterile gloves before sterile procedures
- moving from a contaminated-body site to a clean-body site
- eating during patient care

Perform hand hygiene/decontaminate hands *after*:

- contact with a patient's intact skin
- contact with body fluids or excretions, mucous membranes, nonintact skin, wound dressings, or inanimate objects in the immediate vicinity of the patient
- removing gloves
- using a restroom

If exposure to *Bacillus anthracis* is suspected or confirmed:

- physically washing and rinsing hands under such circumstances is recommended because alcohols, chlorhexidine, iodophors, and other antiseptic agents have poor activity against spores

Gloves

Wear gloves (clean, nonsterile gloves are adequate) when touching blood, body fluids, secretions, excretions, and contaminated items. Put on clean gloves just before touching mucous membranes and nonintact skin. The glove wearer should be careful to never touch herself/himself with a gloved hand.

Change gloves between tasks and procedures on the same patient after contact with material that may contain a high concentration of microorganisms. Remove gloves promptly after use, before touching noncontaminated items and surfaces, and before going to another patient, and wash hands immediately to avoid transfer of microorganisms to other patients or environments.

Mask, Eye Protection, Face Shield

Wear a mask and eye protection or a face shield to protect mucous membranes of the eyes, nose, and mouth during procedures and patient-care activities that are likely to generate splashes or sprays of blood, body fluids, secretions, and excretions.

Gown

Wear a gown (a clean, nonsterile gown is adequate) to protect skin and to prevent soiling of clothing during procedures and patient-care activities that are likely to generate splashes or sprays of blood, body fluids, secretions, or excretions. Select a gown that is appropriate for the activity and amount of fluid likely to be encountered. Remove a soiled gown as promptly as possible and wash hands to avoid transfer of microorganisms to other patients or environments.

Patient-Care Equipment

Handle used patient-care equipment soiled with blood, body fluids, secretions, and excretions in a manner that prevents skin and mucous membrane exposures, contamination of clothing, and transfer of microorganisms to other patients and environments. Ensure that reusable equipment is not used for the care of another patient until it has been cleaned and disinfected or sterilized appropriately. Ensure that single-use items are discarded properly.

Environmental Control

Ensure that the hospital has adequate procedures for the routine care, cleaning, and disinfection of environmental surfaces, beds, bedrails, bedside equipment, and other frequently touched surfaces, and ensure that these procedures are being followed.

Linen

Handle, transport, and process used linen soiled with blood, body fluids, secretions, and excretions in a manner that prevents skin and mucous membrane exposures and contamination of clothing, and that avoids transfer of microorganisms to other patients and environments.

Occupational Health and Bloodborne Pathogens

Take care to prevent injuries when using, cleaning, and disposing of sharp instruments.

Never recap used needles, manipulate them using both hands, or use any other technique that involves directing the point of a needle toward any part of the body. If recapping is necessary, use either a one-handed "scoop" technique or a mechanical device designed for holding the needle sheath.

Do not remove used needles from disposable syringes by hand, and do not bend, break, or otherwise manipulate used needles by hand. Place used sharp items in appropriate puncture-resistant containers.

Use mouthpieces, resuscitation bags, or other ventilation devices as an alternative to mouth-to-mouth resuscitation in areas where the need for resuscitation is predictable.

Patient Placement

Place a patient who contaminates the environment, or who does not (or cannot be expected to) assist in maintaining appropriate hygiene or environmental control, in a private room.

DROPLET PRECAUTIONS

Droplet transmission involves contact of the conjunctivae or the mucous membranes of the nose or mouth of a susceptible person with large-particle droplets (larger than 5 μm in size) containing microorganisms generated from a person who is infected by or who is a carrier of the microorganism. Droplets are generated from the source person primarily during coughing, sneezing, or talking and during the performance of certain procedures such as suctioning and bronchoscopy.

Transmission via large-particle droplets requires close contact between source and recipient persons, because these droplets settle and generally travel only short distances through the air. Because large droplets do not remain suspended in the air, special air handling and ventilation are not required to prevent droplet transmission.

Mask

In addition to wearing a mask as outlined under Standard Precautions, wear a mask when working within 3 feet of the patient. (Logistically, some hospitals may want to implement the wearing of a mask to enter the room.)

Patient Placement

Place the patient in a private room. If a private room is not available, place the patient in a room with a patient(s) who has active infection with the same microorganism but with no other infection (cohorting). When a private room is not available and cohorting is not achievable, maintain spatial separation of at least 3 feet between the infected patient and other patients and visitors. Special air handling and ventilation are not necessary, and the door may remain open.

Patient Transport

Limit the movement and transport of the patient from the room to essential purposes only. If transport or movement is necessary, minimize patient dispersal of droplets by masking the patient.

CONTACT PRECAUTIONS

Direct-contact transmission involves skin-to-skin contact and physical transfer of microorganisms to a susceptible host from an infected or colonized person, such as occurs during patient-care activities that require physical contact. Direct-contact transmission also can occur between two patients (e.g., by hand contact), with one serving as the source of infectious microorganisms and the other as a susceptible host. Indirect-contact transmission involves contact of a susceptible host with a contaminated intermediate object, usually inanimate, in the patient's environment.

Patient Placement

Place the patient in a private room. If a private room is not available, place the patient in a room with a patient(s) who has active infection with the same microorganism but with no other infection (cohorting).

Gloves and Hand Washing

In addition to wearing gloves as outlined under Standard Precautions, wear gloves (clean, nonsterile gloves are adequate) when entering the room.

Change gloves between tasks and procedures on the same patient after contact with material that may contain a high concentration of microorganisms. Remove gloves promptly after use, before touching noncontaminated items and surfaces, and before going to another patient or leaving the room, and wash hands immediately.

After glove removal and hand washing, ensure that hands do not touch potentially contaminated environmental surfaces or items in the patient's room to avoid transfer of microorganisms to other patients or environments.

Gown

In addition to wearing a gown as outlined under Standard Precautions, wear a gown (a clean, nonsterile gown is adequate) when entering the room if you anticipate that your clothing will have substantial contact with the patient, environmental surfaces, or items in the patient's room. Remove the gown before leaving the patient's environment. After gown removal, ensure that clothing does not contact potentially contaminated environmental surfaces to avoid transfer of microorganisms to other patients or environments.

Patient Transport

Limit the movement and transport of the patient from the room to essential purposes only. If the patient is transported out of the room, ensure that precautions are maintained to minimize the risk of transmission of microorganisms to other patients and contamination of environmental surfaces or equipment.

Patient-Care Equipment

When possible, dedicate the use of noncritical patient-care equipment to a single patient (or to a cohort of patients infected or colonized with the pathogen requiring precautions) to avoid sharing between infected and uninfected patients. If use of common equipment or items is unavoidable, then adequately clean and disinfect or sterilize them before use on another patient.

AIRBORNE PRECAUTIONS

Airborne transmission occurs by dissemination of either airborne droplet nuclei (small-particle residue [5 μm or smaller in size] of evaporated droplets that may remain suspended in the air for long periods of time) or dust particles containing the infectious agent. Microorganisms carried in this manner can be dispersed widely by air currents and may become inhaled by or deposited on a susceptible host within the same room or over a longer distance from the source patient, depending on environmental factors; therefore, special air handling and ventilation are required to prevent airborne transmission.

Patient Placement

Place the patient in a private room that has: (1) monitored negative air pressure in relation to the surrounding areas; (2) 6 to 12 air changes per hour; and (3) appropriate discharge of air outdoors or monitored high-efficiency filtration of room air before the air is circulated to other areas in the hospital. Keep the room door closed and the patient in the room. If a private room is not available, place the patient in a room with a patient who has active infection with the same microorganism but with no other infection (unless otherwise recommended).

Respiratory Protection

Wear respiratory protection (such as an N95 respirator or higher level of protection) when entering the room of a patient with known or suspected infection.

Patient Transport

Limit the movement and transport of the patient from the room to essential purposes only. If transport or movement is necessary, minimize patient dispersal of droplet nuclei by placing a surgical mask on the patient, if possible.

REFERENCES

Association for Professionals in Infection Control & Epidemiology (APIC). APIC text of infection control and epidemiology (2nd ed.). Author, 2005.

Centers for Disease Control and Prevention (CDC)/Hospital Infection Control Practices Advisory Committee (HICPAC). Guideline for hand hygiene in health care settings. MMWR 2002 Oct 25;51(RR16):1–44.

Garner JS, Hospital Infection Control Practices Advisory Committee (HICPAC). Guideline for isolation precautions in hospitals. Retrieved February 2007 from http://www.cdc.gov/ncidod/dhqp/gl_isolation_hicpac.html.

Mayhall CG. Hospital epidemiology and infection control (3rd ed.). Baltimore: Lippincott Williams & Wilkins, 2004.

Index

Abdominal pain. *See also* Peritonitis
 differential diagnosis, 56, 56*t*
 imaging, 57*t*, 57–58
 pearls/pitfalls, 57–58
Abendazole, 70*t*
Abruption, 341–342
Abscesses
 brain (*See* Brain abscess)
 breast (*See* Breast abscess)
 clinical features, 217–218, 258
 complications/admission criteria, 261
 epidemiology, 257
 intracranial (*See* Intracranial abscess)
 laboratory/radiologic findings, 259
 liver (*See* Liver abscesses)
 parapharyngeal, 20
 pearls/pitfalls, 261
 penetrating head trauma, 234*t*, 237*t*
 periapical (*See* Periapical abscess)
 peripancreatic (*See* Peripancreatic
  abscesses)
 peritonsillar, 47–48
 postneurosurgery, 234*t*, 237*t*
 retropharyngeal (*See* Retropharyngeal
  abscess)
 splenic (*See* Splenic abscesses)
 subcutaneous (*See* Subcutaneous abscess)
 treatment/prophylaxis, 260, 260*t*
 tubo-ovarian, 56*t*, 340–341
ABthrax (raxibacumab), 427
Acetaminophen, 14*t*
Acetaminophen overdose
 differential diagnosis, 61–62
 pearls/pitfalls, 63
 treatment/prophylaxis, 63
N-Acetylcysteine, acetaminophen overdose,
  63
ACS. *See* Acute chest syndrome (ACS)
Actinomycosis, 45
Activated protein C (APC), 406
Acute acalculous cholecystitis, 68
Acute bacterial cholangitis
 clinical features, 68, 68*t*
 epidemiology, 68
 laboratory/radiologic findings, 68*t*, 69
 treatment, 69, 69*t*
Acute calculous cholecystitis
 clinical features, 65, 66*t*
 complications, 67
 differential diagnosis, 65–66
 gangrenous, 67–68
 laboratory/radiologic findings, 66, 66*t*,
  66*f*
 overview, 65
 pearls/pitfalls, 71
 treatment, 66–67, 67*t*
Acute chest syndrome (ACS)
 clinical features, 411, 411*t*
 differential diagnosis, 411

laboratory/radiologic findings, 411, 411*t*
 overview, 410–411
 pearls/pitfalls, 413–414
 treatment/prophylaxis, 411*t*, 412
Acute cholecystitis, in pregnancy, 340–341
Acute disseminated encephalomyelitis
  (ADEM), 243*t*, 244
Acute fulminant meningococcemia
  (Waterhouse-Friderichsen
  syndrome), 23, 23*t*
Acute infectious diarrhea. *See* Diarrhea,
  acute infectious
Acute mastoiditis, otitis media, 34
Acute necrotizing ulcerative
  gingivostomatitis
 clinical features, 16–17, 17*t*
 complications
  loss of teeth, 19
  osteomyelitis, 19
 differential diagnosis, 18
 pearls/pitfalls, 20
 treatment/admission criteria, 19
Acute paronychia
 clinical features, 123, 124*f*, 124*t*
 differential diagnosis, 123–124, 125
 laboratory/radiologic findings, 124*t*
 overview, 123
 treatment/prophylaxis, 124, 124*t*
Acute prostatitis
 clinical features, 215–216
 pearls/pitfalls, 218
 treatment/prophylaxis, 216–217, 217*t*
Acute respiratory distress syndrome
  (ARDS)
 clinical features, 406, 406*t*
 in SARS, 482–483
 treatment, 406
Acute retinal necrosis (ARN), 165, 165*f*
Acute seroconversion syndrome, 28–29
Acute suppurative parotitis, 51
Acyclovir (Zovirax)
 cautions, 512
 differences/agents, 512
 febrile child treatment, 281*t*
 focal encephalitis, 239*t*
 herpes, 224*t*
 herpes genitalis, 91*t*
 herpetic whitlow, 125*t*
 HSV 1/2, in pregnancy, 345*t*
 keratitis, 161*t*
 neonatal fever/sepsis, 274*t*
 pearls/pitfalls, 513
 properties, 512*t*
 renal function dosage adjustments, 513*t*
 skin/soft-tissue infections, oncology
  patients, 317*t*
 Varicella-zoster infection, 254*t*
 Varicella-zoster virus, in pregnancy, 345*t*
Adamantine derivatives, influenza, 188*t*

ADEM (Acute disseminated
  encephalomyelitis), 243*t*, 244
Adenoiditis, 47–48
Adhesive bowel obstruction, 56*t*
Adverse drug reactions. *See also specific
  drugs*
 clinical features, 31*f*, 31
 differential diagnosis, 62*t*, 61–62
 HIV infection, 29
African tick-bite fever, 358*t*
AIDS, HSV infection, 91
AIG, 427. *See also* HIV infection;
  Immunocompromised patients.
Airborne precautions, infection control, 529
Albendazole
 liver abscesses, 55*t*
 microsporidium, 86*t*, 87
Alcoholism, 51
Alemutuzumab, 315–316, 318*f*
Allegra (fexofenadine), 34*t*
Allergic dermatitis, 38
Allergy, 40
Allograft rejection, 394
Altered mental status/HIV infection
 clinical features, 249–250, 250*t*
 complications/admission criteria, 254
 differential diagnosis
  diffuse cerebral dysfunction, 250, 251*t*
  focal cerebral dysfunction, 250, 251*t*
 epidemiology, 249
 history, 250*t*
 infection control, 254
 laboratory/radiologic findings, 251–252,
  252*t*, 254
 overview, 249
 pearls/pitfalls, 255
 treatment/prophylaxis, 254, 254*t*
Amantadine (Symmetrel)
 avian influenza A (H5N1), 478, 478*t*, 479
 differences/agents, 513
 influenza, 188, 188*t*
 mechanism of action, 513
 pearls/pitfalls, 513–514
 properties, 513
Amikacin
 bacterial meningitis, 229*t*
 endophthalmitis, 166*t*, 167*t*
 properties, 504
 renal function dosage adjustments, 505*t*
Aminoglycosides. *See also specific drugs*
 bacterial meningitis, 229*t*
 cautions, 504
 cystitis/pyelonephritis, in pregnancy,
  337–338
 differences, 504
 infections, oncology patients, 321–322
 mechanism of action, 504
 open fractures, 131–132
 pearls/pitfalls, 504–505